W9-AXS-369

The
HEALTH
NUTRIENT
BIBLE

The Complete
Encyclopedia
of Food as Medicine

LYNN SONBERG

Consulting Editor:
Maureen Callahan, M.S., R.D.

A Fireside Book
PUBLISHED BY
SIMON & SCHUSTER

New York London Toronto
Sydney Tokyo Singapore

FIRESIDE
Rockefeller Center
1230 Avenue of the Americas
New York, NY 10020

Copyright © 1995 by Lynn Sonberg
All rights reserved, including the right of reproduction in whole
or in part in any form.

FIRESIDE and colophon are registered trademarks of Simon &
Schuster Inc.

DESIGNED BY BARBARA M. MARKS

Manufactured in the United States of America

10   9   8   7   6   5   4   3   2   1

Library of Congress Cataloging-in-Publication Data
Sonberg, Lynn.
     The health nutrient bible : the complete encyclopedia of
food as medicine / Lynn Sonberg : consulting editor,
Maureen Callahan.
          p.   cm.
     "A Fireside book".
     Includes bibliographical references and index.
     1. Nutrition.   2. Health.   3. Food—Composition—
Tables.   I. Callahan, Maureen.   II. Title.
RA784.S648   1995
613.2—dc20   95-25139
                                                        CIP

ISBN 0-684-81071-9

Produced by Lynn Sonberg Book Services

Research about human nutrition is constantly evolving.
While the authors have made every effort to include the most
accurate and up-to-date information in this book, there can be
no guarantee that what we know about this complex subject
won't change with time. Please keep in mind that this book is
not intended for the purpose of self-diagnosis or self-treatment.
The reader should consult his or her physician regarding all
health concerns and before undertaking any major dietary
changes.

CONTENTS

Including Calories, Protein, Fat, Saturated Fat, Cholesterol, Carbohydrates, Fiber, Sodium, Potassium, Calcium, Iron, Zinc, Magnesium, Vitamin A, Vitamin C, Thiamine, Riboflavin, Niacin, Vitamin B$_{12}$, Folic Acid

ACKNOWLEDGMENTS

The author wishes to thank Matthew Ostrowski for his invaluable help in researching the nutrient counter portion of this book. She also wishes to thank the many food manufacturers who responded to requests for nutritional information about their products, the United States Department of Agriculture, the Human Nutrition Information Service, and her editor at Fireside Books, Sheila Curry, for her support and encouragement.

INTRODUCTION:
EATING FOR OPTIMUM HEALTH

That good nutrition is important to good health goes without saying. Yet over the last decade researchers studying the connections between diet and health have found that the foods we eat can actually act as preventive medicine! Scientists have identified substances in certain foods that perform as strong protective agents against numerous ailments ranging from heart disease to osteoporosis to premenstrual syndrome (PMS). Indeed, medical report after medical report continues to confirm that what you choose to eat can influence your risk for things as mundane as the common cold or as serious as cancer.

However, sorting through the hundreds of reports that link diet to health, many of them with conflicting opinions, is a cumbersome task at best. With *The Health Nutrient Bible* you can cut right to the heart of new research and glean practical nutrition advice. You'll be presented with the most up-to-date information on diet strategies for each stage of your life and your family's life—infancy, childhood, adolescence, pregnancy, menopause. Plus you'll find all the latest nutrition evidence on how diet influences all sorts of medical concerns, from anemia to weight control. In addition, an unusually comprehensive nutrition counter lets you look at the nutrient profile of more than 9,000 different foods in light of current nutritional concerns: calories, total fat, saturated fat, protein, carbohydrates, fiber, sodium, cholesterol, calcium, iron, zinc, potassium, magnesium, vitamin A, vitamin C, thiamin, riboflavin, niacin, folic acid, and vitamin B_{12}.

Before you read about diet strategies that cover nutritional concerns from A to Z, you'll want to get an overall view of what constitutes a healthy diet. The diet strategies needed to help improve health and fend off illness aren't really that difficult to master. In fact, when you compare the current American diet with the kind of eating style that is recommended by health professionals, it's obvious that the changes you'll need to make aren't overwhelming.

Seven Steps to A Better Diet

While the chart on page 6 gives you a ballpark estimate of how your diet needs to be shaped, the comparisons do reduce diet to a scenario of numbers.

Comparison of Current American Diet to Proposed Healthful Changes

Current Diet	Recommended Diet
Fat 37% of calories	Fat 30% of calories
Protein 12% of calories	Protein 12% of calories
Complex Carbohydrate 22% of calories	Complex Carbohydrate 48% of calories
Sugar 24% of calories	Sugar 10% of calories

Source: U.S. Senate, Select Committee on Nutrition and Human Needs, *Dietary Goals for the United States,* 2nd edition, 1977; United States Department of Agriculture.

The cutoff for cholesterol is listed at 300 milligrams per day. Fat is to be kept at 30 percent of calories or less, and sodium should be limited to about 2,400 milligrams. Luckily, you can easily translate these numbers into real foods. It's as simple as following the practical eating guidelines set forth in the landmark nutrition report called *Diet and Health,* published by the National Academy of Sciences.

That general advice breaks down healthy eating into seven simple strategies, specific guidelines that talk about what kind of foods to eat for good health and how much.

1. *Eat plenty of vegetables and fruits.* Aim for at least five servings of produce (one-half cup cooked) each day. Mix and match selections to get healthy amounts of vitamins A and C.
2. *Fill up on grains at every meal.* Serve yourself six half-cup portions of pasta, brown rice, or cereal each day. Whole grain breads and cereals are preferable as they offer more fiber and nutrients.
3. *Focus on calcium-rich foods.* Rely on obvious sources of calcium such as low-fat dairy products like milk and yogurt. To meet the recommended intake (RDA) for calcium of 800 milligrams per day adults need at least two glasses of low-fat milk (about 300 milligrams of calcium per each eight-ounce glass). Or, they need to include generous portions of the lesser sources of calcium such as canned salmon, tofu, or leafy green vegetables like broccoli and kale.
4. *Reduce salt.* Since diets high in salt have been linked with high blood pressure, the Food and Nutrition Board advocates a sodium intake of no more than 2,400 milligrams (2.4 grams) per day. Interestingly, the body requires less than 500 milligrams of sodium per day, yet most Americans typically eat twenty times that much or more. A recent study shows that more than three-quarters of the sodium most people eat comes from processed foods including such highly salted items as luncheon meats, pickles, snack crackers, and canned foods. Why not limit these foods and spice up meals with other seasonings? Good choices include lemon juice, basil, dill, tarragon, and chili peppers.

5. *Keep fat calories to 30 percent or less.* For most of us, this means cutting back: trimming visible fat from beef, peeling the skin from chicken. Not every food needs to be a certain fat level, however. Balance a fatty burger-and-fries lunch with a broiled fish dinner.

6. *Limit alcohol to one ounce per day,* if you do drink. That amounts to either two cans of beer, two small glasses of wine, or two average cocktails. One caveat: Pregnant women would be wise to avoid alcohol.

7. *Work to maintain weight.* While this book is primarily about diet strategies, controlling weight is a two-part process that involves both a commitment to balanced eating and regular exercise.

Building Meals Pyramid Style

Armed with this general picture of healthy eating for disease prevention, you can then use the new Food Guide Pyramid to build a better diet. Developed by the Department of Agriculture to replace the outdated "Four Food Groups" concept, the pyramid helps convey the message that a healthful diet is one based on grains, fruits, and vegetables with moderate quantities of lean meat and low fat dairy products.

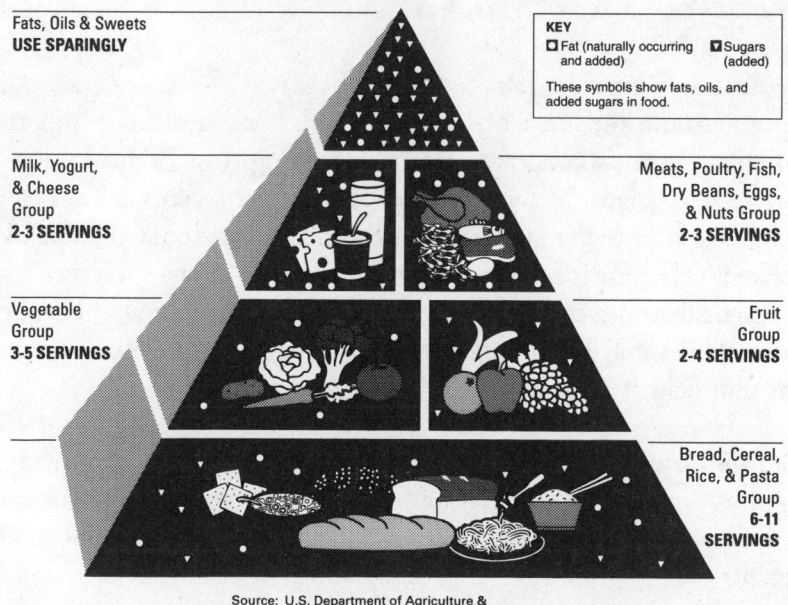

FOOD GUIDE PYRAMID
A Guide to Daily Food Choices

Fats, Oils & Sweets
USE SPARINGLY

KEY
□ Fat (naturally occurring and added)   ▼ Sugars (added)
These symbols show fats, oils, and added sugars in food.

Milk, Yogurt, & Cheese Group
2-3 SERVINGS

Meats, Poultry, Fish, Dry Beans, Eggs, & Nuts Group
2-3 SERVINGS

Vegetable Group
3-5 SERVINGS

Fruit Group
2-4 SERVINGS

Bread, Cereal, Rice, & Pasta Group
6-11 SERVINGS

Source: U.S. Department of Agriculture &
U.S. Department of Health and Human Services

Each of the pyramid's six building blocks houses a separate group of foods. The largest compartment is filled with pictures of pasta, bread, cereals and grains to convey the message that the foundation of a healthful diet is based on grains. Two moderate-size compartments on top of the grain-based section house illustrations of fruits and vegetables. The message is that generous amounts of fruits and vegetables should accompany grains in the diet. The two smaller blocks that sit on top of fruits and vegetables hold meat and dairy foods. While these two food groups supply many critical nutrients, they are needed only in small amounts.

At the tip of the pyramid, a tiny triangle is reserved for fats, oils, and sweets, signifying that although these foods can be a part of the diet they should play a very small role. Circles and triangles sprinkled throughout all compartments are meant to remind you that vegetables can contain added fat (broccoli smothered in cheese sauce, french fries).

Considering Nutrient Density—The pyramid only hints at it, but part of the secret to eating healthfully is to view foods in the context of their nutrient makeup. Nutritionists refer to this concept as *nutrient density.* It's sort of like comparison shopping for foods, but instead of thinking about price, you base your decision on what a food has to offer in the way of nutrition—both the negative and positive aspects. Say you're looking for a good source of calcium. Dairy products come immediately to mind—milk, ice cream, yogurt. Yet whole milk and rich premium ice creams offer that calcium at a high-fat cost. Skim milk, on the other hand, delivers the calcium without added fat and is therefore the better choice.

How to Use This Book

The Nutrition Reference Section

To better understand the impact diet has on health and disease, it sometimes helps to look at each of your nutrition concerns separately. Starting with <u>A</u>dditives and ending with <u>W</u>eight control, we've arranged the most common nutrition concerns and problems alphabetically. You can quickly refer to the nutrition and diet issues that concern you and your family. Under each alphabetical listing is a comprehensive synopsis of all the latest diet research in that area as well as practical strategies on how to put those research results to work for you. One section looks at how diet may affect longevity, another explores how nutrients help build the immune system and make it more efficient at fighting infections.

The Nutrition Counter:

Following the A-to-Z guide you will find the nutrient profiles for more than 9,000 different foods, listing common foods as well as brand-name items such as fast foods and supermarket packaged items.

To look up a food: Nearly all foods are listed in alphabetical order. In other words, *apple* is listed under *a,* not under *fruit; bologna* is under *b,* not under *cold cuts;* and *milk* is under *m,* not under *dairy products.* In a few cases, we did use categories to avoid confusion (for example, baby food, bread, cookies, soup, pudding) but these are definitely the exception rather than the rule.

Calories and nutrient listed: Following each food item, you'll find a calorie count as well as the nutrient content for protein, fat, saturated fat, cholesterol, carbohydrates, fiber, sodium, potassium, calcium, iron, zinc, magnesium, vitamin A, vitamin C, thiamin, riboflavin, niacin, vitamin B_{12}, and folic acid, all expressed as a percentage of the recommended daily intake or daily value (DV).

For ease of use, we decided to provide the nutrient information in one comprehensive table, even though more data exists for the major nutrients than the micronutrients. The big advantage to this format is you only have to look up a given food once to obtain a complete rundown of all available nutrient data on a given food. We have used a dash (—) in instances where data on micronutrients was simply not available from any reliable source. An asterisk (*) means that a given food contains less than 2 percent of the daily value for a particular nutrient.

Give Us Our Daily Values

Now that food labels list the nutrient content of foods in the context of what someone eating a 2,000 calorie diet should be aiming for, the concept of daily values is going to become a more familiar one. Essentially, the daily value for a nutrient is based on what the Food and Nutrition Board of the National Academy of Sciences considers the safe and adequate amount of a nutrient needed by a normal healthy person. You know these recommendations as the RDAs or recommended dietary allowances. The daily values concept simply takes the RDAs and puts them into the context of what experts consider the average diet (a 2,000 calorie plan).

We've arranged the nutrient counter section of the book based on the daily values so that what you read here will be the same type of information you read on food labels. Clearly it's a lot easier to keep track of your nutrient intake using the percent of daily values format than counting out grams and milligrams and then comparing those figures to the RDAs. Don't let yourself get too bogged down in the numbers—the counter section is meant as a reference that you can look at any time you have a question about the nutrient profile of a particular food and how it will fit into your preventive diet plan. For instance, it will give you a chance to look up favorite foods and see if they are a good source of the six nutrients commonly missing from most Americans' diets—folic acid, vitamin B_6, calcium, magnesium, iron, zinc. Or you can just look at the overall nutrient profile of particular foods to compare calorie contents and specific concerns like fat, fiber, vitamins and minerals.

Where We Obtained Nutrient Data—Whenever possible, we used the nutrition information supplied to us directly from food manufacturers and processors of brand-name products. The latest edition of the USDA food tables were another important source. While we made every attempt to provide accurate and up to date information, a certain margin of error is inevitable. Seasonal and regional differences can affect the nutrient content of a given food, and the information supplied may have been rounded off. Also, please keep in mind that product formulations are constantly changing. New products are introduced in new sizes or use different recipes, while older products may be discontinued.

The Major Nutrients

Calories—Experts at the Department of Agriculture estimate that 1,600 calories per day is about the right amount for sedentary women and many seniors. Active women, many children, and teenage girls probably need at least 2,200 calories. Teenage boys and active men may need 2,800 calories. But you won't see these varying caloric requirements on food labels. Experts have taken an average calorie figure, 2,000 calories, and compared the fat and nutrients provided in a food to this recommended level. The nutrition counter will list the calorie value of a food based on realistic portion sizes.

Protein—Most adults need somewhere in the neighborhood of forty-six to sixty-three grams of protein per day. That shouldn't be much of a problem, since surveys show that most Americans eat twice as much protein as they need. The nutrient counter lists the protein content of various foods in grams so that you can add up daily food choices and see if protein needs are being met.

Fat—While fat helps to cushion and protect body organs, acts as a warehouse for fat-soluble vitamins, and performs a number of other critical body functions, you can easily overdo it with this nutrient. Major health organizations, such as the American Heart Association and the National Heart, Lung and Blood Institute, recommend that you limit fat intake to 30 percent of calories or less. On food labels, that means 30 percent of 2,000 calories. However, if you are eating about 1,500 calories per day, a healthy fat budget (30 percent or less of the calories from fat) equates to fifty grams of fat or less. Or since some experts advocate that fat intake be limited to even lower levels, say twenty to twenty-five percent of total calories, you might choose to set a fat budget of thirty-three to forty-two grams per day. (See the section on Heart Health for tips on how to budget fat.)

Saturated Fat—Since saturated fat (found mainly in animal foods like meat, whole milk, and cheese) raises blood cholesterol levels, and its impact is more profound than any other dietary substance, you'll need to limit saturated fat to 10 percent of total calories.

Cholesterol—While it doesn't have as pronounced an impact on blood cholesterol as saturated fat, cholesterol from foods can raise blood cholesterol levels. Aim for less than 300 milligrams of cholesterol per day.

Carbohydrate—Carbohydrates come in both the simple (sugars) and complex (starches) variety. More than half of your calories should come from carbohydrates, preferably the complex variety because they come packaged with healthy amounts of fiber and other nutrients.

Fiber—Most Americans are lucky if they eat a total of eleven grams of fiber per day. Experts at the National Cancer Institute recommend gradually increasing that figure to twenty to thirty-five grams of fiber to help prevent cancer. Preliminary studies suggest that high-fiber diets may help control blood sugar and blood pressure as well as offer protection against certain types of cancer.

Sodium—For people sensitive to sodium, excess amounts of this mineral in the diet can elevate blood pressure. Since there is no convenient test to determine who is and who isn't sodium sensitive, experts recommend limiting sodium to 2,400 milligrams per day or about the amount found in 1 teaspoon of salt. (See the section on High Blood Pressure for more details.)

Potassium—A mineral that helps regulate fluid balance and is involved in muscle contraction, studies suggest that a potassium-rich diet may play a role in managing blood pressure.

The Micronutrients

Vitamin A—Needed for vision, reproduction, growth and repair of body tissue. New reports find that this fat-soluble vitamin may help build immunity and protect you from certain types of cancer. Foods that contain beta-carotene, a compound that can be converted by the body into vitamin A, are an alternate source of the nutrient.

Vitamin C—The role this nutrient may play in helping to prevent heart disease and certain types of cancer makes it something you might want to stock up on. New evidence also suggests vitamin C may play a role in building immunity. That's in addition to the role it plays in helping the body to absorb iron, to synthesize collagen, and to heal injuries.

Thiamin—Critical to the function of the nervous system and a help in energy production, you'll find this B vitamin is widely available in meats, grains, and enriched breads and cereals. There is no evidence that it can offer any specific preventive health benefits, but it is important to overall good health.

Riboflavin—Needed for healthy skin and to promote normal vision, this B vitamin is not being touted for any specific health benefits other than its normal functions. However, older women who exercise regularly may need higher amounts of this nutrient.

Niacin—Needed to keep the digestive system and the skin healthy, this B vitamin is important to the preventive diet simply for its role in promoting overall well-being.

Vitamin B$_{12}$—Found only in animal foods, getting enough of this vitamin may be difficult if you follow too strict a vegetarian diet. This B vitamin is needed to build red blood cells, synthesize genetic material, and to keep the nervous system functioning smoothly.

Folic Acid—One of the hottest new vitamins on the preventive health front, folic acid may help prevent birth defects and certain types of cancer. A diet low in folic acid can result in anemia, which is no surprise since this nutrient is needed for the production of red blood cells.

Calcium—While it plays a major role in bone health, this mineral is also critical to muscle and nerve function and blood clotting. You'll find news about the vital role calcium plays in the preventive diet in several sections, including those on osteoporosis, senior nutrition and menopause. The dietary requirement for calcium is elevated during childhood and up until the age of twenty-four, as these are the critical years for developing dense, strong bones.

Iron—Even though most people realize that this mineral is critical to the production of healthy red blood cells, surveys find that many age groups fall short of meeting dietary needs for this nutrient. Iron deficiency can result in anemia when diets are lacking in sufficient iron, particularly during the times when iron requirements are high: pregnancy, infancy, the teenage years, and a woman's childbearing years. In addition, preliminary reports suggest that iron may play a role in keeping the immune system healthy and strong.

Zinc—Although it has always been crucial to healing, zinc is receiving a lot of attention for the role it may play in building immunity.

Magnesium—Needed to help build strong bones and to help in the normal functioning of nerves and muscles, magnesium is being considered a potential protector against osteoporosis.

Part I

FOOD

AS

MEDICINE

An A to Z Guide

ADDITIVES AND PESTICIDES

There's no doubt that chemicals can pollute the environment and wreak havoc on our health. Pesticides are no exception. Studies have found that the same poisons we use to kill insects, weeds, and fungi are damaging to man as well. Evidence shows that some of these chemicals can cause cancer in the farmers who use them. According to a National Academy of Sciences report, pesticides may also cause cancer in the people who eat fruits and vegetables treated with these chemicals. After looking at twenty-eight different pesticides approved for use on food, the scientists of the National Academy of Sciences estimated that exposure to pesticide residues could result in an extra 20,000 cancer cases each year. But even more cases of cancer would result from *not* eating those same fruits and vegetables.

Additives—chemicals used to preserve and improve processed foods—are not always the safest food ingredients either. Unfortunately, we have become dependent on these chemicals to provide us with a varied and cosmetically attractive food supply. It isn't going to be easy to cut back our dependence on these possibly dangerous chemicals. Granted, it would be simple to immediately eradicate all chemicals and still enjoy an abundant assortment of foods. However, that kind of change may be unrealistic. More important, it can't be made overnight.

In the meantime, you'll have to try to reach some sort of middle ground, learning to tolerate compounds that are safe, yet putting pressure on the government to expose your family to as few chemicals as possible. Part of that effort means learning more about why chemicals are used in foods and what experts say about the safety record of these substances.

Eliminating Pesticide Residues

Over the last decade, food-safety experts have expressed concern about current food safety and pesticide laws, particularly as they apply to young children. Their worry is that the government initially set pesticide residue limits by looking at adult eating patterns. Since children eat similar amounts of food as adults yet have a smaller body size, there is concern that pesticide exposure could be greater among children; the potential danger from pesticide exposure may also be greater since children are still developing.

In a recently released report from the National Academy of Sciences, however, experts conclude that parents should not be overly concerned about pesticides to which their children might be exposed. In fact, the consensus is that the nutritional benefits of feeding children fruits and vegetables far outweigh any risk associated with a minimal exposure to pesticides. Some permissible residue levels are set so high that they already include a wide margin of safety, wide enough to potentially protect children as well as adults.

However, the Food and Drug Administration, the Department of Agriculture, and the Environmental Protection Agency recently came together to propose reforms that would update and improve current pesticide laws. Those proposals include special provisions to protect infants and children from pesticide risks. (Experts plan to identify the foods which children eat frequently and consider these eating habits when setting pesticide tolerance levels for those particular foods.)

The new reforms, the first major changes in pesticide laws since the 1970s, set forth goals for a future that includes better pesticide control methods. Consumers can help too. Since many pesticides are used for cosmetic reasons, consumers could try to learn to live with fruits and vegetables that aren't blemish free and picture perfect. Farmers can do their part by using crop rotation, predator insects (integrated pest management), and biological compounds to help lessen dependence on chemical pesticides. It is hoped that by the year 2000, seventy-five percent of farms will be using fewer pesticides due to these methods.

In the interim, there are some measures you can take to lessen your exposure to pesticides. One option, albeit a costly one, is to buy organically grown produce from a reputable dealer. (See the section on Health Foods, page 81.) Or you could shop for regular produce, but use these handling tips offered by the Food and Drug Administration and Food Marketing Institute:

- Wash fresh fruits and vegetables with water and scrub with a brush when appropriate.
- Throw away the outer leaves of leafy vegetables such as lettuce and cabbage.
- Peel fruits and vegetables when appropriate; remember that some nutrients and fiber are lost when produce is peeled.

The ABC's of Food Additives

"Chemophobia" is how one food-safety expert describes the American reaction to any kind of food additive. It doesn't matter if the substance used has tested as safe or is an ingredient isolated from a real food; many people simply have a fear of anything with a chemical-sounding name. If you understand the rigorous safety tests any new additive must undergo, your unnecessary fears may be alleviated.

In 1958 Congress enacted the Food Additives Amendment (added to the Federal Food, Drug and Cosmetic Act) to make sure that ingredients added to preserve and protect food from spoilage were safe for human consumption. Additives already in use at the time such as nutrients, salt, sugar, and other seasonings were not required to be tested since these additives were already regarded as safe. They automatically went on a list of generally recognized as safe (GRAS) substances.

However, any new additive manufacturers want to use in a food must meet strict testing guidelines. To test an additive for safety, food companies feed large doses of an additive for long periods of time to at least two different types of laboratory animals. This is done to determine if the additive has any toxic effects, could be carcinogenic, or might interfere with nutrition. Results of these tests are then reviewed by the FDA. Companies must also include information showing that the additive is safe for use based on the following criteria.

1. The amount of an additive consumers will be exposed to, or the amount of any other substance that forms in the food secondary to this substance being added.
2. The longterm or cumulative exposure to this substance over the course of a lifetime.
3. The potential for causing cancer or toxicity when eaten by people or animals.

Once a substance is deemed safe, government officials usually set a wide margin of safety. Most of the time that safety margin is one-hundred-fold. This means the FDA considers the highest levels at which an additive fed to test animals did not produce any harm and divides that amount by 100. Food companies can use 1/100th of the amount that tested as safe on animals.

General Types of Additives

Food additives are what keep your bread from molding, your ice cream tasting rich even though it is very low in fat, and your cheese a familiar bright orange. With all these factors, it's no surprise that additives fall into a number of different categories, based on their use.

Emulsifiers   In home baking, the addition of an egg helps to bind water and oil in a muffin or cake batter. In processed foods, from bakery treats to salad dressings, other binding ingredients are used: lecithin, fats (monoglycerides, diglycerides), polysorbate 60, and polysorbate 80.

Thickening Agents   A category of natural substances called *gums* can be added to foods to improve texture and act as binding agents. Most gums come from plants or plant seeds: pectin, xanthan gum, guar gum, locust bean gum, and gum arabic. But gums can be made from food starches like corn, tapioca, or potato and called *modified food starch,* or they can be made from wood pulp (methyl-cellulose and carboxyl-methyl-cellulose).

Chances are you will see gums on the ingredient list of newer fat-free and reduced-fat foods. Gums help bind the water and other ingredients together to give these low-fat foods a creamy texture. One popular gum is made from seaweed: *Carageenan* is the binding ingredient used in many low-fat hamburger products.

Food Colorings   In 1960, the Color Additives Amendment was added to the Federal Food, Drug, and Cosmetic Act to ensure that ingredients used to color foods were safe. Both natural and artificial substances are used as food dyes. Some examples of natural dyes include annato (seeds used to color some cheeses bright orange), turmeric, beet extract, and grape skin. Synthetic dyes include red dye#3, yellow#5 (tartrazine). The latter dye, a known allergen, is the only food coloring that must be listed on food labels. (See the section on questionable additives.)

Preservatives   The main function of preservatives is to extend the shelf life of a food. If a food contains fat, preservatives that prevent fat from *oxidizing* (turning rancid) are used. Other preservatives inhibit the growth of bacteria. Some examples of common preservatives include: calcium propionate, salt, sugar, vitamin C, and two controversial additives—BHA (butylated hydroxyanisole) and BHT (butylated hydroxytoulene).

Questionable Additives

While the majority of food additives are safe, there are some additives which frequently raise cause for concern.

BHA, BHT—Used to slow the process of oxidation which turns fats and oils rancid, BHA (butylated hydroxyanisole) and BHT (butylated hydroxytoulene) are considered controversial food additives. Made from petroleum-based compounds, studies considering the safety of these two preservatives have had mixed results. Some reports find that BHA and BHT can cause tumors in animals. Critics of these reports suggest that the tests don't establish human risk.

To help resolve the issue, the Food and Drug Administration has called on the Federation of the American Societies for Experimental Biology (FASEB) to review the current scientific information on these additives. (Those results are still pending.) It's all part of a larger comprehensive review of additives on the GRAS list. In the meantime, be aware that the GRAS regulations limit the amount of BHA and BHT in a food product to 0.02 percent. That's roughly 200 parts per million.

Sulfites—In 1986, the Food and Drug Administration ruled that sulfite preservatives be listed on the ingredient list so that people allergic to these additives (see the chapter on Allergies and Food Intolerances, page 24) can avoid them. That list includes: sulfur dioxide, sodium sulfite, sodium and potassium bisulfite, and sodium and potassium metabisulfite. It's rare that people have a reaction to sulfites, but the FDA has set the following limits on sulfites in these processed foods.

Sulfite Residue in Foods

Food Item	Maximum residue limit
Baked goods	30 parts per million
Beer	25 ppm
Wine	275 ppm
Tea	90 ppm
Condiments, relishes	30 ppm
Vinegar	75 ppm
Dairy products	200 ppm
Gelatin	40 ppm
Grain products	200 ppm
Fruit juices	300 ppm
Maraschino cherries	150 ppm
Dehydrated potatoes	500 ppm
Sugar	20 ppm
Molasses	300 ppm

Monsodium Glutamate (MSG)—A flavor enhancer that is used in many processed foods, monosodium glutamate is a sodium salt of the amino acid glutamate. In the past, some people complained of symptoms including headaches, tightness in the chest, heart palpitations, and muscular weakness after eating the additive. Since most of the complaints happened after a meal at a Chinese restaurant, where MSG is typically used, the alleged illness was dubbed the *Chinese Restaurant Syndrome*.

To date, researchers have been unable to confirm that MSG is truly responsible for the reported syndrome. (Most of the evidence, at present, is anecdotal.) So while some want to ban the additive, the Food and Drug Administration considers that the evidence doesn't support that the additive is toxic. Granted, some people may be mildly sensitive to MSG, but the ingredient is easily avoided as food labels are required to list MSG when it is used as an ingredient. Foods that could contain MSG include: canned soups, cookies, crackers, snack chips, salad dressing (dry mixes), sausage, and frozen, breaded fish. Keep in mind that hydrolyzed protein (used in canned meats and hot dogs) can also contain MSG.

Tartrazine (Yellow Dye #5) The Food and Drug Administration requires that manufacturers list tartrazine on the ingredient label of both foods and drugs, so that people with an allergy to this food coloring can avoid it. Consumption of the food coloring has been known to cause a runny nose, hives, or symptoms of asthma in certain susceptible people. Estimates are that at least 50,000 Americans are allergic to tartrazine. Foods that typically use this yellow dye include: ice cream, sherbet, gelatins, puddings, salad dressings, cake mixes, and candies.

Nutrients in Disguise

Keep in mind that some of the scariest-sounding chemical names that appear on food labels are actually helpful ingredients. For example ferric orthophosphate or pyridoxine hydrochloride sound foreign but these additives are common nutrients—iron and the B vitamin, pyridoxine—which are added to foods to boost nutritional value. Sometimes nutrients are added to foods to help prevent spoilage. Vitamin C preservatives such as ascorbic acid or ascorbyl palmitate can help to extend shelf life for wine, cured meats, and bakery treats.

Nutrient Additives

Additive Name	Nutrient
Ergocalciferol	Vitamin D
Calcium pantothenate, tricalcium phosphate	Calcium
Sodium riboflavin	Vitamin B_2
Thiamin mononitrate, thiamin hydrochloride	Vitamin B_1
Cyanocobalamine	Vitamin B_{12}
Calcium ascorbate, sodium ascorbate, ascorbyl palmitate, ascorbic acid	Vitamin C
Beta-carotene, beta-apo-8'-carotenal	Vitamin A
Ferric orthophosphate	Iron

The Issue of Irradiation

Now that a company in Florida is irradiating fruits and vegetables, chances are you might come across irradiated produce in the local market. While irradiation doesn't make food radioactive, the facts behind the process often get lost in the charged emotional atmosphere that seems to surround this procedure. Following is a list of the types of food the government currently allows to be irradiated.

Foods Approved for Irradiation

Food	Reason for irradiation
Poultry	To kill salmonella
Pork	To destroy parasites

Fresh fruits	To delay ripening, extend shelf life
Fresh vegetables	To delay ripening, extend shelf life
White potatoes	To inhibit sprouting
Spices	To kill insects
Wheat, wheat flour	To kill insects

To help you make an informed decision about irradiated foods, here are the answers to some popular questions about the process.

What is irradiation?

During the irradiation process, foods are exposed to extremely minute amounts of electromagnetic energy (gamma rays from radioactive cobalt 60 or cesium or X-rays) in order to kill bacteria and prolong shelf life. Tests show that the exposure is not great enough to leave any radiation residue.

Does irradiation change foods in any way?

Yes. A recent report in the *Journal of Food Composition and Analysis* finds that small changes in pH, color, vitamin C, and sugar content can occur when some fruits and vegetables are irradiated, but these changes also commonly result when food is stored for long periods. There are, however, slight molecular changes that occur when foods are irradiated. These molecular changes produce what scientists refer to as *radiolytic compounds*. While there is no evidence that radiolytic compounds are harmful, there is no research to document what the effects of longterm exposure to these substances might be.

What about taste and nutritional value, is that altered in any way?

Studies from the University of Rhode Island find that, at currently used levels, the nutrient content of food exposed to small doses of radiation remains virtually unchanged. Flavor also stays intact.

Why irradiate foods?

Low doses of radiation can destroy bacteria like salmonella that have become an increasingly alarming problem for the chicken and egg industries. It can kill parasites in fish and pork, inhibit sprouting in potatoes, and delay spoilage in fruits like strawberries. Shelf life of foods can be extended, which helps increase the distances that perishable foods can be shipped.

Aren't there other ways to take care of these problems?

Yes. In fact, the American food supply is already one of the safest in the world. Moreover, if you handle foods carefully, risks of food-born illness can be minimized. For instance, cooking chicken and eggs thoroughly can kill salmonella. But proponents of irradiation think Americans need more protection.

Why is that?

The Centers for Disease Control in Atlanta estimates that as many as 10 million cases of food-born illness occur annually. Proponents of irradiation see the process as another useful technology (like pasteurization) that could help make the American food supply even safer.

Do the compounds used to irradiate food pose any safety hazard?

Accidents can happen when you use or transport any potentially hazardous material. Radioactive cobalt 60 and cesium are no exception. On the other hand, companies have been sterilizing medical tools and equipment with irradiation for many years with few dangerous incidents occurring.

How can you spot irradiated produce?

You won't be able to spot a food that has been irradiated visually, but the government requires irradiated foods to carry a label. On the label is a symbol (a broken circle surrounding two petals and a dot) that is the universal sign for irradiation. A statement that explains the food has been irradiated accompanies the symbol.

Milk and Bovine Growth Hormone

Studies show that injections of a growth hormone called *bovine somatotropin* (BST) can boost the milk production of select cattle by ten to twenty-five percent. The hormone, which was recently approved as safe by the FDA, is now used by a limited number of dairy farmers. However, don't expect your milk label to mention the use of BST. Since there are no detectable residues of the growth hormone in the milk produced, milk labels do not state that BST has been used.

Critics, such as the Center for Science in the Public Interest, are up in arms about the missing label information. They feel that consumers have the right to know if the milk they are buying was produced by BST-treated cows. The FDA and many scientists disagree, and contend that BST-treated cows produce safe milk. Chances are this debate will continue. If you are wary about the hormone, you'll need to ask your local dairy or supermarket if they are selling milk produced with BST. Apparently, some supermarket chains are refusing to carry BST-treated milk and some food companies refuse to use the milk as a processed food ingredient.

Reference List

"Three agencies propose pesticide reforms." *FDA Consumer,* January–February, 1994.

"Pesticide report available." *FDA Consumer,* January–February, 1994.

Weisenberger, D.D. "Human health effects of agrichemical use." *Human Pathology;* 24(6): 571–6, 1993.

Marwick, C. "Pesticides pose concern about children's diet." *Journal of the American Medical Association;* 270(7): 802–3, 1993.

Maroni, M., and Fait, A. "Health effects in man from long-term exposure to pesticides." *Toxicology;* 78(1–3): 1–180, 1993.

Abbott, P.J. "Carcinogenic chemicals in food: evaluating the health risk." *Food & Chemical Toxicology;* 30(4): 327–32, 1992.

Krieger, R.I., et al. "Assessing human exposure to pesticides." *Review of Environmental Contamination & Toxicology;* 128: 1–15, 1992.

Mitchell, G.E., et al. "Effect of low dose irradiation on composition of tropical fruits and vegetables." *Journal of Food Composition and Analysis;* 5: 291–311, 1992.

Wessel, J.R. and Yess, N.J. "Pesticide residues in foods imported into the United States." *Reviews of Environmental Contamination & Toxicology;* 120: 83–104, 1991.

"Produce and pesticides: A consumer guide to food quality and safe handling." Food Marketing Institute in cooperation with the Food and Drug Administration.

Botham, P.A. "Are pesticides immunotoxic?" *Adverse Drug Reactions & Acute Poisoning Reviews;* 9(2): 91–101, 1990.

"A primer on food additives." *FDA Consumer,* October, 1988.

Folkenberg, J. "Reporting reactions to food additives." *FDA Consumer,* 1988.

Lecos, C. "The number one food safety problem." *FDA Consumer,* 1988.

Mott, L. and Synder, K. Natural Resources Defense Council. "Pesticide Alert." Sierra Club Books, San Francisco, 1987.

ALLERGIES AND FOOD INTOLERANCES

Are you plagued by stomach cramps or diarrhea after drinking a glass of milk? Do you break out in hives every time you eat strawberries? Is it normal to suffer from migraines and nausea after eating Chinese food? It's easy to blame these kinds of adverse reactions on a food allergy. Some experts say, however, that such symptoms do not always spell food allergy. More than likely they're an intolerance to food. Learning to distinguish between a real food allergy and simply an intolerance to a food is important. The difference is that an intolerance does not involve the immune system and is never life-threatening.

Are You the Victim of Allergy?

True food allergy is rare, according to the American Academy of Allergy and Immunology, affecting less than two percent of Americans. Usually, food allergies strike people who already have a history of allergy such as hay fever or asthma. Close to 25 percent of adults and children with hay fever and asthma report having some type of food allergy. Children, for some reason, are more likely to suffer food allergies than adults. If both parents have allergies, children have a 70 percent chance of being allergic. If only one parent has allergies chances of a child being allergic drop to 25 or 30 percent. Luckily, children usually outgrow food allergies as their immune system matures.

Keep in mind that allergies often don't occur the first time you encounter an offending food. They happen the next time you are exposed; the first exposure sensitizes the body and readies the immune system to respond to the food or food protein as a foreign substance. So, don't try and diagnose a food allergy yourself, particularly if you have had a severe reaction to a food. Doctors can use skin and blood tests to zero in on a problem. An even more effective diagnostic tool is the double-blind food-challenge test used by researchers. With this costly but accurate test, people are alternately fed a placebo and then the offending food (in capsule form or disguised and mixed with another food). The blind challenge is done so that neither you or your doctor have any idea what you are taking. That way any reactions observed will be due to a real reaction to the food rather than a preconceived or suspected response.

Common Causes of Food Allergy

Any food can cause an allergy. But the following list identifies the more common culprits. Why these foods? The immune system mistakes protein particles in these foods for foreign invaders (viruses, bacteria) and the immune system responds by releasing *histamine,* a substance that produces allergy symptoms.

- Milk
- Eggs
- Nuts from trees (walnuts)
- Crustaceans (shrimp, lobsters, crab)
- Shellfish (clams, oysters, scallops)
- Fish
- Legumes (peanuts, soybeans)
- Wheat

Complaints range from migraines to fatigue to hives. Often symptoms occur immediately if the allergy is a severe one; sometimes symptoms are delayed for a few hours. Three types of complaints are most common: gastrointestinal disturbances such as diarrhea, stomach cramps, or nausea; skin reactions; and respiratory reactions. In rare cases, food allergy results in *anaphylactic shock,* a potentially fatal reaction involving the whole body. During anaphylactic shock, blood pressure drops and the throat swells up, causing difficulty breathing. If airways shut completely the result can be fatal.

Common Types of Allergy Complaints

Gastrointestinal
- Abdominal pain
- Nausea
- Vomiting
- Diarrhea
- Gastrointestinal bleeding
- Itchy mouth or throat

Skin complaints
- Hives
- Eczema
- Swollen air passages (angioedema)

- Reddening of the skin (erythema)
- Itching

Respiratory complaints
- Sneezing, runny nose, nasal congestion
- Asthma
- Cough

Systemic (full body) complaints
- Anaphylactic shock

Is It a Food Intolerance?

Some of the same symptoms and complaints that signal a food allergy also indicate a food intolerance. The symptoms of food intolerance are often mild and can easily be avoided by steering clear of or limiting the amount that you eat of the offending food. For instance, some people break out in hives when they eat strawberries. The reaction isn't mediated by the immune system. Simply avoiding strawberries eliminates the negative response, thereby making it unnecessary to seek medical attention.

Flushing and a tightness around the chest are symptoms of a rare intolerance to MSG (monosodium glutamate), a flavor enhancer used in some Chinese restaurants. The most common food intolerance involves an adverse reaction to milk, known as *lactose intolerance.* People with lactose intolerance are missing the enzyme that breaks down and digests milk sugar. Symptoms include gas, bloating, and diarrhea. But unlike food allergy victims, people with lactose intolerance can sometimes tolerate small quantities of milk or milk products. In addition, supermarkets sell milks that have been treated with enzymes that predigest milk sugar. And over-the-counter enzyme tablets (that break down milk sugar) can be swallowed to help digest milk sugars.

Are You Allergic to Sulfites?

While they haven't made headlines lately, six or seven years ago preservatives called *sulfites* created quite a panic in the food industry. It's now known that less than one percent of the population is sensitive to sulfites (usually people with asthma).

After reports of people having severe, and sometimes fatal reactions after ingesting foods treated with sulfiting agents, the government stepped in. Officials at the Food and Drug Administration worked to ensure that food labels divulged the use of sulfites. In addition, many food companies and restaurants replaced sulfites with safer preservatives. The preservatives, commonly sprayed on salad bar greens to keep them fresh, and also used in everything from wine to potato salad, are no longer used as frequently, although the rare person allergic to sulfites needs to carefully scrutinize labels. Sulfites can turn up in unusual places: cereals with dried fruits, cookies with dried fruit fillings such as fig bars, snack crackers, sandwich cookies, and lemon juice concentrate.

Tale of the Disappearing Fish Allergy

As researchers continue to unlock the mysteries of the immune system and how allergies are triggered, scientists from Johns Hopkins Medical Institute in Baltimore offer an unusual new report about fish. When these scientists fed canned tuna to children with known food allergies to fish, the tuna provoked no response. After a food-challenge test (using one-half can of tuna) even children with multiple food allergies showed no symptoms or signs of a problem.

Researchers speculate that the high temperatures and pressures of the canning process break down proteins in the fish into such small particles that they bypass immune-system guards. However, scientists caution parents against feeding tuna to a child with fish allergy. Take your child to a physician for a food-challenge test with canned tuna to make sure he or she is not allergic before packing his or her lunchbox with tuna salad.

Cooking Substitutions

If you or a family member suffers from a food allergy or food intolerance, that doesn't mean recipes from favorite cookbooks have to be avoided. With a few simple ingredient changes you can prepare foods that an allergy or food intolerance sufferer can enjoy easily. However, there is one caveat for allergy sufferers: Be aware that these suggestions are not a substitute for a doctor's advice. If you have a true food allergy, you need to consult with your doctor for guidance as to how to deal with that specific food allergy.

Allergic/intolerant to milk: Use fruit juices or soy milk (purchased in the health food store) in place of milk in baked goods and puddings. The flavor will be slightly different but consistency will stay the same.

Allergic to eggs: Egg substitutes won't always work as replacements since many contain egg whites (allergenic-proteins concentrate in the white). For baked goods, you can make an acceptable binding agent by combining two tablespoons of whole-wheat flour, ½ teaspoon of oil, ½ teaspoon of baking powder and two teaspoons of liquid (water, fruit juice or milk).

Allergic to chocolate: Carob makes a good stand-in. Carob powder, sold in health food stores, can be used to replace cocoa powder. Or mix three tablespoons of carob powder with two tablespoons of margarine as a substitute for one square of baking unsweetened chocolate.

Allergic to corn: Since most baking powder contains cornstarch, recipes for baked goods will need a corn-free leavening agent such as baking soda. Or, mix one-quarter teaspoon of cream of tartar with one-half teaspoon of baking soda to equal one teaspoon of baking powder. With puddings or sauces that call for cornstarch, substitute equal amounts of either arrowroot or potato starch.

Allergic to wheat: Wheat flour is used in most bakery and bread products including crackers, cookies, and cereals. If you bake from scratch, acceptable substitutes include rye flour, oats, oat flour, and buckwheat or barley flour.

Allergic to soy: Check labels carefully as soy is used in many foods and can appear on the ingredient list as hydrolyzed vegetable protein, textured vegetable protein or vegetable protein, soybeans, soy flour, soy milk, soy sauce, miso, tempeh, and tofu (soybean curd). Soy oil is the only soy product that can be safely eaten by individuals with soy allergy, and then only if it is free of soy protein. Since most of us don't use soy products at home, substitutions aren't usually necessary. Other vegetable oils and wheat flour can be easily substituted for soy products. There is no substitute for tofu.

Food Allergy Shopping Sleuth

Since convenience foods are part of most people's lifestyle, give yourself plenty of extra time at the supermarket to read the fine print on labels. Sometimes the food you are allergic to can turn up where you least expect it. A person allergic to corn will need to avoid peanut butter made with corn syrup, for example. A good substitute is natural peanut butter made with ground peanuts only and no added sweeteners. A person allergic to eggs, milk, or wheat needs to know that these foods can be listed as an ingredient in a number of different ways.

Eggs—can be listed as albumin, egg white solids, egg yolk, yolks.
Milk—can be listed as milk solids, cream, curds, whey, whey solids, lactalbumin, casein, caseinate, sodium caseinate, lactose.
Wheat—can be listed as flour, durum flour, semolina, wheat bran, wheat germ, wheat starch, gluten, graham flour, modified food starch, vegetable gums, vegetable starch, hydrolyzed vegetable protein.

CAUTION: Anyone with a history of anaphylactic reactions (swelling of the throat, asthma-like difficulty with breathing) to a food needs to take extreme caution with packaged and restaurant foods. New labeling laws require all packaged foods to list their ingredients, and most restaurants can tell a patron how the chef prepares a dish. Remember that sometimes food manufacturers and chefs change the recipe. Don't hesitate to ask. And if you are in doubt about a food or dish, don't eat it.

Reference List

Herian, A.M., et al. "Allergenic reactivity of various soybean products as determined by RAST inhibition." *Journal of Food Science;* 58: 385–88, 1993.

Metcalfe, D.D. "Food allergy." *Current Opinion in Immunology;* 3(6): 881–6, 1991.

Metcalfe, D.D. "Diseases of food hypersensitivity." *The New England Journal of Medicine;* 321: 255, 1989.

Pastorella, E.A. "Role of the elimination diet in adults with food allergy." *Journal of Allergy and Clinical Immunology;* 84: 475, 1989.

Taylor, S.L., et al. "Sensitivity to sulfited foods among sulfite sensitive subjects with asthma." *Journal of Allergy and Clinical Immunology;* 81: 1159, 1988.

Novembre, E., et al. "Foods and respiratory allergy." *Journal of Allergy and Clinical Immunology;* 81: 1059, 1988.

Bahna, S.L. "Milk allergy in infancy." *Annals of Allergy;* 59: 131, 1987.

Bock, S.A. "Prospective appraisal of complaints of adverse reactions to foods in children during the first three years of life." *Pediatrics;* 79: 683, 1987.

Taylor, S.L. "Food allergies and sensitivities." *Journal of the American Dietetic Association;* 86: 599, 1986.

Bock, S.A. "A critical evaluation of clinical trials in adverse reactions to foods in children." *Journal of Allergy and Clinical Immunology;* 78:165, 1986.

Bush, R.K., et al. "A critical evaluation of clinical trials in reactions to sulfites." *Journal of Allergy and Clinical Immunology;* 78:191, 1986.

Bush, R.K., et al. "Prevalence of sensitivity to sulfiting agents in asthmatic patients." *American Journal of Medicine;* 81:816, 1986.

Butkus, S.N., et al. "Food allergies: Immunological reactions to foods." *Journal of the American Dietetic Association;* 86: 601, 1986.

Mansfield, L.E., et al. "Food allergy and adult migraine. Double blind and mediator confirmation of allergic etiology." *Annals of Allergy;* 55: 126, 1985.

Bock, S.A. "Natural history of severe reactions to foods in young children." *Journal of Pediatrics;* 107:676, 1985.

Atkins, F.M., et al. "Evaluation of immediate adverse reactions to foods in adult patients: A detailed analysis of reaction patterns during oral food challenge." *Journal of Allergy and Clinical Immunology;* 75: 356, 1985.

American Academy of Allergy and Immunology, Committee on Adverse Reactions to Foods. NIH Publication No. 84-2442, 1984.

Egger, J., et al. "Is migraine food allergy?" *Lancet;* 2: 805, 1983.

Bernstein, M., et al. "Double blind food challenge in the diagnosis of food sensitivity in the adult." *Journal of Allergy and Clinical Immunology;* 70: 205, 1982.

Bernhisel-Broadbent, J., et al. "Cross allergenicity in the legume botanical family in children with food hypersensitivity." *Journal of Allergy and Clinical Immunology;* 70: 205, 1982.

Minford, A.M.B., et al. "Food intolerance and food allergy in children: A review of 68 cases." *Archives Diseases of Childhood;* 57: 742, 1982.

Bock, S.A. "The natural history of food sensitivity." *Journal of Allergy and Clinical Immunology;* 69: 173, 1982.

ANEMIA

Apathetic, irritable, or having trouble concentrating at work? Your problem could be related to stress, depression, or just moodiness—then again, you might be suffering from an iron deficiency. Studies confirm that even a marginal deficiency of this trace mineral can hinder work performance and learning ability in both adults and children. It's also been suggested that too little iron in the diet can depress immune function and make it more difficult to fight off infection.

When iron levels in the diet are too low, that deficiency can result in *iron-deficiency anemia.* Another type of nutritional anemia can develop when the diet lacks recommended amounts of the B-vitamin folic acid. Even though both conditions are easily corrected through diet, recent studies indicate that nutritional anemias are still a common problem in this country, particularly for women and children. Unfortunately, deficiencies are often mild enough to go unnoticed. For example, in a recent report, researchers point out that while severe iron deficiency has been virtually eradicated in this country, borderline deficiencies of the mineral are common among children.

Groups Most At Risk for Iron Deficiency

While iron-deficiency anemia—a condition marked by fewer red blood cells and a lower blood hemoglobin concentration—can be caused by a rare genetic disorder or blood loss, the more likely cause of this medical problem is usually a diet lacking in iron-rich foods. Women and children, because they have higher iron requirements than men, are more susceptible to iron-deficiency anemia. For example, the recommended dietary allowance (RDA) for iron is only ten milligrams per day for men; women require fifteen milligrams. The following groups are at risk for iron deficiency:

- Children, ages six months to four years. During periods of rapid growth the body requires more iron. But the iron content of milk, a major food in a child's diet, is low.
- Teenagers, particularly girls. Another rapid growth phase; iron requirements are elevated during the early adolescent years. Girls are most at risk due to their lower calorie intakes and a cultural obsession with dieting.

- Young adult women. During the reproductive years iron is lost each month due to blood lost during the menstrual cycle.
- Pregnant women. Demands of the fetus and an expanding blood volume create a need for more iron during pregnancy. Blood loss during childbirth lowers iron stores.

Pumping Iron

Not only does iron carry oxygen through the body, this mineral is also involved in many important body functions. It's a component of many of the key enzymes that regulate body reactions. In addition, new research suggests that iron may prove crucial in helping the body fight infection by keeping the immune system healthy (see the section on Immunity, page 100). Recent studies find that iron-poor diets can impair cognitive performance and make it more difficult for children to exercise and keep active. The major symptom of iron deficiency in both adults and children is unexplained fatigue.

Estimates are that most Americans eat around six milligrams of iron with each 1,000 calories of food. Since most men eat 2,000 or more calories per day, they can easily meet their recommended dietary allowance (RDA) for iron of 10 milligrams. A bowl of chili (one cup kidney beans, three ounces of meat) at lunch and a baked potato at dinner easily meets the ten milligram requirement. The only time men need higher amounts of iron is when they lose major amounts of blood due to injury or illness.

While the RDA for women is higher than for men, it recently dropped from 18 milligrams to 15 milligrams of iron per day. Of course, that doesn't mean American women are getting enough iron. Heavy blood loss during menstruation and childbirth can deplete stores of iron. If a woman is dieting or eating only 1200 to 1500 calories each day, chances are she is taking in only seven to nine milligrams of iron, far less than the 15 milligrams she needs. (If you become pregnant, iron needs will double. See the section on Pregnancy, page 151.)

If a woman were to follow the same meal pattern mentioned above for men (a bowl of chili at lunch, a baked potato at dinner) she would also need to add two slices of whole wheat toast at breakfast and one half cup of cooked spinach to meet the 15 milligram mark. A vegetarian could eat meatless chili, but to make up for the iron lost from omitting the three ounces of meat it would be necessary to add another one-half cup of cooked spinach at supper.

Don't count on cast-iron pots and pans to help boost iron intake. Even though acidic foods (tomato sauce) do leach iron from the cookware into food, scientists report that little of this iron is available to the body. Food is still the best source of this key mineral.

Food Sources of Iron

Heme Iron   is a readily absorbed form of iron found in meats and animal food.

Food	milligrams of iron
Clams, 4 large or 9 small	11.9
Oysters, 6 medium	5.6
Sirloin steak, 3 oz.	2.8
Roast beef, 3 oz.	2.5
Lean hamburger, 3 oz.	1.8
Chicken, light meat, 3 oz.	1.0
Chicken, dark meat, 3 oz.	.9

Non-Heme Iron   comes from vegetable foods; not as easily absorbed as the iron from meats.

Vegetables	milligrams of iron
Spinach, ½ cup cooked	3.2
Potato, baked with skin	2.8
Kidney beans, ½ cup cooked	2.6
Lima beans, ½ cup cooked	2.6
Navy beans, ½ cup cooked	2.3
Green peas, ½ cup cooked	1.1
Tomato juice, 6 ounces	1.0
Broccoli, ½ cup cooked	.9
Brussels sprouts, ½ cup cooked	.9

Grains	
Fortified cereal, 1 cup	4.4
Oatmeal, 1 cup cooked	1.6
Whole wheat bread, 1 slice	.9

Fruits	
Raisins, ½ cup	1.9
Apricots, dried, 5 halves	.8
Raspberries, 1 cup	.7
Strawberries, 1 cup	.6

Improving Iron Absorption

Even if you are not a vegetarian, most of the iron you eat is likely to come from the less available vegetable sources. Both vegetarians and nonvegetarians can employ two diet tricks guaranteed to help improve iron absorption from plant foods. Keep in mind that tea, antacids, and some high-fiber foods, such as whole-grain breads and cereals, wheat germ, bran, dried fruits, and legumes, contain compounds that can decrease non-heme iron absorption by substantial amounts.

Vitamin C　Recent research finds that adding seventy-five milligrams of vitamin C (oranges, tomatoes, papaya) to a meal improves absorption of non-heme iron.

Foods with 75 milligrams or more of vitamin C

	Serving size
Orange juice	6 oz.
Strawberries	1 cup
Broccoli	¾ cup
Kiwifruit	1 medium
Red pepper	½ large
Cantaloupe	1 cup cubes

The meat factor:　Research documents that adding three ounces of meat, chicken, or fish to a non-heme meal can help double iron absorption. Scientists aren't sure if it's the heme iron in meat that aids absorption or some other factor.

Is It Possible to Overdo It on Iron?

When Finnish researchers noticed a link between high blood levels of iron and heart-attack risk in men (see the Heart Health section, page 85) news stories hinted that it might be wise to cut back on iron-rich foods. But experts say it's far too soon to be thinking along these lines. Almost the only people who run into toxicity problems with iron are people who have a rare genetic disorder that makes them absorb iron too efficiently. Children can also develop problems with iron overload when they have access to their parents' iron supplement tablets. (Every year, United States doctors see approximately 2,000 cases of iron poisoning, mainly among youngsters who mistake iron supplements for candy.) The lethal dose of ferrous sulfate for a two-year-old is approximately three grams.

The Other Kind of Nutritional Anemia

Now that folic acid is in the news as a protector against certain types of birth defects (see Pregnancy and Breastfeeding, page 151) and cancer (see Cancer, page 47), you probably are more aware of this B vitamin. Yet nutritionists say that the folacin (folic acid) content of most diets in this country is fairly low. If folacin levels plummet far enough, red blood cells are damaged and anemia can develop fairly quickly.

A vitamin B_{12} deficiency (pernicious anemia) can produce symptoms similar to those of a folacin deficiency. That's because both of these B vitamins are involved in the production of red blood cells. But be aware that the anemia caused by a B_{12} deficiency is not usually diet related. The problem is created by an inability of the digestive tract to absorb this nutrient. (Regular injections of B_{12} can correct the problem.)

Symptoms of a Folacin Deficiency

It can be difficult to pinpoint a folic-acid deficiency relying on symptoms alone. That's because the signs of a potential folic acid deficiency are common complaints caused by any number of different problems, such as:

- Fatigue
- Irritability
- Forgetfulness
- Poor appetite
- Diarrhea

Foods Rich in Folic Acid

Even though the nutrient is widely available in many foods, it's easily destroyed by long storage, overcooking, and processing. Shop for the freshest produce and foods that are minimally processed as they tend to be your best sources of folacin.

RDA: 4 micrograms

Food	micrograms of folic acid
Spinach, 1 cup cooked	262
Asparagus, 1 cup cooked	176
Lima beans, 1 cup cooked	156
Broccoli, 1 cup cooked	108
Wheat germ, ¼ cup	106
Beets, 1 cup cooked	90
Cauliflower, 1 cup cooked	64

Orange (navel), 1 medium	47
Cantaloupe, ½ melon	46
Cabbage, 1 cup raw	40
Tofu, firm, ½ cup	37

Reference List

Oski, F.I. "Iron deficiency in infancy and childhood." NEJM; 329: 190–193, 1993.

Gray, A.B., et al. "The effect of intense interval exercise on iron status parameters in trained men." *Medicine & Science in Sports and Exercise;* 25: 778–82, 1993.

Telford, R.D., et al. "Iron status and diet in athletes." *Medicine & Science in Sports and Exercise;* 25: 796–800, 1993.

Recommended Dietary Allowances, 10th edition. Washington D.C., 1989: National Academy Press.

Lozoff, B. and Brittenham, G.M. "Behavioral aspects of iron deficiency." *Clinics in Haematology;* 14: 23–53, 1986.

Merhav, H. "Tea drinking and microcytic anemia in infants." *American Journal of Clinical Nutrition;* 41: 1210–1213, 1985.

Dallman, P.R., et al. "Prevalence and causes of anemia in the United States, 1976–1980." *American Journal of Clinical Nutrition;* 39: 437–45, 1984.

Gillooly, M., et al. "The effects of organic acids, phytates and polyphenols on the absorption of iron from vegetables." *British Journal of Nutrition;* 49: 331–42, 1983.

Monsen, E.R., et al. "Estimation of available dietary iron." *American Journal of Clinical Nutrition;* 31: 134–141, 1978.

Cook, J.D. and Monsen, E.R. "Food iron absorption in human subjects: Comparisons of the effect of animal proteins on nonheme iron absorption." *American Journal of Clinical Nutrition:* 29: 859–67, 1976.

Viteri, F.E. and Torun, B. "Anaemia and physical work capacity." *Clinics in Haematology;* 3: 609–26, 1974.

ARTHRITIS

If you're one of the nearly forty million Americans plagued by arthritis, you'd no doubt love to read news of a cure. Since that is not yet possible, the next best strategy is to find ways to relieve your symptoms. Fortunately, great advances are being made in the management and treatment of the more than 100 different disorders that fall under the umbrella heading of arthritis. Diet, which was once considered an unlikely therapy, is now high on the list of treatment tools being carefully studied.

It's too soon to make firm promises, but convincing new studies hint that diet is effective at relieving some of the debilitating symptoms that accompany many types of arthritis. Studies continue to look at the oils from fatty fish, vegetarian diets, and a little known trace mineral called *boron* as potential weapons in the arsenal against arthritis.

The Anti-Arthritis Diet

There is no one specific diet that helps relieve arthritis. In fact, the type of diet strategies currently under study vary depending on the type of arthritic disorder being treated. Currently, the bulk of arthritis research focuses on the two most common rheumatic illnesses, rheumatoid arthritis (RA) and osteoarthritis. These are the two areas where diet therapy is considered a promising part of the treatment regimen.

Rheumatoid arthritis—Typically the more painful of the two most common rheumatic illnesses, rheumatoid arthritis afflicts 2.1 million Americans, most of them women. Common symptoms include fatigue, malaise, pain that doesn't go away with rest, and low-grade fever. Treatment varies depending on the acuteness of the illness. Preliminary dietary studies find potential benefits for a number of foods and eating styles.

- *Fatty fish*   Several studies find that some people with RA find at least a small amount of relief from painful symptoms when their diets contain omega-3 fatty acids, the polyunsaturated oils found in fatty fish. (For a complete list of the fish that contain these oils refer to the section on Heart Health, page 85.)

- *Fasting regimens*   Early reports find that fasting can help relieve pain and symptoms for many RA sufferers. The problem is that once food is reintroduced, the pain and symptoms reappear.
- *Vegetarian diets*   Several research groups have tested strict and moderate vegetarian eating regimens on RA sufferers. In one recent study, 27 people fasted, then followed a vegan (no animal products) diet and then progressed to a lacto-ovovegetarian (dairy products and eggs) (see the section on Vegetarianism, page 197, to learn more about the distinctions between these different types of vegetarian diets) regime. After the first four weeks symptoms lessened. But the results were short-lived.

Osteoarthritis—Nicknamed the "wear-and-tear" disease, osteoarthritis claims nearly sixteen million sufferers. There is a gradual loss of the cartilage that cushions the bones of joints. This type of arthritis is generally limited to only a few joints and is less disabling than rheumatoid arthritis. Most people over sixty, male or female, have some degree of osteoarthritis, but women are three times more likely to suffer from this illness than men. Joints commonly affected are usually weight-bearing joints like the hip or knee.

If you are overweight, losing weight is one of the best diet therapies for this type of arthritis. (See the section on Weight Control, page 203, for tips on how to lose weight.) As a general strategy, the Arthritis Foundation recommends that all arthritis sufferers eat a well-balanced diet. The theory is that you will do better with arthritis treatments and therapies if you are well-nourished.

Bring on the Boron

Seldom mentioned as a tool to fight arthritis, the trace mineral boron is beginning to gain some recognition as a potential dietary weapon. It's already known that low levels of boron in the diet can interfere with the metabolism of calcium and so may indirectly impact on osteoporosis. (See the section on Osteoporosis, page 145.) But one recent study suggests that diets low in boron may be linked to arthritis as well. Over the last fifty years, these researchers note, boron levels in the diets of Americans have gone down and the incidence of arthritis has gone up. In countries like Israel, where diets contain high levels of boron, the incidence of arthritis is low.

These findings do not show cause and effect between dietary levels of boron and arthritis; rather, they hint that there may be some association. In the meantime, there's no harm in enjoying boron-rich foods since most of them harbor plenty of other beneficial ingredients. Foods rich in boron include apples, grapes, peaches, legumes, almonds, cashews, and other nuts.

Reference List

Kjeldsen-Kragh, M., et al. "Controlled trial of fasting and one-year vegetarian diet in rheumatoid arthritis." *Lancet;* 338: 899–902, 1991.

Kremer, J.M. "Clinical studies of omega-3 fatty acid supplementation in patients with rheumatoid arthritis." *Rheumatic Disorders Clinics of North America;* 17: 391–402, 1991.

Belch, J. "Fish oil and rheumatoid arthritis: Does a herring a day keep rheumatologists away?" *Annals of Rheumatic Diseases;* 49: 71–72, 1990.

White-O'Connor B., et al. "Dietary habits, weight history, and vitamin supplement use in elderly osteoarthritis patients." *Journal of the American Dietetic Association;* 89: 378–84, 1989.

Tougher-Decker, R. "Nutritional considerations in rheumatoid arthritis." *Journal of the American Dietetic Association;* 88: 327–31, 1988.

Kremer, J.M., et al. "Fish-oil fatty acid supplementation in active rheumatic arthritis." *Annals of Internal Medicine;* 106: 497–501, 1987.

Wolman, P.G. "Management of patients using unproven regimens for arthritis." *Journal of the American Dietetic Association;* 87: 1211–13, 1987.

Panusch, R.S. "Controversial arthritis remedies." *Bulletin of Rheumatic Diseases;* 34(5): 1, 1983.

Parke, A.L., et al. "Rheumatoid arthritis and food: A case study." *British Medical Journal;* 282: 2027–30, 1981.

Baur, W. "What should the patient with arthritis eat?" *Journal of the American Medical Association;* 104:1, 1935.

CAFFEINE & ALCOHOL

One day you drink your coffee with little concern; the next, a new scientific study blasts this morning's brew as detrimental to health and links it to all kinds of ills like PMS, heart disease, or infertility. Ditto for alcohol. While some scientists talk about alcohol protecting against heart disease, others suggest it may encourage the development of certain types of cancer. Don't let conflicting reports about the health hazards of these two beverages confuse you—despite all the media hoopla, medical experts contend that both beverages are relatively safe in moderate amounts. Of course, you'll need to know what constitutes "moderate" and become familiar with the studies that led researchers to conclude that a moderate dose is safe.

Heartening Findings on Caffeine

With heart disease the nation's number one killer, it makes sense that any food or lifestyle factor contributing to risk for this disease would make headlines. Since caffeine is a potent stimulant, concerns were that the drug might damage the heart. A large, multigenerational heart study underway in Framingham, Massachusetts seems to dismiss that concern. Several years ago, after analyzing the coffee-drinking habits of more than 6,000 men and women, Framingham researchers announced that there was no significant link between coffee and heart-disease risk. Now, after studying the second generation of Framingham families (another 4,000 men and women), there still appears to be *no* connection.

It's been suggested that past studies finding a connection between coffee drinking and heart disease might have been influenced by other lifestyle factors, yet it's difficult for scientists to separate out the effects of poor lifestyle habits. However, a new study from the University of California at San Diego found that people who drink coffee tend to eat more cholesterol and more saturated fat than those who don't drink coffee. Coffee drinkers also tend to smoke more cigarettes.

Highlighting Other Concerns

In the past, scientific reports have suggested a link between caffeine and problems such as infertility, cancer, breast disease, and high blood pressure. Here's a brief review of these issues.

- *Breast disease*—In the midseventies, a small study found a link between fibrocystic breast disease and caffeine consumption. However, larger studies, including a major report from the National Cancer Institute, have failed to confirm the finding. Most experts feel that there is no need to eliminate caffeine from the diet unless you're one of the rare women who has breast sensitivity to this stimulant.
- *Cancer*—Numerous studies from around the world have looked at dietary practices and carefully studied the way people eat in an effort to establish how foods might affect cancer risk. According to the American Cancer Society: "There is no indication that caffeine, a natural component of both coffee and tea, is a risk factor in human cancer."
- *High blood pressure*—Based on a review of the results of seventeen different caffeine and blood pressure studies, scientists reporting in the *Archives of Internal Medicine* found that caffeinated beverages don't elevate the blood pressure, at least not on a permanent basis. People who are sensitive to caffeine may experience a small jump in blood pressure. Comparatively speaking, it's no more than the rise a person would experience from climbing some stairs or engaging in some other mild activity.
- *Infertility*—After numerous conflicting reports, researchers at Harvard Medical School and the Centers for Disease Control decided to thoroughly investigate the connection between caffeine and infertility. Their published efforts, a massive report that studied nearly 3,000 women, found no connection between caffeine and fertility problems. Now a new study with close to 5,000 Canadian and American women (1,050 cases with primary infertility, 3,833 controls) finds that high intakes of caffeine seem to increase risk of infertility due to tubal disease or endometriosis. Women in the upper levels of caffeine consumption—five to seven grams of caffeine per month—were at significantly higher risk. While this sounds like a large amount of caffeine it breaks down to about two cups of coffee per day, an amount usually considered moderate.
- *Pregnancy*—Once women become pregnant, the health risks of caffeine again pose a concern because caffeine does cross the placenta. However, health professionals see no harm for women partaking of moderate amounts of caffeine-containing beverages; but in this case moderate may mean less than the usual two cups per day. To play it safe, you may want to limit yourself to one cup of coffee per day or less. Scientists are uncertain of the health risks a heavy caffeine user places on her unborn child.

Caffeine: Deciding Your Dose

To most experts, moderation is defined as one or two cups of coffee or a similar dose of a caffeine-rich beverage per day. However, as people react to doses of caffeine differently, moderation is something you'll need to define individually. Bear in mind that caffeine is a powerful stimulant. Some people are so sensitive to caffeine that one cup of cola or coffee keeps them awake or overstimulates them. Others can drink three or four strong cups of coffee and then sleep soundly.

A dose of about 200 to 240 milligrams of caffeine is necessary to produce stimulatory effects and increase alertnesss in most people. A few words of caution: Don't fool around with caffeine if you have a medical condition that will be adversely affected by stimulants. In fact, if you have ulcers or any medical problems, consult with your physician to determine if caffeine will aggravate the condition. Also, don't rely on caffeine as a regular pick-me-up that substitutes for sleep. Remember, caffeine is a powerful drug and you can become addicted.

Caffeine Content of Foods and Beverages—While chocolate does contain some caffeine, the bigger doses of this stimulant come from beverages. If you'd like to cut back on caffeine, try decaffeinated coffees and teas, or herbal teas. Make sure your switch to decaffeinated products is gradual, however. Cutting back too suddenly on caffeine can cause withdrawal headaches.

Beverage Type	Milligrams caffeine
Coffee: 5-oz cup	
Brewed, drip method	115
Brewed, percolator	80
Instant	65
Decaffeinated	3
Tea: 5-oz cup	
Iced tea, 12-oz glass	70
Brewed, imported brands	60
Brewed, major US brands	40
Instant	30
Cola, 12-oz can	40
Baker's chocolate, 1 oz	26
Dark chocolate, 1 oz	20
Milk chocolate, 1 oz	6
Chocolate milk, 8 oz	5
Chocolate flavored syrup, 1 oz	4

Source: Food Additive Chemistry and Evaluation Branch, The Food and Drug Administration.

Alcohol: Dietary Protector or Villain?

For years, moderate drinking—about one or two drinks per day—has been ranked as one of the few dietary habits that might actually be beneficial to health. Most of the research centered on how wine and other spirits might offer protection against heart disease. Now come studies that implicate alcohol as a risk factor for everything from osteoporosis to breast cancer. As the issue of whether or not to imbibe grows more complicated, one factor is clear. The right attitude toward alcohol is one that takes into account your individual health and other medical conditions.

Intriguing new studies find that women absorb and process alcohol differently from men, something they must consider when deciding whether or not to drink. Weighing the pluses and minuses of alcohol requires acknowledging both your genetic risk for chronic illness and your current lifestyle habits.

- *Heart disease*—Harvard researchers recently reported that one or two drinks a day can lower the risk of heart attack, stroke, and fatal heart disease by 26 percent in men and up to 50 percent in women. Scientists reached that conclusion after two to four years of follow-up on more than 150,000 men and women. Speculation is that alcohol raises blood levels of HDL, the "good" cholesterol that doesn't clog arteries. Nonetheless, health professionals don't want nondrinkers to adopt drinking as a strategy to protect their hearts. Low-fat diets (see Heart Health, page 85) and exercise are more powerful ways to lessen heart disease risk.
- *Breast cancer*—Opinions are mixed about the effects of alcohol on breast cancer risk, because prominent research institutions offer studies with conflicting results. Several years ago a large study from Harvard found an increased risk for breast cancer among women who drink. On the heels of that study came another one, this time from the Centers for Disease Control in Atlanta, that found no association between alcohol and breast cancer. While more studies seem to agree with the Harvard research, scientists want to have more conclusive evidence before making any public-health recommendations. Until that time, moderation is probably the safest course.
- *Osteoporosis*—Alcohol can be a risk factor for the brittle-bone disease of old age, osteoporosis. It's not certain how alcohol causes problems, but excessive intake may be toxic to osteoblasts, cells that develop into bone. Moderate intake of alcohol is probably not harmful.
- *Fetal alcohol syndrome*—The Surgeon General advises women to avoid alcohol during pregnancy because of the risk of birth defects. Pregnant women who are heavy drinkers are more likely to deliver babies with a devastating condition called *fetal alcohol syndrome* (FAS). Infants born with FAS suffer severe health consequences including men-

tal retardation, heart defects, and hyperactivity. They may also be born with damage to the face and limbs. Since research can't document what constitutes a safe level of alcohol during pregnancy, abstinence is the best policy.

Women React Differently to Alcohol—New research confirms that it takes a smaller dose of alcohol to intoxicate a woman than it takes to intoxicate a man. There are two reasons. First, a woman's body contains proportionately less water than a man's. It has to do with body composition; muscles hold more water than fat. (Women have a higher fat content; men are more muscular.) That extra water that men store helps dilute the effects of alcohol. Alcohol in a woman's blood is not watered down, but stays at more concentrated levels.

Second, recent studies find that the enzyme which helps break down alcohol in the stomach acts more sluggishly in women. Scientists speculate that these differences may help to explain why women suffer the effects of alcoholism (liver disease) at lower levels of alcohol intake.

What Is It about Red Wine?—Speculation surrounding why the French have a lower rate of heart disease than Americans (they have about a third as many heart attacks as we do) is focusing on diet. And many researchers wonder if red wine, rather than any particular food, may be the cause. Evidence presented at a recent American Heart Association conference suggested that red wine (California Burgundy and French Bordeaux were the two types tested) may offer protection against heart disease because it contains non-nutrient compounds called *polyphenols.*

Polyphenols, found in grape stems, skins, and seeds (as well as other fruits and vegetables) keep sticky platelets in the blood from clumping together and clogging arteries. White wines don't have as high a polyphenol content as red wines because the skins and seeds are removed early in the fermentation process. The Wisconsin researchers that reported these new findings have expanded their research to include beer (which contains some of the same polyphenols found in wine) in order to determine its effect on blood platelets.

What Does Moderate Drinking Mean?

While the American Heart Association and other health organizations don't recommend that nondrinkers start drinking alcohol as a way to prevent heart disease, they do accept the fact that many Americans drink. The consensus is that moderate amounts of alcohol are probably not harmful and may put a person at lower risk for heart attack.

Since moderate to one man might mean downing a six-pack of beer in one sitting and moderate to another could equate to one martini, the AHA offers its own limits for alcohol intake. If you do drink, says the AHA, limit yourself to one to two ounces of alcohol a day. The U.S. Department of Agriculture's Dietary Guidelines for Americans is less generous to women. It defines moderate drinking for women to be no more than one drink per day. For men, moderate equates to no more than two drinks per day.

One drink counts as
- 12 ounces of beer
- 5 ounces of wine
- 1½ ounces of hard liquor (80 proof)

A Few Words of Warning

Not to be lost in the shuffle with guidelines about moderate drinking is the fact that alcohol provides no nutrients to the body. It is simply a source of calories. More important, excessive amounts of alcohol can interfere with the body's absorption of nutrients. In fact, continued abuse of alcohol can lead to malnutrition as empty calories from liquor take the place of more nutritious foods.

Although the warning label on bottles of wine, beer, and hard liquor is vague and the print is fine, the message bears repeating: *Consumption of alcoholic beverages impairs your ability to drive a car or operate machinery and may cause health problems.*

Reference List

Folts, J.D. "Spirits, spice, sticky platelets and heart attack." The American Heart Association's 21st Science Writers Forum, 1994.

Grodstein, F., et al. "Relation of female infertility to consumption of caffeinated beverages." *American Journal of Epidemiology;* 138: 1353–60, 1993.

Anderson, J.B. and Metz, J.A. "Contributions of dietary calcium and physical activity to primary prevention of osteoporosis in females." *Journal of the American College of Nutrition;* 12: 387–93, 1993.

Larroque, B., et al. "Effects on birth weight of alcohol and caffeine consumption during pregnancy." *American Journal of Epidemiology;* 137: 941–50, 1993.

Holbrook, T.L. and Barrett-Connor, E. "A prospective study of alcohol consumption and bone mineral density." *British Medical Journal* 306: 1506–1509, 1993.

The Healthy Heart Handbook. U.S. Department of Health and Human Services, National Institutes of Health, 1992.

Stavric, B. "An update on research with coffee/caffeine." *Food & Chemical Toxicology;* 30 (60): 533–55, 1992.

Dlugosz, L. and Bracken, M.B. "Reproductive effects of caffeine: a review and theoretical analysis." *Epidemiology Reviews;* 14: 83–100, 1992.

Myers, M.G. "Caffeine and cardiac arrhythmias." *Annals of Internal Medicine;* 114(2): 147–50, 1991.

Grobbee, D.E., et al. "Coffee, caffeine, and cardiovascular disease in men." *The New England Journal of Medicine;* 323: 1026–32, 1990.

Klatsky, A.L., et al. "Coffee use prior to myocardial infarction restudied: heavier intake may increase risk." *American Journal of Epidemiology;* 132: 479–88, 1990.

Dietary Guidelines for Americans, third edition. U.S. Department of Health and Human Services, 1990.

LaVecchia, C., et al. "Coffee consumption and myocardial infarction in women." *American Journal of Epidemiology;* 130: 481–85, 1988.

Leonard, T., et al. "The Effects of Caffeine on Various Body Systems: A Review." *Journal of the American Dietetic Association;* 87: 1048, 1987.

Massey, L.K., et al. "The effect of dietary caffeine on urinary excretion of calcium, magnesium, sodium and potassium in healthy young females." *Nutrition Research*; 4: 43, 1984.

CANCER

Almost every time you pick up a newspaper, there's a new report about some substance or behavior that might cause cancer. Foods are no exception. Studies implicate diet, particularly a diet high in fat and low in fiber, as a potential contributor to cancer risk. Yet the overwhelming bulk of current diet/cancer research centers on how certain foods, or the ingredients they contain, seem to foil the growth of cancer cells. Researchers are carefully studying everything from tea to carrots to tomato paste to figure out how certain foods may act as weapons in the battle against cancer.

The Strongest Diet Protectors

More than 175 different reports have analyzed the relationship between fruits and vegetables and cancer risk, and the evidence is both overwhelming and consistent. Diets high in fruits and vegetables appear to lower the risk for at least fifteen different types of cancer. Scientists cite a number of different protective nutrients and diet ingredients as responsible: antioxidants (vitamin C, beta-carotene), fiber, folic acid, and substances called *phytochemicals.*

In one recent study, women who frequently eat dark green or yellow vegetables and fruit juices were found to have a lower risk for cervical cancer. The probable protector, according to researchers, is folic acid. Foods high in folic acid include leafy greens such as spinach, kale, and broccoli; dried beans such as kidney beans, black-eyed peas, and split peas; citrus fruits including oranges and grapefruit.

Beta-carotene: Bonus or Problem?

While numerous studies confirm that beta-carotene may offer protection against many types of cancer, particularly cancer of the lung, a new Finnish study raises concern about beta-carotene supplements. When Finnish researchers assigned a group of 29,000 middle-aged smokers to supplementation with beta-carotene, vitamin E, both supplements, or neither, they noticed that risk for lung cancer actually increased 18 percent in the beta-carotene supplement group.

Interestingly, the dose of beta-carotene these volunteers took was 20 milligrams per day, an amount previously considered nontoxic. Researchers are unsure what to make of the new findings. After all, it is only one negative study amid numerous positive reports suggesting a protective link between beta-carotene and cancer risk. Some scientists speculate that beta-carotene may not have appeared protective against lung cancer in this study because cancer is a slow-growing, progressive disease that probably takes decades to develop. Taking supplements at a late stage in the development of cancer may not offer the same extent of protection as if the nutrient were taken earlier.

Clearly, the Finnish study has raised a lot of new concerns for researchers to explore. Keep in mind that the study tested the benefits of beta-carotene supplements, not beta-carotene-rich foods. The bottom line: There is plenty of evidence suggesting that diets rich in fruits and vegetables, including the beta-carotene-rich variety, may offer protection against various cancers. Foods high in beta-carotene include bright orange-colored fruits and vegetables such as cantaloupe, sweet potatoes, and carrots; leafy green vegetables (chlorophyll masks the orange pigment) such as spinach, kale, and broccoli.

Phytochemicals: Agents That Fight Cancer

There's more to fruits and vegetables than nutrients, however. As part of its $20 million research endeavor, the Experimental Food Program, the National Cancer Institute is working to isolate specific cancer-fighting chemicals (phytochemicals) in foods that appear to offer protection against cancer. The five foods currently being studied include garlic; the umbelliferous vegetable family which includes carrots, parsnips, and parsley; licorice root extract; soybeans; and flaxseed—a grain high in omega-3 fatty acids that is typically baked into breads and crackers in Europe.

The ultimate goal of the project, according to the agency, is to single out which compounds in plants can protect against cancer. At Johns Hopkins College of Medicine, scientists recently identified a phytochemical in broccoli that appears to boost the activity of enzymes that fight cancer. Called *sulforaphane,* this substance is only one ingredient in broccoli that may help protect against cancer. Studies from many years ago suggest that broccoli and other members of the cruciferous vegetable family contain compounds called *indoles* which might be capable of blocking tumor growth. Cruciferous vegetables, members of the mustard family, also include brussels sprouts, cabbage, cauliflower, collard greens, mustard greens, kale, radishes, rutabagas, and turnips.

Is It Fat or Is It Fiber?

For years, research has implicated a high-fat diet as a potential risk factor for cancer, particularly breast cancer. The problem is the findings have never been consistent. In fact, a brand new report from Harvard Medical School created quite a stir when it documented no connection between fat and risk for breast cancer. These findings contradict other reports which have found a link between fat and breast cancer. According to an unrelated medical report, it could be the type of fat (not the total amount) that is related to cancer risk.

In that study scientists saw a definite link between saturated fat intake and lung-cancer risk. (Smoking is responsible for the majority of lung-cancer cases, but this report looks at the potential causes of lung cancer among nonsmokers.) Among a group of nonsmoking women, those who ate the highest levels of saturated fat were five times more likely to develop lung cancer than women who ate less.

Similarly, researchers from Harvard Medical School in Boston discovered that women who ate red meat (beef, pork, lamb) on a daily basis had more than twice the risk for colon cancer as women who ate meat only once a month. Scientists speculate that animal fat (which is more highly saturated than most vegetable fats) itself may increase cancer risk. The issue of animal and vegetable fat is a confusing one. Even the Harvard researchers admit that eating large amounts of vegetable fat might be just as hazardous as eating large amounts of animal fat.

All this leads to the theory that maybe it's not simply fat that creates a cancer risk but a lack of fiber in the diet. In one intriguing study, scientists found that men who ate very little fiber and large amounts of saturated fat were almost four times as likely to develop colon polyps—growths that are liable to develop into cancer—as men who ate a high-fiber, low-saturated fat diet.

Studies of Seventh Day Adventists (SDA), a group of people whose religion dictates eating a vegetarian diet, appear to prove the theory that fiber may be protective against cancer. Overall, Adventists have about half the risk of developing colon cancer as the average American. However, vegetarian diets that include milk products are not always healthy. Researchers studying the eating habits of 35,000 Adventists found a solid link between risk of colon cancer and higher levels of animal fat intake. Remember that while vegetables and whole grains help keep vegetarian diets high in fiber, you have to be careful to keep preparation and cooking techniques low fat. Vegetarians who add large amounts of fats, oils, and whole-milk dairy products (cheese, cream cheese, butter, whole milk) to their meals may negate the cancer protective benefits of a high-fiber intake.

Unlikely Helpers in the Cancer Battle

While too much fat and too little fiber are obvious culprits in the dietary saga surrounding diet and cancer, researchers aren't ruling out other dietary substances as potential protectors. It's possible that a certain food, nutrient, or phytochemical may be important at one cancer site while another is important somewhere else. Or protective substances might substitute for each other or work in tandem to reinforce one another.

In other words, there is still a lot to be learned about how diet can protect against cancer. In fact, some of today's preliminary findings may turn out to be tomorrow's preventive medicine.

Green Tea—At the first International Symposium on the physiological and pharmacological effects of camellia sinensis (tea), scientists from around the world reported findings confirming that green-leaf teas may inhibit certain types of cancerous growths. (Green is the color of unprocessed tea leaves. Many Oriental teas use green leaves but most American tea leaves are processed, which turns tea leaves black.) Speculation is that a chemical in green tea, *epigallocatechin gallata,* confers the protection. Studies are currently underway in both China and Japan to determine if green teas can act as anticarcinogens for people.

Fish Oils—According to studies at Boston University School of Medicine, fish oils could offer protection against colon cancer. When scientists implanted cancer cells into the colons of lab animals and then fed these animals fish oils, cancer development was inhibited. Interestingly, if tumor-forming cells are implanted into another area of the body, the skin or leg, fish oils do not slow tumor growth, leading researchers to speculate that the protective effects of fish oils are site-specific.

Herbs and Spices—A recent study suggests that three popular spices—cumin, basil, and poppy seed—may be able to impede the development of stomach cancer. Researchers who fed laboratory animals (who were previously given a chemical known to cause stomach tumors) large amounts of these spices found that cancer growth was inhibited 60 to 80 percent. However, the amounts used were much higher than most people would use in cooking. While you wait for more research to be completed in this area, it can't hurt to use these seasonings liberally. (For more details on the health benefits of spices turn to the section on Diabetes, page 61.)

Putting It All Into Perspective

In a recent Australian study, researchers found that skin-cancer free subjects ate much larger amounts of legumes (beans, lentils), fish, and vegetables (particularly those rich in vitamin C or beta-carotene) than those suffering from skin cancer. Rather than attempt to single out each and every protective ingredient in studies such as these, many experts are content to talk about preventing cancer in terms of an overall diet.

Speculation is that the overall quality of your diet may be even more important to cancer prevention than any one single food or ingredient. That's why experts at the National Cancer Institute encourage you to take a broad approach to an anticancer diet. The diet strategies they propose, interestingly, are virtually identical to the recommendations for a diet to help prevent or treat other chronic diseases such as heart disease, diabetes, and high blood pressure.

- Maintain a healthy weight.
- Limit the amount of fat you eat.
- Increase fiber intake to twenty to thirty-five grams per day. Eating more whole grains (oats, whole-wheat bread, and whole-grain cereals) can help boost fiber levels in the diet.
- Increase intake of fruits and vegetables. That can help contribute needed fiber as well as protective nutrients to your diet.
- Limit alcohol to moderate levels. Reports are mixed on what role alcohol plays in cancer risk. Some studies hint that high levels of alcohol may increase breast-cancer risk for some women. (For more details on how to moderate alcohol intake refer to the section on Heart Health, p. 85.)
- Limit intake of smoked, pickled, and salt-cured foods. International research suggests a connection between diets rich in smoked foods and gastric and esophageal cancer. When foods are smoked (smoked salmon, smoked turkey, smoked nuts) the process can produce substances that might cause cancer. This is also true for the pickling and curing process. However, if you eat these foods infrequently there is no cause for alarm.

Reference List

The Alpha-Tocopherol, Beta-Carotene Cancer Prevention Study Group. "The effect on vitamin E and beta-carotene on the incidence of lung cancer and other cancers in male smokers." *The New England Journal of Medicine;* 330: 1029–35, 1994.

Hennekens, C.H., et al. "Antioxidant vitamins—benefits not yet proved." *The New England Journal of Medicine;* 330: 1080–81, 1994.

Sandler, R.S., et al. "Diet and the risk of colorectal adenomas: Macronutrients, cholesterol and fiber." *Journal of the National Cancer Institute;* 85: 884–91, 1993.

Butterworth, C.E., et al. "Folate deficiency and cervical dysplasia." *Journal of the American Medical Association;* 267: 528–33, 1992.

Byers, T. and Perry, G. "Dietary carotenes, vitamin C and protective antioxidants in human cancers." *Annual Reviews of Nutrition;* 12: 139–159, 1992.

Block, G., et al. "Fruit, vegetables and cancer prevention: A review of the epidemiological evidence." *Nutrition and Cancer;* 18: 1–29, 1992.

Ziegler, R. "A review of epidemiological evidence that carotenoids reduce the risk of cancer." *Journal of Nutrition;* 119: 116–22, 1989.

Kritchevsky, D. "Diet, nutrition and cancer: The role of fiber." *Cancer;* 58: 1830–36, 1989.

Subar, A.F., et al. "Folate intake and food sources in the U.S. population." *American Journal of Clinical Nutrition;* 50: 508–16, 1989.

Hennekens, C.H. "Micronutrients and cancer prevention." *The New England Journal of Medicine;* 315: 1288–89, 1986.

Hennekens, C.H. and Eberlein, K. "A randomized trial of aspirin and beta-carotene among U.S. physicians." *Preventive Medicine;* 14: 165–68, 1985.

Hennekens, C.H., et al. "Micronutrients and cancer chemoprevention." *Cancer Detection and Prevention;* 7: 147–58, 1984.

Diet, nutrition and cancer: The National Research Council, National Academy Press, Washington D.C., 1982.

CHILDHOOD NUTRITION

Once children pass the age of two, their diet needs mimic those of adults. They need the same variety of foods—fruits, vegetables, whole grains, lean meats, low-fat dairy foods. And, just like adults, their calorie needs vary. Preschoolers generally require about 1,600 calories per day. Most older children need about 2,200 calories per day. That's the same amount of energy required by most active women and many sedentary men.

About the only different dietary advice experts recommend for a child involves the bone-strengthening mineral, calcium. Since children's bones are growing rapidly, requirements for calcium are higher in children. Currently, recommendations advise that children have at least three servings from the milk group each day. (See the Food Guide Pyramid, page 7.) New research indicates that the amount of calcium needed by children may be higher than what is currently advised. Fascinating new studies are turning the tables on beliefs about childhood dietary villains like sugar and cholesterol. In fact, sorting through what and how much to feed a child today can be quite a challenge.

Feeding the Pint-Sized Palate

In their first year, babies usually triple their weight. By age one, the growth spurt is already slowing down and so is a child's appetite. A one-year-old needs about 1,000 calories a day. By age three, only about 300 to 500 more calories per day are necessary. In fact, a good rule of thumb about child-sized portions is to give one tablespoon of food—meat, fruit, vegetable, or grain—for each year of a child's age. For a four-year-old, a serving of mashed potatoes would be about four tablespoons, or one-quarter cup.

While calorie needs vary for youngsters, nutrient needs are consistent no matter what the age. In fact, the average four-year-old has the same requirements for calcium, phosphorus, vitamin C and vitamin D as a ten-year-old. It's important to consider what you give your child to meet these nutritional needs. Kids don't eat as much food as adults but their nutrient needs are high. You can use the Food Pyramid as a guide (see introduction, page 7) to feeding your child. But experts recommend smaller servings sizes.

Pyramid Food Groups: Servings For Children

While the Department of Agriculture's Food Guide Pyramid recommends a range in the number of servings from different food groups, experts have more definite ideas in mind about the amount of food that children need. For instance, the grain group, at the base of the pyramid and the base on any healthy diet, lists six to eleven servings per day as the recommended amount. Children fit into the lower part of the range; six grain/bread servings per day are sufficient. Also, children have a greater need for calcium (for growing bones), so the top of the range for the milk group—three servings—is recommended. This list presents the number of servings children need from each of the pyramid food groups.

Food group	Number of servings	Some healthy choices	Nutrients supplied
Breads, cereals, pasta	6	1–2 slices whole grain bread, ½ cup hot or cold cereal, rice, pasta or noodles, bagel, rice cake	B vitamins, iron, fiber, carbohydrate
Fruits, vegetables	5	½ cup citrus fruit, berries, tomatoes; ¼ cup, raw or cooked, broccoli, carrots, squash, sweet potato	Vitamin C, Vitamin A
Milk, yogurt, cheese	3	8 ounces low-fat milk or yogurt, 1½ oz low-fat cheese	Calcium, riboflavin, protein
Meat, poultry, fish, eggs, dried beans	2	2 to 3 ounces lean meat, fish or chicken, one egg, 2 tablespoons peanut butter, ¾ (after cooking) cup dried beans	Protein, iron, thiamin
Fats, oils, salad dressing, sugar, soft drinks, candy, desserts		Use sparingly	Source mainly of calories, few nutrients

Clearing up Some Confusion

Not only do children come in a variety of shapes and sizes but each of them is likely to have his or her own set of health problems. According to a recent survey, nearly one out of four American children (aged five to eight) have risk factors that significantly increase their chance of heart disease including high blood pressure, sedentary lifestyle, and obesity. That last condition, obesity, is growing at such an alarming pace that one researcher claims that American parents are raising a nation of butterballs.

Despite these findings, experts urge parents not to be too strict about a child's diet. Several research studies find that if you are too stringent with a child's diet, you can stunt growth.

Myth: All kids need to eat a low-fat diet.

Fact: Low-fat diets are not recommended before the age of two, since children need fat and cholesterol to help the brain and nervous system develop properly. If you eliminate too much fat from your child's diet, you may set him back both physically and emotionally. Once youngsters pass that age, it's safe to begin acquainting them with the same heart-healthy diet (see the section on Heart Health, p. 85) and lifestyle adults should follow. If you instill the right attitude early, kids will follow a healthful diet path much more readily.

Myth: Sugar makes youngsters hyperactive.

Fact: Past studies seemed neither to strongly confirm nor deny that sugar has an adverse affect on behavior. A new report from Vanderbilt University, however, seems to clear sugar as a dietary villain. When these scientists fed a group of forty-eight supposedly sugar-sensitive children diets that included sugar or artificial sweeteners there was no evidence that any sweetener had an adverse effect on behavior. Three-week stints on sugar, aspartame, and saccharin did not make children more jumpy, inattentive, or aggressive.

Myth: Kids need three complete meals a day.

Fact: Food jags and changing appetites make it hard to feed kids on any kind of rigid schedule. Give kids the structure of mealtimes, but don't fret about the quantities and types of foods they eat. Concentrate on offering your child a variety of nutritious foods and snacks. Recent studies from the University of Illinois show that children, if faced with a variety of nutritious food choices, have an innate sense of what they need to eat to grow.

Myth: Kids should be taught to like all foods.

Fact: Try to be realistic. Did you like everything you were served as a child? Food preferences are individual. It's not necessary for a child to like every vegetable, fruit, or fish you place in front of them. However, research shows that familiarity often brings acceptance. It may take as many as ten attempts (so hang in there and be patient) but eventually children who are afraid to try a new food may actually learn to accept it.

Myth: There are good and bad foods.

Fact: It's not foods that are good or bad, but diets. You don't need to deny kids hot dogs, potato chips, and hot-fudge sundaes. (A healthy diet allows leeway for indulgence in favorite foods; these foods should just be eaten less frequently.) In fact, banning junk foods from the diet often tends to make kids crave them more. It may also set the stage for future weight problems and eating disorders.

Are You Raising a Butterball?

Statistics reveal that one out of every four children in the United States is overweight. Heredity can be blamed to some extent: If you and your spouse are both overweight, there is an 80 percent chance your child will have a weight problem. (With one overweight parent, the chance is 40 percent.) But lifestyle—how a child lives and eats—may be an even more influential factor.

Perhaps the biggest factor, the one that sets many a child up for weight gain, is a sedentary lifestyle. Youngsters today are much less active than kids of fifteen or twenty years ago. They're seldom active at school—only 10 percent of elementary schools even require physical education classes. At home, television and computers are rapidly edging out active pursuits like bike riding, sports, and other outdoor play.

Recent studies find that children who watch four hours of television per day are twice as likely to be fat as are kids who watch less often. The combination of inactivity and high-fat snacking while watching television may help explain some of the weight gain. Experts say to resist the temptation to cut back on your overweight child's food. Food deprivation can backfire and youngsters may become more preoccupied with food—afraid they won't get enough to eat, children deprived of food are often prone to overeat when given the chance.

Medical consensus is that growing children should not be put on strict diets. Before you put your child on any kind of weight control plan, talk with your physician. Chances are the advice you will receive is to cut back on fat in the family diet. Being prudent about fat is healthy for the heart as well as an easy way to trim calories and lose weight gradually. In fact, a new study finds that there is a direct correlation between the amount of body fat a child carries (the body-fat percentage) and the amount of fat he or she eats, rather than the total calories.

Carefully Limiting the Fat—Walking the fine line between how much fat is healthy and how much is too much for children to eat isn't so difficult. Studies show that American children probably get about 35 percent of their calories from fat. To drop down to 30 percent fat, the new recommendation for children over the age of two, requires no drastic changes. It's simply a matter of giving fresh fruits, vegetables, whole grains, and lean meats a prime place in the diet, highlighting these foods as day-to-day choices. Help your kids learn to enjoy higher-fat foods (hot fudge sundaes, french fries) in smaller portions and less frequently.

One of the best ways to steer children toward low-fat foods is to get them involved with shopping, planning, and cooking meals. At younger ages, it's enough to let children be around while you cook. Later, let them help with food preparation. Children learn by example; if you are interested in low-fat foods, they will be too. You'll probably want to make changes slowly and without any major announcements. Indeed, school-lunch cooks find that when they trim the fat in inconspicuous ways, kids don't even notice.

Handing Out Healthy Snacks

While children need lots of calories to help them grow, a small stomach capacity limits what they can eat at one sitting. That's why snacks tend to contribute a big percentage of a child's total calorie intake. Keeping these snacks healthy is paramount to good health. Here are a few child-pleasing suggestions.

- Yogurt parfait (low-fat yogurt layered with fruit)
- Cut-up fresh melon, strawberries
- Dried fruit mix: apricots, raisins, papaya
- Air-popped popcorn
- Low-fat cookies: fig bars, vanilla wafers, gingersnaps, animal crackers
- Pretzels, no-fat tortilla chips
- Graham crackers with apple butter
- Part-skim string cheese
- Toasted bagel half with jam
- Frozen fruit and juice bars
- Rainbow sherbet, fruit ices
- Turkey in a pita pocket
- Lean ham and lettuce rolled in a tortilla

Filling in the Gaps

Studies continue to show that kids are not getting enough of some of the vitamins and minerals critical to growth. For example, a new report finds that although severe iron-deficiency is no longer a problem for children (as it was ten years ago), mild iron deficiency is still common among kids. In addition, a group of Indiana researchers find that youngsters who take in higher amounts of calcium than currently recommended end up having denser bones than children who get less calcium. Unfortunately, most children eat far less than is recommended, according to scientists from the University of Minnesota. These researchers also point out that children today are being shortchanged of vitamin B_6 and zinc. It's important to highlight these problem nutrients in your child's diet.

Iron—Too little iron in a child's diet can alter cognitive performance, impair motor function, and cause a number of other serious health problems.

The RDA: 10 milligrams (12 mgs for boys 11–12)

Top Five Kid-Pleasing Sources of Iron

Food	milligrams iron
Kidney beans (chili), 1 cup cooked	8.8
Lean hamburger (sirloin), 3 oz	2.8
Baked potato	2.8
Broccoli, 1 cup cooked	1.8
Chicken, 3 oz	1

Zinc—This mineral is critical to a child's growth in many ways. Kids with a zinc deficiency can fail to grow and mature sexually. Loss of appetite (taste) and impaired wound healing are also problems.

The RDA: 10 milligrams

Top Five Kid-Pleasing Sources of Zinc

Food	milligrams zinc
Lean hamburger, 3 oz	18.2
Beef (pot roast), 3 oz	4.7
Peanuts, oil-roasted, 2 oz	3.7
Baked beans (no meat), ½ cup	3.6
Turkey, 3 oz	2.6

Calcium—Everyone knows that calcium helps build and maintain bones and teeth. What you might not realize is that new studies find that children not only eat far less than the RDA for this mineral, but the RDA may be set too low. Researchers in Indiana find that children eating more than the RDA for calcium have denser bones.

The RDA: 800 milligrams (for ages 1 to 10)
            1200 milligrams (for ages 11 to 12)

Top Five Kid-Pleasing Sources of Calcium

Food	milligrams calcium
Low-fat yogurt, 8 oz	415
Skim milk, 8 oz	302
1% chocolate milk, 8 oz	287
Part-skim mozzarella, 1 oz	183
Broccoli, 1 cup cooked	178

Vitamin B$_6$—This B vitamin plays an important role in helping to keep both the nervous system and the muscles working properly. It's also needed for the production of red blood cells and antibodies. Childhood requirements for the nutrient rise with age.

The RDA 1.0 milligrams (for ages 1 to 3)

1.1 milligrams (for ages 4 to 6)

1.4 milligrams (ages 7–10, girls 11–12)

1.7 milligrams (for boys ages 11 to 12)

Top Five Kid-Pleasing Sources of B$_6$

Food	milligrams B$_6$
Banana	.70
Chicken breast, 3 oz	.50
Sirloin steak, 3 oz	.40
Baked potato (with skin), ½	.35
Sweet potato, ½ cup mashed	.24

Reference List

Gazzaniga, J.M. and Burns, T.L. "Relationship between diet composition and body fatness with adjustment for resting energy expenditure and physical activity in preadolescent children." *American Journal of Clinical Nutrition;* 58: 21–28, 1993.

Birch, L.L., et al. "Effects of a nonenergy fat substitute on children's energy and macronutrient intake." *American Journal of Clinical Nutrition;* 58: 326–33, 1993.

Oski, F.A. "Iron deficiency in infancy and childhood." *The New England Journal of Medicine;* 329: 190–193, 1993.

Kaplan, R.M. and Toshima, M.T. "Does a reduced fat diet cause retardation in child growth?" *Preventive Medicine;* 21(1): 33–52, 1992.

Lifshitz, F. "Children on adult diets: is it harmful? Is it healthful?" *Journal of the American College of Nutrition;* 11(Suppl): 84S–90S, 1992.

"The Food Guide Pyramid." *Home and Garden Bulletin* No. 252; U.S. Department of Health and Human Services, 1992.

Birch, L.L., et al. "The variability of young children's energy intake." *The New England Journal of Medicine;* 324: 232–5, 1991.

Recommended Dietary Allowances: 10th edition. Washington, D.C.: National Academy Press, 1989.

Birch, L.L., et al. "Caloric compensation and sensory specific satiety: evidence for self-regulation of food intake by young children." *Appetite;* 7: 323–31, 1986.

Davis, C.M. "Self-selection of diet by newly weaned infants: an experimental study." *American Journal of Diseases of Childhood;* 36:651–79, 1928.

DIABETES

If you think taking care of diabetes is as simple as avoiding sugary-sweet foods, experts now say your attitude is quite outdated. A whole wealth of new research is bringing to light other ways in which diet can influence the development and progression of diabetes. Scientists at the U.S. Department of Agriculture find that common household spices like cinnamon and turmeric can triple the effectiveness of insulin, the hormone that helps control blood sugar. University of Kentucky researchers document a strong role for soluble fiber—apples, oats, dried beans—in lowering blood-sugar levels. Colorado scientists find that fatty diets can triple your risk of developing diabetes. And one researcher is singling out the mineral chromium as a significant previously unrecognized regulator of blood sugar.

Rather than make the diabetic diet more complicated to follow, these new findings are allowing more freedom. The result is diabetic meal plans that are more appetizing and less rigid. New findings have also led experts to dramatically change their attitude about simple sugars and sweets, foods once forbidden on the diabetic diet. If you are diabetic, or at risk for developing diabetes, it's important to learn how the dietary treatment of diabetes is changing. The first step is to determine your risk profile.

Are You at Risk for Diabetes?

There are two types of diabetes: insulin-dependent diabetes mellitus (IDDM) which is also referred to as Type I or juvenile onset diabetes, and noninsulin dependent diabetes mellitus (NIDDM), also called adult-onset diabetes or Type II. Of the roughly seven million diabetics in this country, more than 80 percent fall into the second category. Extra weight and a sedentary lifestyle tends to put them there.

Type I diabetes—This is a chronic illness that develops when the pancreas does not produce enough insulin to regulate blood sugar adequately. Onset occurs early in life, usually in childhood, and requires injections of synthetic insulin to keep blood sugar stable.

Type II diabetes—This chronic disease results from the body's inability to use some or all of the insulin produced by the pancreas. It typically occurs in adults, some time after the age of forty. The risk factors for Type II diabetes are:

- Family members or relatives with diabetes
- Overweight
- Over 40 years of age
- Sedentary
- Female

If you want to forestall or prevent adult onset diabetes, experts now realize that exercising and maintaining a healthy weight may be your two most important strategies. Diet, because it plays a role in controlling both weight and blood sugar, may be the most important tool.

Diabetic Diets: Just Well-Balanced Eating Plans

Whether you are at risk for diabetes or already have it, the basic principles of the diabetic diet form a good foundation for healthy eating, a diet that is easy to follow. The goal of a diabetic diet is to keep blood sugar on an even keel. When blood sugar is too high (hyperglycemia) it can create minor problems such as excessive thirst, headaches, and fatigue. If left uncorrected, damage becomes more severe. High levels of sugar in the blood can injure body organs—the kidneys, the arteries, and the blood vessels in your eyes.

Results of a 1,400-participant National Institutes of Health Study recently offered firm proof that tight blood-sugar control can help protect against diseases aggravated by high blood sugar (atherosclerosis or heart disease, kidney failure, glaucoma). In general, diabetics achieve better blood sugar control with an eating style that emphasizes complex carbohydrates (starchy foods) and fiber.

Rather than simply encouraging diabetics to eat more starch and less fat, experts at the American Diabetes Association and the American Dietetic Association have come up with a flexible prescription for the right balance of carbohydrate, protein, and fat that will control blood sugar. Keep in mind that the new emphasis is on individualizing the diet. Rather than mandatory percentages of protein, fat, and carbohydrate, the new diet plan calls for 10 to 20 percent of total calories as protein. The rest of the daily calorie allotment is then divided between carbohydrate and fat, but the amounts of these two dietary components vary depending on individual goals for blood sugar and fat levels and weight. Remember that the diabetic diet can work for dieters and people who want to develop a healthy eating style.

Carbohydrate—Contrary to popular belief, eating a lot of candy, cake, cookies, or other sugary sweets won't increase your risk of developing diabetes. Simple and complex sugars *do* play a role in regulating blood sugar levels. Meal plans for diabetics include 55 to 60 percent of their calories from carbohydrates, mostly the complex variety. In the past, simple sugar foods were avoided as it was believed they caused a rapid rise in blood sugar. However, the attitude toward simple sugars (table sugar, candy, sweet confections) has changed radically. New guidelines from the American Diabetes Association allow for the inclusion of simple sugars as part of the carbohydrate total, as long as these sugars are included with the meal. They must also be substituted for other carbohydrates, so that the total amount of carbohydrate at the meal stays constant. The reason for the change in thinking is that new studies document that the total amount of carbohydrate a person eats may be more important than its source when it comes to controlling blood sugar.

Nevertheless, complex carbohydrates—whole grain breads and cereals, rice, pasta, potatoes, and other starchy foods—are still the best source for the bulk of carbohydrate calories since these foods typically contain more nutrients than simple sugars. For instance, studies confirm that whole grains and other fiber-rich carbohydrates help regulate blood sugar. Longtime fiber researcher James Anderson of the University of Kentucky College of Medicine continues to find evidence that foods high in water-soluble fiber (apples, dried beans, barley, and oats) lower blood sugar just as effectively as they lower blood-cholesterol levels.

Soluble fiber appears to let the body absorb other sugars more slowly, helping insulin to keep blood sugar on an even keel. In recent studies done in Korea, researchers find that buckwheat, a grain native to Central Asia, is capable of leveling out blood sugar levels and may help curb the urge to snack. For other sources of soluble fiber, this list will help.

Good Sources of Soluble Fiber

Item	Grams of soluble fiber
Butter beans, ½ cup cooked	2.7
Baked beans, ½ cup cooked	2.6
Black beans, ½ cup cooked	2.4
Kidney beans, ½ cup cooked	2.0
Brussels sprouts, ½ cup cooked	2.0
Apricots, 4 fresh	1.8
Mango, ½ small	1.7
Oatmeal, ⅓ cup uncooked	1.3
Peas, ½ cup cooked	1.3

Fat—Since diabetics are at higher risk for heart disease than the general population, the diabetic diet strictly follows the fat guidelines promoted by the American Heart Association. Researchers at the University of Colorado Health Sciences Center recently uncovered yet another reason why excessive fat can be harmful. Fatty diets, they say, may triple your risk of developing diabetes.

You can find more information about a low-fat diet in the chapter on Heart Health (p. 85). In a nutshell, the diet calls for 30 percent or less of the total calories to come from fat. (Experts favor 20 to 25 percent fat for diabetics who have heart disease or risk factors for heart disease such as an elevated blood-cholesterol level.) Saturated fats, like those found in fatty meats, cheese and whole milk dairy products, make up no more than ten percent of the calories or one-third of the total fat allowance. (Keep in mind that saturated fats raise blood cholesterol levels.) Polyunsaturated and monounsaturated fats round out the difference. But be aware that preliminary reports indicate that monounsaturated fats—like those found in olive oil, avocados, and many nuts—may be particularly beneficial for controlling diabetes.

In fact, the diabetic diet is similar to the diet recommended to lower risk for heart disease. That's important, considering that diabetics have two to three times the risk of developing heart disease as does the general population. Indeed, studies show that diabetics are not only more likely to suffer heart attacks and strokes, but they suffer from these diseases at a much earlier age.

Protein—Protein requirements for the diabetic are the same as for any healthy adult, 0.8 grams for each kilogram of body weight (or roughly 0.36 grams for each pound). Using these guidelines, a 120-pound woman would need 43 grams of protein. Someone 150 pounds would need 54 grams, someone weighing 175 pounds would need 63 grams, and so on. Protein can account for 10 to 20 percent of total calories in the diabetic diet.

Planning Meals by the Exchange Method

Although the general prescription for a diabetic diet is loosely based on percentages of fat, protein, and carbohydrate, you don't need to do any calculations. Nutritionists have developed an easy approach to diet called the *food exchange system,* which groups foods together that are similar in protein, carbohydrate, and fat content much the way many weight-loss plans do. Diet prescriptions are developed based on the number of calories an individual needs to maintain their current weight. For an 1800-calorie diet, a diabetic would be encouraged to eat two, three, four, or however many servings from each of the six different groups during the course of the day.

Starch/Bread List—This food list contains a wide variety of starchy foods—cereals, grains, some vegetables—that contain roughly fifteen grams of carbohydrate, three grams of protein, and eighty calories per serving. Obvious selections are bread—one slice or one ounce constitutes a serving—and one-half cup serving of starchy foods such as cereal, potatoes, or pasta. Other starchy items with a similar nutrient profile can be substituted for these selections. These include:

Kidney beans—⅓ cup
Wheat germ—3 tablespoons
Peas—½ cup

Winter squash—1 cup
Tortilla, 6″ across—one whole
Popcorn, air popped—3 cups
Pretzels—¾ oz
Animal crackers—8

Meat List—One exchange, or one meat serving, is equal to one ounce of cooked meat, fish, or poultry. (Most diabetics are allowed three to four ounces of meat per meal, an amount that fits snugly into the palm of a small hand.) That serving size contains roughly seven grams of protein. Fat content of meats vary widely so this group is split into three different categories: lean meats, medium-fat meats, and high-fat meats. Lean and medium-fat meats are better choices. High-fat protein selections (hot dogs, or high-protein meat substitutes such as peanut butter and cheese) are limited to three times per week or less. A few other items that are considered one meat serving include:

Cottage cheese—¼ cup
Oysters—6
Egg—1 whole
Tofu—4 oz
Luncheon meat (86% fat free)—1 oz

Vegetable List—One-half cup of cooked vegetable, or one cup raw, contains a small amount of protein (2 grams) and about five grams of carbohydrate. That makes it very easy for diabetics to regulate vegetable portions. However, some vegetables, because they contain very few calories, are considered "free" foods for diabetics. For example, lettuce and salad greens can be eaten in any quantities. With other "free" vegetables, amounts are limited to one cup raw of cabbage, Chinese cabbage, cucumber, green onion, mushrooms, radishes, and zucchini.

Fruit List—In general, ½ cup of juice or fresh fruit is considered one serving of most fruits. One exception is dried fruits. Since they have more sugar per ounce, the serving size is ¼ cup. In addition, whether you are diabetic or just counting calories, you might want to steer clear of canned or frozen fruits packed in sugar syrup as they are much higher in calories. Here are some serving sizes for some commonly eaten whole fruits:

Grapes, small—15 grapes
Figs, fresh—2 figs
Kiwi, large—1 kiwi
Mandarin oranges—¾ cup
Watermelon cubes—1¼ cups

Milk List—Foods in the milk group contain about the same amount of protein as one meat serving, but they also contain twelve grams of carbohydrate. Milk products, like meats, vary in fat content. Skim and low-fat dairy products are recommended with one cup or eight ounces the standard serving size.

Skim milk—1 cup
Evaporated skim milk—½ cup
Plain nonfat yogurt—8 oz

Fat List—Perhaps the most important food group to measure carefully, one serving of fat carries five grams of fat and forty-five calories. When you consider that one pat of margarine is one fat serving, it's easy to see how fat calories can rapidly add up. A diabetic who eats too much fat risks a rise in blood sugar and weight. Be aware that fats come in forms other than oil and margarine.

Avocado—⅛ medium
Mayonnaise—1 tsp
Peanuts—20 small
Sunflower seeds—1 tbsp
Olives—5 large
Salad dressing—2 tsp
Bacon—1 slice
Cream cheese—1 tbsp
Sour cream—2 tbsp
Coconut, shredded—2 tbsp

When Foods Don't Fit into Categories

While it may seem as if the exchange system requires diabetics to eat separate servings of meats, potatoes, and vegetables, diets don't need to be that rigid. Combination foods such as pizza, chow mein, and chili are considered appropriate food choices. If you know the ingredients that go into a particular recipe it is easy to figure out how those items convert into food exchanges. For example, a new exchange list for combination foods estimates that one cup of commercial chili with beans is equivalent to 2 starch servings (beans), 2 medium-fat meat (ground beef) and 2 fat servings (oil used for cooking).

Frozen entrees and many other convenience foods offer information about diabetic exchanges on their nutrition labels. Some fast-food restaurants also list diabetic food exchanges for their menu items.

How Much Do You Really Eat?

It's obvious from the exchange list system that controlling portions is critical for diabetics. It's the perfect way to help regulate blood sugar and also an excellent way to manage weight. Interesting new research points out that some dieters underestimate, albeit unintentionally, how much food they actually eat over the course of a day. Think about it. Do you know exactly what a three-ounce hamburger patty looks like? Or how many ounces of roast beef the deli packs on your sandwich? Does a one-half cup serving of rice fit into an average cereal bowl or custard dish?

When researchers at Ohio University tested a group of 200 students on their food portion knowledge, results were surprising. On the whole, participants who received training (a ten-minute session with plastic food models depicting standard portions of ten different foods) did better than people who had no training on portion size. Even so, some guesses of amounts were off as much as 84 percent.

That could indicate that most of us need to sharpen our knowledge of what constitutes a realistic portion of food, whether we are diabetic or not. For instance, a three-ounce helping of meat is about the size of a deck of cards, not a slab that fills half the plate. An average serving when it comes to fruits, vegetables, and whole grains is about one-half cup. For milk or yogurt, a serving is one full cup.

In the past, food labels have been notorious for setting unrealistic serving sizes (to keep calories low). New labeling changes are eliminating these kinds of problems.

How Sugars and Substitutes Affect Blood Sugar

Sugar substitutes such as aspartame, saccharine, and acesulfame K are considered free foods on the diabetic diet since they contain no nutrients and thus have no effect on blood-sugar levels. Regular sugars such as table sugar, honey, and fruit sugar (fructose) are a different story. Scientists know that the body digests and absorbs different types of carbohydrates at different rates. Potatoes, for instance, cause a more rapid rise in blood sugar than a bowl of kidney beans. Experts measure those rates in terms of what they call the *glycemic index* of a food.

But experts don't want these minor discrepancies to cause undue concern. In fact, new studies document that the total amount of carbohydrate a person eats may be more important than the source when it comes to controlling blood sugar. When the diabetic food exchange lists were recently revised, new plans allowed for small amounts of simple sugars to be substituted for other carbohydrates at a meal. Small substitutions like this are not likely to elevate blood sugar.

Cakes, cookies, and frozen yogurt are just some of the sweets allowed on a list of Foods For Occasional Use. Some of the other foods that diabetics can eat on occasion include:

Food	Exchange Equivalent
Angel food cake, 1/12 cake	2 starch
Cake, no icing, 3" square	2 starch, 2 fat
Cookies, 2 small	1 starch, 1 fat
Frozen fruit-yogurt, 1/3 cup	1 starch
Ice cream, 1/2 cup	1 starch, 2 fat
Sherbet, 1/4 cup	1 starch

Some Unusual Blood-Sugar-Lowering Agents

As scientists continue to determine how different foods affect blood sugar, the diabetic diet is likely to undergo changes. Two provocative new findings come out of the U.S. Department of Agriculture's Beltsville, Maryland, lab. Scientist Richard Anderson finds that spices and foods like broccoli may aid in blood-sugar control. In preliminary unpublished studies, Anderson finds that cinnamon, cloves, turmeric, and bay leaves triple the effectiveness of insulin. However, those results are from laboratory test-tube studies and have yet to be demonstrated in people.

Unrelated research, also by Anderson, indicates that the trace mineral *chromium* (found in foods such as whole grains, broccoli, and mushrooms) may also improve insulin's power.

The Protective Powers of Exercise

Doctors have always encouraged diabetics to keep active: Exercise helps regulate blood sugar. Now, new studies find that exercise may actually help prevent the illness. Several major reports, including a large-scale study from Harvard Medical School, indicate a strong protective role for exercise. Harvard scientists find that nurses who exercise and keep body weight at healthy levels are less likely to develop diabetes than those who are overweight and sedentary. If adult-onset diabetes runs in your family, it's something to keep in mind.

References

The American Dietetic Association. "Position of the American Dietetic Association: Use of nutritive and nonnutritive sweeteners." *Journal of the American Dietetic Association;* 93(7): 816–818, 1993.

Exchange Lists For Meal Planning. American Diabetes Association, 1989.

Jenkins, D.J.A. "Starchy foods and glycemic index." *Diabetes Care* 11: 149, 1988.

Weinstock, R.S., et al. "The role of dietary fiber in the management of diabetes mellitus." *Nutrition* 4: 187, 1988.

Crapo, P.A. "Use of alternative sweeteners in the diabetic diet." *Diabetes Care* 11:174, 1988.

Anderson, J.W., et al. "Dietary fiber and diabetes: A comprehensive review and practical application." *Journal of the American Dietetic Association* 87(9): 1189, 1987.

Franz, M.J. "Exercise and the management of diabetes mellitus." *Journal of the American Dietetic Association* 87(7): 872, 1987.

Laine, D.C., et al. "Comparison of predictive capabilities of diabetic exchange lists and glycemic index of foods." *Diabetes Care* 10:387, 1987.

Morley, J.E., et al. "Diabetes mellitus in elderly patients: Is it different?" *American Journal of Medicine* 83:533, 1987.

National Institutes of Health: "Consensus development conference on diet and exercise in non-insulin-dependent mellitus." *Diabetes Care* 10:639, 1987.

Kovar, M.G., et al. "The scope of diabetes in the United States population." *American Journal of Public Health* 77: 1549, 1987.

Jenkins, D.J.A., et al. "Simple and complex carbohydrates." *Nutrition Reviews* 44: 173–180, 1986.

Jenkins, D.J.A. "The glycemic response to carbohydrate foods." *Lancet* 2:388, 1984.

DIGESTIVE HEALTH

While you can't blame every digestive complaint on diet and lifestyle, chances are you can probably avoid a good percentage of minor digestive woes and maybe even stave off major problems like colon cancer, if you pay a little more attention to what you eat. New research continues to outline how diet, particularly a diet high in fiber, acts as strong preventive medicine. Indeed, if you keep plenty of fiber in your diet, stay active, and drink lots of fluid, your digestive tract will operate so smoothly you'll probably forget that it's even at work.

Curing Constipation

Constipation, the top digestive complaint doctors treat, can sometimes be a sign of serious illness such as an intestinal obstruction or tumor. More often, however, it is due to dietary and lifestyle factors. Common causes of constipation include diet (inadequate fiber, too little fluid), stress, lack of exercise, illness, pregnancy, and poorly tolerated medications.

When you eat very little fiber and drink very little fluid (fluid helps soften the stool) stools become hard and difficult to pass. Fiber, say scientists, is the broom that helps to move digested food materials through your intestines quickly. Luckily, if you find yourself plagued by constipation, the remedy is simple. Just add more high-fiber foods to your meals—whole-grain breads and cereals, fruits, vegetables, legumes—and drink plenty of liquid, at least eight glasses per day.

Keep in mind that if you neglect the fluid part of the prescription you are setting the stage for other digestive ills. If stools are too hard to pass and constipation is causing you to strain, hemorrhoids—a bulging of the muscles inside and outside the rectum—can result. Inadequate fiber and inadequate fluid can also increase your chances of developing diverticuli, outpouchings in the wall of the intestine that if infected can cause a great deal of pain.

Your chances of developing diverticulosis (many pouchings of diverticuli) increases with age. A low-fiber diet seems to be at the crux of the illness. Ironically, when diverticuli become inflamed, the resulting illness—diverticulitis—can be aggravated by a high-fiber diet. That's why prevention, in the form of a diet rich in fiber, is so important.

Finding the Fiber

Most Americans eat around eleven grams of fiber per day, less than half of what is recommended. Following is a list of common foods and their fiber content. You might be surprised to find that foods like lettuce are virtually devoid of fiber, while legumes are loaded with it.

Food	Grams of Fiber
Breads	
Pumpernickel, 1 slice	2.7
Cracked wheat, 1 slice	1.9
Rye, 1 slice	1.8
Corn tortilla, 1	1.4
French bread, 1 slice	0.9
English muffin, ½	0.8
Bagel, ½	0.7
Flour tortilla, 1	0.7
Waffle, 1	0.7
Biscuit, 1	0.5
Pita bread, ½ pocket	0.5
Saltines, 6 crackers	0.5
Cereals	
Oatbran, ¾ cup cooked	4.0
Wheat germ, 3 tbsp	3.9
Shredded wheat, ⅔ cup	3.5
Grapenuts, ¼ cup	2.8
Oatmeal, ⅓ cup uncooked	2.7
Wheat flakes, ¾ cup	2.3
Popcorn, 3 cups popped	2.0
Cornflakes, 1 cup	0.5
Puffed rice, 1 cup	0.2
Fruits	
Apricots, 4	3.5
Pear w/skin, 1 small	2.9
Strawberries, 1¼ cups	2.8
Apple, 1 small	2.3
Banana, 1 small	2.2

Applesauce, ½ cup	2.0
Fruit cocktail, ½ cup	2.0
Peach w/skin, 1 medium	2.0
Prunes, 3 medium	1.7
Blueberries, ¾ cup	1.4
Pineapple, ⅛ cup canned	1.4
Raisins, 2 tbsp	0.4
Orange juice, ½ cup	0.1

Vegetables

Brussels sprouts, ½ cup	3.8
Kale, ½ cup	2.5
Broccoli, ½ cup cooked	2.4
Green peas, ½ cup cooked	2.4
Carrot, 1 large	2.3
Beets, ½ cup	2.2
Green beans, ½ cup	2.0
Onion, ½ cup chopped	2.0
Asparagus, ½ cup cooked	1.8
Eggplant, 1 cup	1.8
Celery, 1 cup chopped	1.7
Bean sprouts, 1 cup	1.6
Corn, ½ cup	1.6
Mushroom, 1 cup	0.8
Cucumber, 1 cup	0.5
Iceberg lettuce, 1 cup	0.5

Legumes

Kidney beans, ½ cup cooked	6.9
Navy beans, ½ cup cooked	6.5
Black beans, ½ cup cooked	6.1
Pinto beans, ½ cup cooked	5.9
Lentils, ½ cup cooked	5.2
Black-eyed peas, ½ cup	4.7
Chick peas, ½ cup	4.3
Lima beans, ½ cup	4.3
Split peas, ½ cup cooked	3.1

Source: "Plant fiber in foods." James W. Anderson; HCF Nutrition Research Foundation, Inc, 1990.

If It Gives You Gas . . .

Take care to add high-fiber foods to your diet gradually. Too much fiber too fast can cause excess gas, indigestion, and cramping. The digestive tract expels gas an average of thirteen times a day, usually in small quantities that measure up to about 700 cc (1000 cc equals about a quart) in volume by day's end. That's normal. Gas is the digestive tract's response to indigestible compounds. Usually the offending culprits are carbohydrates, such as the sugars in milk or dried beans. For example, if you lack the enzyme needed to digest milk sugar (See lactose intolerance in the Allergies and Food Intolerances chapter, page 24), intestinal bacteria will ferment the undigested sugar. Gas is merely a by-product of that fermentation process.

Dried beans like pinto, navy, and kidney beans can be gas causing for much the same reason. *Raffinose* and *stachyose,* two hard-to-digest carbohydrates found in dried beans, cannot be broken down by digestion completely. Luckily, soaking dried beans overnight helps to break down some of these indigestible compounds. *Sorbitol,* a sweetener used in many sugar free candies, is also likely to cause gas if eaten in large quantities.

Many of the other foods blamed for causing gas (onions, broccoli, brussels sprouts) are more likely the result of your individual intolerance to a food rather than a uniform occurrence. The easiest way to minimize gas from offending foods, whatever they are, is to avoid the foods or to eat only small quantities. Some people find relief with an over-the-counter product that is added to gassy foods. If none of these remedies seems to help and you feel you pass abnormally large amounts of gas, it's probably time to visit the doctor. Excessive gas can be a sign of malabsorption problems.

Help for Heartburn

Even more aggravating than flatulence to some people is heartburn: the nagging, burning sensation in the chest caused by indigestion. Actually, heartburn is not really a true digestive complaint but a symptom. In most cases, heartburn is caused by gastroesophageal reflux, a back-up of acid from the stomach. Under normal conditions, a tight sphincter muscle at the entrance to your stomach keeps stomach contents from regurgitating backwards into the esophagus. Many environmental factors, however, can weaken the sphincter muscle. Certain foods—chocolate, coffee (caffeine), alcohol—loosen it. Being pregnant or overweight weakens it, too. Like many other body parts, the muscle relaxes a little too much with age.

Whether you suffer from occasional heartburn that lasts only a few minutes or are a chronic sufferer who bears with excruciating pain for as long as a few hours at a time, doctors say a few simple strategies should help you find relief.

- Limit caffeine and alcoholic beverages, as they can relax the sphincter and stimulate the stomach to produce more acid.
- Avoid spicy, fatty, and acidic foods (tomatoes, citrus fruits) as they can also result in weakening of the sphincter.
- Don't overeat at mealtime. Too much food in the stomach creates pressure, which also weakens the lower esophageal sphincter muscle. (Some people find that smaller, more frequent meals are helpful.)
- Reduce weight if overweight. Being overweight increases pressure on the abdomen, which can aggravate reflux.
- Stop smoking. Nicotine can bring on or aggravate reflux.
- Don't lie down right after a meal. Wait at least two or three hours before reclining. This allows time for the stomach to empty.
- Elevate the head of your bed at least four to six inches. This helps alleviate nocturnal reflux. (Keeping the head and upper chest elevated will help combat the forces of gravity that allow acid to flow back into the esophagus when you lie down flat.)
- If none of these measures work, have your doctor check out the problem. Left untreated, refluxed acids can damage or ulcerate the lining of the esophagus.

Over-the-Counter Digestive Aids

Bulking agents made with natural fibers such as bran or psyllium can help the digestive tract keep regular without doing any harm. Chemical laxatives and antacids are a different story. Many doctors find that people overuse these compounds.

Chemical Laxatives—The problem with these compounds is that they cause the bowel muscle to become dependent on chemical stimulation. The muscle then "forgets" how to act on its own. Some experts contend that no one really needs a laxative.

Antacids—Antacids can be beneficial to some people as they help neutralize stomach acid. However, a recent report in *The New England Journal of Medicine* finds that "indiscriminate" or "inappropriate" use of antacids can alter bowel habits. Aluminum-containing antacids can cause constipation in some people; magnesium-containing antacids may cause diarrhea.

Keeping the digestive tract running smoothly is best done with fiber and fluid. Then, too, there are natural food laxatives such as those found in prunes. An old digestive standby, prunes carry a substance called *dihydroxyphenylisotin,* a compound that stimulates movement or motility along your GI tract. (A constipation prevention tip: drink your prune juice at night so that the gastrointestinal tract has time to work on the juice overnight. After a light breakfast, your bowels should move easily.)

Signs of More Serious Trouble

Doctors say that a change in bowel habits (suddenly becoming constipated or prolonged bouts of diarrhea) and rectal bleeding are the two major warning signs that a digestive complaint could be serious. It's true that rectal bleeding may be caused by hemorrhoids. However, since bleeding is also an early warning sign of cancer, make sure to have any rectal bleeding investigated. (About one time out of every ten, bleeding turns out to be due to cancer.) Early detection and treatment of cancer improves your chances of survival.

Digestive Health and Cancer

You can prevent or at least delay the development of colon cancer with careful attention to diet and lifestyle. Numerous studies link a diet high in fiber with a lower risk for colorectal cancer. Scientists are still puzzling over whether or not that link is due to a high intake of fiber or whether it is the result of a diet low in fat. (Most high-fiber diets tend to be low in fat and high-fiber foods—fruits, vegetables, whole grains—are naturally low in fat.)

Newer research also hints that there could be other protective components in high-fiber foods. In studies with animals, scientists find that cruciferous vegetables such as brussels sprouts and broccoli offer some protection against colon cancer.

Getting the Cruciferous Crunch

Plants in the mustard family are called cruciferous because of their cross-shaped blossoms. On that list:

- Bok choy (Chinese cabbage)
- Broccoli
- Brussels sprouts
- Cabbage
- Cauliflower
- Collard greens
- Kale
- Mustard greens
- Radishes
- Rutabagas
- Turnips

Rather than worry about specific families of vegetables or foods that act as anticarcinogens, health professionals stress the need for a wide variety of high-fiber foods. The National Cancer Institute recommends increasing intake to twenty to thirty-five grams of fiber per day.

Reference List

Devroede, G. "Constipation: mechanisms and management." *Gastrointestinal Disease: Pathophysiology, Diagnosis and Management, 4th edition;* W.B. Saunders, 1989.

"Dietary fiber and health." Council on Scientific Affairs, The American Medical Association. *Journal of the American Medical Association* 262: 542–53, 1989.

"Diet and health: implications for reducing chronic disease risk." National Research Council, National Academy of Sciences, 1989.

"Position of The American Dietetic Association: health implications of dietary fiber." *Journal of the American Dietetic Association;* 88: 216–19, 1988.

Bright-See, E. "Dietary fiber and cancer." *Nutrition Today;* 23(4): 4–10, 1988.

Surgeon General's Report on Nutrition and Health. USDHHS Publication No. 88-50210, Public Health Service, 1988.

Lanza, E., et al. "Dietary fiber intake in the U.S. population." *American Journal of Clinical Nutrition;* 46: 790–93, 1987.

Joint Committee on Diet as Related to Gastrointestinal Function of The American Dietetic Association and the American Medical Association. "Diet as related to gastrointestinal function." *Journal of the American Dietetic Association;* 38: 425–36, 1961.

FAST FOOD

Just about everyone eats fast-food meals on occasion. They're quick, and convenient, which makes them appealing to the overworked, the harried, or the just plain frazzled. However, chances are you feel a twinge of guilt about all the grease that comes with your fast-food fare. After all, the typical fast-food meal—burger, french fries, and a milkshake—racks up around 1300 calories according to one recent medical report. About 40 to 55 percent of those calories come from fat.

Another problem: A steady diet of many fast-food menu items lacks adequate amounts of key diet components like fiber and vitamins A and C. Fortunately, menus at the bigger fast-food chains—McDonald's, Arby's, and Kentucky Fried Chicken, are showcasing a handful of lean and low-fat additions. Small fresh green salads, carrot and celery sticks, roasted or grilled chicken, low-fat milkshakes, bagels, and broiled fish are just a few of the healthful foods finding their niche in the fast-food repertoire. If you build a meal around these lower-fat choices it's actually possible to cut fat levels of the traditional fast-food meal by as much as half.

Figuring out What's Healthiest

If you want to go by the numbers, most fast-food restaurants will be happy to provide nutritional information on their products. (Some nutritionists would like to see that information right on the food label. For now, you'll have to be content to ask for brochures or flyers that list this information.) Use the numbers to let yourself do some comparison shopping.

For example, compare chicken sandwiches. Burger King's nutritional chart would show you that the BK Broiler Chicken Sandwich (379 calories; 162 from fat) is a much leaner choice than the regular chicken sandwich (685 calories; 360 from fat). At Wendy's, the grilled chicken sandwich with 340 calories (117 from fat) is leaner than the Chicken Club Sandwich (506 calories; 225 from fat).

After doing chart comparisons for a while, you'll find that scrutinizing the numbers isn't always necessary. In fact, you can spot the leaner choices just as easily by zeroing in on preparation techniques and ingredients. Leaner choices follow a central theme. Sandwiches come grilled (not breaded and fried); toppings are fat-free condiments like catsup and mustard. Cheese, which can add ten grams of fat or more to a burger or salad, is nowhere to be found. If you keep these points in mind when reviewing fast-food menus, ordering a low-fat meal will become much easier.

General Low-Fat Strategies

- Opt for small plain burgers instead of sandwiches with the "works." Special sauces (which generally contain mayonnaise) and large amounts of meat make these sandwiches high in fat and calories.
- Skip the cheese. One ounce of cheese adds eight to ten grams of fat to your sandwich or salad. A new study from *Consumer Reports* finds that many fast food items have as much as 20 percent more fat than companies estimate, usually because servers are too liberal with cheese and fatty sauces.
- Choose salads, plain rolls, and baked potatoes as your side dish instead of french fries.
- Choose sandwich spreads or sauces that are low in fat—mustard, catsup, and salsa, instead of salad dressings, tartar sauce, and mayonnaise. If you leave the mayonnaise off a Burger King Whopper you will save 210 calories and twenty-three grams of fat.
- Skip the "extra crispy" at KFC. Extra fat is what makes it crispier and calories can be as much as 100 more per piece.
- Keep a baked potato lean by topping it with vegetarian chili and salsa rather than cheese or sour cream.
- Satisfy a sweet tooth with low-fat frozen yogurt rather than a fried pie.

Can A Fast-Food Breakfast Be Healthful?

Checking on ingredients and preparation techniques is probably even more important at breakfast, where high-fat choices are more common than lean cuisine. From buttery croissants laden with eggs, cheese, and sausage to french-toast sticks that carry more fat than a hamburger, quick food drive-thrus package a morning menu that is guaranteed to make you sluggish. Even the bread items—giant-sized muffins, biscuits, croissants, and danish—tend to be fatty. You can't see the fat, but set them aside on a napkin (or in a brown paper bag) and before long grease leaches out onto the paper.

Better breakfast choices are those that contain more carbohydrate fuel than heavy fat calories. On that list: fat-free muffins, bagels, English muffins with jam, cereal with low-fat milk, pancakes with syrup. Judging from the small number of low-fat selections, it's obvious that breakfast is one meal that's probably quicker and healthier eaten at home. If you need to munch your meal in the car, why not spread a bagel or English muffin with reduced-fat cream cheese or jam before you leave home?

If What You Really Crave Is High Fat

If you're craving fried fish, you're not going to care that Long John Silver's is expanding its line of broiled seafood items yet again. If you're craving a burger, grilled chicken may seem a less than satisfying substitute. And there is nothing wrong with splurging on the occasional high-fat meal. That is, as long as you learn to balance those high-fat meals with lower-fat items so that over the course of a day or the week your diet is moderately low in fat.

Of course, to do an adequate balancing job, you'll need to have some idea how your favorite fast foods stack up when it comes to fat. In the past, nutrition experts focused on brands, comparing burgers at McDonald's to those at Burger King. But a better strategy is for you to get an overall picture of fast foods in general. For while it's true that a McDonald's milkshake has only one gram of fat and a Wendy's Frosty has 13 grams, the majority of fast-food items are not dramatically different when it comes to fat content.

If you learn the generic nutrient profiles of some of your favorite fast foods, you can budget fat and calories without worrying so much about the specific numbers and how they vary from restaurant to restaurant. (If you really want the exact nutrient profile for a particular food at a particular restaurant, you can find that information in nutrient tables in the back of this book.)

Item	Calories	Cal from fat
Entree		
Burrito, bean	224	72
Enchilada, cheese & beef	324	162
Plain hamburger	275	108
Cheeseburger	295	126
Bacon cheeseburger	464	243
Double cheeseburger	457	261
Fried chicken, leg & thigh	430	243
Fried chicken nuggets, 6	290	162
Chicken fillet sandwich	515	270
Chili, one cup	254	72
Corndog	460	171
Fried fish sandwich	431	207
Cheese pizza, small slice	140	27
Pepperoni pizza, small slice	181	63
Ham and cheese sandwich	353	144
Roast beef sandwich	346	126
Submarine sandwich	456	171

Side dish		
Baked potato, plain	250	18
French fries, regular order	237	108
Onion rings, 8–9	275	144
Coleslaw, ¾ cup	147	99
Vanilla milkshake	314	72
Fried fruit pie	266	126

Source: Figures adapted from Bowes & Church's Food Values of Portions Commonly Used, 16th edition, J.B. Lippincott Company, 1994.

References

Pennington, J.A.T. *Bowes and Church's Food Values of Portions Commonly Used,* 16th edition. Philadelphia: J.B. Lippincott Company, 1994.

Consumer Reports. "Fast food for fat-watchers." *Consumer Reports Magazine;* 574–578, Sept, 1993.

Product Information. Arby's Inc. Atlanta, GA, 1993.

Product Information. Burger King. Miami, FL, 1993.

Product Information. Kentucky Fried Chicken. Louisville, KY, 1993.

Product Information. Long John Silver's. Lexington, KY, 1993.

Product Information. McDonald's. Oakbrook, IL, 1993.

Product Information. Taco Bell Corporation. Irvine, CA, 1993.

Product Information. Wendy's International Inc. Dublin, OH, 1993.

HEALTH FOODS

Anyone who cares about good health cares about the nutritional quality of the foods they eat. Proponents of health foods contend that the healthiest foods are organically grown, free of additives and preservatives, and brimming with a fresh supply of nature's nutrients. With scares about food contamination from pesticides and additives frequently in the news (See chapter on Additives and Pesticides, page 15) you might be wondering if they are right.

What Is a Health Food?

Health-food stores are a permanent part of the shopping landscape. Some sell a complete line of groceries (organic milk, free-range chicken, organically grown produce). Others sell mostly nutrition supplements and canned or dried goods (soy crackers, lecithin, granola bars). Advertisements attempt to convince shoppers that the merchandise in these stores is superior to the ordinary products sold in supermarkets, but nutritionists say that's debatable.

When the New York City Department of Consumer Affairs compared foods from health-food stores with those from the regular supermarket, the main difference they found was in the price tag. Health-food store items can cost twice as much (sometimes more) than comparable foods bought at the local supermarket. What do you get for that higher price tag? Less than you might think. Apparently, the health foods studied did not differ significantly from conventional foods in terms of nutritional values, appearance, or taste.

Part of the problem with the whole concept of health foods is that the terminology and the movement is loosely defined.

Health food—A confusing term, *health food* has no legal definition, but it is usually used to refer to organically grown or natural foods. In general, health foods are purported to be superior to foods that are not labeled as such. Nutritionists say that the virtues of these foods are often exaggerated, however. In reality, all foods can contribute to health when eaten in the context of a healthy diet.

Organically grown—To the health food movement, the term *organic* has come to describe a food that is grown in soil enriched with animal or vegetable fertilizers—manure, compost, bone meal. No pesticides, herbicides, or inorganic fertilizers are used. Over the last decade, many states have worked diligently to establish legal definitions for the term organic and certification programs exist for these foods in twenty states. However, at present, there is no test that can differentiate organically grown foods from similar commercially grown products. That means you will need to rely on the integrity of growers and distributors to ensure that foods have been grown organically. (See the section on Additives and Pesticides, page 15).

Natural—Webster's may define *natural* as "produced or existing in nature: not artificial or manufactured." There is, however, no legal definition for the term as it appears on food labels. It's more of a selling tool for manufacturers since many consumers equate natural to mean healthier.

Dispelling Health-Food Hype

There is nothing wrong with wanting to eat foods that are free of pesticides and are not highly processed. In fact, the concept of organically grown foods is a good one, particularly for the environment. Instead of throwing away garbage and using chemicals that might pollute the land and water, garbage (compost, manure) is recycled to fertilize soil.

On the other hand, it is important to realize that organically grown produce is not nutritionally superior to crops grown with chemical fertilizers. As many positive things as there are to say about organically grown and minimally processed foods, there is a lot of hype and misinformation connected with the health-food movement. It's important to separate fact from fiction.

Myth: Honey is better than sugar.
Fact: Honey has some vitamins, but the amount is minuscule. In fact, to derive any nutritional advantage from honey you would need to eat it by the cupful, hardly a realistic amount. More importantly, both table sugar (sucrose) and honey are digested by the body and broken down into the same two simple sugars—glucose and fructose. Once digested, the body can not distinguish between these energy fuels.

Myth: White bread has very little nutritional value.
Fact: Back in the nineteen-seventies, some researchers fed a group of lab animals white bread and water for thirteen weeks straight. By the end of the study, animals were sick and losing their hair. While this may sound like proof that white bread is bad for health, don't jump to conclusions. All the study really points out is that white bread, by itself, doesn't carry every nutrient needed for good health. Neither does any other food. In fact, when these same re-

searchers fed animals a steady diet of hamburger and water, all but one of the animals were dead by the end of the thirteenth week.

In the end, the important point to remember is that both white bread or whole-wheat bread can fit into a healthy diet. But if your diet is low in fiber, like most Americans, breads made from whole wheat or other whole grains are preferable to white bread.

Myth: Snacks sold in health-food stores are more nutritious than supermarket snacks.

Fact: Buying your snack chips or sweet indulgences from a health-food store probably won't make much nutritional difference. A potato chip made with organic potatoes and sea salt is still a potato chip and carries a hefty amount of fat. And granola bars, often touted as a healthful alternative to candy bars, often contain as much or more fat and sugar than the candy they are supposed to replace. (You might not realize how high that sugar content is because the ingredient list slips many different forms of sugar into the recipe—honey, brown sugar, molasses, fructose, maltose—rather than just one type.)

Is Juice Really Better?

Within the health movement is a minimovement of self-appointed practitioners who are emphasizing the miraculous health benefits of fresh-squeezed fruit and vegetable juices. Popular juicing instruction books rave about the delicious taste of fresh-squeezed juices. They also sell improved health as a big motive for juicing. One of the books proposes that a glass of fresh squeezed carrot-apple juice can lower cholesterol, boost energy levels, make hair shinier, and promote weight loss.

That same author also writes that ". . . when fruits and vegetables are consumed as juice the vitamins and minerals are quickly released into the bloodstream directly to cells requiring them the most." Nutritionists see these promises as a bit far-fetched. Your body gets nutrients from whole foods (fresh carrots and apples) just as quickly as from juice. More important, the whole foods offer more nutritional benefits. Juicing fruits and vegetables eliminates the fiber and perhaps other beneficial compounds that may be combined with that fiber.

Proponents of juicing recommend using the leftover juice pulp (it takes four cups of raw chopped carrot to produce eight ounces of juice) as compost for your garden. But if it makes your garden plants grow strong and healthy, doesn't it make sense that you might be throwing out some beneficial ingredients when you discard the pulp? It's likely that the juicing movement is another passing food fad. There's nothing wrong with enjoying fresh-squeezed fruit and vegetable juices. Just don't make them your sole diet and don't expect them to be nutritional cure-alls.

Reference List

Price, C.C., et al. "Organic certification programs." *National Food Review;* 15: 31–32, 1991.

Institute of Food Technologists' expert panel on food safety and nutrition. "The effects of food processing on nutrient values: A scientific status summary." *Food Technology;* 40: 109–16, 1986.

Gourdine, S.P., et al. "Health food stores investigation." *Journal of the American Dietetic Association;* 83: 285–290, 1983.

Handbook of Clinical Dietetics: The American Dietetic Association. New Haven, CT; Yale University, 1981.

"Nutrition misinformation and food faddism." *Nutrition Reviews;* 32(S1), 1974.

Hegsted, D.M., et al. "Whole foods and some not so scientific experiments." *Nutrition Today;* 13; 22–25, 1973.

HEART HEALTH

In the battle against heart disease, the nation's number-one killer, diet has always been a critical prevention strategy. Initially, much of the advice centered on limiting certain foods that might be damaging to heart health. But now researchers have found a whole arsenal of dietary ingredients that may actually protect the heart, foods that you can *add* to your diet. For example, new evidence confirms that certain nutrients—vitamin E, beta-carotene, and vitamin C—may protect the heart from damage. Garlic, wine, margarine, and iron-rich foods also influence the health of your heart.

While these findings are exciting, you must not forget that fat and cholesterol still play a major dietary role in heart health. More important, cutting-edge research confirms that the right kind of low-fat diet may actually help reverse cardiovascular disease by helping to unplug clogged arteries.

Figuring Out the Role of Fat

While it's not an earth-shattering diet strategy, lowering the total amount of fat and saturated fat in your diet can help lower blood cholesterol levels. (See Low-Fat Eating, page 131 and Labels on Food, page 118). Study after study proves that diets rich in saturated fat and cholesterol can elevate blood cholesterol. And high-blood cholesterol levels, along with high blood pressure, smoking, and inactivity, are the major controllable risk factors for heart disease.

Astonishing new research finds that people with severe coronary heart disease can sometimes reverse their disease with stricter dietary fat limits—a mostly vegetarian diet with less than 10 percent of the calories from fat—and other healthful lifestyle changes. Four years into this very low-fat diet strategy, participants in the Lifestyle Heart Trial still continue to show signs that their arteries are gradually unplugging. For people who don't suffer from coronary artery disease, however, this new approach may be too restrictive.

Health professionals recommend a diet with 30 percent or less of total calories from fat as a starting point to help protect against heart disease. Eventually try to lower fat to 20 to 25 percent of total calories or less. Many experts feel that the 25 percent range is healthier for the heart. (Less than 20 percent fat calories may be too restrictive; talk with your physician before limiting fat to the 10 percent level being tested on volunteers in some research projects.)

While some people have taken the recommendation for the 25 percent or 30 percent rule as one that applies to single foods (and so eat only foods that contain 25 percent or 30 percent or less of their calories as fat) that's not how the advice is intended. The percent rule doesn't apply to individual foods. The idea is to balance high- and low-fat food choices so that the daily or weekly overall total is 25 or 30 percent. Perhaps the easiest way to reach that goal is to establish your own personal fat "budget."

Based on total calories, a budget helps you keep within fat limits by counting grams of fat rather than figuring out percentages for every food. A woman who eats 1,500 calories or so per day, would have a daily fat budget of 50 grams. (Thirty percent of 1,500 calories equals 450 calories of fat. Since fat carries nine calories per gram, divide 450 by nine to equal 50 grams.) Arriving at 50 grams of fat by day's end could allow for many different food combinations.

If you eat . . .	Your fat budget is . . .		
	30%	25%	20%
1,500 calories	50 grams	42 grams	33 grams
1,600 calories	53 grams	44 grams	36 grams
1,700 calories	57 grams	47 grams	38 grams
1,800 calories	60 grams	50 grams	40 grams
1,900 calories	63 grams	53 grams	42 grams
2,000 calories	67 grams	55 grams	44 grams
2,100 calories	70 grams	58 grams	47 grams
2,400 calories	80 grams	67 grams	53 grams

The Right Kind of Fat

Once you're able to trim the total fat in your diet to healthy levels, experts recommend keeping an eye on the types of fat you eat. There are three types of fats (fatty acids) that occur naturally in foods: saturated, polyunsaturated, and monounsaturated. For heart health, experts recommend equally dividing fat intake between the three types. Keeping saturated fat levels to less than 10 percent of total calories should be your first priority. Mountains of research supports that these fats are harmful to the heart. Unsaturated fats can also influence heart disease risk.

Saturated Fats—Small quantities of saturated fat won't damage the heart. The problem sets in when you eat too much saturated fat. These fatty acids, which are solid at room temperature, can adhere to the walls of your arteries and narrow them. As build-up increases, arteries can become totally clogged, precipitating a heart attack or stroke. Animal foods are high in saturated fat: meat, whole milk, cream, butter.

Polyunsaturated Fats—One of two types of unsaturated fats, polyunsaturated fatty acids appear capable of lowering blood cholesterol levels when these fats are substituted for saturated fats in the diet. Plants and vegetables are the primary sources of polyunsaturated fat: corn oil, cottonseed oil, sunflower oil, soybean oil. Fatty fish like salmon and mackerel are high in polyunsaturated fats called omega-3 fatty acids. Studies find that these fats can lower blood cholesterol too.

Monounsaturated Fats—Studies from the Mediterranean suggest that monounsaturated fats may help protect against heart disease. Found mainly in olives (olive oil), peanuts, and canola oil, these fats used to be considered neutral to heart health. Avocados are also high in this type of fat.

Cholesterol-Busting Foods

Once you have fat under control, there are some dietary changes, actually additions to your diet, that may improve your heart-disease risk profile. Scientists find that the soluble fiber and other compounds found in many fruits, vegetables, and whole grains can go a long way toward lowering cholesterol. (Remember, a high blood-cholesterol level is a major controllable risk factor for heart disease.) Here's some of the newest fighters in the anticholesterol brigade.

Barley—Blood cholesterol levels dropped an average of fourteen points when participants in one study included *either* foods cooked with barley or oat flour in their daily diets, according to scientists at Montana State University. Since barley flour isn't widely available, these researchers recommend you look for pearl barley. A dried grain that is cooked like pasta, barley is sold in the legume section of the supermarket alongside the dried beans and split peas. Use it in soups and casseroles.

Garlic—At a recent American Heart Association conference, a University of Wisconsin researcher presented more evidence to confirm that garlic offers strong protection against heart attacks.

Garlic contains compounds—quercitin, ajouene—that help prevent platelets in the blood from clumping together and building up on artery walls. Since most of the research to date has used large quantities of raw garlic, scientists must now grapple with the question of the protective benefits of smaller quantities of garlic (one or two cloves) and how cooking influences those benefits.

Grapefruit—University of Florida researchers find that grapefruit may be able to slow the development of atherosclerosis. It seems that grapefruit pectin, a soluble fiber concentrated in the white membrane coating of grapefruit sections, causes total cholesterol and harmful LDL levels to drop. So far the studies have been done only with lab animals. We hope that future research will test the concept with studies on people.

Oats—Numerous studies confirm that the soluble fiber in oats is capable of lowering blood cholesterol. But the effect is small, and oats do not negate the effects of a high-fat diet. Include oats as part of a low-fat diet to glean the most benefits.

Prunes—When scientists from the University of California at Davis recently fed men with high cholesterol levels a dozen prunes a day, heart-harmful LDL cholesterol levels dropped. The drop wasn't dramatic, but may be explainable. More than half the fiber in prunes comes from the soluble fiber *pectin,* a fiber already known to be capable of lowering cholesterol levels.

Rice Bran—Speculation is that the oil that is warehoused in the outer shell (bran layer) of the rice grain might be a powerful cholesterol-lowering agent. Studies from abroad and at Louisiana State University confirm that rice-bran oil can lower blood-cholesterol levels in both animals and people. Many supermarkets now carry the oil. Or you can tap into a dose of potential protection every time you eat brown rice. (Brown rice contains 10 percent bran.) As an added plus, one-half cup of brown rice delivers two grams of fiber.

Shellfish—Oysters, crabs, and clams are rich in the same omega-3 fatty acids found in fatty fish like salmon and mackerel. Despite the fact that these shellfish also harbor small amounts of cholesterol, recent studies show that they contain enough of the omega-3s to help lower total- and LDL-cholesterol levels. Shrimp, you'll notice, is not on the protective list. Even though it contains omega-3s, studies find that shrimp don't seem to lower blood cholesterol—on the other hand, they don't seem to raise it either.

Wine—A recent report from researchers in Wisconsin has identified compounds in red wine known as *polyphenols* that help to keep platelets in the blood from sticking together and thereby may help prevent arteries from clogging. (See the section on Caffeine and Alcohol, page 40.) Beer, white wine, and pineapple juice contain these same substances, but in much smaller quantities.

Antioxidants Rescue the Heart

Cutting back on fat and eating foods that lower your cholesterol level is one way to help lessen the risk for heart disease. Scientists today are even more surprised at the strong role that antioxidant nutrients like vitamin E, vitamin C and beta-carotene seem to play in heart health. Recent studies from Tufts University in Boston find that people who eat plenty of vitamin C-rich foods have lower blood pressure and higher levels of HDL, the heart-healthy cholesterol, than people with very little vitamin C in their diet.

Vitamin C-rich Foods

Food	Milligrams C
Papaya, 1 medium	188
Guava, 1 medium	165
Orange juice, 8 oz	97
Strawberries, 1 cup	85
Navel orange, 1 medium	80
Kiwifruit, 1 medium	75
Grapefruit juice, 8 oz	72
Cantaloupe, 1 cup	68
Mango, 1 medium	57
Elderberries, 1 cup	52
Cherimoya, 1 medium	49
Pink grapefruit, ½ medium	47
Tomato juice, 6 oz	33

According to preliminary new reports from Harvard Medical School, fruits and vegetables rich in beta-carotene, the pigment-like substance that colors fruits and vegetables bright orange, might also be a hedge against heart disease. In one study, physicians with heart disease who took 50 milligrams of beta-carotene (about the amount in two cups of cooked carrots) every other day had almost half as many heart attacks, strokes, and death related to heart disease as those who did not. In another recent report, older adults eating large quantities of beta-carotene-rich foods had a lower risk of death from heart disease than their counterparts who ate less.

Two new reports from Harvard Medical School confirm a similar benefit from vitamin E, which is perhaps the strongest of the antioxidant nutrients. This new research confirms that women and men with higher intakes of vitamin E are at a lesser risk for heart disease. (For more information on antioxidant nutrients and foods that contain these protective agents refer to the chapter on Immunity, p. 100.)

A New Role for B Vitamins

Low dietary intake of two B vitamins—folic acid and vitamin B_6—could put you at risk for heart disease and stroke, according to a new report published in *The Journal of The*

American Medical Association. When scientists studied a group of older adults (aged sixty-seven to ninety-six), they found that people who ate the least amounts and had the lowest levels of these B vitamins in their blood had the highest levels of homocysteine. High levels of homocysteine have been linked with increased heart-disease risk.

Conversely, adults who consumed large levels of the nutrients, about double what is currently recommended, had the lowest risk of heart attack.

Food Sources of Folic Acid
- Green leafy vegetables
- Asparagus
- Lima beans
- Black-eyed peas
- Beets
- Sunflower seeds
- Cantaloupe
- Kidney or pinto beans
- Winter squash
- Cauliflower
- Wheat germ

Food Sources of Vitamin B$_6$
- Lean red meat
- Navy beans
- Potatoes
- Bananas
- Chicken
- Salmon and other fish
- Pork
- Spinach
- Whole grains

Margarine versus Butter

When it comes to calories and total fat content, margarine and butter have always been of equal standing. Each tablespoon of margarine and each tablespoon of butter contain the same 11.5 grams of fat and 100 calories. Where the two spreads differ is in the type of fat they are made from. Butter contains large amounts of saturated fat, the kind of fat that can raise blood-cholesterol levels. Margarine, because it is high in polyunsaturated fats, fats that don't raise blood cholesterol, has long been touted as a healthy substitute for butter.

But new studies have caused some researchers to speculate that margarine may not be as healthy as once suspected. Apparently, processing liquid vegetable oils to make margarine produces an altered type of fat—trans-fatty acids. While technically a polyunsaturated fat, trans-fatty acids are altered enough in processing that they behave differently. One new study suggests that trans fats can raise blood cholesterol levels and so may increase heart disease risk. However, this is probably not cause for alarm.

Estimates are that most Americans eat very little trans-fat, probably less than 5 percent of total calories. In fact, the consensus is that margarine is still a better spread than butter (butter contains cholesterol; margarine does not). However, if you want to minimize your exposure to trans-fats, opt for liquid or tub margarines. Softer margarines are processed less and so have fewer of the trans-fats. You can also cut down on trans-fats by using liquid vegetable oils in cooking and in baking.

Establishing a Copper Connection

For years, research from the USDA Human Nutrition Research Center in Grand Forks, North Dakota, has linked diets low in copper to elevated blood-cholesterol levels. In one of the most recent reports, scientists find that the combination of stress and a low-copper diet is even more damaging. When researchers subjected lab animals to "shift stress" (scientists used light and dark cycles to mimic shift work) cholesterol levels jumped dramatically. It is known that shift workers have higher rates of cardiovascular disease; what was surprising about the new study is that a combination of shift stress and low levels of copper in the diet more than doubled the cholesterol damage. Cholesterol levels jumped a whopping 70 percent when these two factors were combined.

Much more research is required to determine the precise role copper may play in heart health. Yet, some researchers contend that you may be able to lower heart-disease risk by seeking out copper-rich foods. On that list are oysters, nuts and seeds, and whole grains.

A Question of Iron

A few years ago, Finnish researchers noticed a link between high blood levels of iron and increased risk for heart attack. Specifically, men with high blood-iron stores had twice the risk for heart attack as those who had low stores. Not long after their report, however, three new studies failed to confirm this iron–heart disease connection. For now, experts feel it's too soon to make any dietary recommendations based on these conflicting results. It's not clear if high-iron stores are the real culprit when it comes to increased risk, or if some other factor is responsible. More important, the studies were done with men. Women, due to monthly blood loss from menstruation, are not likely to suffer with high blood levels of iron. In fact, studies show that most women in this country don't get enough iron in their diets.

In addition, both men and women need to be aware that iron performs many critical functions. It helps transport oxygen throughout the body. Iron is a component of key enzymes that control body reactions. It also may play a valuable role in fighting off infection. (See the chapter on Immunity, p. 100.) Until researchers understand more about the effects of iron on the heart, it's wise for both sexes to eat plenty of iron-rich foods. (See the chapter on Anemia, p. 31.)

Sources of Iron
Meats and meat substitutes: Beef, lamb, poultry, fish, oysters, clams, dried beans.
Grains: Whole grains, enriched breads, cereals.
Vegetables: Dark, green leafy vegetables, dried beans, asparagus, lima beans, brussels sprouts, black-eyed peas, tomato juice.
Fruits: Strawberries, blueberries, watermelon, dried fruits such as apricots, dates, prunes.

Reference List

Folts, D. "Spirits, spice, sticky platelets, and heart attack." American Heart Association's 21st Science Writer's Forum, Jan. 1994.

Selhub, J., et al. "Vitamin status and intake as primary determinants of homocysteinemia in an elderly population." *Journal of the American Medical Association;* 270(22): 2693–98, 1993.

Stampfer, M.J. and Willet, W.C. "Homocysteine and marginal vitamin deficiency: The importance of adequate vitamin intake." *Journal of the American Medical Association;* 270(22): 2726–27, 1993.

Manson, J.E., et al. "Antioxidant and cardiovascular disease: A review." *Journal of the American College of Nutrition;* 12: 426–32, 1993.

Ornish, D., et al. "Can lifestyle changes reverse coronary atherosclerosis?" *Circulation;* 88 (Suppl): 1–385 abstract, 1993.

Rimm, E.B., et al. "Vitamin E consumption and the risk of coronary heart disease in men." *The New England Journal of Medicine;* 328(20): 1450–6, 1993.

Kris-Etherton, P.M. and Krummel, D. "Role of nutrition in the prevention and treatment of coronary heart disease in women." *Journal of the American Dietetic Association;* 93(9): 987–93, 1993.

Feskens, E.J. and Kromhout, D. "Epidemiologic studies on Eskimos and fish intake." *Annals of the New York Academy of Sciences;* 683: 9–15, 1993.

Connor, W.E., et al. "N-3 fatty acids from fish oil. Effects on plasma lipoproteins and hyper-triglyceridemic patients." *Annals of the New York Academy of Sciences;* 683: 16–34, 1993.

Woodard, D.A. and Limacher, M.C. "The impact of diet on coronary heart disease." *Medical Clinics of North America;* 77(4): 849–62, 1993.

Von Beresteijn, E.C.H., et al. "Perimenopausal increase in serum cholesterol: A 10-year longitudinal study." *American Journal of Epidemiology;* 37: 383–92, 1993.

Barrett-Connor, E. and Friedlander, N.J. "Dietary fat, calories and the risk of breast cancer in postmenopausal women: A prospective population based study." *Journal of the American College of Nutrition;* 12: 390–99, 1993.

Anderson, J.W. "Diets, lipids and cardiovascular disease in women." *Journal of the American College of Nutrition;* 12: 433–37, 1993.

Stampfer, M.J., Rimm, E.B., and Walsh, D.C. "Commentary: alcohol, the heart and public policy." *American Journal of Public Health;* 83(6): 801–4, 1993.

Grobbee, D.E., et al. "Coffee, caffeine and cardiovascular disease in men." *The New England Journal of Medicine;* 323(15): 1026–32, 1990.

Willett, W.C., et al. "Intake of trans fatty acids and risk of coronary heart disease among women." *Lancet;* 341(8845): 581–5, 1993.

HIGH BLOOD PRESSURE

High blood pressure kills thousands of Americans every year and contributes to the deaths of thousands more. The American Heart Association estimates that one out of every four adults has high blood pressure (about 50 million Americans); many don't realize it. Studies show that during early and middle adult years men are more likely to suffer from hypertension. In later years, more women than men develop high blood pressure.

Scientists have yet to determine what causes high blood pressure or why the risks change over the course of a lifetime. Exciting new research is honing in on how diet can play a role in preventing and treating mild and more severe cases of high blood pressure. Researchers are exploring specific foods, including everything from fatty fish to salt (sodium) to potassium, in order to determine how these dietary ingredients affect blood pressure readings. In addition, evidence proves that excess weight can negatively influence blood pressure.

Take Off the Weight

In a recent study from the National Heart, Lung and Blood Institute, researchers confirm (and not for the first time) that weight loss can reduce blood pressure. When a group of overweight adults aged thirty to fifty-four were randomly assigned to follow a weight-loss diet (they were further divided into either a diet-alone or a diet-plus-medication group) or left to follow their regular patterns for blood-pressure control, it was the weight-loss group that was more successful. Weight loss reduced blood pressure. The more weight a person lost, the bigger the drop in blood pressure reading.

Another new study, the Trial of Antihypertensive Intervention and Management, reports more success in treating blood pressure when overweight hypertensives shed excess pounds. In this study, scientists noticed a 23 percent drop in treatment failure when hypertensives were following a weight-loss diet. In other words, taking weight off helps keep blood pressure under control.

It's studies like these that helped the National High Blood Pressure Education Program Working Group to rank weight loss (along with reductions in sodium and alcohol) as dietary measures that help treat high blood pressure. In fact, reducing sodium levels in your diet is a much more powerful treatment for most people than supplementing the diet with potassium-rich foods.

To Salt or Not to Salt?

The body actually requires only about 200 milligrams of sodium (one-tenth of a teaspoon of salt). Yet on a typical day, you probably eat around two or three teaspoons' worth of salt, or about thirty times as much sodium as is necessary. For years, health organizations like the American Heart Association and the National Heart, Lung and Blood Institute have been recommending that Americans cut back on salt and high-sodium foods. Experts say 2,400 milligrams of sodium per day, about a third of what we eat, is more than enough.

However, these recommendations are based on the fact that salt, or more specifically the sodium it contains, might aggravate high blood pressure. Yet recent studies find that not everyone's blood pressure is sensitive to salt. Estimates are that one-third to one-half of the population is salt sensitive. The trouble is that there's no inexpensive way to test for salt sensitivity. More important, many researchers feel that sensitivity may change as your weight increases or as you get older, making it wiser for everyone to learn to keep sodium intake moderate.

How do you cut back? Well, don't throw out the salt shaker. When scientists from the Monell Chemical Senses Center in Philadelphia studied the amount of salt people sprinkled on foods at the table and during cooking, researchers found that these two practices accounted for only 11 percent of a person's total sodium intake. Processed foods such as canned soups, salty chips, and frozen dinners account for more than three-fourths of the sodium most people eat. If you start downplaying processed foods and highlighting fresh fruits, vegetables, and lean meats, sodium levels will drop dramatically. Make sure to read labels on processed foods carefully to find products that are low sodium as not all high-sodium foods taste salty.

High-Sodium Processed Foods

Cucumbers are very low in sodium. Cure them into pickles, however, and sodium content jumps more than 800 percent. The same principle applies to meats, vegetables, spices, and sauces. All of the following foods are high in sodium due to processing with salt.

- *Deli or smoked meats:* Bologna, corned beef, pastrami, ham, liverwurst, hot dogs, sausage, salt pork, smoked turkey.
- *Prepared sauces:* Worcestershire, soy, barbecue.
- *Soups:* Instant mixes, bouillon cubes, canned varieties like chicken noodle or cream of mushroom.
- *Cheeses:* All varieties, particularly processed cheese foods and spreads.

- *Smoked or canned fish:* Anchovies, caviar, pickled herring, smoked salmon.
- *Snacks:* Potato chips, pretzels, salted popcorn, salted nuts, crackers.
- *Miscellaneous:* Sea or kosher salt, canned vegetables, T.V. dinners, olives.

Sodium Labeling Sense

Law requires that processed foods making claims about sodium content follow these guidelines. (For more help deciphering nutrition information on food packages see the chapter on Labels on Food, p. 118.)

Sodium free—five milligrams per serving or less.
Very low sodium—35 milligrams per serving or less.
Low sodium—140 milligrams per serving or less.
Reduced sodium—processed so that usual amount of sodium is cut by 75 percent.
Salt free—processed without salt; may contain sodium in the form of other preservatives.

Stand-Ins for Salt

Although processed foods are probably the biggest source of sodium, it helps to try and cut back on salt in cooking, too. Learn to be creative with fresh or dried herbs and you'll never miss the salt.

- Stir dill into low-fat yogurt for a dip, or use it as a sauce to coat cucumber or poached salmon.
- Mix allspice, cinnamon, or cloves into sweet potatoes or winter squash for a hint of sweetness.
- Sprinkle cumin, red pepper flakes, garlic, and ginger into a stir-fry to fire it up.
- Slip sprigs of fresh rosemary or basil leaves under the skin of a chicken before baking to infuse it with a different flavor.
- Compile your own seasoning blends. Italian spice mix is made with a mixture of seasonings such as oregano, rosemary, basil, and thyme.
- Add a splash of wine, sherry, citrus juice, or flavored vinegars to finish off a dish with a tart or sweet flavor.

The Power of Potassium

Doctors often tell patients with high blood pressure to eat bananas, orange juice, and other potassium-rich foods. The reason has more to do with medication than with the treatment of blood pressure. Some diuretics used to lower blood pressure work by helping rid the body of excess sodium, which also depletes potassium stores. When doctors prescribe potassium-rich foods this is usually the reason.

However, preliminary reports suggest that potassium may help lower blood pressure on its own. The hitch is that it seems to work only for certain population groups, most notably African Americans. Yet when you consider the following list of potassium-rich foods, there's no reason not to include these nutrient-dense gems in your daily diet.

Food Sources of Potassium

Food	Milligrams of potassium
Skim milk, 8 oz	247
Potato, baked w/skin	115
Potato, baked w/o skin	78
Orange juice, 8 oz	53
Spinach, ½ cup cooked	50
Zucchini, ½ cup cooked	36
Tomato juice, 6 oz	34
Prunes, 5 dried	33
Raisins, ⅓ cup	32
Cantaloupe, 1 cup	27
Banana, 1 medium	22
Winter squash, ½ cup	20

Provocative New Findings

Every once in a while studies come along that suggest other nutrients may be helpful in controlling blood pressure. Fish oils, calcium, and magnesium are three frequently talked about examples. Scientists say findings are far too preliminary to make any practical dietary recommendations. The thinking is that eating plenty of fruits, vegetables, whole grains, fish, low-fat dairy products, and lean meats—a healthy diet—is probably your best strategy for preventing high blood pressure.

Indeed, there could be any number of protective substances in these foods that help ward off not just high blood pressure but other chronic ills as well. For example, a new study from Harvard finds that diets rich in fruit fiber may help prevent high blood pressure. Looking at eating habits of a group of more than 30,000 men, researchers found that men who ate the least fiber (less than eleven grams per day) had a 46 percent higher risk of developing high blood pressure than men with the highest fiber diets (twenty-five grams of fiber or more).

Can Fatty Fish Lower Pressure?

Perhaps the most controversial of dietary treatments for high blood pressure is the use of fish-oil supplements. Preliminary research results appear mixed on whether or not these polyunsaturated fats can actually lower blood pressure. In a recent double-blind, placebo-controlled crossover study (the gold standard of clinical trials because neither the researcher nor the participant knows which treatment is being used, and both treatments are tried on each participant), fish oils showed little promise as a treatment for hypertension.

Specifically, researchers fed a group of hypertensive and normotensive men either a capsule with twenty grams of fish oil or a placebo capsule with the same amount of safflower oil. After a four week washout period during which there is no treatment at all so the body clears out any remaining residue, treatments were switched. Blood pressure values were not significantly different with either treatment. These kind of negative results may be why experts from the National High Blood Pressure Education Group recently concluded that there is not enough solid evidence to recommend fish oils as a treatment for high blood pressure.

The story on fish oils is far from complete. An even newer report, published in the heart journal *Circulation* suggests that fish oils are an effective treatment, at least for some people. When these scientists analyzed thirty-one different controlled dietary trials using fish oils they noticed that people with hypertension or atherosclerosis were more likely to benefit from the oils. However, the oils don't have any impact on the blood pressure readings of healthy normotensive people.

Another new report pools evidence from seventeen different fish-oil diet trials and reaches much the same conclusion. That is, the magnitude of blood-pressure reduction with fish oils is greater for people who already have high blood pressure. However, fish-oil supplements are still not something most physicians want to recommend as a treatment for hypertension. The capsules are oil, and that oil has calories as well as unpleasant side effects. In the meantime, a better approach to lowering blood pressure with fish oils is to go to the source: fatty fish. Fatty fish contain plenty of the oils—rich in omega-3 fatty acids—that may lower blood pressure. These are also the same fats that appear to help lower heart disease risk and alleviate some of the suffering among people with rheumatoid arthritis. (See Arthritis, p. 37.)

Fatty Fish That Are Rich in Omega-3s

Type of fish	Grams of Omega-3 fats
Atlantic mackerel	5.0
King mackerel	4.5
Pacific herring	4.0
Albacore tuna	3.0
Atlantic salmon	3.0
Bluefin tuna	3.0

Chinook salmon	3.0
Norwegian sardines	3.0
Sockeye salmon	2.5

Portion Size: 7 ounces raw; 5 ounces cooked

Source: *Journal of the American Dietetic Association.*

References

Heart and Stroke Facts: 1994 Statistical Supplement. The American Heart Association, 1994.

Appel, L.J., et al. "Does supplementation of diet with 'fish oil' reduce blood pressure." *Archives of Internal Medicine;* 153: 1429–38, 1993.

Lofgren, R.P., et al. "The effects of fish oil supplements on blood pressure." *American Journal of Public Health;* 83: 267–69, 1993.

The Fifth Report of the Joint National Committee on Detection, Evaluation, and Treatment of High Blood Pressure. *Archives of Internal Medicine;* 153: 154–83, 1993.

Neaton, J.D., et al. "Treatment of Mild Hypertension Study: Final results." *Journal of the American Medical Association;* 270: 713–24, 1993.

Morris, M.C., et al. "Does fish oil lower blood pressure? A meta-analysis of controlled trials." *Circulation;* 88: 523–33, 1993.

Davis, B.R., et al. "Reduction in long-term antihypertensive medication requirements: Effects of weight reduction by dietary intervention in overweight persons with mild hypertension." *Archives of Internal Medicine;* 153: 1773–82, 1993.

Hepburn, F., et al. "Provisional tables on the context of Omega-3 fatty acids and other fat components of selected foods." *Journal of the American Dietetic Association;* 86: 788–97, 1986.

IMMUNITY

It's no secret that good nutrition is crucial to helping the body fight infection. Indeed, the cells of the body's immune system need adequate nourishment just like any other cells. Surprisingly, the immune system seems extraordinarily sensitive to certain nutrients. Early nutrition research proved that adequate calories and adequate protein were key to healthy immune function. (Scientists have long known that malnourished people have weaker immune defenses.) New reports, findings that are generating excitement in the medical community, zero in on other nutrients, such as vitamin A, beta-carotene and vitamin B_6 and the role they seem to play in improving immune response.

For example, production of *interleukin 2,* a substance secreted by immune cells to fight off foreign invaders, can become impaired when you shortchange your body of vitamin B_6. Neglect to eat beta-carotene-rich foods like carrots, cantaloupe, or broccoli, and you risk shortchanging yourself of a powerful antioxidant that helps stimulate natural killer (NK) cells, the immune warriors that recognize and destroy viruses and tumors. Indeed, the list of ways nutrients can influence how your immune system functions just continues to grow.

If you learn to select the right diet, you can help activate your own powerful internal defense arsenal and keep it working at top efficiency. Conversely, if your eating habits are haphazard, it might be harder for your body to fend off illness. Studies of people with eating disorders suggest that it's not only overt malnutrition that compromises immune function. Borderline nutrient deficiencies and dietary excess may impair immune defenses too, particularly as you get older.

Revitalizing an Aging Immune System

It's hard to pin down a specific age when decline occurs, but immune responses naturally tend to weaken as you get older, making it harder and harder to fight off even minor infections like the common cold. Part of the problem is that your immune system produces fewer of the T and B lymphocytes fundamental to your defense against foreign invaders. Luckily, these changes in immunity are not inevitable.

Promising new research suggests that at least two vitamins have the ability to rejuvenate an aging immune system, or at the very least slow down its aging. When scientists gave a group of older adults daily supplements of vitamin E (800 milligrams), certain key immune responses improved. Since the recommended dietary allowance (RDA) for vitamin E is only ten milligrams, researchers are debating if the RDA for vitamin E might need to be raised. Some feel there is enough convincing data to warrant cautious use of vitamin E supplements (100 to 400 milligrams a day) and take small daily doses of the vitamin themselves. However, others remain unconvinced since the findings are at present only preliminary. It's wise to discuss any supplements you plan to take with your doctor.

Interestingly, the amount of vitamin B_6 needed to protect immune function appears also to be well above the current RDA. United States Department of Agriculture (USDA) scientists have already reported that the optimal dose of vitamin B_6 for older adults appears to be three milligrams, one milligram more than currently recommended. When these researchers deprived older adults of vitamin B_6, they found that all the volunteers had measurably lower levels of interleukin 2, a T cell growth factor. Lymphocyte responsiveness was also depressed. But as soon as vitamin B_6 was replaced (using supplements) immune response rebounded to original levels.

To better understand the critical role these two vitamins and other nutrients play in immune health over the course of a lifetime, you should have some idea how the body mounts a battle against illness. The system is complex, but researchers have unraveled at least a few of the mysteries behind how this powerful internal defense arsenal works.

Members of the Immune Defense Team

An accidental finger cut, a nasty flu "bug," or a run-in with the bacteria that cause food poisoning—no matter what the injury, your body's immune system comes rapidly to your defense. Dispersed throughout the body, its microscopic network of cells continuously mounts ruthless attacks on poisons, microorganisms, foreign particles, and diseased cells.

Two basic levels of immune defense are continuously at play: innate immunity and acquired immunity.

Innate Immunity—Sometimes referred to as *natural immunity,* your body has a whole host of chemical and physical barriers that start defending you immediately after birth. Your skin, the mucous membranes in your mouth, throat, eyes, intestines, and urinary tract all act as the first line of defense against foreign invaders. If a foreign toxin does slip through one of these barriers, *phagocytes,* cells that devour foreign substances, attempt to destroy it. Another innate component, known as the *complement system,* also works to destroy invading viruses and microorganisms.

Acquired Immunity—The body's second line of defense is a bit more complicated and not as well understood. It consists of numerous cells and substances that not only battle foreign substances but help you to recognize and catalog them for future reference. Crucial to this type of immunity is the body's ability to distinguish foreign substances (non-self) from its own body tissues (self). If, at forty-five, you are exposed to a strain of influenza that you battled back in your early twenties, your immune system will still carry the memory and the weapons to fight that virus. You could say your immune system learns from experience, a memory that is carried throughout life.

Primary warriors in this acquired immunity battle are two types of *lymphocytes* (white blood cells) which scientists refer to as *T cells* and *B cells*. While all lymphocytes are produced in the bone marrow (along with red blood cells), the T cells travel to an organ near the heart, the thymus, to mature and train. Their primary job is to learn to battle against viruses, parasites, and perhaps cancer. T cells also communicate with B cells, the lymphocytes that produce antibodies against foreign substances.

B-lymphocytes battle mainly bacterial invaders. When the immune system recognizes a foreign invader, specific B cells immediately begin cloning themselves and producing large quantities of antibodies to battle the invaders (*antigens*). These antibodies lock on to various antigens to circumvent the damage they cause to cells. Next, phagocytes come in and clean up the mess, gobbling the whole antigen-antibody complex and destroying it. In reality, of course, it's a little bit more complicated. At any step along the way there are numerous reactions and signals that involve a vast number of substances. Researchers have yet to untangle the whole system. However, it's apparent that diet does play a role in modulating or helping to turn on and off some of these different reactions.

It's likely that each of the forty nutrients play some role in maintaining a healthy immune system. Yet, as research is now proving, some dietary ingredients stand out as particularly potent medicine. Make a point to include foods rich in these nutrients in your daily diet, and your chances of warding off minor ailments such as a cold or the flu and perhaps more serious illnesses like cancer, could dramatically improve.

Immune-Boosting Foods

Nutrients, particularly vitamins and minerals, seem to influence your immune system on many levels. In various metabolic pathways, they appear to act as critical cofactors that help regulate (turn on and off) the functioning of a variety of immune cells. Sometimes they appear to have their own direct effect. However, it's important to keep in mind that the whole field of nutrition immunology is still in its infancy by scientific standards. Much of the research that supports a link between nutrition and immune function has been carried out in the lab or with animal studies. Yet, as the field grows researchers are beginning to test their theories on people.

Positive roles are being uncovered for several trace minerals and for some of the B vitamins, most notably B_6 (pyridoxine). But singled out as particularly helpful to immune defenses are the antioxidant nutrients, vitamins E and C and beta-carotene, a precursor of Vitamin A.

The Power of Antioxidants

Damaging substances called *free radicals* cause abnormal changes in cells that may induce heart disease, cataracts, and certain types of cancer. Antioxidants like beta-carotene and vitamin E and C can trap and destroy these dangerous compounds. Because they bind to free radicals and inactivate them, antioxidants are being studied for their ability to help prevent a host of different chronic illnesses. Theory has it that free radicals may be at the root of many of the changes we chalk up to aging.

Beta-Carotene

Carrots, cantaloupe, and dark green vegetables contain generous amounts of this plant pigment that not only has vitamin A but also appears to stimulate immune function. Specifically, beta-carotene helps to regulate natural killer (NK) cells, the T and B lymphocytes, and *macrophages,* the white blood cells that engulf and digest microorganisms and foreign debris. Studies hint that beta-carotene's antioxidant capabilities are critical to healthy immune function. Most research finds that it takes only small amounts, fifteen to thirty milligrams (the amount found in one or two carrots) to create an immune benefit.

Larger doses are also being tested. In one new study, "helper" T cell activity increased when people infected with the human immunodeficiency virus (HIV) were given 180 milligrams of beta-carotene each day. Other reports find an increased need for this compound among smokers and people exposed to large quantities of long-wave ultraviolet (UV-A) radiation. Apparently, beta-carotene blocks the suppression of immune function that is caused by exposure to UV-A.

Potential for Toxicity   Although it's still considered nontoxic (large doses may color the skin yellow), a new study from Finland finds that large doses of beta-carotene supplements could be carcinogenic. A group of 29,000 middle-aged smokers who took beta-carotene supplements (twenty milligrams per day for five to eight years) did not appear to gain protection from lung cancer with the supplements but actually appeared at slightly higher risk for the illness. It's too soon for scientists to draw any firm conclusions from this puzzling new finding. It may be that the smokers started taking beta-carotene supplements too late in the cancer process (cancers grow slowly over the course of decades) to notice any protective benefits. Moreover, since numerous studies find protective health benefits derived from beta-carotene, health experts encourage Americans to eat beta-carotene rich foods.

Food sources: If you munch on a couple of large carrots per day, you can boost beta-carotene by fifteen milligrams, an amount research shows to be beneficial. Other options are to sprinkle chopped dried apricots into a bowl of cereal or a favorite muffin recipe; slip a spinach leaf or two into a sandwich. Or include these other beta-carotene-rich foods at as many meals as possible: cantaloupe, sweet potato, winter squash, papaya, mango, turnip greens, and broccoli.

Vitamin A

Right after it was discovered, scientists labeled vitamin A the *anti-infection vitamin.* Early on, doctors noticed a higher infection rate in people with vitamin A-deficient diets. However, vitamin A appears most effective at fighting off respiratory infections. When there is a deficiency, greater numbers of bacteria are able to cling to cells of the respiratory tract. In addition, fewer T and B lymphocytes are produced in response to certain foreign invaders. And the thymus, a small gland near the heart that turns lymphocytes into disease-fighting T cells, begins to atrophy.

Potential for toxicity: Too much vitamin A can impair immune function. An overdose can also cause other serious side effects, including liver and kidney damage. Researchers say it's difficult to overdose on vitamin A-rich foods, but supplements can pose a real problem.

Food sources: Most milks and dairy products are supplemented with vitamin A. Make sure to choose the low-fat versions. If you don't like milk, the body can convert beta-carotene-rich fruits and vegetables (mentioned above) into vitamin A.

Vitamin E

This antioxidant vitamin is the primary defense against potentially harmful substances called *free radicals.* Other antioxidants, vitamin C, and selenium play a supporting role. For some reason, vitamin E stores seem to decline with age. In one short-term study, elderly adults who took a daily vitamin E supplement (800 milligrams) were able to boost certain aspects of immune function. Scientists are working now to see if they can achieve the same results with smaller doses over longer periods.

Potential for toxicity: Compared to other fat-soluble vitamins, vitamin E is relatively nontoxic. Several reports find no problems with the large doses used in studies. Since the RDA is set at 10 milligrams, many scientists consider amounts in excess of 100 milligrams to be a druglike dose, so caution is advised.

Food sources: The most concentrated sources of vitamin E are polyunsaturated vegetable oils (corn, safflower, and so on), and margarines made with these oils. However, because it is important to limit fat (of any kind) to keep the immune system healthy, don't use oils as your primary source of vitamin E. Other sources include wheat germ, nuts, and green leafy vegetables.

Vitamin C

Experts can't agree on whether or not vitamin C cures the common cold. But they will tell you that too little vitamin C in the diet can elevate your chances of developing an infection. In one recent study, marathon runners taking vitamin C supplements (600 milligrams) for three weeks prior to a race were better able to fight off postrace upper-respiratory tract infections compared with those taking a placebo. (A sedentary control group that was also taking vitamin C complained of fewer symptoms and their infections lasted fewer days.)

Another report finds that 500 milligrams of vitamin C on a daily basis can boost the concentration of other important antioxidant defense mechanisms. The beneficial dose of vitamin C could range anywhere from 100 to 500 milligrams.

Potential for toxicity: A water-soluble vitamin, the body generally excretes excess amounts of vitamin C. While many scientists suspect it's possible to overdose, solid evidence is lacking. In rare cases, excess vitamin C may increase the risk of developing kidney stones in certain susceptible people. Symptoms that may accompany an excess include nausea, abdominal cramps, and diarrhea.

Food sources: One eight-ounce glass of orange juice at breakfast puts you right near the 100 milligram mark for vitamin C. So does one cup of fresh or frozen strawberries, a cup of broccoli, or eight brussels sprouts. A medium-sized papaya offers almost double that amount. If you can't eat these items whole, try citrus juices or vegetable juices. Other sources of C include: cranberry juice, tomatoes, potatoes, green pepper, and kiwi fruit.

Vitamin B_6

Of all the B vitamins, B_6 (pyridoxine) seems to have the strongest influence on immune function. Several studies find it critical to maintaining normal immune responsiveness. When healthy older adults are put on vitamin B_6-deficient diets, immune response is immediately dampened. Fewer lymphocytes are manufactured and the production of interleukin 2, a substance secreted by immune cells to help fight foreign invaders, is impaired. Fortunately, once researchers correct the deficiency, immune responsiveness returns to prestudy levels. Speculation is that older adults may need at least three milligrams of vitamin B$_6$ daily to keep the immune system functioning smoothly. Earlier in life, two milligrams is probably sufficient.

Potential for toxicity: Experts warn against too casual an attitude toward this vitamin. While it is water soluble, overdosing on vitamin B$_6$ (200 milligrams or more per day) has been known to cause serious nerve damage.

Food sources: Many foods contain small quantities of this vitamin so you'll need to mix and match to reach the two to three milligram goal. Good sources include: navy beans, potatoes, salmon, bananas, canned tuna, chicken, turkey, lean ground beef, lean pork, and soybeans. Try to keep the skin on baked potatoes—vitamin content of potatoes eaten with the skin on is 4.7 milligrams—without the skin it's only 0.7 milligrams.

Iron

This essential mineral presents a dilemma to immunologists. While studies find that people with iron deficiency anemia are more likely to suffer infections and have impaired immune responses, taking extra iron doesn't cure the problem. In fact, excess iron can dampen the immune response. Part of the problem may be that many bacteria need iron to grow and multiply.

Still, when the diet is deficient in iron, fewer antibodies are produced, natural killer cells are less destructive, and *phagocytosis,* the process by which white blood cells gobble up toxins and debris, slows measurably. The current recommended dietary allowance (RDA) for this mineral, fifteen milligrams, appears sufficient for healthy immune function.

Potential for toxicity: Excess iron can weaken immune defenses. Certain people are at risk for iron overload due to a rare genetic disorder. However, toxicity is rare in general population unless iron supplements are abused.

Food sources: Lean red meats, poultry, and fish are the best sources of iron. Eating a small serving of red meat (about two to three ounces) twice a week and chicken and fish two or three times per week should help you meet recommended iron levels. If you eat whole grains, enriched cereals, and breads or dried beans as your protein source, keep in mind that this iron isn't as easily absorbed by the body. You can boost the amount absorbed by drinking orange juice or eating a vitamin C-rich food with your vegetarian meal.

Zinc

Crucial for healing wounds, a deficiency of zinc interferes with both repair and growth of new cells. Research suggests zinc may act on immune function at several levels. A deficiency can lead to abnormalities in T-lymphocyte and *neutrophils* (fast-acting cells that engulf and destroy foreign toxins), and may interfere with activation and signaling of immune responses. In animal studies, even a diet that was only marginally low in zinc resulted in a 20 to 30 percent drop in immune responsiveness. You would be wise to try to meet the RDA for zinc, twelve to fifteen milligrams, in order to help protect immune response.

Potential for toxicity: Excess amounts of zinc depress immune function. Men taking daily supplements of 150 milligrams (10 times the recommended dose) produced fewer lymphocytes and showed impaired ability to engulf and destroy foreign invaders (phagocytosis). Healthy adults taking twenty times the recommended dose (300 milligrams) for one month also saw a drop in immune responsiveness. Excess zinc interferes with the absorption of copper.

Food sources: Three oysters provide more than double the RDA for zinc, although it's unlikely you can make them a regular habit. Instead, a small portion of lean red meat, poultry, or fish will provide about half the needed amount of zinc. Make up the difference by choosing whole grain cereals and breads, green vegetables, legumes, and nuts to round out each meal.

Copper

Although most of the preliminary work has been done with animals, scientists feel that copper may have a profound impact on immune function. Copper deficiency is rare, but too little copper does seem to weaken response to antigens and interfere with proper maintenance of the immune system. A deficiency can also lead to decreased activity of natural killer cells, the immune defenders that recognize and destroy viruses and tumor cells. A copper deficiency can result from overzealous use of zinc supplements. Zinc interferes with the absorption of copper.

Potential for toxicity: It's fairly rare for someone to overdose on copper. There is no RDA for this trace mineral, but experts estimate that people can safely take in five milligrams of copper per day without any harmful side effects.

Food sources: Lean red meat, poultry, fish, seafoods, whole grain cereals and breads, green vegetables, legumes, and nuts.

Selenium

Obtained primarily from grains, preliminary reports suggest that this trace mineral may have anticancer and antitumor properties. How it works is unclear, but if selenium proves to be toxic to tumor cells, scientists may be able to use the mineral to modify or slow down their growth. In laboratory studies, a selenium deficiency can impair natural killer cells and T-lymphocytes. A known antioxidant, selenium works along with vitamin E to make it more effective.

Potential for toxicity: Large doses of selenium have an adverse effect on immune response. Excessive supplementation with selenium (five milligrams per day) can result in hair and nail loss.

Food sources: Lean red meat, low-fat milk, fish, seafood, and whole grain cereals and breads.

Two More Dietary Factors To Consider

Keep in mind that vitamins and minerals are not the only substances that affect immune response. Other dietary components can influence disease-fighting ability, sometimes in a negative way. For instance, too much alcohol in the diet can dampen immune response. Excess fat, particularly polyunsaturated fat, seems to do the same. To keep the immune system strong, moderation is key with both of these dietary components.

Fat
Generally speaking, obese adults and adolescents are more likely to suffer with infections than their normal-weight counterparts. Studies find that it's the type and amount of fat you eat that probably has the biggest influence on immune response. To date, most of the research has been done with animals. For instance, scientists find that natural killer cell and lymphocyte activity is sluggish in obese animals. Polyunsaturated fats, the kind of fats found in vegetable oils like corn oil and safflower oil, seem to wreak more havoc on the immune system than saturates (animal fats) or monounsaturates (olive oil).

Polyunsaturated fat—Excess levels of this fat dampen immune response. Lymphocytes respond sluggishly to antigens and cells that engulf and destroy foreign invaders are less efficient. This is not cause to avoid polyunsaturated fats completely. It's well known that diets that lack essential fatty acids (two polyunsaturated fatty acids the body cannot make so must rely on food to provide) tend to suppress immune function. The key word with polyunsaturated fats is moderation.

Omega-3 fatty acids—The oils in fatty fish like mackerel and salmon contain a type of polyunsaturated fat called omega 3. Scientists find that these oils may help relieve some of the symptoms of rheumatoid arthritis, an autoimmune disorder in which the body's immune system turns on itself and attacks its own tissues as if they were foreign invaders. Since much more work needs to be done with these fats, experts caution against fish-oil supplements. The best source of these fats are fatty fish: salmon, mackerel, herring, sablefish, whitefish, anchovies, and tuna. Also good choices are bass, bluefish, halibut, perch, pollack, and trout.

Cholesterol—Laboratory studies find that high levels of cholesterol suppress immune function. It's far too soon to say how these results will apply to the average person, however, it can't hurt to limit cholesterol-rich foods like meats, milk, and cheese as this can help ward off heart disease, the country's number-one killer.

Alcohol

When alcohol is consumed in excess it can act to weaken immune defenses in two different ways. First, alcohol is capable of exerting a direct toxic effect on cells and organs. Prolonged exposure to excessive amounts of alcohol can damage the liver and other tissues perhaps including those of the immune system. Studies show that chronic alcohol consumption can depress production of certain immune cells. The inability to produce these cells could put alcoholics at increased risk when they are challenged by a severe infection.

The second problem is that alcohol interferes with diet. Alcohol impairs absorption, utilization, storage, and excretion of nutrients, particularly the B vitamins. That alone might be enough to create borderline nutrient deficiencies that could weaken immune defenses. But the fact that high alcohol intake is usually accompanied by low food intake (skipped or partly eaten meals) is probably what is really responsible for alcoholic malnutrition. Scientists caution that these implications, if they do prove correct, relate to the alcoholic or excessive drinker. Moderate amounts of alcohol probably do not have much effect on immune function.

Are Supplements the Answer?

After taking a daily multivitamin (with extra vitamin E and beta-carotene) for one year, Canadian senior citizens ended up getting sick only half as often as those that took a placebo. Moreover, if they did become sick, infections lasted half as long and required less treatment. With all this solid evidence that individual nutrients can play a role in fighting infection, you might be tempted to take supplements, particularly single dose pills of the key immune-boosting dietary components.

As promising as these findings seem, scientists feel they are still a long way from knowing the optimal amounts of nutrients needed for immune function. Still, many experts are calling into question the recommended dietary allowances (RDAs). Set early in the 1940s, the RDAs were first established to help prevent vitamin-deficiency diseases like scurvy (vitamin C deficiency) and rickets (vitamin D deficiency), problems that no longer plague this country. Instead, we have to contend with chronic ills like heart disease and cancer, diseases that may be prevented by certain nutrients.

Some scientists feel that single supplements of most of the antioxidant nutrients (beta-carotene, vitamin E, and vitamin C) may be safe and helpful to preventing these illnesses. On the other hand, many experts are cautious about prescribing any kind of single nutrient supplements as a way to boost immune function. Since megadoses of some single nutrient can impair immune defenses, they feel your best infection-fighting diet strategies lie in making use of nutrient-rich foods. If you are worried about haphazard eating habits, a daily multivitamin might help fill in the gap. Be careful that it doesn't provide more than 100 percent of the RDA for any single nutrient.

General Diet Strategies to Strengthen Immune Function

Most nutrition research focuses on how single nutrients affect immune function, but scientists agree that the best infection fighting program is one that employs general diet strategies.

- Eat at least five servings of fruits and vegetables a day. Focus on including both vitamin C- and beta-carotene-rich items as often as possible. Slip tomato slices into a sandwich for a dose of vitamin C. Microwave a potato (vitamin C, B_6) for lunch and top with salsa or low fat cheese. Chop up carrots, green pepper, and other vegetables and mix them into meatloaf.
- Limit fatty foods. A good rule of thumb is to eat no more than 30 percent of your total calories as fat. If you don't want to track numbers, fill up on fruits, vegetables, and whole grains and eat small servings of lean meat or low-fat dairy foods. Cook with limited amounts of oil (or use vegetable-oil cooking sprays and nonstick pans). Flavored vinegars and chicken broth make good low-fat cooking mediums.
- Include fish regularly in your diet. Fatty fish such as salmon and mackerel contain omega-3 fatty acids, which appear to enhance immune function and protect against heart disease. Eating fish two or three times per week can lower your risk of heart disease, according to one landmark study.
- Fill up on whole grains and starchy foods (pasta, bread, and potatoes). Experts recommend you aim for at least six to eleven servings of the starch/whole grain group each day. Since one-half cup or one slice of bread is considered a serving you'll need at least two starchy foods at each meal. They can help you become used to eating less fat, plus they can provide nutrients that may enhance immune function such as the B_6 vitamin pyridoxine, and the trace mineral selenium.
- If you do drink, limit yourself to moderate quantities of alcohol. The AHA says moderate means one cocktail, four ounces of wine or one twelve-ounce beer per day.
- Keep your weight at a healthy level. People who are considerably overweight have more trouble fighting off infections.

Reference List

The Alpha-Tocopherol, Beta-Carotene Cancer Prevention Study Group. "The effect of vitamin E and beta-carotene on the incidence of lung cancer and other cancers in male smokers." *The New England Journal of Medicine;* 330: 1029–35, 1994.

Meydani, S.N. and Blumberg, J.B. "Vitamin E and the Immune Response" in: *Nutrient Modulation of the Immune Response,* S. Cunningham-Rundles (ed). New York: Marcel Dekker, Inc, 223–38, 1993.

Johnston, C.S., et al. "Vitamin C elevates red blood cell glutathione in healthy adults." *American Journal of Clinical Nutrition;* 58: 103–5, 1993.

Russell, R.M., et al. "Vitamin requirements of elderly people: an update." *American Journal of Clinical Nutrition;* 58: 4–14, 1993.

Peters, E.M., et al. "Vitamin C supplementation reduces the incidence of postrace symptoms of upper-respiratory tract infection in ultramarathon runners." *American Journal of Clinical Nutrition;* 57: 170–4, 1993.

Prince, M.R., et al. "Beta-carotene accumulation in serum and skin." *American Journal of Clinical Nutrition;* 57: 175–81, 1993.

Mangels, A.R., et al. "Carotenoid content of fruits and vegetables. An evaluation of analytic data." *Journal of the American Dietetic Association;* 93(3): 284–296, 1993.

Marcos, A., Varela, P., Santacruz, I., and Munoz-Velez, A. "Evaluation of immunocompetence and nutritional status in patients with bulimia nervosa." *American Journal of Clinical Nutrition;* 57(1): 65–9, 1993.

Chandra, R.K. "Effect of vitamin and trace-element supplementation on immune responses and infection in elderly subjects." *Lancet;* 340: 1124–1127, 1992.

Sherman, A.R. "Zinc, copper, and iron nutriture and immunity." *Journal of Nutrition;* 122(3 Suppl): 604–9, 1992.

Maki, P.A. and Newberne, P.M. "Dietary lipids and immune function." *Journal of Nutrition;* 122(3 Suppl): 610–4, 1992.

Fuller, C.J., et al. "Effect of beta-carotene supplementation on photosuppression of delayed-type hypersensitivity in normal young men." *American Journal of Clinical Nutrition;* 56: 684–90, 1992.

Beisel, W.R. "History of nutritional immunology: introduction and overview." *Journal of Nutrition;* 122 (3 Suppl): 591–6, 1992.

Chandra, R.K. "Nutrition and immunoregulation: Significance for host resistance to tumors and infectious diseases in humans and rodents." *Journal of Nutrition;* 122 (3 Suppl): 754–7, 1992.

Katz, M. "Malnutrition and immunity (letter)." *Journal of Infectious Diseases;* 166(6): 1458, 1992.

West, C.E., et al. "Vitamin A and immune function." *Proceedings of Nutrition Society;* 50(2): 251–62, 1991.

Chandra, R.K. "Nutrition and immunity: lessons from the past and new insights into the future." *American Journal of Clinical Nutrition;* 53(5): 1087–101, 1991.

Field, C.J., Gougeon, R., and Marliss, E.B. "Changes in circulating leukocytes and mitogen responses during very-low-energy-all-protein reducing diets." *American Journal of Clinical Nutrition;* 54(1): 123–9, 1991.

Meyandi, S.N., et al. "Vitamin B-6 deficiency impairs interleukin 2 production and lymphocyte proliferation in elderly adults." *American Journal of Clinical Nutrition;* 53(5): 1275–80, 1991.

Blumberg, J.B. "Considerations of the recommended dietary allowances for older adults." *Clinical Applied Nutrition;* 1(4): 9–18, 1991.

Cerra, F.B. "Nutrient modulation of inflammatory and immune function." *American Journal of Surgery;* 161(2): 230–4, 1991.

Kelley, D.S., et al. "Dietary alpha-linolenic acid and immunocompetence in humans." *American Journal of Clinical Nutrition;* 53(1): 40–6, 1991.

Ribaya-Mercado, J.D. et al. "Vitamin B6 requirements of elderly men and women." *Journal of Nutrition;* 121: 1062–1074, 1991.

Stites, D.P. and Terr, A.I. (eds.) *Basic Human Immunology.* Norwalk, CT: Appleton & Lange, 1991.

Alexander, J.W.; and Gottschlich, M.M. "Nutritional immunomodulation in burn patients." *Critical Care Medicine;* 18(2 Suppl): S149-53, 1990.

Payette, H., Rola-Pleszczynski, and M. Ghadirian, P. "Nutrition factors in relation to cellular and regulatory immune variables in a free-living elderly population." *American Journal of Clinical Nutrition;* 52(5): 927–32, 1990.

Meydani, S.N., et al. "Vitamin E supplementation enhances cell-mediated immunity in healthy elderly subjects." *American Journal of Clinical Nutrition;* 52(3): 557–63, 1990.

Kendler, B.S. "AIDS, nutrition, and infection (letter.)" *Annals of Internal Medicine;* 113(5): 409–10, 1990.

Block, G. "Vitamin C status and cancer: epidemiologic evidence of reduced risk." *Annals of New York Academy of Sciences;* 669: 280–292, 1993.

NRC (National Research Council). *Recommended Dietary Allowances, 10th revised ed.* Washington, D.C.: National Academy Press, 1989.

Bendich, A. "Vitamin C and immune responses." *Food Technology;* 41: 112–14, 1987.

Bowman, B.B. and Rosenberg, I.H. "Assessment of the nutritional status of the elderly." *American Journal of Clinical Nutrition;* 35: 1142–1151, 1982.

Beisel, W.R. "Single nutrients and immunity." *American Journal of Clinical Nutrition;* 35L 417–463, 1982.

INFANT NUTRITION

Infancy is a time of rapid growth and high nutritional demands. Babies double their birthweight in the first four months of life and triple it by the end of the first year. Still, advice about feeding remains fairly simple, because the most crucial factor—how much to feed your baby—is very easy to figure out. All parents need to do is follow an infant's lead. Babies are good at letting you know when they are hungry, as well as when they've had enough to eat.

Of course, the question of whether to bottle or breast feed, as always, deserves careful consideration. New research finds advantages for both methods of feeding. Surprising new guidelines offer parents a safe way to heat formula in the microwave. When it is time to introduce your infant to solid foods, there are a few new points to bear in mind.

Feeding with Bottle or Breast?

With immature gastrointestinal tracts and underdeveloped kidneys, babies need dilute, easy-to-digest fuel. Breast milk and infant formula both fit that bill, making it easy for babies to thrive and grow on either type of feeding. There are distinct advantages and disadvantages to the two methods. You'll need to weigh the options and figure out which choice is right for you.

Making the Choice to Breastfeed

Breast milk is an excellent way to meet the nutritional requirements of an infant. Experts cite one big advantage of breast milk over bottle feedings: Breast milk contains antibodies that help babies fight infection. In the first few days of milk production, breasts produce a watery fluid called *colostrum* that contains special substances that help build immunity to several diseases.

In addition, preliminary studies with animals suggest that breast milk harbors a generous supply of hormones and growth factors, substances that direct behavior, sexual development, and the maturation of an infant's brain and other tissues. Speculation is that a nursing woman's breast tissue directly manufactures the needed hormones to ensure an abundant supply. Other plusses to breastfeeding include the ease of feeding. There is no messy formula to mix or clean up after. Babies decide how much to drink and breasts produce that supply in light of the demand. If these plusses outweigh the minuses (frequent feedings, tender breasts, the need to pump breasts if the mother will be absent for a length of time) in your mind, here are some common questions you'll want answered.

Should I avoid spicy or gassy foods while breastfeeding?

Some moms worry that babies will suffer with gas or indigestion if they themselves eat the wrong foods. Unless you have a lot of food intolerances (or a strong family history of intolerances), your baby probably can tolerate whatever diet you are used to eating. If an infant can't, you will know.

Can I drink coffee while breastfeeding?

Caffeine is a powerful stimulant. However, sensitivity to the drug varies from individual to individual. Skip the coffee if you sense your infant is overstimulated whenever you drink the brew. Or you could drink coffee after you breastfeed; caffeine levels will diminish somewhat by the next feeding. (Stimulant effects of caffeine are strongest in the first hour after ingestion.)

Do I need to drink a glass of beer to improve the flow of breast milk?

Probably not. Scientists have found no compounds in beer or any type of alcohol that are capable of making breast milk flow more easily. In addition, some alcohol may pass on to your baby through the breast milk. Yes, there is some speculation that alcohol probably acts as a relaxant for some mothers (and relaxed moms let down more milk). Obviously, you can learn to relax without alcohol.

How can I improve the quality of my breast milk?

If you are eating a nutritious diet (see the chapter on pregnancy) and are in good nutritional shape (no nutrient deficiencies due to poor eating habits), the breast milk you produce will be high in quality. As a back-up: If something is lacking in your current diet, your body will dip into nutrient reserves so that breast milk remains nutrient-dense.

How much more food (calories) do I need while breastfeeding?

While estimates are that most breastfeeding moms need about 500 extra calories a day, remember that this is an average. How many calories you need depends on two factors: the amount of milk you produce, and how much body fat you have stored. If you feed on demand (about every two or three hours), chances are you're producing a quart of milk per day. That level of production requires 850–900 calories, some of which can come from foods and some from fat stores around your hips and thighs. If you feed less frequently or smaller amounts (which is the case for many moms) you probably won't require as many extra calories.

Making the Decision to Formula Feed

Sometimes infants do not take to breastfeeding. They can't suckle strongly enough, perhaps because they are too tiny (premature) or because their mouth is not yet well-developed. In other cases, it's mothers who don't have the desire or time to breastfeed: Babies need to be breastfed about once every two to three hours; each feeding session requires about 30 minutes. This kind of schedule is not easy and sometimes not even feasible for mothers who work outside the home.

Whatever the reason, moms who bottle feed should realize that they can bond just as easily with a child as moms who breastfeed; babies don't need to suckle at the breast to sense that they are loved. Cuddling and interacting with infants is what helps establish a bond.

Perhaps the only health disadvantage of formulas is that they cannot confer the immunological protection found in breast milk. However, as most of those immunological benefits are transferred mother to child in the first six weeks of breastfeeding, it's possible to breastfeed for a short time (say, while on maternity leave from work) and then switch to the bottle. Rest assured that commercial formulas do offer a baby everything it needs for good nutrition. In fact, the majority are modeled after breast milk, providing nearly the same amount of nutrients, in much the same quantities, as the real thing.

While whole cow's milk is not recommended for the first six months of life, the primary ingredient of most popular formulas is an altered version of cow's milk. Heat processing alters milk protein (*casein*) making it easier to digest. Butterfat is removed and replaced with polyunsaturated vegetable oils, and vitamins and minerals are added to mimic those found naturally in breast milk. Formulas are also made with soy protein for babies who can't tolerate casein.

Bear in mind that you should use commercial formulas as your pediatrician prescribes. One recent study found that infants can fail to grow when well-meaning parents water down the formula, thinking that this strategy may help prevent obesity or heart disease in their growing child.

One of the biggest advantages of the formula-feeding route is that supply is unlimited. In addition, it allows mothers to share feeding responsibilities with other family members, often freeing up more time in a busy schedule. With the advance of microwaves, warming up formula no longer takes forever.

Heating Formula in The Microwave

Only a few years ago, pediatricians advised parents against heating infant formula in the microwave for two reasons. First, there was the risk of accidental burns from unevenly heated liquid. Second, it was unclear whether microwaving might destroy some of the nutrients in formula. New research from Pennsylvania State University puts these concerns to rest. Researchers confirm that formula can be heated safely in any size microwave with no loss of nutritional quality as long as parents follow these guidelines.

- Heat only refrigerated formula. The colder formula is to start, the less chance there is of overheating.
- Use only plastic bottles. Glass can crack; disposable plastic liners might explode.
- Uncap the bottle before heating. Lids and nipples trap heat.
- Keep bottles upright. Don't cap a bottle and lay it on its side.
- Heat eight-ounce bottles at full power for no more than forty-five seconds; heat four-ounce bottles for no more than thirty seconds.
- Don't heat less than half a bottle of formula because temperatures are hard to control when amounts are this small.
- Cap the bottle after heating, and gently shake it to help even out temperature. (Gentle shaking is equivalent to inverting the bottle about ten times.)
- Always test formula on the tongue or the top of the hand. (Wrists are not as sensitive to heat.) It should feel cool. Warm temperatures indicate that formula is hotter than body temperature and requires cooling.

New Thinking about Introducing Solid Food

About ten or fifteen years ago, some doctors encouraged parents to start feeding infants solid food as early as possible. Health professionals now realize that the introduction of cereals, applesauce, and chunky food mixtures is something that should be tied to physical development. Along about the time a baby can sit up straight, usually at six months, he or she is becoming developmentally capable of learning to swallow solid foods.

Keep in mind that the practice of starting solid foods at the age of six months is not carved in stone. Each child grows at a different pace. As a parent, you need to watch and learn from your infant. Just as your baby knew how much and when he or she wanted to suckle on liquids, expect your child to let you know when and how much solid food he or she needs. Iron-fortified cereals are the preferred soft solid to begin feeding babies, because at about the sixth-month mark an infant is running low on body stores of iron (breast milk is low in iron). Cereals provide an easy-to-swallow dietary source of the mineral.

What follows are some general guidelines as to when to introduce different solids. Remember, they are only guidelines. Sometime between the ages of six months and twelve months most babies progress from soft solids to table food. Some children progress rapidly from cereals to pureed foods to table foods; others take much longer. Trust your child to go at the right pace.

Age	Solid Foods to Introduce
6 months	Infant is learning to swallow and take food from a spoon. Try iron-fortified rice cereal (babies have difficulty digesting wheat at this age) mixed with milk.
7 to 10 months	Babies are learning to gum foods and to move foods around in their mouths. Try pureed and fork-mashed fruits and vegetables, and finger foods that are easy to chew like cereal, breads, and crackers.
8 to 12 months	Babies are learning to chew. Finely chopped meats, any kind of soft table foods such as cooked carrots, boiled potatoes, pasta, or yogurt.

Reference List

Howie, P.W., et al. "Protective effect of breast feeding against infection." *British Journal of Medicine;* 300: 11–14, 1990.

Pugliese, M.T., et al. "Parental health beliefs as a cause of nonorganic failure to thrive." *Pediatrics;* 80: 175–182, 1987.

Story, M. and Brown, J.E. "Do You children instinctively know what to eat." *The New England Journal of Medicine;* 316: 1–3–110, 1987.

Fomon, S.J. "Reflections on infant feeding in the 1970's and 1980's." *American Journal of Clinical Nutrition;* 46: 171–79, 1987.

Committee on Nutrition, American Academy of Pediatrics: "Follow-up on weaning formulas." *Pediatrics;* 83: 1067–69, 1989.

Committee on Nutrition, American Academy of Pediatrics: "Recommendations for use in infant feeding." *Pediatrics;* 72: 359–62, 1983.

Committee on Nutrition, American Academy of Pediatrics: "The use of whole cow's milk in infancy." *Pediatrics;* 72: 253, 1983.

Committee on Nutrition, American Academy of Pediatrics: "On the feeding of supplemental foods to infants." *Pediatrics;* 65: 1178–81, 1980.

Beal, V.A. "On the acceptance of solid foods and other food patterns of infants and children." *Pediatrics;* 28: 448–56, 1957.

LABELS ON FOOD

Ever since Congress passed tough new labeling legislation, understanding the language on food packages has become easier. Called the Nutrition Labeling and Education Act of 1990, these new label laws give the Food and Drug Administration power to enforce a whole gamut of regulations. Labels now list fourteen nutrients, including fat, fiber, and protein. And use of terms like *light* and *reduced fat* is strictly defined. Health claims (such as "may help reduce risk of osteoporosis") must be backed up by solid scientific evidence. As an added bonus, the new regulations don't apply solely to packaged foods. Nutrition information will be displayed near bins and display cases of fresh foods like fruits, vegetables, and fresh seafood. In addition, serving sizes of similar products have been standardized.

Portion Size

For years, manufacturers have manipulated serving sizes of foods to make them seem more nutritionally appealing. By cutting standard portion size in half (or sometimes even more), cakes, cookies, and ice creams could be made to appear lower in fat and calories. Not anymore. Serving sizes from one brand of frozen yogurt to the next will be uniform even if the containers hold different amounts. Specifically, one serving of frozen yogurt equals four ounces or one-half cup. (In the past some companies called a serving size three ounces in order to make the calories and fat profile of their frozen yogurt appear lower.)

The FDA has defined serving sizes for 139 food product categories. Now you can easily compare the nutrient profiles of different brands of breads, cereals, cookies, and so on without using a calculator. Since portion sizes are uniform, you can quickly spot the product that is lowest in sodium, lowest in calories, or that meets your nutritional concerns.

Conquering the New Terminology

In addition to providing new and useful information, the NLEA agenda sets standard definitions for terms like *high fiber, light,* and *low cholesterol.* In the past these terms meant different things depending on the food company, making it very difficult to compare food products. General language *(high, good source of)* must also meet strict guidelines.

However, before you start scrutinizing new labels, it helps to understand what new labeling terms really mean. Newer terms like *Daily Values* and familiar phrases like *low sodium* all have precise definitions.

General Terms

The new labels work to put each particular food into the context of a healthy diet. They can let you know if a food is high or low in certain nutrients. In addition, nutrition guidelines, called *Daily Values,* help you compare the nutrient and fiber profile of a food to current dietary requirements.

- *Daily values*—A general term that replaces the U.S. RDA's. Daily Values are based on the Recommended Dietary Allowances. The Daily Values section of the label is used to reveal what a food offers in terms of your nutrient needs. Daily Values (DVs) are listed not just for vitamins and minerals but also for dietary ingredients that are major health concerns: fat, saturated fat, cholesterol, and fiber. To individualize the concept, DVs for a nutrient are listed as percentages of a 2,000 calorie diet (for most women and older adults) and a 2,500 calorie diet (for most men). Keep in mind that these two calorie levels are meant only as general guidelines.
- *High*—This labeling term describes a food that contains 20 percent or more of the Daily Value for a key nutrient such as calcium or vitamin C. Food companies may substitute *rich in* or *excellent source of* for the term *high.*
- *Good source*—Identifies a food that contains 10 to 19 percent of the Daily Value (DV) for a specific nutrient. A cereal label might claim that one serving is a "good source of fiber." Since the DV for fiber is twenty-three grams (per 2,000 calories) a "good source" would need to contain 2.3 to 4.4 grams of fiber per serving.
- *More*—Contains 10 percent more of a nutrient per serving than the traditional food. Most foods that use this claim are typically fortified or enriched with specific nutrients. On that list are foods such as breads or cereals (enriched with B vitamin and iron) and milk (fortified with extra calcium or protein.) The terminology does not cover such claims as a product having more raisins, or more caffeine; it is solely used in reference to nutrients.
- *Low*—Denotes a food that contains small amounts of major nutrients of concern—fat, saturated fat, cholesterol, sodium, or calories. The term means something different for each different nutrient. (See specific definition under each of these general categories below.)

Revealing the Truth about Fat and Cholesterol

For years, food companies have been fooling consumers about the fat content of foods, by making the portion size unusually small so that the amount of fat per serving seemed minuscule. For instance, one tablespoon of salad dressing used to be listed as a serving, so when you looked up the fat grams in a serving of salad dressing it might have said three grams; chances are you ended up thinking the dressing was moderately low in fat.

In reality most Americans use at least one quarter cup of salad dressing per salad. In other words, a typical serving really amounted to twelve grams of fat. Since new regulations set more realistic portion sizes for foods (based on what most people actually eat) companies can't hide the fat content under the guise of smaller portions.

- *Low-fat*—three grams of fat or less per serving or 100 grams (three and one-half ounces) of food.
- *Low cholesterol*—20 milligrams of cholesterol or less per serving or 100 grams of food; two grams or less of saturated fat.
- *Low saturated fat*—One gram of saturated fat or less per serving. In addition, no more than 15 percent of the calories come from saturated fat.
- *Fat-free*—Less than 0.5 grams of fat per serving. Serving size is now set by the FDA, not food companies.

Is It Really Low Calorie?

During the years that the FDA didn't have a legal definition for terms like *light,* a food company might shave a few calories from a traditional product and call the new version *light.* That has changed.

- *Low Calorie*—Contains forty calories or less per serving. Appropriate serving size varies depending on food; portions are set by the FDA.
- *Calorie-free*—Contains fewer than five calories per serving. Serving size is set by the FDA.
- *Sugar-free*—Contains less than 0.5 grams of sugar per serving.
- *Light or lite*—Contains one-third fewer calories than the regular product. If light is used to describe texture or color complete details are required such as the terms *light in color* or *light in texture.*
- *Less*—Twenty-five percent less sodium, fat, calories, or cholesterol than the original version of a food.

Revelations about Sodium

Regulations defining sodium have changed very little, but, with portion sizes now more realistic, some products can no longer fit into the category of low or very low sodium.

- *Low in sodium*—Contains 140 milligrams of sodium, or less, per serving. Serving size is set by the FDA.
- *Very low sodium*—Contains thirty-five milligrams of sodium, or less, per serving.
- *Less sodium*—Twenty-five percent less sodium, fat, calories, or cholesterol than the original version of a food.

Reading the New Food Label

To give you an idea as to how all this new information fits on the food label, the FDA offers this sample label. You'll notice that after a listing of serving size, calories and calories from fat are the most prominent features of the new label. This underlines the fact that overconsumption, particularly of fat, is one of the nation's number-one nutrition problems.

The New Food Label at a Glance

The new food label will carry an up-to-date, easier-to-use nutrition information guide, to be required on almost all packaged foods (compared to about 60 percent of products up till now.) The guide will serve as a key to help in planning a healthy diet.*

Serving sizes are now more consistent across product lines, stated in both household and metric measures, and reflect the amounts people actually eat.

The list of **nutrients** covers those most important to the health of today's consumers, most of whom need to worry about getting *too much* of certain items (fat, for example), rather than too few vitamins or minerals, as in the past.

The label will now tell the number of calories per gram of fat, carbohydrates, and protein.

New title signals that the label contains the newly required information.

Calories from fat are now shown on the label to help consumers meet dietary guidelines that recommend people get no more than 30 percent of their calories from fat.

% Daily Value shows how a food fits into the overall daily diet.

Daily values are also something new. Some are maximums, as with fat (65 grams *or less*); others are minimums, as with carbohydrates (300 grams *or more*). The daily values on the label are based on a daily diet of 2,000 and 2,500 calories. Individuals should adjust the values to fit their own calorie intake.

Nutrition Facts

Serving Size ½ cup (114g)
Servings Per Container 4

Amount Per Serving

Calories 90   Calories from Fat 30

	% Daily Value*
Total Fat 3g	5%
Saturated Fat 0g	0%
Cholesterol 0 mg	0%
Sodium 300g	13%
Total Carbohydrate 13g	4%
Dietary Fiber 3g	12%
Sugars 3g	
Protein 3g	

Vitamin A 80%	■	Vitamin C 60%
Calcium 4%	■	Iron 4%

*Percent Daily Values are based on a 2,000 calorie diet. Your daily values may be higher or lower depending on your calorie needs:

	Calories:	2,000	2,500
Total Fat	Less than	65g	80g
Sat Fat	Less than	20g	25g
Cholesterol	Less than	300mg	300mg
Sodium	Less than	2,400mg	2,400mg
Total Carbohydrate		300g	375g
Dietary Fiber		25g	30g

Calories per gram:
Fat 9   ■   Carbohydrates 4   ■   Protein 4

*This label is only a sample. Exact specifications are in the final rules.
Source: Food and Drug Administration 1992

Label-Reading Shortcut

Chances are you won't always have time to peruse every bit of information on the new food labels, but there is a quick way to tell if the food you want to buy is a nutritional bargain. Skip the front of the package labels (stickers or advertising hype don't tell the real nutrition story), and proceed right to the nutrient panel. Focus on just the major nutrition concerns: fat, fiber, and sodium. Note the amounts of these nutrients in a serving and what they contribute to daily needs. Remember, you are trying to minimize your fat and sodium intake while getting as much fiber as possible.

Next, look to the ingredient list. Are there any items you are trying to avoid? If the product meets your needs, buy it, and then review the rest of the nutrient information when you have more time.

Should Food Labels Make Health Claims?

When studies first showed that oats might help lower blood cholesterol levels many food companies highlighted these findings on cereal and bakery labels. Officials at the Food and Drug Administration don't want food manufacturers to use this "food as medicine" sales pitch too loosely. New legislation allows food manufacturers to make diet/health claims only if the claims are supported by solid scientific evidence. According to the agency, six food/health relationships seem solid enough to warrant use on food labels.

1. Fat and heart disease—Plenty of scientific evidence supports the fact that foods low in saturated fat and cholesterol may help reduce the risk of heart disease. To make a claim about lower heart disease risk, a food has to meet the standards for low saturated fat, low fat, or low cholesterol.
2. Fiber and cancer—A diet low in fat and high in fiber might reduce your risk of developing certain types of cancer. Besides meeting the definition for "a good source of fiber," a food must also be low in fat to make this claim. In addition, only fruits, vegetables, whole grains, or foods that contain one of these ingredients can claim the diet–cancer connection.
3. Sodium and high blood pressure—Studies show that restricting sodium (salt) may help prevent high blood pressure. Foods that meet the guidelines for low sodium or very low sodium may make this claim.
4. Calcium and osteoporosis—Scientists know that eating calcium-rich foods might help ward off the bone crippling disease osteoporosis. To make this claim a food must contain at least 20 percent of the Daily Value for calcium (200 milligrams) per serving.
5. Fiber and cardiovascular disease—New evidence finds that water-soluble fiber (apples, oats) can help to lower blood cholesterol levels. To make this claim, a food must naturally contain at least 0.6 grams of soluble fiber. At the same time it must meet stan-

dards for low fat, low saturated fat, and low cholesterol. The latter guidelines help to make sure that a food which is high in soluble fiber but also high in fat doesn't boast about the fiber.

6. Fat and cancer—Numerous reports suggest that a diet low in fat can reduce the risk for certain types of cancer. To make this claim a food must meet the standards for low fat.

Special Exceptions to Labeling Laws

Small food companies (bakeries, vending-machine operators) do not have to comply with new labeling legislation. In addition, fresh meat and poultry, which is monitored by the Department of Agriculture and so is not under FDA jurisdiction, will not have to carry nutrition labeling either. However, the Department of Agriculture has issued labeling regulations for processed meat products (luncheon meats, turkey franks, and so on).

Reference List

Kurtzweil, P. "'Daily Values' encourage healthy diet." *FDA Consumer.* May: 28–32, 1993.

Cassell, J.A. "A nutrition label the public can understand and count on." *Topics in Clinical Nutrition;* 8: 51–56, 1993.

"The New Food Label: FDA Backgrounder, Current and Useful Information from the Food and Drug Administration." Bethesda, Maryland: FDA Press Office, 1992.

Porter, D.V. and Earl, R.O. (eds.) *Food Labeling.* Committee on State Food Labeling, Washington D.C.: Institute of Medicine, National Academy Press, 1992.

Porter, D.V. and Earl, R.O. (eds.) *Nutrition Labeling: Issues and Directions for the 1990's.* Washington D.C.: Institute of Medicine, National Academy Press, 1990.

Hutt, P.B. "Regulating the misbranding of food." *Food Technology;* 43(9): 288–93, 1989.

Lewis, C.J., et al. "Serving size issues in estimating dietary exposure to food substances." *Journal of the American Dietetic Association;* 88:1545–52, 1988.

Pao, E.M., et al. "Foods commonly eaten by individuals: Amount per day and per eating occasion." Home Economics Research Report No. 44; Human Nutrition Information Service, Department of Agriculture, Washington D.C., 1982.

LONGEVITY

Whether or not you live to fiftysomething, sixtysomething, or ninetysomething is partially programmed by genes and partially influenced by lifestyle. An overwhelming amount of new evidence seems to suggest that foods and nutrients can turn back the aging clock and may act as the ultimate antiaging elixirs. Common foods like carrots, oranges, and wheat germ are turning out to be potential weapons against everything from cataracts to heart disease to declining immune function. Scientists cite prime nutritional powerhouses like vitamin C, vitamin E, and beta-carotene as the most potent protection factors and have a plausible explanation as to how they work their magic.

How Antioxidant Nutrients Fight Aging

One widely accepted theory on aging is based on the speculation that *free radicals,* highly reactive compounds formed when fats are metabolized, and in response to stresses like environmental contaminants, can wreak havoc on body tissues. Normally, the body has mechanisms that cope with free radicals, but if build-up is too great, that system can be overwhelmed. Left unchecked, free radical (oxidative) damage might then set the stage for chronic illnesses like heart disease, cancer, or cataracts.

Nutrients like vitamin C, vitamin E, and vitamin A precursor beta-carotene, because they can hook up with free radicals and neutralize them, could prevent damage. This capacity to quell free radicals gives these vitamins the label antioxidant. Numerous studies are pointing to antioxidants as prime candidates for turning back the aging clock in a number of ways.

The Vitamin C Factor

There's some evidence that high plasma levels of vitamin C equate with lower risk for cardiovascular disease. New findings from the Baltimore Longitudinal Study, a large research project that is tracking the diet and lifestyle patterns of 1,000 adults (ages twenty to ninety-five), show a positive correlation between blood levels of vitamin C and HDL, the good cholesterol.

Cutting-edge research at Tufts University sees a similar connection between vitamin C and HDL. It also suggests an influential role for vitamin C in regulating two heart disease risk factors: high blood pressure and LDL cholesterol levels. In three separate studies, people who had the highest blood levels of vitamin C had more of the heart-protective HDL, and less of the heart-harmful LDL. They were also less likely to have high blood pressure. Besides helping protect the body against infection and promoting the absorption of iron, vitamin C may now be a candidate for staving off heart disease, the nation's number-one killer.

Some Notable Food Sources of Vitamin C

Item	Milligrams of Vitamin C
Red pepper, 1 cup chopped	190
Papaya, 1 whole	188
Orange juice, 1 cup	124
Broccoli, 1 cup cooked	98
Strawberries, 1 cup	85
Kiwifruit, 1 whole	75
Cauliflower, 1 cup cooked	72
Cantaloupe, 1 cup	68
Tomato juice, 1 cup	60
Cabbage, 1 cup raw	34
Baked potato	31
Tomato, 1 whole	24

Protecting the Heart, Prolonging Lifespan

Beta-carotene, a plant pigment that the body converts to vitamin A, is winning attention as a protector against heart disease. In a recent Harvard Medical School study, researchers found that eating higher amounts of antioxidant nutrients like beta-carotene and vitamin E can put women at less risk for developing heart disease. An earlier study from Harvard resulted in a similar finding for men. Physicians with heart disease were given either a placebo or a supplement of fifty milligrams of beta-carotene (about the amount in two cups of cooked carrots). The supplement group had nearly half the risk of heart attack, stroke, and early death from heart disease as the placebo group.

Eating lots of beta-carotene-rich plant foods like cantaloupe, sweet potatoes, and broccoli might also prevent or delay cataracts, an age-related change that is the number one cause of blindness in later years. Studies at Tufts University find that people who eat fewer than three and one-half servings from the vegetable/fruit group have nearly six times the risk of developing cataracts as people who eat more. Tufts researcher Paul Jacques speculates that beta-carotene and vitamin C protect the lens of the eye against oxidative damage.

Where to Find Beta-carotene

Since beta-carotene is a coloring pigment that turns plants orange, yellow, or red, it's easy to spot fruits and vegetables rich in this vitamin A precursor. A good rule of thumb: the deeper the color, the higher the concentration of beta-carotene. One exception is leafy green vegetables like spinach, where chlorophyll masks the pigment.

Vegetable sources include: Sweet potato, carrot, pumpkin, winter squash (butternut, acorn), dark leafy greens like broccoli, kale, beet greens, and spinach.

Fruit sources include: cantaloupe, mangoes, papaya, apricots, peaches, guava, carambola (star fruit), nectarines, and tangerines.

Vitamin E Fights Cataracts and Infections

Researchers at the Wilmer Eye Institute in Baltimore find that high plasma levels of another antioxidant, vitamin E, show a protective effect on both cataracts and macular degeneration, an age-related change in the eyes that impairs vision.

Vitamin E also seems capable of bolstering immune response. Research from the Department of Agriculture's Human Nutrition Center on Aging at Tufts University finds that healthy elderly adults who add vitamin-E supplements to their diets (800 units of vitamin E for thirty consecutive days) demonstrate much better immune responsiveness than participants taking a placebo. It's known that as most people get older the immune system goes into a slow decline, making it more difficult to fight off even common ailments like colds or the flu.

Vitamin E, long known to protect the integrity of cell membrances, appears to shield immune cells from oxygen damage and thereby helps preserve immune capacity, according to researchers at the antioxidant research lab and Aging Center at Tufts University. The hitch, however, is that the levels of vitamin E used in these new experiments are much higher than most people eat or could eat even if they stocked up on almonds, wheat germ, and other vita-

Food Sources of Vitamin E

Item	Milligrams (as alpha tocopherol)
Sunflower seeds, 1 oz	14.2
Sweet potato, 1 medium	5.9
Wheat germ, ¼ cup	4.1
Peanut butter, 2 tbsp	3.0
Mango, 1 medium	2.3
Asparagus, 8 spears cooked	1.6
Pasta, 1 cup enriched	1.0

min-E rich foods. Fortunately, preliminary evidence seems to suggest that smaller amounts over longer periods might be just as helpful. Look for studies to confirm these findings sometime in the next few years.

Can Eating Less Lengthen the Lifespan?

A small but vocal group of researchers think that another potential factor in the antiaging equation may lie in how much food you eat—your daily calorie intake. Numerous studies of animals show that depriving small animals of adequate calories (but keeping nutrient levels adequate) can lengthen lifespan. Specifically, cutting a laboratory rat's food by half or more can stretch its lifespan as much as 40 to 50 percent. Of course, laboratory rats are a far cry biologically from humans.

Studies are currently underway at the National Institute on Aging to find out if the calorie-deprivation theory works on larger animals like monkeys, who are more biologically similar to people. It's already obvious that underfeeding monkeys can slow down the maturation process, say researchers. Monkeys on a lower-calorie diet mature an average of one year later than those on a regular feeding regimen. Yet whether delayed maturation will equate to a longer lifespan won't be known until studies are complete.

In the meantime, you should know that most scientists are skeptical of calorie deprivation as an antiaging tool. Many consider the concept far too sketchy to make any kind of current diet recommendations. A major concern is that people who make a dramatic cutback in calories could end up shortchanging themselves of critical nutrients needed for the body to function. In addition, less food is likely to equate to less of the antioxidant chemicals and other protective substances in foods, compounds that are only now being realized as potential weapons in the battle to slow the aging process.

Putting Together the Optimum Eating Program to Slow Aging

While studies can point out how much and what types of food and nutrients might slow aging, you'll need to apply general strategies within the context of your lifestyle.

- Do you smoke? If you do, keep in mind that smoking increases your requirements for antioxidant nutrients.
- Are you living in a big city with large amounts of pollutants? High levels of ozone and other environmental contaminants can also put a demand on the body for more antioxidants.

- Finally, what are your eating habits like? If fruits, vegetables, and whole grains are missing at your meals, make an attempt to include more of these foods.

Of course, there is no harm in taking a multivitamin supplement to help boost your intake of protective nutrients, but opinions are mixed as to whether single nutrient supplements of each of the antioxidant vitamins are wise. Some scientists suggest that foods may not be capable of providing the quantities of antioxidants needed to promote longevity, and think that careful and prudent use of antioxidant supplements might be the answer to meeting the demands of aging. Others see the evidence linking these vitamins to longevity as compelling but conclude that food is still the best source of these nutrients.

In the meantime, most of the diet advice offered by major health organizations to ward off chronic ills like heart disease and certain types of cancer is the same strategy for slowing down the biological time clock.

1. Eat less fat. Health experts recommend limiting fat to 30 percent of total calories or less. Choose lean meats and low-fat dairy products, cook with less fat by sprinkling spices and splashing flavored vinegars and low-fat broths onto foods.
2. Focus on high fiber. The National Cancer Institute recommends aiming for twenty to thirty-five grams of fiber per day. Switch to whole-grain breads and cereals; wheat germ is an excellent source of antioxidant vitamin E.
3. Give fruits and vegetables a high five. Eating plenty of produce supplies the body with key vitamins and nutrients. Zero in on antioxidant-rich items: citrus, tomatoes, and kiwi for vitamin C; for betacarotene choose carrots, cantaloupe, leafy greens, and sweet potatoes.

How Exercise Can Slow Aging

Any discussion of how healthful eating might slow aging should include an addendum about exercise. Ongoing research at the Department of Agriculture's Center on Aging finds that many of the effects of aging can be slowed or even reversed through exercise. Strength or weight training is especially important in controlling the loss of muscle mass and bone density that begins to occur after age thirty.

In yet another study looking at fitness and mortality, scientists are uncovering health benefits for even small amounts of exercise. According to the Dallas researchers, an unfit woman who exercises to become fit might expect to reduce her risk of early death by almost fifty percent. With all this positive news about diet and exercise, it's clear that helping to slow down the biological time clock could be as simple as stocking up on vitamin-rich fruits, vegetables, and whole grains and keeping active.

References

Rimm, E., et al. "Vitamin E consumption and the risk of coronary heart disease in men." *The New England Journal of Medicine;* 328: 1450–59, 1993.

Stampher, M., et al. "Vitamin E consumption and the risk of coronary heart disease in women." *The New England Journal of Medicine;* 328: 1444–49.

Hunter, D.J., et al. "A prospective study of the intake of vitamins C, E and A and the risk of breast cancer." *The New England Journal of Medicine;* 329: 234–40, 1993.

Meyandi, S.N., and Blumberg, J.B. "Vitamin E and the immune response" in: *Nutrient modulation of the immune response,* S. Cunningham Rundles (ed). New York: Marcel Dekker, Inc, 223–38, 1993.

Russell, R.M., et al. "Vitamin requirements of elderly people: an update." *American Journal of Clinical Nutrition;* 58: 4–14, 1993.

Ames B.N., Shigena M.K., and Hagen T.M. "Oxidants, antioxidants, and the degenerative diseases of aging." Proceedings of the National Academy of Sciences; 90(17)L 7915–22, 1993.

Chandra, R.K. "Effect of vitamin and trace-element supplementation on immune responses and infection in elderly subjects." *Lancet;* 340: 1124–27, 1992.

Chandra, D.B., et al. "Vitamin C in the human aqueous humor and cataracts. *International Journal of Vitamin Nutrition Research;* 56: 165–68, 1986.

Jacques, P.F., et al. "Nutritional status in persons with and without senile cataract. *Archives of Opthalmology;* 106: 337–40, 1988.

Jacques, P.F., et al. "Epidemiological evidence of a role for the antioxidant vitamins and carotenoids in cataract prevention." *American Journal of Clinical Nutrition;* 53: S352–55, 1991.

Cadet, J.L. "The potential use of vitamin E and selenium in Parkinsonism." *Medical Hypothesis;* 20: 87–94, 1986.

Fahn S. "The endogenous toxin hypothesis of the etiology of Parkinson's disease and a pilot trial of high-dosage antioxidants in an attempt to slow the progression of the illness." *Annals of New York Academy of Sciences;* 70: 186–96, 1989.

Burr, M.E., et al. "Vitamin C and cholesterol in the elderly." *Human Nutrition Clinics in Nutrition;* 39C: 387–88, 1985.

Peterson, V.E., et al. "Quantification of plasma cholesterol and triglyceride levels in hypercholesterolemic subjects receiving ascorbic acid supplements." *American Journal of Clinical Nutrition;* 584–87, 1975.

Dallal, G.E., et al. "Ascorbic acid, HDL cholesterol and apolipoprotein A-1 in an elderly Chinese population in Boston." *Journal of the American College of Nutrition;* 8(1): 69–74, 1989.

Jacques, P.F., et al. "Ascorbic acid, HDL, and total plasma cholesterol in the elderly." *Journal of the American College of Nutrition;* 6: 169–74, 1987.

Gaziano, J.M., et al. "Beta-carotene therapy for chronic stable angina." *Supplement to Circulation;* 82 (4): III–201, 1990.

Manson, J.E., et al. "A prospective study of antioxidant vitamins and incidence of coronary heart disease in women." *Supplement to Circulation;* 84 (4): II–546, 1991.

Meyandi, S.N., et al. "Vitamin E supplementation enhances cell-mediated immunity in healthy elderly subjects." *American Journal of Clinical Nutrition;* 52 (3): 557–63, 1990.

LOW-FAT EATING

There's no question that cutting back on fat is important to health. Unfortunately, if you're like most people, the thought of giving up your favorite foods and rearranging eating habits in an effort to limit fat is definitely an unpleasant one. Surprisingly, changing your eating habits doesn't have to be that difficult. According to new findings from scientists at Pennsylvania State University, two small changes—switching to skim milk instead of whole and using lean cuts of meat—would be enough to bring fat levels in the current American diet to within recommended levels. More importantly, a recent discovery from Philadelphia researchers confirms that it's actually possible to train your tastebuds to enjoy and even prefer a low-fat style of eating.

Learning to Like It Low-Fat

It may sound hard to believe, but an intriguing report from scientists at the Monell Chemical Senses Institute in Philadelphia showed that normal, healthy men (none of whom had any desire to cut back on fat) could be switched to a diet low in fat and like it. As part of a fat preference study, these scientists placed volunteers into three groups. One group received a low-fat diet with no added fats such as salad dressing, margarine, or mayonnaise. A second group followed a low-fat diet using modified fat foods such as reduced-fat mayonnaise and diet margarine. A control group paid no attention to dietary fat.

At the end of twelve weeks, scientists asked participants to rate preference of common foods; foods were doctored so that fat content varied. It seems that men on the low-fat diets didn't like puddings, chocolate milk, and cream soups that were high in fat. They showed a clear preference for low-fat versions of these foods, leading researchers to suggest that high-fat foods are an acquired taste, one that can be unlearned.

Just as people who cut back on salt eventually find they don't like the taste of overly salty foods, people who cut back on fat tend to find that greasy, fried foods taste too rich. So, if you can hang in there during the initial eight or twelve weeks of a low-fat diet, chances are you will grow to like this style of eating.

Trim Some of the Fat, But Not All

An important point about low-fat eating, one that many people misunderstand, is that low-fat doesn't mean no fat. There is no reason to totally eliminate fat from your diet. In fact, that approach is unhealthy. Fat is a necessary nutrient that performs critical body functions. It cushions and protects vital organs. Fat also acts as a storage facility for fat soluble vitamins and gives integrity and strength to cell walls.

The hitch is that it takes only small amounts of fat to perform these functions. Any extra fat you consume is going to have to be stored. These extra fat stores, particularly if they result in obesity or lodge around your middle, can cause health problems. So rather than eliminate fat from your diet, learn to balance low-and high-fat foods so that your fat intake stays below 30 percent of total calories or less. Many experts believe that lowering fat intake to less than 20 to 25 percent of total calories is even better.

Tracking Fat in The Diet

Fried chicken, fast food, and rich, premium ice creams are just some of the foods that keep the fat level in American diets at an unhealthy 37 percent. To make sure you're not over-doing it with high-fat foods, keep tabs on fat intake for a few days.

Playing the Percentages.

Health professionals encourage you to aim for 30 percent or less of total calories from fat. Keep in mind that the 30 percent rule doesn't apply to every single food you eat. A few potato chips, the occasional slice of cheesecake, or a pastrami sandwich won't destroy an otherwise low in fat diet. The point is to balance choices over the course of a day or a few days so that you average out to 30 percent or less. (The same balancing act also applies if you cut your fat intake to 20 to 25 percent of total calories.) Use the food charts in the back of the book to help fill you in on fat content of favorite foods.

Fat Mathematics:

Determining the percentage of calories that come from fat isn't difficult. Since each gram of fat has nine calories, you can multiply the number of grams of fat in a food by nine. That will tell you the number of calories that come from fat. Divide the number of calories that come from fat by the total amount of calories to figure out the percentage of calories that come from fat. In other words, if a bran muffin contains 200 calories and five grams of fat, you would multiply $5 \times 9 = 45$. That means 45 of the 200 calories come from fat. Divide 45 by 200 = 0.22 (or 22% fat calories). Luckily, food labels already compute these percentages for packaged foods.

Budgeting Fat by Grams

Another way to look at advice to eat 30 percent or less of calories from fat is to convert percentages into total grams of fat. The chart below uses some typical calorie levels and converts the recommendation for 30 percent, 25 percent, and 20 percent fat into grams of fat. You can use this budgeting method as a starting point for helping you assess current fat intake and where you need to make changes. Or you can budget fat on a daily basis, adding up the grams of fat of each food you eat.

If you eat	Your fat allowance is . . .		
	30%	*25%*	*20%*
1,200 calories	40 grams	33 grams	27 grams
1,500 calories	50 grams	42 grams	33 grams
1,800 calories	60 grams	50 grams	40 grams
2,100 calories	70 grams	58 grams	47 grams
2,400 calories	80 grams	67 grams	53 grams
2,600 calories	87 grams	72 grams	58 grams
2,800 calories	93 grams	78 grams	62 grams
3,000 calories	100 grams	83 grams	67 grams

"Good" Fats versus "Bad" Fats

Now that you have an idea about how much fat is healthy, the next step is to think about "good" and "bad" fats. Scientists identify three major types of fat in foods: saturated, monounsaturated, and polyunsaturated. It's really not necessary to delve into the biochemistry of these dietary fats. Simply keep in mind that saturated fats—concentrated in animal foods like meats, whole milk, and butter—raise blood cholesterol levels. Polyunsaturated vegetable fats like corn oil and safflower oil, and monounsaturated fats like olive oil do not. In fact, these unsaturated fats may help to lower it. (For more detailed information on good fats and bad fats, turn to the chapter on Heart Health, page 85.)

Cooking with Less Fat

Taking the leap from being concerned about eating less fat to cutting back on fat in cooking is a much easier task when you break the project down into small steps. Little by little, these gradual changes will add up to an eating style that is low in fat.

134 THE HEALTH NUTRIENT BIBLE

Remodel Packaged Mixes—Start skimming fat from the recipes for instant potatoes, rice mixes, and packaged pastas. For example, a dried macaroni and cheese mix can be made with less fat than the label suggests. Simply substitute skim or 1% milk (for whole) and cut down on added fat (butter or margarine) by half or more. Instant potatoes and many rice mixes can be made without any fat.

Bake with Less Fat—Replace the fat in brownie and cake mixes with low-fat yogurt or pureed fruits (banana, pumpkin, or applesauce). Substitute equal amounts of the fruit or yogurt for oil or shortening. Use two egg whites to replace each egg.

Add Low-Fat Meals—Serve one low-fat meal per week to your family. Then gradually increase it to two low-fat meals, and so on. One noted heart researcher is fond of mentioning that most families eat the same ten meals over and over again. If you work at finding acceptable replacements for favorite meals that are high in fat, your diet can become low in fat within a few months.

Revamp Favorite Recipes—Try substituting lower-fat ingredients for higher-fat ones in your family recipes. Start with these examples:

Substituting Low-Fat Ingredients

Instead of . . .	Switch to	Fat Calories Saved
Sour cream, ½ cup	Low fat yogurt	162
Ricotta cheese, ½ cup	1% Cottage cheese	126
Whole milk, 1 cup	Skim milk	72
Cheddar cheese, 1 oz	Skim mozzarella	36
Fudge sauce, 2 tbsp	Chocolate syrup	36
Cream cheese, 1 oz	Neufchatel cheese	27

Stock the Pantry with Low-Fat Condiments—Switching to low-fat condiments for sandwiches, salads, and spreads can add up to big fat savings. One tablespoon of mayonnaise delivers eleven grams of fat and ninety-nine fat calories. Any of the following condiments add spice to food yet carry less than one gram of fat and very few calories.

Try One Tablespoon of:

Condiment	Calories	Grams fat
Sweet & sour sauce	22	0
Barbecue sauce	20	0
Chili sauce	20	0

Pickle relish	20	0
Catsup	15	0
Dijon mustard	15	0
Horseradish	10	0
Enchilada sauce	6	0
Picante sauce	6	0
Salsa	6	0
Soy sauce	6	0
Teriyaki sauce	5	0
Worcestershire	5	0

Low-Fat, High Flavor Cooking Techniques

Broiling or roasting meats yields a lower-fat end product than frying. Fat can drip away during the first two methods; the latter method retains and even adds fat. Sauteeing in a non-stick pan with a quick spritz of vegetable-oil spray uses less fat than sauteeing in a few tablespoons of oil or butter. Employing low-fat cooking methods is only one part of low-fat cuisine. To make foods tasty, you'll need to go one step further and find spices and flavoring ingredients that can fill in for the fat you've removed.

Take a cue from professional chefs who experiment with using fresh and dried herbs, wines, and other flavoring agents to help enhance the flavor of foods. It's going to take a bit of trial and error to find out which flavoring agents and spices you and your family like. Here are a few ideas to help you get started:

- Season fresh, cooked vegetables with lemon juice. (You can mix lemon juice with a small bit of margarine at first to get used to the switch.)
- Add small amounts of an acidic liquid—balsamic vinegar, apple cider, wine—to low-fat soups, stews, and other dishes to give them an extra zing. These acids round out flavor by helping balance salty and sweet tastes.
- Top pudding or custard made with skim milk with a dash of cinnamon or nutmeg.
- Oven-roast vegetables (sweet potatoes, eggplant, asparagus) to concentrate flavor. Spray sliced vegetables with a light coating of vegetable-oil spray to keep them from drying out.
- Drizzle some citrus juice (orange, lemon, lime) onto grilled chicken to boost flavor.
- Marinate chicken, lean meats, and fish in low-fat liquids such as reduced fat Italian salad dressing, or wine before grilling.

Snacking on Less Fat

Just as important as trimming the fat at meals is trimming the fat from snacks. Sweets, desserts, and snack chips can carry large amount of hidden fats. One scoop of premium ice cream can carry as much as sixteen grams of fat; a pint might carry sixty-four grams of fat—more than most people's daily fat allotment. Granted, food companies are offering more and more reduced-fat snacks. But many of these reduced-fat foods are high in sugar and calories. Why not try some naturally low-fat substitutes for favorite snacks?

Instead of . . .	Switch to . . .
Gourmet ice cream	Ice milk, frozen yogurt, sherbet, fruit ices
Chocolate milkshake	1% chocolate milk, skim milk mixed with cocoa and sugar.
Butter cookies, sandwich cookies	Animal crackers, fig bars, gingersnaps, vanilla wafers
Bakery brownies	Homemade brownies made with applesauce or low-fat yogurt instead of oil.
Danish pastry	Bagel with jam, English muffin with apple butter.
Potato chips, corn chips	Pretzels, air-popped popcorn

Are Manufactured Fat-Free Foods Necessary?

Food industry giants have gone off the deep end with fat-free and reduced-fat foods, supplying many more choices than you probably need to keep your fat intake in line. There are fat-free mayonnaise, fat-free ice cream, fat-free cream cheese, fat-free potato chips, and fat-free breakfast pastries, just to name a few. Some of the products are quite tasty and offer acceptable substitutes for high-fat foods. Others definitely need to go back to the drawing board for improved taste and texture.

How, and if, you decide to use these foods as part of your low-fat diet is up to you. But do realize that the terms fat-free and low-fat don't make a food a nutritional star. For example, fat-free coffeecakes often contain large amounts of sugar and calories. One of the ways manufacturers keep fat content low is to bulk up the food with extra amounts of sweeteners and carbohydrates (to replace the fat). Even though you won't overdo it on fat with these cakes, the extra calories from sugar will add up, particularly if you eat two, three, or four servings.

In addition, keep in mind that many of these fat-free concoctions turn out to be low in fiber and nutrients. In fact, in a lot of cases you'll be better off (and so will your pocketbook) if you simply choose foods that are naturally low in fat. That is, if you crave a low-fat dessert, opt for ice milk, sherbet, fudge pops, angel food cake, and so on. (See the section Snacking on Less Fat, page 136.)

Where Do High-Cholesterol Foods Fit In?

Most animal foods—meat, milk, butter, cheese—that are high in fat are also high in cholesterol. Cholesterol is not a fat, but a waxy fatlike substance. Research finds that cholesterol-rich foods can raise blood cholesterol levels in some people. Be aware that dietary cholesterol doesn't have as strong an impact on blood cholesterol levels as saturated fat. The American Heart Association advises Americans to limit cholesterol to no more than 300 milligrams per day.

Keep in mind that all animal foods contain cholesterol. Plant foods do not. Be careful to limit organ meats such as liver, kidney, and brains, since they are also high in cholesterol. Three ounces of cooked liver contains 331 milligrams of cholesterol. One egg yolk caries 213 milligrams of cholesterol or more than two-thirds the daily limit. Whenever you can, substitute two egg whites for a whole egg in cooking.

MENOPAUSE

While women typically live longer than men, they don't escape the debilitating ravages of chronic illnesses such as heart disease, high blood pressure, osteoporosis, and diabetes. In fact, the risk for these diseases rapidly escalates during menopausal years, making good nutrition more crucial than ever. Keep in mind that as a woman's body adapts to the hormonal alterations which accompany menopause, nutritional requirements can change in profound ways.

Luckily, scientists are discovering dietary strategies that could help women adjust to and sail more smoothly through this nutritionally demanding stage of life. It's not just minerals like calcium that are important. New findings establish vital roles for vitamin E, beta-carotene, and a host of other dietary components. These nutrient superstars seem to act as protectors against disease, including the number one killer of women—heart disease.

Taming the Wild Cholesterol

You've probably heard that blood-cholesterol levels rise during menopausal years due to a drop in levels of the female hormone *estrogen*. The magnitude of that change may be more than you realize. A new study from the Netherlands documents a 19 percent jump in blood-cholesterol levels among women during the period at and around menopause. In numerical terms that could mean a jump of about thirty-eight points. If your cholesterol level hovers at a healthful 200 at age thirty-five, a 19 percent rise will equate to a cholesterol reading of 238 (borderline high) during menopausal years.

In the Netherlands study, which covered from two years before to six years after menopause, total cholesterol levels rose an average of one point per year. (After that, increases level off and are fairly minor.) Perhaps the more important finding, however, was the role diet played in mediating this hike in cholesterol. Researchers noticed that the rise in serum cholesterol was significantly lower in women who increased their intake of polyunsaturated fatty acids (vegetable fats such as corn, safflower, and soybean oil), compared with women who decreased their intake of these fats.

More work needs to be done to test the precise impact of dietary changes on cholesterol levels. But these experts feel that a prudent low-fat diet (lots of fruits, vegetables, and grains;

and only small quantities of lean meat and low fat dairy products) is even more important for women as they grow older than for men. (For more details on how diet can help ward off heart disease turn to Heart Health, page 85.)

Making a Case for Antioxidants

Antioxidant nutrients like vitamin E and beta-carotene may also be an important part of a heart-healthy diet during menopausal years. Recent research done with women, clearly implicates these nutrients as vital to warding off heart attack and stroke. A recent study from Harvard finds that women who eat fifteen milligrams of beta-carotene each day have a 40 percent lower risk of stroke and a 22 percent lower risk of heart attack than women who eat less.

Food Sources of Beta-Carotene

Food	Milligrams Beta-carotene
Sweet potato, ½ cup cooked	16.8
Pumpkin, ½ cup	16.1
Carrot, 1 raw	12.1
Spinach, 1 cup cooked	8.8
Mango, 1 medium	4.8
Spinach, 1 cup raw	4.4
Papaya, 1 medium	3.7
Cantaloupe, ¼ medium	3.1
Winter squash, ½ cup cooked	2.2
Mustard greens, ½ cup boiled	2.0
Apricots, 3 medium	1.7
Avocado, 1 medium	1.1
Broccoli, ½ cup cooked	1.1

Another new study finds that nurses who take in the most vitamin E (100 or more milligrams daily) have a 36 percent lower risk of heart attack and a 23 percent lower risk of stroke than women who take in the lesser amounts of the vitamin. While it's difficult to reach the 100 milligram level through diet (these women used supplements), you can emphasize foods high in vitamin E.

Good Food Sources of Vitamin E
Vitamin E is readily found in vegetable oils and other high-fat foods like nuts and seeds. However, you can obtain small amounts of this potent antioxidant from vegetables without increasing fat or calorie intake.

Food	Milligrams Vitamin E as Alpha Tocopherol
Sunflower seeds, 1 oz	14.2
Almonds, dried, 24 nuts	6.7
Sweet potato, 1 medium cooked	5.9
Wheat germ, ¼ cup	4.1
Peanut butter, 2 tbsp	3.0
Avocado, raw, 1 medium	2.3
Mango, 1 medium	2.3
Brussels sprouts, 12 cooked	2.0
Corn oil, 1 tsp	1.0
Apple, 1 medium with skin	0.8

Warding off Osteoporosis

Besides being potentially damaging to the heart, the drop in estrogen levels that occurs with menopause can be damaging to bone as well. In fact, in the first few years after menopause the body breaks down bone at a rapid pace in order to meet calcium demands. Estrogen-replacement therapy can help slow that loss; so can increased amounts of calcium and other bone-strengthening minerals in the diet. Recent studies find that as you grow older, bones still need a generous supply of vitamin D (the sunshine vitamin), magnesium, calcium, and boron.

Although that last dietary substance, boron, is a trace mineral, it is not considered a nutrient. Promising new studies from the Department of Agriculture's Human Nutrition Research Center in Grand Forks, North Dakota have found that women with boron-rich diets are less likely to fall victim to osteoporosis. Good food sources of boron include most fruits and vegetables, particularly apples.

Confusion About Calcium

Opinions are mixed about whether caffeine consumption is a risk factor for osteoporosis (For other health risks of coffee see the section on Caffeine, page 40.) An unusual new finding hints that any risk posed by caffeine or coffee may be negated when women drink plenty of milk. Specifically, researchers at the University of California at San Diego find that women who drink two or more cups of coffee per day throughout life end up with less dense bones in later years. However, that risk seems to be canceled out if women drink at least one glass of milk per day.

This is all the more reason not to make the mistake of foregoing dairy foods. Contrary to popular belief, all dairy foods are not high in fat and cholesterol. More important, reduced-fat and fat-free versions of many dairy products make excellent sources of calcium. Although many vegetables also contain calcium, quantities of the mineral are much smaller. Spinach, once touted as one of the best vegetable sources of the nutrient, is no longer considered a good source of calcium. Compounds called *oxalates* bind the calcium in spinach so that the body is unable to absorb it.

Food	Milligrams Calcium
Dairy	
Low-fat yogurt, 8 oz	415
Parmesan, 1 oz	336
Skim milk, 8 oz	302
1% Milk, 8 oz	300
Cheddar cheese, 1 oz	204
Part-skim mozzarella, 1 oz	183
Part-skim ricotta, ½ cup	141
1% Cottage cheese, ½ cup	138
Light cream cheese, 1 oz	38
Nondairy	
Salmon, canned w/bone 3 oz	203
Kale, 1 cup cooked	180
Broccoli, 1 cup cooked	178
Chinese cabbage, 1 cup cooked	158
Amaranth, ½ cup boiled	138
Navy beans, 1 cup cooked	128
Great Northern beans, 1 cup	121
Swiss chard, 1 cup cooked	102
Chick peas, 1 cup cooked	80
Brussels sprouts, 8	56
Kidney beans, 1 cup cooked	50
Artichoke, 1 medium boiled	47
Black beans, 1 cup boiled	47

Dealing With An Inflated Diabetes Risk

Some experts refer to diabetes as a "woman's disease" since after the age of forty-five, about twice as many women as men develop the illness. This has many serious complications.

The most problematic for menopausal women is an elevated risk for heart disease. Just as estrogen levels are dropping and heart-disease risk is rising, the development of diabetes worsens the risk picture. High blood-sugar levels damage blood vessels (in both women and men). But for some unknown reason the risk of heart disease and heart-related deaths is higher for diabetic women than diabetic men.

Since 80 percent of adult-onset diabetics are at least 20 percent overweight, weight control is a big issue during menopausal years. (See the section on Weight Control on page 203 for tips on managing weight if you are overweight. You might also want to look at the chapter on Diabetes, page 61, to understand more about dietary preventive strategies.) However, the same diet that helps ward off heart disease, cancer, and other chronic ills is the one that will keep diabetes at bay: A low-fat, high-fiber diet that emphasizes fruits, vegetables, whole grains, lean meats, and low-fat dairy products.

Zooming Blood Pressure

High blood pressure is often called a silent killer because it wreaks havoc on heart vessels without making people feel sick. While both men and women need to have their blood pressure checked regularly, as women grow older the risk for hypertension increases. More than half of all women over the age of fifty-five have high blood pressure.

Among African-American women, the illness is even more common and more severe. Experts report that African-American women are 24 percent more likely to die of coronary heart disease than Caucasian women. Of course, medications can help control blood pressure. But even if blood pressure is normal, diet and lifestyle strategies can help ward off future problems. (See the section on High Blood Pressure, page 94.) One of the newest studies finds a role for fruit fiber in helping to ward off high blood pressure. Scientists are unsure why fruit fiber seems protective. It is hoped that future research will be able to duplicate these preliminary results and offer scientists some insight into why fruit fiber is so beneficial. In the meantime, here's a list of some fruits and their fiber content:

Fiber Content of Various Fruits

Type of Fruit	Grams of Fiber
Blackberries, fresh, ¾ cup	3.7
Orange, fresh, 1 small	2.9
Pear, fresh w/skin, 1 small	2.9
Apple, 1 small	2.8
Strawberries, fresh, 1¼ cups	2.8
Banana, 1 small	2.2
Applesauce, ½ cup	2.0

Fruit cocktail, canned, ½ cup	2.0
Peach, fresh w/skin, 1 medium	2.0
Cherries, red fresh, ½ cup	1.8
Dates, dried, 5 medium	1.8
Nectarine, w/skin, 1 medium	1.8
Kiwifruit, 1 large	1.7
Grapefruit, fresh, ½ medium	1.6
Blueberries, fresh, ¾ cup	1.4
Pineapple, canned, ⅓ cup	1.4
Melon, cantaloupe, 1 cup	1.1

Serving size: 3½ ounces

Source: "Plant Fiber in Foods." James W. Anderson, HCF Research Foundation, 1990.

Reference List

Von Beresteijn, E.C.H., et al. "Perimenopausal increase in serum cholesterol: A 10-year longitudinal study." *American Journal of Epidemiology;* 137: 383–92, 1993.

Barrett-Connor, E. and Friedlander, N.J. "Dietary fat, calories and the risk of breast cancer in postmenopausal women: A prospective population based study." *Journal of the American College of Nutrition;* 12: 390–99, 1993.

Manson, J.E., et al. "Antioxidant and cardiovascular disease: A review." *Journal of the American College of Nutrition;* 12: 426–32, 1993.

Ju, H.F., et al. "Dietary calcium and bone density among middle-aged and elderly women in China." *Journal of the American College of Nutrition;* 58: 219–27, 1993.

Bostick, R.M., et al. "Relation of calcium, vitamin D, and dairy food intakes to incidence of colon cancer among older women: the Iowa Women's Health Study." *American Journal of Epidemiology;* 137: 1302–17, 1993.

Morley, J.E. "Nutrition and the older female: a review." *Journal of the American College of Nutrition;* 12: 337–43, 1993.

Nelson, M.E., et al. "A one-year walking program and increased dietary calcium in postmenoupauseal women: effects on bone." *Medicine and Science in Sports & Exercise;* S: 377, 1990.

Gavaler, J.S. "Alcohol and nutrition in postmenopausal women." *Journal of the American College of Nutrition;* 12: 349–56, 1993.

Duazo, F. and Khachadurian, A.K. "Prevention and treatment of osteoporosis in the elderly." *Topics in Clinical Nutrition;* 8: 9–15, 1993.

Anderson, J.W. "Diets, lipids and cardiovascular disease in women." *Journal of the American College of Nutrition;* 12: 433–37, 1993.

Anderson, J.J.B. and Metz, J.A. "Contributions of dietary calcium and physical activity to primary prevention of osteoporosis in females." *Journal of the American College of Nutrition;* 12: 378–83, 1993.

Nelson, M.E., et al. "Hormone and bone mineral status in endurance trained and sedentary postmenopausal women." *Journal of Clinical Endocrinology and Metabolism;* 66: 927–33, 1988.

Saltman, P.D. and Strause, L.G. "The role of trace minerals in osteoporosis." *Journal of the American College of Nutrition;* 12: 384–89, 1993.

Dawson-Hughes, B., et al. "Dietary calcium intake and bone loss from the spine in healthy postmenopausal women." *American Journal of Clinical Nutrition;* 46: 68–87, 1987.

OSTEOPOROSIS

Recent medical research confirms that the amount of bone amassed during early adulthood—the teens and twenties—plays a pivotal role in bone health during senior years. Yet along about the time you should be thinking about preventing osteoporosis, a crippling disease of old age characterized by brittle bones, it's probably the furthest thing from your mind. While you can't go back and redo your growing years, there are still strategies you can use to lessen the risk of osteoporosis.

A new study from Boston confirms the practicality of a multilevel approach to prevention using both changes in diet and lifestyle. Researchers find that a calcium-rich diet coupled with exercise slows bone loss and increases bone density. The interesting twist, according to researchers, is that exercise helps boost bone density in certain areas; calcium works in others.

Perhaps there will be even more exciting news in the near future as the National Institutes of Health is directing a massive amount of research money into a new project that will look for a better understanding of osteoporosis and how to treat it. At the same time, the NIH is awarding research funds to a group of scientists in Wisconsin who plan to study levels of the male hormone testosterone and its effect on bone health in men over the age of sixty-five.

Doing a Remodeling Job on Bones

For some reason, parents have no trouble nagging youngsters to drink their milk, but as most Americans slip into adulthood and middle age, chances are they will neglect milk and eat fewer calcium-rich dairy foods. Even though bones stop growing in length and width when you become an adult, bone is living tissue that needs to be constantly nourished and replenished.

You can do a lot to help protect the integrity and strength of the bone tissue you already have by paying careful attention to what you eat and how you live. Both diet and exercise can effect the rate and extent of bone loss. Eating a well-balanced diet with adequate amounts of calcium and vitamin D is of prime importance. New studies suggest that the trace minerals boron and magnesium also seem to be potentially important dietary components.

Counting on More Than Calcium

In the early nineteen-eighties, calcium was hyped as something of a cure for osteoporosis. Scientists never meant that people should think that calcium was the only dietary ingredient involved in keeping bones strong. Before reviewing your calcium needs, look at some of the other nutrients that affect bone health.

Sunshine and Vitamin D

Studies show that without vitamin D, the sunshine vitamin, bones will not harden. As you grow older, however, it's more difficult for the skin to manufacture vitamin D from sunlight. In studies at the Human Nutrition Research Center on Aging at Tufts University in Boston, researchers noticed that bone mass decreased during the winter months in women who were not getting at least 500 I.U. of Vitamin D a day.

Unfortunately, it's difficult to get an extra 400 I.U. of vitamin D from foods. You would have to drink about a quart of fortified milk (eight ounces of milk contains 100 I.U. of vitamin D) or eat a generous serving of salmon or other fatty fish to meet daily demand. Of course, some multivitamin supplements can cover your vitamin D needs. Be careful about single dose supplements of the nutrient. Strange as it may seem, the right dose of this vitamin can keep bones strong, but too much vitamin D does just the opposite, actually weakening bones so that they end up breaking more easily.

Boron—Ten years ago this trace mineral was not even mentioned in the same breath with osteoporosis. Two different studies conducted on people find that diets low in boron can interfere with the absorption of calcium. In one promising new report, scientists find that postmenopausal women who boost their dietary boron intake to three grams a day (by eating more fruits, legumes, and nuts) can help prevent calcium loss. Notable sources of boron include apples, pears, peaches, grapes, raisins, legumes, and nuts.

Magnesium—Numerous biochemical reactions in the body are regulated by magnesium, so it really isn't surprising that magnesium is involved in the bone-remodeling process. In a recent scientific report, researchers speculate that if your diet is both low in magnesium and low in boron, that lack could significantly damage bones. Whole grains are an excellent source of magnesium. More than 80 percent of magnesium is lost when processing peels the outer layer and germ from any whole grain, so opt for bread products made with whole grains rather than refined flours. Notable sources of magnesium include the following foods:

Food	Milligrams magnesium
Spinach, 1 cup cooked	158
Broccoli, 1 cup cooked	94
Kale, 1 cup cooked	94
Almonds, 1 oz	86
Cashews, 1 oz	74
Oatmeal, 1 cup cooked	40
Sunflower seeds, 1 oz	37
Whole wheat bread, 1 slice	23

Calcium—Although the RDA for calcium is 800 milligrams for women and men over the age of twenty-five, a 1984 NIH Consensus Conference encouraged premenopausal women to aim for 1,000 milligrams of calcium per day. Women past the age of fifty were told to aim for a daily calcium dose of 1,500 milligrams. Low-fat dairy products are your best source of calcium. However, keep in mind that some seafoods and leafy green vegetables also contain appreciable amounts of the mineral. One caveat: Steer clear of spinach. Compounds called oxalates bind the calcium in spinach so that it's not available to the body.

Food	Milligrams Calcium
Low-fat yogurt, 8 oz	415
Skim milk, 1 cup	302
Swiss cheese, 1 oz	272
Sardines with bones, 2 oz	230
Kale, 1 cup cooked	180
Broccoli, 1 cup cooked	178
Bok choy, 1 cup cooked	158
Salmon, canned with bones, 2 oz	136
Tofu, ½ cup	130
American cheese, 1 oz	124
Mustard greens, 1 cup cooked	104
Frozen yogurt, ½ cup	100
Clams, 3 oz cooked	78
Ice milk, ½ cup	78
Oysters, 3 oz cooked	76

Picking a Calcium Supplement

Food is preferable to supplements because foods contain other nutrients—magnesium, phosphorous, vitamin D—that are useful in building and maintaining bone. In addition, the calcium in many foods is more available than the calcium in some supplements. But if you do find it necessary to use supplements, take time to make your selection carefully. Some products are formulated poorly (See Shopping Tips in the section on supplements, page 186.)

You can tell if the calcium in a supplement is available to the body by dropping the tablet in a few ounces of plain vinegar. Stir occasionally over the next thirty minutes. A well-formulated supplement will break up or start to disintegrate in the vinegar just as easily as it would in the acidic environment of the stomach. (It doesn't need to dissolve totally.)

Be aware too that calcium supplements come in several different chemical forms. Calcium lactate, calcium gluconate, and calcium citrate (the form of calcium once used to fortify orange juice) are organic salts. Speculation is that these organic salts are much easier to absorb, particularly for older people, than inorganic salts like calcium carbonate and calcium phosphate. Another thing to keep in mind is that each calcium salt—inorganic or organic—can have a different amount of calcium. Calcium carbonate is about 40 percent calcium; calcium gluconate contains less than 10 percent calcium. That means you will need to take many more calcium gluconate tablets to reach a level of 1,000 milligrams of calcium than you would calcium carbonate tablets.

Considering Other Protective Measures

When it comes to lifestyle, smoking and large amounts of caffeine or alcohol can weaken bone. (See the chapter on Caffeine and Alcohol for more about the health risks of these two drugs, page 40.) Exercise and estrogen replacement therapy can also play a vital role in helping to minimize bone loss.

Alcohol and Caffeine—Although one new study of premenopausal women suggests that moderate amounts of alcohol may actually help to protect bone, most experts feel that curbing intake of this drug, or at least taking in only small amounts, is probably a wise preventive strategy. This is also true of caffeine. (For more detailed information on the health risks of coffee turn to the section on caffeine, page 40.)

Note: There were too few participants in this study who drank only decaffeinated coffee (throughout their life) for researchers to draw any conclusions about decaf's impact on bone density. It's entirely possible that some ingredient in coffee other than caffeine could be associated with bone loss. But current research seems to point to caffeine as the culprit.

Estrogen Replacement Therapy—About one in three women have extensive enough bone loss that they require supplemental estrogen. Several studies show replacement estrogen can cut the risk of hip fracture dramatically for women, as well as lowering the risk for ischemic heart disease. Some controversy surrounds estrogen replacement as preliminary reports link ERT with a higher risk for certain types of cancer. Due to the controversy, it's definitely a good idea to discuss the benefits of ERT against the risks with your physician. (See the chapter on Menopause to learn more about the health risks posed by dropping estrogen levels, page 138.)

Exercise—Exercise stimulates the formation of new bone. Studies of tennis players show that they have about one-third more cortical bone in their dominant arm than in the nondominant one. Impact exercises that generate load on the bones and weight-lifting exercises that strengthen muscles are best for maintaining bone health. On that list are brisk walking, tennis, square dancing, cycling, and weight lifting. The Osteoporosis Foundation emphasizes that exercise must be done at least three times per week for at least thirty minutes to have any benefit.

Reference List

Barret-Connor, E. "Coffee-associated osteoporosis offset by daily milk consumption: The Rancho Bernardo Study." *Journal of the American Medical Association;* 271(4): 280–83, 1994.

Ju, H.F., et al. "Dietary calcium and bone density among middle-aged and elderly women in China." *American Journal of Clinical Nutrition;* 58: 219–27, 1993.

Wardlaw, G.M. "Putting osteoporosis in perspective." *Journal of the American Dietetic Association;* 93(9): 1000–6, 1993.

Bickle, D.D. "Alcohol-induced bone disease." *world Review of Nutrition & Diet;* 73: 53–79, 1993.

Bostick, R.M., et al. "Relation of calcium, vitamin D, and dairy food intakes to incidence of colon cancer among older women: The Iowa Women's Health Study." *American Journal of Epidemiology;* 137: 1302–17, 1993.

Morley, J.E. "Nutrition and the older female: A review." *Journal of the American College of Nutrition;* 12: 337–43, 1993.

Gavaler, J.S. "Alcohol and nutrition in postmenopausal women." *Journal of the American College of Nutrition;* 12: 349–56, 1993.

Massey L.K. and Whiting S.J. "Caffeine, urinary calcium, calcium metabolism and bone." *Journal of Nutrition;* 123(9): 1611–4, 1993.

Duazo, F. and Khachadurian, A.K. "Prevention and treatment of osteoporosis in the elderly." *Topics in Clinical Nutrition;* 8: 9–15, 1993.

Beattie, J.H. "The metabolic fate of (3H) estradiol in relation to dietary intake of boron in ovariectomized rats." *Journal of Steroid Biochemistry & Molecular Biology;* 45(6): 549–54, 1993.

Anderson, J.J.B. and Metz, J.A. "Contributions of dietary calcium and physical activity to primary prevention of osteoporosis in females." *Journal of the American College of Nutrition;* 12: 378–83, 1993.

Lloyd, T., et al. "Urinary hormonal concentrations and spinal bone densities of premenopausal vegetarian and nonvegetarian women." *American Journal of Clinical Nutrition;* 54(6): 1005–10, 1991.

Nielsen, F.H. "Studies on the relationship between boron and magnesium which possibly affects the formation and maintenance of bones." *Magnesium & Trace Elements;* 9(2): 61–9, 1990.

Nelson, M.E., et al. "A one-year walking program and increased dietary calcium in postmenopausal women: effects on bone." *Medicine and Science in Sports & Exercise;* S: 377, 1990.

Nielsen, F.H. "New essential trace elements for the life sciences." *Biological Trace Element Resources;* 26/27: 599–611, 1990.

Nelson, M.E., et al. "Hormone and bone mineral status in endurance trained and sedentary postmenopausal women." *Journal of Clinical Endocrinology and Metabolism;* 66: 927–33, 1988.

Saltman, P.D. and Strause, L.G. "The role of trace minerals in osteoporosis." *Journal of the American College of Nutrition;* 12: 384–89, 1993.

Dawson-Hughes, B., et al. "Dietary calcium intake and bone loss form the spine in healthy postmenopausal women." *American Journal of Clinical Nutrition;* 46: 68–87, 1987.

PREGNANCY AND BREASTFEEDING

While the term "eating for two" is a bit of an exaggeration, nutrient and calorie needs do increase considerably during pregnancy and while a new mother is breastfeeding. Particularly important are nutrients like protein, calcium, iron, and B vitamins, nutrients growing babies need in plentiful supply. If you are pregnant, rather than focus on a few particular nutrients, you'll want to follow the general guidelines for good eating set by the Department of Agriculture's Food Guide Pyramid (see page 7). That means a diet based on fruits, vegetables, whole grains, lean meats, and low-fat dairy foods.

While there are not many new studies looking at diet during pregnancy, a recent government report has created new guidelines about appropriate weight gain and nutrient supplementation during pregnancy that spell a major shift in the thinking bout these two subjects. (The guidelines will be presented later in this section.) Perhaps the real cutting-edge scientific news for women who are pregnant is the impact of diet during the preconception phase. Numerous studies suggest that the amount of folic-acid rich foods you eat before you even become pregnant can have a huge impact on the health of your baby. Speculation is that the overall quality of the diet prior to pregnancy may be just as important, if not more so, than what you eat during pregnancy.

Preconception Diet Planning

It's well known that a poor diet (malnutrition) during pregnancy can hinder a child's capacity to learn and have a negative impact on a newborn's behavior. Yet little research has been done to learn about how diet influences health prior to pregnancy and in the first few weeks of a pregnancy, when many women aren't even aware of their condition. There are a few preliminary findings.

For instance, one recent study finds that a heavy alcohol intake prior to conception can result in a lower-birth-weight baby. (Lower-birth-weight babies can be plagued with learning and growth problems.) Numerous reports link a diet low in folacin to increased risk for neural tube birth defects such as spina bifida.

Foods High in Folic Acid

Food	Milligrams of Folic Acid
Spinach, 1 cup cooked	262
Asparagus, 1 cup cooked	176
Lima beans, 1 cup	156
Broccoli, 1 cup cooked	108
Wheat germ, ¼ cup	106
Beets, 1 cup cooked	90
Cauliflower, 1 cup cooked	64
Orange, navel, 1 medium	47
Cantaloupe, ½ melon	46
Cabbage, 1 cup raw	40
Tofu, firm, ½ cup	37

All the Right Foods

While pregnant women need to eat the same kind of foods that the rest of us do, they do need a little bit more of certain nutrients.

Protein—Although protein needs jump from forty-six to fifty grams prior to pregnancy to sixty grams (during pregnancy) and sixty-five grams (while breastfeeding), most women already eat these higher levels of protein. (Americans tend to eat double the RDA for protein.) However, the difference, which amounts to about ten to fifteen grams for most women is easily met by adding an extra one and a half ounces of lean meat or twelve ounces of milk each day.

Calcium—Calcium needs jump an extra 400 milligrams during pregnancy and lactation. An extra glass of low-fat milk (which provides about 300 milligrams of calcium) almost meets this extra demand. See the chapter on Osteoporosis (beginning on page 145) for a list of calcium-rich dairy foods and calcium-rich vegetables.

Vitamin A—Vitamin A is required for growth and normal development of the fetus. Studies suggest that the nutrient is also critical to the healthy immune system (see the chapter on Immunity, page 100). However, your requirements for this fat-soluble vitamin don't change during pregnancy. They do increase from 800 micrograms (retinol equivalents) to 1,300 while you are breastfeeding. Fortified milk and eggs are good sources of vitamin A. In addition, the beta-carotene found in plants (bright orange fruits and vegetables such as carrots and cantaloupe; dark leafy greens such as broccoli and spinach) can be converted by the body to vitamin A.

Vitamin C—Important to wound healing and healthy immune function, vitamin C requirements increase slightly during pregnancy; needs are even higher during lactation. These increases are easily met with vitamin-C-rich foods such as citrus fruit, strawberries, broccoli, and potatoes.

B Vitamins—Your need for these B vitamins—thiamin, riboflavin, niacin, and vitamins B and B_{12}—is slightly higher during pregnancy and lactation. Rather than focus on each of these vitamins, which are widely available in foods, you can meet the increased demands by boosting your intake of fruits, vegetables, and whole grains. Fortified breads and cereals often contain several of these B vitamins.

Vitamin E—Important for normal neurological development, vitamin E requirements increase only slightly during pregnancy. A fat-soluble vitamin found in vegetable oils, whole grains, nuts, and dark, leafy green vegetables, vitamin E appears important to the healthy immune system. (See the chapter on Immunity, page 100.)

Vitamin D—Since vitamin D is needed for skeletal growth (strong bones), it's no surprise that requirements for this nutrient are higher during pregnancy and lactation. If your skin is regularly exposed to small amounts of sunlight, the body can manufacture enough vitamin D to meet these needs. Vitamin D can also be obtained from fortified milk and dairy products; make sure to choose the low or reduced fat variety.

Zinc—Critical for immune function, zinc is important during pregnancy and lactation. Your requirements will increase from twelve milligrams per day to fifteen milligrams per day during pregnancy. Requirements increase to nineteen milligrams during lactation. If you are eating lean meats and poultry, seafood, eggs, milk, and whole grains (see the chapter on Immunity, page 100 for a complete list of zinc-rich foods), it should be easy to meet these increased needs.

Iron—Your need for iron doubles during pregnancy (from fifteen milligrams per day to thirty milligrams). Some doctors prescribe iron supplements to help meet these requirements but you can boost your intake with iron-rich foods. Iron from meat is more readily absorbed than iron from vegetables (see the section on Anemia, page 31 and the section on Immunity, page 100 for tips on which foods are rich in iron and how to improve iron absorption).

Phosphorous—The mineral phosphorous is another nutrient critical for normal skeletal formation. It works in tandem with calcium and other nutrients such as magnesium to create strong bones, which is why needs increase during pregnancy and lactation. Good sources of phosphorous include dairy products, lean meats and poultry, fish, and whole grains.

Magnesium—Critical to strong bones, magnesium is also needed for normal muscle function and nerve transmission. Your needs will increase only slightly during pregnancy and lactation. The extra requirements are easily met though low-fat milk, meat, legumes, green vegetables, and whole grains.

The Matter of Weight Gain

Women who gain generous amounts of weight over the course of their pregnancy seem more likely to deliver healthier babies. One recent study links higher levels of weight gain in mothers to lower rates of both infant mortality and low birth weight. (Average weight gain for pregnant women in the study was twenty-three-and-one-half pounds; babies weighed in at about seven-and-one-quarter pounds.) The American College of Obstetricians and Gynecologists now recommends a weight gain range of somewhere between twenty-two and twenty-seven pounds.

Weight gains of as much as thirty-five pounds don't seem out of line, say experts. In a recent National Center for Health Statistics report reviewing 10,000 live births, moms who gained this much weight were still able to deliver healthy babies. In fact, generous weight gain seems most important for first-time mothers (particularly teenagers), underweight women, and women under the age of thirty. Weight gains of over thirty-five pounds, however, seemed to be slightly more risky.

The usual pattern of weight gain during pregnancy is a three-to-four pound gain in the first trimester. In the months that follow, women typically gain three pounds per month. Caloriewise, that amounts to an extra 150 calories (about six ounces of low-fat yogurt or one small whole-wheat bagel) a day during the first trimester. Later, 350 calories, or a little over double that amount, is sufficient.

Battling Morning Sickness

A large majority of women find that they can survive the nausea and vomiting brought on by morning sickness in the early days of pregnancy with a few simple strategies. Experts at the American Dietetic Association offer the following ideas.

- Switch to smaller, more frequent meals. It can help limit both nausea and heartburn (see the section on Digestive Health, page 70, for more about how to relieve heartburn).
- Avoid fluids at meal time; drink fluids in between meals instead.
- Choose bland instead of spicy foods.

- Enjoy more fruits and complex carbohydrates such as pasta, potatoes, and crackers. Queasy stomachs find them easy to tolerate.
- Take prenatal vitamin/mineral supplements later in the day rather than in the morning.
- Get out of bed slowly in the morning. Keep some plain crackers or dry cereal on your bedside table to quiet nausea.

If these strategies don't seem to help, talk with your doctor about how to deal with your individual symptoms. A recent report hints that some women suffer with more severe morning sickness and may need nontraditional treatments devised by their doctor or dietitian.

Should You Take Prenatal Supplements?

A comprehensive report issued recently by the National Academy of Sciences offers some specific guidelines about the use of nutritional supplements during pregnancy. You should be aware that the new recommendations discourage routine across-the-board supplementation without first assessing the diet of a pregnant woman, except in the case of iron and sometimes folic acid.

Iron Supplements—Since it is very difficult to meet increased iron demands through diet alone, the new guidelines suggest that most pregnant women would benefit from a daily supplement of ferous iron during both the second and third trimesters. You can reach this level of ferrous iron with either 150 milligrams of ferrous sulfate, 300 milligrams of ferrous gluconate, or 100 milligrams of ferrous fumarate. Some caveats: Take iron supplements on an empty stomach (between meals or at bedtime) to promote absorption. Don't bother with vitamin C; while the vitamin increases your absorption of iron from vegetable foods it can't improve the absorption of ferrous iron.

Folic Acid—The U.S. Public Health Service now recommends that pregnant women receive supplements of 400 micrograms (0.4 mg) of folic acid each day to prevent birth defects. It's possible, however, to boost your folic acid intake to these levels with diet alone.

Multivitamin/Mineral Supplements—If you are eating a well-balanced diet a MVI supplement is not necessary. But if you eat haphazardly or fall into the high-risk pregnancy category, doctors may prescribe a MVI. The National Academy of Sciences recommends that it contain the following nutrients:

Iron	30 milligrams	Vitamin B_6	2 milligrams
Zinc	15 milligrams	Folate	300 micrograms
Copper	2 milligrams	Vitamin C	50 milligrams
Calcium	250 milligrams	Vitamin D	5 micrograms

Nutritional Demands of Breastfeeding

Nutritionists find that the amount of calories and nutrients you will need during breast-feeding is directly related to the amount of milk you produce. Estimates are that it takes about one calorie to produce each cc of breast milk. To produce 500 cc (about one-half quart) of breast milk you will need 500 calories of energy. If you produce only 300 cc of breast milk, you will need only 300 extra calories. Fat stores built up during pregnancy can contribute to that increased energy demand.

As for the increased nutrient demands, keep in mind that you will essentially need additional amounts of the same nutrients that you needed during pregnancy. The exception is calcium. The need for this mineral increases to 400–500 milligrams, making it extremely important that low-fat dairy products are a regular part of the diet. One glass of skim milk contains about 300 milligrams of calcium. (For a list of foods high in calcium refer to the chapter on Osteoporosis, page 145.) Rather than focus on any other nutrients, breastfeeding moms need to think in terms of choosing extra calories wisely. Stock up on nutrient-dense selections, foods that carry a wide variety of nutrients (fruits, low-fat yogurt, whole grains) rather than empty-calorie junk foods.

Reference List

Block, G. and Abrams, B. "Vitamin and mineral status of women of childbearing potential." *Annals of the New York Academy of Sciences;* 678: 244–54, 1993.

Committee on Genetics: American Academy of Pediatrics. "Folic acid for the prevention of neural tube defects." Pediatrics; 92(3): 493–94, 1993.

The Centers for Disease Control and Prevention. "Recommendations for use of folic acid to reduce number of spina bifida cases and other neural tube defects." *Journal of the American Medical Association;* 269(10): 1233–38, 1993.

Willet, W.C. "Folic acid and neural tube defect: Can't we come to closure?" *American Journal of Public Health;* 82: 666–68, 1992.

MRC Vitamin Research Study Group. "Prevention of neural tube defects: Results of the Medical Research Council Vitamin Study." *Lancet;* 338: 131–37, 1991.

Butte, N.F., et al. "Effect of maternal diet and body composition on lactational performance." *American Journal of Clinical Nutrition;* 39: 296–306, 1984.

American Medical Association. "Fetal effects of maternal alcohol use." *Journal of the American Medical Association;* 249(18): 2517–21, 1983.

Hackman, E., et al. "Maternal birth weight and subsequent pregnancy outcome." *Journal of the American Medical Association;* 250(15): 2016–19, 1983.

Linn, S., et al. "No association between coffee consumption and adverse outcomes of pregnancy." *The New England Journal of Medicine;* 306: 141–45, 1982.

Committee on Nutrition, American Academy of Pediatrics: "Nutrition and lactation." *Pediatrics;* 68: 435–43, 1981.

Lecos, C. "Caution light on caffeine." *FDA Consumer;* October, 1980.

PREMENSTRUAL SYNDROME

On the one hand, it almost seems too soon to talk about successful treatments for premenstrual syndrome (PMS) when scientists still can't agree on how to define this disorder. Yet, if you suffer with any of the symptoms of PMS—irritability, breast tenderness, bloating, headache, change in appetite, fatigue, mood swings (alternating between sadness and anger), oversensitivity (episodes of crying), social withdrawal, depression—chances are you would try just about anything to get relief, particularly if your symptoms are severe.

Currently, experts define PMS as a disorder with both psychological and biological components. However, PMS, which was first identified in 1931, isn't an illness that's been subject to rigorous scientific scrutiny. It's suspected that the disorder is somehow tied to the cyclic hormonal changes (estrogen and progesterone) all premenstrual women experience as symptoms tend to recur during the same phase of the menstrual cycle. How these hormonal fluctuations impact on other body systems, particularly neurotransmitters like serotonin, could, in part, help explain PMS.

New evidence suggests that satisfying menstrual food cravings with carbohydrate-rich snacks might help alleviate symptoms. Other reports single out caffeine, various supplements, and vitamin E for the dietary role they play in influencing PMS.

Finding Effective Treatments

Since so little is known about what causes PMS and the more than 150 symptoms that plague sufferers are common ones which mimic other health problems, most experts favor a conservative line of dietary treatment. For instance, you might want to try cutting back on salt during the luteal phase (five days prior to menses when most women begin to experience PMS symptoms) of your cycle, if bloating is one of your symptoms. Cutting back on nutrient-poor foods such as sweets and alcohol could also be beneficial.

In fact, many experts encourage women who suffer with PMS to focus on building a diet that is nutrient-dense. It's entirely possible that PMS symptoms are exacerbated by haphazard styles of eating and marginal nutritional deficiencies rather than any one specific food. Still, even though it's still too soon to offer any real remedies, there are a few promising strategies worth considering.

Unproven But Promising

Symptoms and the degree of severity of PMS is dramatically different from one woman to the next. That's why it makes sense that some dietary strategies may help one woman and not another. Some of the following treatments have met with some success in preliminary studies. But much more research is needed.

Caffeine—Considering that individual response to caffeine varies widely, it's no surprise that studies attempting to link caffeine to PMS have had mixed results. A new report from Oregon State University bears out this concept. Researchers noticed that some female college students could drink caffeine-containing beverages (coffee, tea, cola) without suffering PMS. With others, as little as one caffeine-containing beverage per day seemed to make them more susceptible. Interestingly, the connection appears dose-related. As caffeine intake increased, PMS symptoms among students worsened. If you suffer from PMS, there is no harm in trying to forego caffeine for a few months to see if this stimulant has any impact on your symptoms.

Sources of Caffeine—Over-the-counter cold remedies, pain relievers, stimulants, and weight-control aids can contain caffeine. For most people, beverages are the biggest source of the stimulant. Brewing time varies the caffeine content of hot beverages like coffee and tea.

Food	*Milligrams Caffeine*
Coffee, 5-oz cup	
Brewed by drip method	110–150
Brewed w/percolator	64–124
Instant	40–108
Decaffeinated	1–5
Tea, 5-oz cup	
Brewed, domestic	20–90
Brewed, imported	25–110
Instant	25–50
Soft drinks, 12-oz can	
Cola	30–46
Mountain Dew	52
Cocoa, 5 oz	2–20
Milk chocolate, 1 oz	1–15
Dark chocolate, 1 oz	5–35

Source: The Food and Drug Administration.

Vitamin E—Preliminary reports from a recent controlled diet study find that 300 to 600 I.U. of vitamin E per day helped improve symptoms for PMS sufferers. The problem with this finding is that the amounts of vitamin E used for treatment are 30 times that which is recommended. (The RDA for vitamin E is ten I.U.) While many studies show these levels are probably safe, the practice is something you will want to talk over with your physician. Unfortunately, it would be difficult to obtain these quantities of vitamin E from diet alone. Food sources of vitamin E include: wheat germ, spinach, kale, collard greens, nuts and seeds, whole grains, fortified cereals, and vegetable oils.

The Pyridoxine Dilemma

Not so long ago, the popular press reported successful treatment of PMS with supplements of vitamin B_6 (pyridoxine). Some physicians even recommended supplements of the vitamin to their patients. Unfortunately, daily doses of two to three grams of pyridoxine (the amount commonly recommended) can be neurotoxic. Medical reports document neurological difficulties (numbness in the hands and feet). Concern is that this nerve damage could be irreversible. If you want to try vitamin B therapy concentrate on foods rich in this nutrient.

Vitamin B_6 (Pyridoxine)-Rich Foods—Meats, dried beans, grains, fruits, and vegetables all contain some vitamin B_6. But vegetables deliver the largest amount of the nutrient at the lowest calorie cost.

Food	Milligrams Vitamin B6
Banana, 1 medium	.70
Potato, w/skin	.70
Breast of chicken, baked, 3.5 oz	.58
Pork tenderloin, lean, 3.5 oz cooked	.53
Potato, w/o skin	.50
Sirloin steak, 3.5 oz cooked	.50
Tomato paste, ½ cup	.50
Spinach, 1 cup cooked	.40
Green peas, 1 cup cooked	.34
Ground turkey, 3 oz cooked	.33
Canned tuna, water pack 3 oz	.32
Miso, ½ cup	.30
Navy beans, 1 cup cooked	.30
Green or red (bell) pepper, 1 large	.24

| Sweet potato, ½ cup mashed | .24 |
| Watermelon, 1 cup | .23 |

Carbohydrates, Cravings, and Serotonin

Food cravings aren't unusual. But when they are for carbohydrate-rich foods, the craving could be your body's way of relieving PMS symptoms. At least that is the speculation of a small group of researchers. Recently, an intriguing new study found that women with PMS who ate a carbohydrate-rich (protein-poor) evening test meal during the late luteal phase of their menstrual cycle noticed an improvement in their symptoms. Researchers propose that the improved mood and lessening symptoms may be tied to an increase in the production of *serotonin*, a brain neurotransmitter that has a calming effect on the body.

Studies show that a meal rich in carbohydrates increases serotonin synthesis. (Meals rich in protein (meat, eggs, cheese and crackers) do not. Researchers at Massachusetts Institute of Technology suggest that high levels of serotonin in the blood also help to normalize food intake. Critics say these findings are preliminary and are more theory than fact, but this is one time you don't have to wait for further research before making a diet change. You can test the food-and-mood concept on yourself without any kind of serious nutritional repercussions. Since nutritionists already recommend complex carbohydrate foods (bagels, pasta with tomato sauce, whole-grain breads) as much healthier snacks than high-fat munchies like potato chips, french fries, and chocolate, it obviously makes sense to eat these snacks during PMS days as well as all month long.

Don't Try It, It Won't Help

In the early days of research, loose definitions of PMS and uncontrolled open trials made it difficult to draw firm conclusions about what kind of therapy could help. But scientists have been able to rule out two popular treatments for PMS that don't work and might be harmful.

- *Evening primrose oil*—Perhaps one of the most widely touted treatments for PMS, scientists find no conclusive proof that supplements of this oil effectively relieve PMS symptoms.
- *Vitamin and Mineral Supplements*—Researchers have tested everything from vitamin A to calcium to zinc in an effort to find a nutritional cure for PMS. A recent review of dietary supplement studies finds critical problems with the way these studies were conducted. More important, single dose supplements, particularly of fat-soluble nutrients

like vitamin A, could have potentially toxic effects. Rather than zero in on any one supplement, the wise strategy is a diet approach that includes a healthy amount of a wide variety of nutrient-dense foods.

Reference List

Chuong, C.J. and Dawson E.B. "Critical evaluation of nutritional factors in the pathophysiology and treatment of premenstrual syndrome." *Clinical Obstetrics & Gynecology;* 35(3):679–94, 1992.

Rapkin, M.D. "The role of serotonin in premenstrual syndrome." *Clinical Obstetrics & Gynecology;* 35(3): 629–38, 1992.

Mortola, J.F. "Issues in the diagnosis and research of premenstrual syndrome." *Clinical Obstetrics & Gynecology;* 35(3): 587–92, 1992.

Mortola, J.F. "Assessment and management of premenstrual syndrome." *Current Opinion in Obstetrics & Gynecology;* 4(6): 877–85, 1992.

Tucker, J.S., and Whalen R.E. "Premenstrual syndrome." *International Journal of Psychology in Medicine;* 21(4): 311–41, 1991.

Wurtman, J.J. "Carbohydrate craving. Relationship between carbohydrate intake and disorders of mood." *Drugs;* 39 (Suppl 3): 49–52, 1990.

Robinson, G.E. and Garfinkel, P.E. "Problems in the treatment of premenstrual syndrome." *Canadian Journal of Psychology;* 35(3): 199–206, 1990.

Machlin, L.J. "Use and safety of elevated dosages of vitamin E in adults." *International Journal of Vitamin & Nutrition Research;* 30 (Suppl): 56–68, 1989.

Parry, G.J. and Bredesen, D.E. "Sensory neuropathy with low dose pyridoxine." Neurology: 35: 1466–68, 1985.

Schaumburg, H.J., et al. "Sensory neuropathy from pyridoxine abuse: A new megavitamin syndrome." *The New England Journal of Medicine;* 309: 445–48, 1983.

SENIOR NUTRITION

Nutrient requirements change throughout life. The specific nature of these differences in the over-fifty population has been more speculation than science until recently. New findings now offer solid proof that the requirements for a handful of key dietary components from vitamin D to folic acid to calcium change with increasing age. Keeping on top of this changing nutritional agenda is important not only for maintaining good health but as a way to stave off some of the chronic ills of old age. Diet may also play a role in helping to prolong life as well.

Biological Changes, Altered Nutrient Needs

As your body ages major biological changes will become apparent. For instance, the liver, kidneys, and pancreas will begin to function a bit more sluggishly; efficiency levels drop. Body-fat levels increase as lean body mass (muscle) is replaced by fat stores. The stomach, at least in many older adults, has difficulty producing enough hydrochloric acid. All of these little changes conspire to alter nutrient requirements, sometimes profoundly, sometimes only by miniscule amounts.

Less acid in the stomach means problems with absorption for certain nutrients. Folic acid, vitamin B_{12}, calcium, and iron seem to be most affected. Older adults seem to need more of these nutrients, although just how much more is yet to be precisely determined. Conversely, biological changes can significantly lessen the need for some nutrients. In fact, some experts believe that the RDA for vitamin A might be set a little too high for seniors. Medical reports suggest that older adults absorb vitamin A more efficiently, a factor which could create a risk of a toxic build-up of this fat soluble vitamin.

Rethinking the RDAs

As scientists try to determine how these changes translate into specific dietary recommendations, it's apparent that there is a lack of consensus about how to interpret the latest research. Experts at the National Academy of Science's Food and Nutrition Board, in the latest edition of Recommended Dietary Allowances are still basing nutrient needs for older adults on studies done with young people.

Many researchers feel that the new research more than indicates that it's time to update the RDAs as they apply to older adults. At the forefront are scientists from the Department of Agriculture's Human Nutrition Research Center on Aging in Boston. These researchers find a lot of evidence that nutrient needs for the following dietary components vary with age.

Vitamin B$_6$—For some reason, vitamin B$_6$ requirements increase with age. In a study at the USDA Aging Center, scientists found that older men require a daily dose of 1.96 milligrams of this vitamin; older women need 1.90 milligrams. While the current RDA is set at 2 milligrams per day for men, it's only set at 1.6 milligrams for women. Good sources of the nutrient include chicken, fish, pork, eggs, and organ meats like liver. Also rich in B$_6$ are brown rice, soy beans, oats, whole wheat products, peanuts, and walnuts.

Calcium—Not only do requirements for calcium increase as people grow older, but the body also has trouble absorbing calcium from the diet. (See the section on Osteoporosis, page 145.) Low-fat dairy products like yogurt and skim milk are the best sources of this mineral. Also notable are deep green vegetables like kale, collard greens, and broccoli.

Vitamin D—Convincing scientific evidence indicates that your skin makes less vitamin D from sunshine as you grow older. Dairy products fortified with this vitamin—low-fat milk and margarine—are major food sources of vitamin D. One 8-ounce glass of milk contains 100 I.U. of the vitamin. Fatty fish like salmon and mackerel are even better sources.

Vitamin B$_{12}$—Although the evidence is limited, there is some indication that B$_{12}$ requirements rise in later years. Good sources include animal foods such as lean meats of any kind, fish, milk, and eggs.

Folic Acid—There are only a few studies to suggest that folic acid needs rise with age, but many researchers support this suggestion. In fact, folic acid is becoming well known for its protective role against certain types of cancer. Leafy green vegetables such as spinach, legumes (dried beans, lentils, soybeans), and citrus fruits are rich sources of this vitamin.

Beta-carotene—Compelling research suggests that beta-carotene and other antioxidants may help ward off or, at the very least, delay the onset of illnesses like heart disease, cataracts, and certain types of cancer. Speculation is that antioxidants work to neutralize damaging substances in the body called *free radicals*, substances that scientists speculate could cause or complicate some of the changes that occur with aging. (See the chapter on Longevity, beginning on page 124, to learn more about antioxidants.)

Generous amounts of this antioxidant are widely available from fruits and vegetables. The list includes most orange and yellow vegetables such as carrots, winter squash, sweet potatoes, and cantaloupe. Dark-green leafy vegetables such as broccoli and spinach are also good sources.

Vitamin E—Promising new research from the USDA Human Nutrition Research Center on Aging in Boston finds that an extra dose of vitamin E helps boost immune function in older adults. (See the chapter on Immunity, page 100.) It is too soon to make recommendations as to the amount of vitamin E that is necessary for good health, but many researchers think it's certain that the amount will probably be higher than the current recommended allowances. Good sources of the vitamin include wheat germ, nuts, and vegetable oils. Green leafy vegetables also contain small amounts of vitamin E.

Vitamin C—Studies suggest that another of the antioxidant nutrients, vitamin C, may play a role in warding off heart disease (see the chapter on Heart Health, page 85) as well as some types of cancer (see the Cancer chapter, page 47.) In addition to citrus fruits, good sources of this vitamin include broccoli, green peppers, tomatoes, potatoes, and strawberries.

In Search of Nutrient Density

Nutrient requirements aren't the only thing that can change with age. Calorie or energy requirements are also different. Fattier bodies (fat requires less energy to maintain than muscle) mean lower energy demands. Estimates are that you will end up eating about 600 fewer calories per day in your senior years than you did when you were younger. The problem is that with this 25 percent drop in calories, you can expect a drop in the quality of your diet unless you make a concentrated effort to choose foods wisely.

Nutritionists refer to wise food choices as nutrient-dense foods. That is, foods that contain large amounts of a variety of nutrients at a low or moderate calorie cost. On that list are lean meats, low-fat dairy products, whole grains, fruits, and vegetables. Unfortunately, in an effort to cut back on fat, many people shun meat and dairy foods. That eliminates some of the best sources of trace minerals like copper, zinc, and chromium, as well as calcium. Rather than avoid animal foods, the better strategy is to make leaner selections.

Drug–Nutrient Interactions

Just as important as including nutrient-dense foods in your diet in senior years is having an understanding of how medications influence diet and appetite. Drugs can often increase or decrease appetite, and can also have an indirect impact on nutritional health by interfering with your absorption of certain nutrients. The more medications you take, the more likely your diet may be shortchanged by a drug–nutrient interaction.

Even a common drug like aspirin can deplete nutrient supplies. Salicylates (including aspirin) can cause the body to lose iron. Laxatives can interfere with the absorption of fat-soluble vitamins such as vitamin A, D, and E. Some diuretics prescribed to treat high blood pressure cause the body to lose potassium. (See the chapter on High Blood Pressure for potassium-rich foods, page 94.) Medications like L-dopa, a drug used to treat Parkinson's disease, can depress appetite.

While doctors are aware of most of these potential interactions and side effects, you can take a few steps to help minimize drug–nutrient interactions.

- To improve drug absorption, experts recommend you take pills at least one hour prior to a meal or two hours after. That way food won't interfere with your body's uptake of the drug.
- However, if taking a drug on an empty stomach causes gastrointestinal distress, you might want to try a eating a carbohydrate-rich snack such as fruit, cereal, or toast with your medication.

Do Supplements Help?

When you consider how medications, the need for fewer calories, and altering nutrient requirements can all influence your nutritional health in later years, vitamin/mineral supplements might seem like a good idea. Consider, too, a recent Canadian study which found that older adults taking a multivitamin with extra amounts of beta-carotene (see the chapter on Immunity, page 100) were sick less often than their counterparts who didn't take a supplement.

Experts are reluctant to prescribe any kind of special supplement product for seniors. Much of the research on nutrient needs for older adults is still in the preliminary stages. A regular multivitamin preparation with no more than 100 to 150 percent of the RDA for any one nutrient is a better choice if you want to cover your bases and keep your diet nutrient rich. (See the chapter on Supplements for more tips on selecting an appropriate supplement, page 186.) Granted, you might need more calcium (see the chapter on Osteoporosis, page 145) to keep bones strong. As far as the other vitamins and minerals discussed, health professionals advocate focusing on food as your primary source. Instead of popping a pill, concentrate on making good food selections based on a generous nutrient profile, and spend your fewer food calories more wisely.

Reference list

Russell, R.M., et al. "Vitamin requirements of elderly people: An update." *American Journal of Clinical Nutrition;* 58: 4–14, 1993.

Ames, B.N., Shigena, M.K. and Hagen, T.M. "Oxidants, antioxidants, and the degenerative diseases of aging." *Proceedings of the National Academy of Sciences;* 90(17)L 7915–22, 1993.

Rimm, E., et al. "Vitamin E consumption and the risk of coronary heart disease in men." *The New England Journal of Medicine;* 328: 1450–59, 1993.

Stampher, M., et al. "Vitamin E consumption and the risk of coronary heart disease in women." *The New England Journal of Medicine;* 328: 1444–49, 1993.

Meyandi, S.N. and Blumberg, J.B. "Vitamin E and the immune response" in: *Nutrient modulation of the immune response:* S. Cunningham Rundles (ed). New York: Marcel Dekker, Inc, 1993, 223–38.

Chandra, R.K. "Effect of vitamin and trace-element supplementation on immune responses and infection in elderly subjects." *Lancet;* 340: 1124–27, 1992.

Nielsen, F.H. "Studies on the relationship between boron and magnesium which possibly affects the formation and maintenance of bones." *Magnesium and Trace Element Research;* 9(2): 61–9, 1990.

Chandra, D.B., et al. "Vitamin C in the human aqueous humor and cataracts." *International Journal of Vitamin and Nutrition Research;* 56: 165–68, 1986.

Jacques, P.F., et al. "Nutritional status in persons with and without senile cataract." *Archives of Ophthalmology;* 106: 337–40, 1988.

Jacques, P.F., et al. "Epidemiological evidence of a role for the antioxidant vitamins and carotenoids in cataract prevention." *American Journal of Clinical Nutrition;* 53: S352–55, 1991.

Cadet, J.L. "The potential use of vitamin E and selenium in Parkinsonism." *Medical Hypothesis;* 20: 87–94, 1986.

Fahn S. "The endogenous toxin hypothesis of the etiology of Parkinson's disease and a pilot trial of high-dosage antioxidants in an attempt to slow the progression of the illness." *Annals of New York Academy of Sciences;* 70: 186–96, 1989.

Burr, M.E., et al. "Vitamin C and cholesterol in the elderly." *Human Nutrition in Clinical Nutrition;* 39C: 387–88, 1985.

Peterson, V.E., et al. "Quantification of plasma cholesterol and triglyceride levels in hypercholesterolemic subjects receiving ascorbic acid supplements." *American Journal of Clinical Nutrition;* 584–87, 1975.

Dallal, G.E., et al. "Ascorbic acid, HDL cholesterol and apolipoprotein A-1 in an elderly Chinese population in Boston." *Journal of the American College of Nutrition;* 8(1): 69–74, 1989.

Jacques, P.F., et al. "Ascorbic acid, HDL, and total plasma cholesterol in the elderly." *Journal of the American College of Nutrition;* 6: 169–74, 1987.

Gaziano, J.M., et al. "Beta-carotene therapy for chronic stable angina." *Supplement to Circulation;* 82 (4): III–201, 1990.

Manson, J.E., et al. "A prospective study of antioxidant vitamins and incidence of coronary heart disease in women." *Supplement to Circulation;* 84 (4): II–546, 1991.

Meyandi, S.N., et al. "Vitamin E supplementation enhances cell-mediated immunity in healthy elderly subjects." *American Journal of Clinical Nutrition;* 52 (3): 557–63, 1990.

SHOPPING FOR GOOD HEALTH

With more than 25,000 different items in the average supermarket, it is difficult to isolate the healthful selections without being fooled by advertising hype. Assuming your plan is to cook more nutritious meals, the first place to start is to stock up on all the right staples and ingredients. It helps to become proficient at reading labels (See the chapter Labels on Food, page 118.) Even if you don't have time to agonize over each and every nutrition information panel, there are some shopping shortcuts.

First, zero in on the fat information. (New food labels list the calories from fat and grams of fat in a prominent place at the top of nutrition information panels. Fat percentages are located in the Daily Values section of the nutrient panel.) Besides having more than twice the calories of carbohydrates and protein, excess amounts of fat can be unhealthy for the body. Keep in mind that no more than 30 percent of total calories should come from fat over the course of a day. For example, if you are eating 1,800 calories per day, that amounts to no more than sixty grams of fat per day.

At the same time, you'll want to spend shopping dollars so that you end up with as many nutrients as possible. Concentrate on filing your grocery cart with nutrient-dense foods such as fresh fruits, vegetables, lean meats, and whole grains. Not only do these foods offer high-quality fuel to the body, but that fuel comes packaged with a number of important vitamins and minerals. All it takes is a quick scan of the nutrition panel to see if nutrients are in generous supply.

However, if even that sounds complicated, keep in mind that shopping with an eye toward a variety of minimally processed foods is probably the easiest way to keep the nutritional quality of your diet high. Purchasing a variety of foods is also the best way to make up for any nutrients that might be missing.

Stockpiling Missing Nutrients

Recent government surveys find that many Americans fall short of meeting requirements for four important nutrients: folic acid, magnesium, vitamin B_6, and zinc. If you are a woman, chances are you're not getting enough calcium or iron either. To remedy that shortfall, keep this shopping list in mind when you're packing items into your grocery cart.

Folic acid—Leafy green vegetables such as spinach, and asparagus, green peas, legumes, sunflower seeds, and wheat germ.

Magnesium—Nuts and seeds, peanut butter, legumes, fish, shrimp, oysters, spinach, potatoes, wheat germ, whole grains.

Vitamin B$_6$—Fish, lean red meat, poultry, soybeans, bananas, potatoes, wheat germ, whole grains.

Zinc—Oysters, lean red meat, poultry, clams, low-fat yogurt, sesame seeds, pecans, wheat germ.

Calcium—Skim or low-fat milk, low-fat yogurt, low-fat cheeses, canned salmon with bones, tofu.

Iron—Lean red meats, poultry, fish, shellfish, dried beans, enriched breads and cereals.

Stocking the Low-Fat Pantry

As you conquer the concept of nutrient density, keep in mind that fat continues to be an important shopping issue. In fact, having a pantry and refrigerator stocked with low-fat staples is a good foundation for any healthful diet. If you start with nutritious basics in the cupboard, then all you'll need is a quick trip to the supermarket or farmer's market once a week for fresh seasonal vegetables, fresh fish, poultry, and meats. Build your healthy pantry with these versatile ingredients.

Dried Goods

Grains: Pasta and noodles (spinach fettuccini, spaghetti), brown rice, dried beans (navy, pinto, kidney), split peas, barley, lentils, oats, flour, unprocessed bran.

Condiments: Vinegars (balsamic, red wine, rice, cider), Sherry, wine, defatted chicken stock, oil (olive, corn), mustard (Dijon, grainy), canned tomatoes, tomato paste.

Herbs and Spices: Basil, bay leaves, dill, garlic, ginger, oregano, onions, soy sauce (low sodium), chili powder, curry powder, cloves, cinnamon, nutmeg.

Perishables

In the Refrigerator: Low-fat yogurt, low-fat cottage cheese, low-fat sour cream, skim milk, fresh lemons, fresh limes.

In the Freezer: Frozen apple juice concentrate, frozen vegetables (corn, peas, broccoli, spinach, winter squash), ice milk or low-fat frozen yogurt.

Filling the Cart with Less Fat

If you could only make one change in your diet, health experts unanimously agree that cutting back on fat is the most important health strategy. A well-stocked low-fat pantry is only the beginning. It's easy to gradually cut back on fat by shopping for the leanest foods in each supermarket aisle. For instance, you can concentrate first on foods that are naturally low in fat: fresh fruits, vegetables, pasta, and whole grains.

Next, look for reduced-fat versions of everyday and favorite foods. For example, if mayonnaise is on your shopping list pick up the low-fat variety. It carries only five grams of fat per tablespoon (regular has eleven grams). That means you can save about fifty-four fat calories each time you make a sandwich. Savings grow even more rapidly when you start substituting the reduced fat dressing in a batch of potato, tuna, or chicken salad.

Every time you let reduced-fat products (skim milk, low-fat cheese, fat-free sour cream, low-fat snack crackers) stand in for the full-fat variety you trim another bit of fat from your diet. Before you know it, all these little changes add up to a big difference in total fat levels. Make it your goal to find acceptable low-fat substitutes for as many of your favorite everyday foods as possible. Then, when you feel the urge to snack, the cupboards will be lined with tasty, good-for-you munchies like pretzels, popcorn, and fig bars. Or when you need to throw together a quick meal, all the right ingredients will be on hand.

Of course, shopping for low-fat cuisine involves personal preference. In their zeal to produce a myriad of fat-free and reduced-fat products, some manufacturers are coming up with foods that are not so wonderful when it comes to flavor. You'll have to do some sampling to determine what reduced-fat foods are acceptable to you. You might decide that fat-free cream cheese is excellent when it comes to making a low-fat cheesecake, but that it just doesn't cut it as a spread for bagels and sandwiches. The point is to make the substitutions that are acceptable. (High-fat foods that have no acceptable substitutes can be eaten on occasion, as long as you balance them with lower-fat fare.)

Gradual Changes Aisle by Aisle

Faced with thousands of food choices, the task of searching out low-fat items may seem overwhelming at times. Don't worry about the fresh produce aisle. With the exception of avocados and coconut, everything else is pretty much low in fat and nutrient-dense. To get through the other supermarket aisles, it helps to break down choices category by category until the concept of healthful selections is easier to master.

Breads and Cereals

Breads—Rye bread, bagels, and English muffins have similar nutrient profiles. In fact, most bread products differ only when it comes to fiber; products made with whole grains are richer sources of fiber. Still, do pay attention to fat.

Buying Strategy: Consider one or two grams of fat per serving acceptable. Limit breads that contain larger amounts of fat: biscuits, croissants, Danish pastry, doughnuts, scones.

Cereals—With the exception of granolas, most cereals are low in fat. Fiber content, however, varies widely. So, too, does sugar content.

Buying strategy: Consider one or two grams of fat per serving acceptable. Aim for cereals that are high in fiber (at least three to five grams per serving) and not too sugary (less than six grams of sugar per serving.)

Desserts, Snacks, and Cookies

Snack Crackers—Fat content of chips and snack crackers ranges across the board from fat-free to buttery rich. Fatty crackers are easy to spot when you let them sit on a napkin or in a brown paper bag—they leave big grease marks.

Buying Strategy: Aim for crackers that offer less than two grams of fat per serving (usually one ounce, or three or four crackers). Pretzels, air-popped popcorn, soda crackers, and rice cakes all fit into the low-fat category. Fat-free tortilla chips and salsa are a nice lean indulgence.

Cookies—Cookies are another item with widely varying fat levels. It all depends on the recipe. Some recipes are naturally low in fat, like gingersnaps, fig bars, vanilla wafers, animal crackers.

Buying Strategy: Look for cookies with only one or two grams of fat per serving.

Cakes, Pies, Desserts—Most desserts contain generous amounts of fat. There are some items that are naturally low in fat such as angel food cake (top it with fresh fruit). Plus, there is a plethora of reduced-fat selections. Keep in mind that the while these new treats are low in fat, they often contain large amounts of sugar and are definitely not calorie-free.

Buying Strategy: Purchases in this category will most likely be an occasional indulgence so there is no set limit. You'll need to figure out how big a dent you want to make in your daily fat budget and then choose items accordingly. For instance, a slice of lemon meringue pie (five grams of fat) is a leaner choice than a slice of pecan pie (thirteen grams of fat). Check the food charts at the back of the book and read food labels to help budget your selections. Look for and try reduced fat products that carry only a few grams of fat per serving; keep an eye on calories per serving too.

The Dairy Case

Butter—High in saturated fat, butter is not a good everyday spread for toast and vegetables. However, on special occasions or in limited amounts, you can get away with eating small quantities of this dairy fat.

Buying Strategy: Purchase butter in limited amounts, preferably for special occasions. Whipped butters (whipped with air and water) and "light" stick butters have less fat than regular solid sticks. Butter/margarine blends, while not lower in fat than butter, are lower in saturated fat.

Cheese—Food companies are experimenting with the fat content of cheeses with mixed results. Some imitation and fat-free products lack flavor and texture. Others, particularly the reduced fat cheeses, are quite acceptable.

Buying Strategy: Look for hard cheeses that carry five grams of fat or less per ounce. (Many part-skim mozzarella cheeses have always fit into this category.) Buy 1 percent cottage cheese or the nonfat variety, or part-skim variety of ricotta cheese.

Margarine—Concerns about margarine (see Heart Health chapter, page 85) aside, most health professionals still recommend margarine as a substitute for butter. An endless variety of choices, however, can confuse even the smartest shopper.

Buying Strategy: Choose liquid or tub margarines over sticks since they have less saturated fat. Look for a ratio of two to one for polyunsaturated versus saturated fat. You don't really need to buy diet margarines if you're using only small amounts. Higher water content makes them difficult to bake or cook with.

Milk—While the difference between 1 percent, 2 percent and 3.5 percent (whole) milks may seem slight, it isn't. These numbers denote fat content by weight. Translated to percentages, whole milk delivers more than 50 percent of its calories as fat.

Buying Strategy: Choose skim or 1 percent milk, and buttermilk or chocolate milks made with these lower-fat milks. Remember, even children as young as two years old benefit from drinking 1 percent milk. If you and your family are currently drinking whole milk, you might want to make the switch gradually by mixing 2 percent milk with whole milk, then 2 percent milk with 1 percent milk, until you finally work your way down to skim milk. Even if you find you prefer 1 percent milk over skim, use skim milk in cooking. Ditto for yogurt. Buy the nonfat or low-fat varieties.

The Butcher Case

Beef—Beef is graded by fat content with *prime* representing the fattiest cuts and *select* representing the leanest. Unfortunately, not many supermarkets carry select meats. Butcher shops usually carry these leaner cuts, however.

Buying Strategy: Choose select grade beef over prime or choice if it is available. If your market sells only choice-grade meats, stick to the leanest cuts; eye of round, round, sirloin. Trim beef of all visible fat before cooking.

Chicken, Turkey—White meat is lower in fat than dark meat, but the biggest fat savings comes when you pull the skin off poultry. Researchers find that leaving the skin on chicken while it is cooking doesn't add to the fat content but does keep the meat moist. Just be sure to remove the skin before serving.

Buying Strategy: Buy any types of light or dark meat poultry; remove the skin before eating. (See deli section in this chapter for discussion of luncheon meats made from poultry.)

Fish—Fresh fish can vary in fat content but even the fattiest varieties (salmon, mackerel) are healthful.

Buying Strategy: Buy any type of fresh fish or shellfish; most are low in fat and low in saturated fat. Purchase tuna or other canned fish that is packed in water, not oil.

Pork—While pork is growing leaner, many cuts are still high in fat. The tenderloin, although an expensive cut, is comparable in fat to skinless white-meat chicken.

Buying Strategy: Purchase lean cuts such as tenderloin or center loin. Most ham is also very lean, although it may be high in salt.

Frozen Foods

Entrees, Dinners—A huge selection of low-fat, low-calorie frozen meals makes it easy to find healthful options in the freezer case. Be careful about sodium; some frozen foods are loaded with salt.

Buying Strategy: Look for products that emphasize their low-fat content and contain only modest amounts of sodium (less than 750 milligrams per meal, preferably less). Realize that portion size is usually small and that meals need to be rounded out by adding side dishes such as a small salad, roll, and fruit.

Desserts—Aside from fresh fruit, most packaged desserts are combinations of fat and sugar. Neither ingredient is something you should eat in large quantities, although sugar is not a major health problem except when it comes to fostering tooth decay.

Buying Strategy: Opt for ice milk, sherbet and Italian ices or sorbets. Frozen yogurts, yogurt, and frozen-fruit bars and fudge pops are also usually low in fat. Check the label to make sure.

Vegetables—Most vegetables are flash-frozen right after picking which keeps nutrient content high. Very few have salt added.

Buying Strategy: Stick to plain frozen vegetables. Limit vegetables that are breaded, fried, or covered with fatty cream or cheese sauces.

Deli and Takeout

Luncheon meats—Traditional luncheon meats like bologna, salami, and liverwurst are loaded with fat and sodium. Even when these products are made with chicken or turkey (turkey hot dogs, turkey bologna) they are still quite high in fat and sodium.

Buying Strategy: Limit your intake of fresh deli-sliced luncheon meats like bologna, salami, and pastrami. Buy lean ham or roasted turkey instead, preferably the low-salt variety. With prepackaged meats, be sure to read the label. Aim for meats that carry five grams of fat or less per ounce.

Prepared Salads—Since you can't subtract the mayonnaise from already-prepared potato, macaroni, or chicken salad, try to limit these items. Instead, buy prepared vegetables and mix low-fat dressings using reduced-fat mayo, low-fat yogurt, and spices. Or use one of the many bottled low-fat dressings that are available.

Buying Strategy: Look for salad bars where you can make a salad from scratch, prepackaged salad mixes that contain only vegetables (no dressing), and reduced-fat salad dressings.

Prepared Meats—Rotisserie cooked chickens, fried chicken, and meatloaf are just some of the selections in the hot-food-to-go section of the deli. Most of the items are high in fat even without the gravies and sauces served alongside them.

Buying Strategy: Stick to the whole chicken that is broiled or roasted. You can remove the skin at home.

Canned Foods, Convenience Mixes

Canned Soups—While most canned soups are high in sodium, many are low in fat. Chicken broth or a tomato base is a good sign that products will be low in fat.

Buying Strategy: Stay away from creamed soups (you could make them with skim milk but they are still high in fat). Make your own chicken broth or vegetable broth. Or stock up on the canned variety. You can defat the broth by putting it in the refrigerator. When chilled, fat will rise to the top and form a layer that can easily be removed. Use this defatted broth as a base for your own homemade soups, or buy low-fat soup varieties like chicken noodle, lentil, minestrone, or all-vegetable soup.

Canned Vegetables—You can lower the sodium content of canned vegetables by draining and rinsing them. You are better off buying frozen or fresh vegetables if you want to keep sodium levels low.

Buying Strategy: Most vegetables are canned with salt and water although there are a limited number of low-sodium canned products. Fat content is minimal, so you don't need to look for any special varieties.

Convenience Mixes—Macaroni and cheese, hamburger and noodles, and main-dish rice mixes often call for the addition of meat. Some call for added fat, too.

Buying Strategy: You can add lean meats like low-fat ground turkey or low-fat hamburger, or substitute chicken or water-packed tuna for beef. As for added fats like margarine or oil, try skipping them altogether or at least cutting down on the amount you use. Remember, it doesn't take that long to cook pasta from scratch and then add a low-fat tomato or spaghetti sauce for a quick low-fat meal.

Guided Supermarket Tours

We've given you the basics for healthful shopping. If you'd like a little bit of extra help, consider taking a supermarket tour with a nutrition professional. All around the country, registered dietitians are helping consumers find foods for special diets or become smarter shoppers when it comes to nutrition. Tours take shoppers through the supermarket aisle by aisle, reviewing food choices and answering questions.

For example, there will be a stop by the dairy case to discuss the merits of skim versus 1 percent versus 2 percent milk. Then you'll learn how to select the heart-healthiest margarine. In short, you'll be benefiting from the keen eye and insights of a nutrition expert while learning to shop for your special needs. Some tours are free; others cost a minimal amount. To locate a tour in your neighborhood, contact your local dietetic association (listed in the phone book). Or put in a request to the director of consumer affairs in the store where you shop.

SPORTS NUTRITION

Competitive athletes learn quickly that diet plays a role in performance. Faced with the choice of fueling up on complex carbohydrates (bagels, bread, pasta) or a fatty steak, Olympic and professional athletes now choose carbohydrates. The prime reason: research confirms that high-fat meals slow the body down. To gain a competitive edge, athletes need a more efficient fuel—carbohydrate. Fluid and protein are also critical. In addition, exciting new research hints that vitamin E, riboflavin, and iron may have a strong impact on physical performance.

So whether you are just fitness walking or training seriously for a marathon, take a cue from the professionals. Learn the ins and outs of how foods and nutrients influence energy level and help you achieve peak performance. A recent report written by dietitians who specialize in sports nutrition lays down some general diet advice for active people. Newer research findings continue to build on these recommendations.

- Drink plenty of water before, during, and after exercise. Dehydration can hinder performance.
- Use sport replacement drinks when strenuous activity lasts longer than one hour. The extra sugar they contain helps maintain blood-sugar levels when workouts are extensive.
- Include iron-rich foods (red meat, fish, chicken, dried beans, leafy greens, enriched breads, and cereals) in your daily diet. Adequate iron stores help prevent fatigue.
- Eat more carbohydrates and less fat. Starchy foods like pasta and bread are important to fuel both workouts and competitive events. They help prevent performance problems due to low-blood sugar.

Four Special Nutrients for Active People

While all forty nutrients are needed to keep the body healthy, surprising new evidence suggests that riboflavin and vitamin E may play particularly important roles for active people. In addition, scientists have long known that nutrients like iron and vitamin C play a critical part in keeping athletes healthy.

Vitamin E—Findings from the Department of Agriculture's Human Nutrition Research Center on Aging in Boston show that vitamin E can help repair the muscle damage that normally occurs with exercise in older adults. Notable food sources of vitamin E include: Vegetable oils, almonds, sunflower seeds, leafy green vegetables.

Riboflavin—A recent report suggests that older women who exercise may need slightly higher amounts of the B vitamin riboflavin. Notable food sources of riboflavin include: Lean red meats, low-fat milk, low-fat yogurt, mushrooms, broccoli, asparagus, enriched breads and cereals.

Iron—Strenuous exercise or physical activity won't increase iron needs, according to a new report from the U.S. Army Research Institute. But it's known that too little iron in the diet can lead to fatigue. Notable food sources of iron include: lean red meat, poultry, oysters, kidney beans, black-eyed peas, dried beans, spinach.

Vitamin C—Already a known immune system enhancer, a new South African study finds that extra vitamin C may help ultramarathon runners fend off upper-respiratory infections that commonly occur after a race. Notable food sources of vitamin C: Citrus fruits and juices, tomatoes, kiwifruit, broccoli, cantaloupe, papaya, green pepper, strawberries, cauliflower.

Carbohydrates: Choosing the Right Kind

When sports nutritionists emphasize the fuel efficiency of carbohydrates, realize that they're referring to complex carbohydrates. Simple sugars like candy or cola are not a good choice to fuel activity.

Simple Carbohydrates—The term *simple* in carbohydrate language means sweet foods such as honey, brown sugar, and maple syrup. These sugars, either single molecules *(monosaccharides)* or double sugars *(disaccharides),* are easily digested and act as primary fuel for the brain, nervous system, and body cells.

Unfortunately, simple sugar doesn't provide the kind of high-octane fuel that will help you last through a grueling aerobics session or an evening jog. If you were to eat a handful of table sugar the body would digest it so quickly that within one to five minutes blood sugar levels would rise. Before long blood sugar levels would plummet, often to lower than normal levels.

Another problem with simple-sugar foods (candy bars, cola) is that they tend to crowd out more nutritious calories. If you absolutely must have something sugary before you work out, why not satisfy your sweet tooth with foods that carry some nutrients. Some suggestions: frozen yogurt (rich in calcium, riboflavin, protein), fresh fruit (rich in fiber, vitamins A or C), dried fruit. Better yet, why not munch on a cinnamon raisin bagel, a sweet-tasting complex carbohydrate food.

Complex Carbohydrates—Cereal, mashed potatoes, and pasta are some of the starchy foods that nutritionists call *complex carbohydrates*. Structurally speaking, these foods are made up of simple sugars. But those sugars are tightly linked (anywhere from ten to hundreds of sugar molecules) in a large starch network. Part of what makes complex carbohydrates so appealing nutritionally is this chain network.

Digestion breaks down the chain into glucose, but the process is a slow one that allows blood sugar to stay on an even keel (rather than the roller coaster effect that comes with rapid digestion of simple sugars). You might say that complex carbohydrates provide a time-released source of energy. It doesn't hurt that these starchy foods typically come packaged with healthy doses of fiber and many other nutrients. About the only way to negate the fuel efficiency of potatoes, pasta, and other complex carbs is to slather on high-fat toppings—butter, cheese sauce or sour cream.

How Much Carbohydrate Is Healthy?

You'll be sufficiently fueled for activity if around 60 to 65 percent of your calories come from carbohydrates. Not surprisingly, these diet recommendations, along with the overall diet advice for athletes, mimics the recommendations set forth in the Dietary Guidelines and Food Guide Pyramid. (See the section on Healthy Eating, page 5.) To reach the sixty carb level without calculating percentages, downplay meat and fill up on potatoes, pasta, and whole-grain breads.

Sometimes it helps to picture your plate as a pie. Two-thirds of that pie is filled with starches (potatoes, pastas, whole-grain breads). The other third carries a small portion of meat. Instead of a meat-and-potatoes diet, the emphasis should be on potatoes or pasta with a little meat.

Prior to intense endurance events you might need to increase carbohydrate amounts to 65 to 70 percent of total calories. The extra carbohydrate helps to load muscles with easily utilized fuel.

Do You Need to Carbohydrate Load?

About three days prior to a big event, some endurance athletes slowly curtail their practice schedule and begin fueling up on pasta, whole grains, and other high-carbohydrate foods. The idea is to pump muscles full of glycogen—the storage form of carbohydrate—that can be called on during intense activity. A diet with 60 percent carbohydrate calories does load muscles with glycogen. But endurance athletes like to bring carbohydrate calories up to 70 percent of the total hoping to add more fuel to those stores.

Fitness experts recommend carbohydrate loading only if endurance activities are going to last more than ninety minutes. If you decide to try carbohydrate loading, keep in mind that you will need to taper your training one week before a competitive event. Complete rest is essential the day before. Three days before the competition begin loading up on carbohydrates, about 500 to 800 grams per day. Those massive quantities require generous servings of breads, cereals, pasta, and produce. Consider the carb content of these foods: one cup of spaghetti noodles or legumes contains about forty to forty-five grams of carbohydrate, one slice of bread or one cup of cereal has about fifteen grams of carbohydrate, one cup of skim milk has twelve grams of carbohydrate, and one-half cup of vegetables has about four grams. To meet the 500 gram carbohydrate mark you could have two cups of cereal at breakfast with one cup of milk and one medium banana, four slices of toast with jam. At lunch you could load your plate with one cup of red beans and two cups of rice cooked with a one-cup mixture of tomatoes, green peppers and onions. At supper you'll need at least two plates of pasta and red sauce (two cups of noodles on each plate). And then for a snack at night you could eat two bagels (60 grams of carb) with jam.

On the day of the event a small carbohydrate-rich meal (85 to 200 grams of carbohydrate) two to six hours before you compete is also important. Some athletes like to take this carbohydrate as liquid to prevent gastric distress. Solid foods work just fine for some people. For example:

2 cups cornflakes	50 gms Carb
1 cup skim milk	12 gms Carb
1 medium banana	27 gms Carb
Total	89 gms Carb

Be careful to keep track of fat when carbohydrate loading. Hidden fats can negate the benefits of extra carbohydrate. Fatty breakfast pastries and croissants (27 gms carb, 11.8 gms fat) will slow you down. Better choices are bagels (31 gms carb, 1.4 gms fat), or English muffins (26 gms carb, 1.1 gms of fat). It's better to top pancakes with syrup instead of butter. Trade hamburgers for pasta with red sauce. Try topping a baked potato with salsa or low-fat yogurt instead of sour cream.

Fluids that Fuel Activity

Aside from carbohydrate, water is perhaps the most important nutrient for the athlete. The body can go long periods without many nutrients, but it can only survive a few days without water. According to the American Running and Fitness Association, active people will start noticing a drop in performance when body fluid levels drop only 2 percent. (Your body is about 60 to 70 percent water; the more muscular you are, the higher the water content.)

One recent study finds that a drop of 3 percent body water will cause muscle endurance to drop 30 percent. If fluid losses rise above eight percent, and the fluid is not replaced, resulting dehydration can cause mental confusion and loss of concentration. In hot summer weather, dehydration coupled with heat exhaustion can lead to loss of consciousness and heat stroke. That is why it's important to drink plenty of fluid before, during, and after any kind of physical activity. Individual requirements can vary. If you're taking a simple walk or bicycle ride around the neighborhood you might want to try drinking a glass of water ten or fifteen minutes before you leave and then another drink when you return. (It doesn't hurt to carry a water bottle and replenish fluids every fifteen minutes or as needed.)

One way to tell if you are replacing fluid adequately is to weigh yourself before and after exercise and subtract the difference. Ideally, you need to drink enough fluids so that your weight does not change. Keep increasing fluid intake until you reach the right level for your body. Don't forget that watery foods can contribute needed fluid. Many fruits and vegetables are 80 to 95 percent water.

Water-Rich Foods

Food	Percentage Water by weight
Cucumber	95
Celery	94
Tomato	93
Broccoli	90
Carrot	87
Lettuce	87
Orange	86
Apple	83
Banana	74

Source: Adapted from *Bowes & Church's Food Values of Portions Commonly Used,* 16th Edition, 1994.

Fluid Requirements for Competitive Athletes

Strenuous activities and competitive events tend to create larger fluid demands. The American Dietetic Association offers these guidelines for endurance events.

Prior to endurance/competitive event
Two hours before: Drink two cups of fluid
Fifteen to twenty minutes before: Drink another two cups
During Event: Drink small amounts (four to six ounces) of cool water

Do You Need a Sports Beverage?

Fitness experts say cool water is the best fluid replacement since the stomach empties cool liquids much faster than warm ones. However, if you are exercising for more than one hour or sweating profusely due to extremely hot and humid conditions, a sports drink may be helpful. Look for a beverage with about 6 to 8 percent sugar (glucose, sucrose, or glucose polymer) and small amounts of sodium. Small quantities of sugar are absorbed quickly and help keep blood sugar on an even keel. (Beverages sweetened with fructose are not as quickly absorbed and can cause gastric distress for some athletes.) Small amounts of sodium help replace mineral loss due to sweating.

Pouring on the Potassium

When you sweat and lose fluids, your body also loses electrolytes like sodium and potassium. It's true that you can replace these minerals with sports beverages, but foods are an even richer source of the nutrients. If you aren't familiar with high-potassium foods, the following list should help. Potassium, a mineral critical to maintaining a regular heartbeat, is also good for regulating blood pressure. (See the chapter on High Blood Pressure and diet, page 94.)

High-Potassium Foods

Food	Milligrams of Potassium
Skim milk, 8 oz	247
Potato, baked with skin	115
Orange juice, 8 oz	53
Spinach, ½ cup cooked	50
Tomato juice, 6 oz	34
Prunes, 5 dried	33

Raisins, ⅓ cup	32
Cantaloupe, 1 cup	27
Banana, 1 medium	22

Figuring out Protein Needs

Contrary to popular belief, athletes don't need massive quantities of protein because protein doesn't fuel muscle. Carbohydrate is the preferred muscle fuel. It's also incorrect to assume that large amounts of protein are needed to build muscle. Exercise builds muscle. To fuel that muscle-building process the body needs extra calories (energy does not need to come from protein).

The RDA for protein is 0.8 milligrams per kilogram body weight. Healthy, active adults should do fine with these protein levels, which amount to about forty-five to sixty-three grams of protein per day. However, some fitness experts believe that intense activity could elevate protein requirements to as high as 1.0 to 1.5 grams of protein per kilogram of body weight. When you consider that most American currently eat twice as much protein as they need, athletes are already exceeding any needed increase. If you want to calculate your protein needs, follow this simple formula. First, you need to convert your weight into the metric weight measurement—kilograms.

How to Figure Protein Needs

1. To convert weight to kilograms, divide by 2.2
   If you are 165 pounds ÷ 2.2 = 75 kilograms
2. Multiply 75 kgs by 0.8 gms (RDA)
   75 × 0.8 = 60 grams protein
3. Athletes can multiply 75 kgs by 1.0 gm
   75 × 1.0 = 75 grams protein

Reference List

Pennington, J.A.T. *Bowes & Church's Food Values of Portions Commonly Used, 16th Edition.* Philadelphia: J.B. Lippincott Company, 1994.

Meydani, M., et al. "Protective effect of vitamin E on exercise-induced oxidative damage in young and older adults." *American Journal of Physiology;* 264 (5 part 2): R992–8, 1993.

"Position of The American Dietetic Association and The Canadian Dietetic Association: Nutrition for physical fitness and athletic performance for adults." *Journal of the American Dietetic Association;* 93: 691–96, 1993.

Grandjean, A.C. "Practices and recommendations of sports nutritionists." *International Journal of Sports Nutrition;* 3(2): 232–42, 1993.

Peters, E.M., et al. "Vitamin C supplementation reduces the incidence of postrace symptoms of upper-respiratory-tract infection in ultramarathon runners." *American Journal of Clinical Nutrition;* 57: 170–4, 1993.

Moore, R.J., et al. "Maintenance of iron status in healthy men during an extended period of stress and physical activity." *American Journal of Clinical Nutrition;* 58: 923–7, 1993.

Evans, W.J. "Muscle damage: nutritional considerations." *International Journal of Sports Medicine;* 1 30: 214–24, 1991.

Clark, N. *Nancy Clark's Sports Nutrition Guidebook. Eating to Fuel Your Active Lifestyle.* Champaign, IL: Leisure Press, 1990.

Recommended Dietary Allowances, 10th edition. Washington D.C.: National Academy Press, 1989.

Paul, G.L. "Dietary protein requirements for physically active individuals." *Sports Medicine;* 8: 154–76, 1987.

Murray, R. "The effects of consuming carbohydrate-electrolyte beverages on gastric emptying and fluid absorption during and following exercise." *Sports Medicine;* 4: 322–51, 1987.

National Research Council, National Academy of Sciences. "Water deprivation and performance of athletes." *Nutrition Reviews;* 32 (10): 314–15, 1974.

SUPPLEMENTS

Health experts still consider food to be the best source of nutrients, but if you're like most Americans, your diet is not always well-balanced. Vitamin and mineral supplements seem to be a tempting way to fill in the missing gaps. At the same time, a wealth of new studies support a role for certain nutrients in warding off everything from common infections to serious ailments like heart disease, cancer, and cataracts. In light of provocative new research, you might wonder if you should start taking certain supplements as preventive medicine against chronic illnesses.

Since the protection/prevention angle is somewhat uncharted scientific territory, there are no firm answers. How you should use supplements is an open question, one that you'll want to discuss with your doctor or health-care professional. The first thing you'll learn is that attitudes are changing toward multivitamin supplements and that doctors routinely prescribe supplements in certain special circumstances.

Figuring Out Your Supplement Needs

Experts concur that a daily multivitamin supplement, as long as it doesn't contain more than 100 to 150 percent of the recommended allowance for a nutrient, can do little harm. In addition, physicians recognize that nutrient needs can change enough in some special situations to warrant the use of certain supplements. Here are some situations you might want to consider.

Pregnant women—To help prevent birth defects, the U.S. Public Health Service recently began recommending women of childbearing age and pregnant women take in 0.4 milligrams of the B vitamin folic acid. A multivitamin-mineral supplement can help meet those and any other special requirements. Also, a recent report from the National Academy of Sciences calls for low-dose iron supplements (thirty milligrams) since it is difficult to meet the iron needs of pregnancy through diet alone.

Vegetarians—Since only animal foods contain vitamin B_{12}, a supplement of this nutrient is a must for strict vegetarians. Vegetarian diets can also fall short of calcium, iron, and zinc. These needs can be met with a multivitamin preparation.

Smokers—It is known that smokers have higher requirements for Vitamin C. Experts recommend 100 milligrams of this nutrient per day, or nearly twice the amount needed by nonsmokers.

Newborn Infants—Newborns will require a one-time injection of vitamin K. As their digestive tract matures, it will begin to produce this nutrient.

Dieters—Those who are following stringent weight-loss plans (1,200 calories or less) can get shortchanged of a number of different nutrients. Many teenage girls fall into this group, and the fact that they are still growing complicates the problem even further. A multivitamin helps offer insurance.

Older people—Seniors may actually need more of some nutrients as they age, according to preliminary new research. On that list are vitamins B_6, B_{12}, D, folic acid, and calcium. One exciting new finding shows that a multivitamin with added antioxidant nutrients (beta-carotene) can help older adults ward off infections. Men and women taking the supplement were half as likely to get sick as those taking an inactive placebo. When they did get sick, the duration of illness was cut in half.

Sickness—Many illnesses can alter nutrient needs. For example, doctors often prescribe both calcium and vitamin D supplements to women suffering from osteoporosis. Studies show that the additional calcium can help strengthen bones, although not all calcium supplements are absorbed equally well. Research finds that supplements made with calcium citrate are the most efficiently absorbed. For more information on calcium supplements you can refer to the chapter on Osteoporosis, page 145.

Making Your Decision about Preventive Medicine

While most nutritionists have come to accept multivitamin preparations, opinions are mixed about whether healthy adults benefit from supplements as preventive medicine. In one camp are scientists who remind us that the Food and Nutrition Board updates the Recommended Dietary allowances for nutrients about every five years. These recommendations are based on the amount of a nutrient a normal, healthy person might need to prevent a vitamin or mineral deficiency.

In the other camp are researchers who talk about the fact that chronic diseases, not deficiencies, are today's number-one health problem. Shouldn't the RDAs address the issue of preventive medicine? For example, in a recent Harvard Medical School report, researchers point out that women with the highest vitamin E intakes (100 milligrams or ten times the RDA) have the lowest risk for heart disease. Another study links use of multivitamin and vitamin C supplements with a reduced risk of oral cancer. Canadian researchers find that people taking vitamin E and vitamin C supplements have a lower risk for cataracts than people who do not use these supplements. In fact, the unsupplemented group had a two to four times greater risk of developing cataracts than the supplement users.

Of course, it's very easy to get swept up in the excitement of all this new research. Don't forget that these reports are preliminary. Even the researchers involved, while they may admit to taking supplements themselves, don't feel ready to make public-health recommendations. Instead, they recommend that you make individual decisions about supplements based on your lifestyle and a physician's prescription.

Taking Supplements Safely

Despite the fact you have access to hundreds of different kinds of supplements, don't be complacent about these substances. Supplements are not 100 percent safe, particularly when used incorrectly. Two important questions to keep in mind: how toxic is the nutrient in large doses and what do health experts consider a safe dose. When you take most vitamins or minerals in large druglike doses (ten times the RDA) you may end up with druglike side effects.

It's even possible to overdo it with multivitamin/mineral formulations. One recent report finds that four out of five MVI supplements contain levels of nutrients in excess of 200 times the RDA. Another company is marketing a multivitamin supplement product that offers six times the recommended levels of one nutrient. The only way to steer clear of these potential problems is to carefully read labels.

What Is the Right Dose?

Scientists categorize vitamins based on whether they dissolve in water or fat. Nine vitamins are soluble (dissolve readily) in water: vitamin C; and the B vitamins thiamin, riboflavin, niacin, vitamin B_6, pantothenic acid, and biotin. Fragile nutrients, these vitamins are stored in the water-filled compartments of the body. They are easily excreted when their concentration in the body and blood becomes too high, so it's unlikely that you would overdose on these nutrients—but it's not impossible.

People who have taken large doses of vitamin C, for instance, can have such symptoms as nausea and abdominal cramps. It's suspected that megadoses of vitamin C can precipitate the formation of kidney stones in certain susceptible people.

Fat-soluble vitamins (A, D, E, and K) can be even more toxic since the body stores any excess in the liver and in fat tissues. Vitamin D is the most toxic of the fat-soluble vitamins. As little as four or five times the recommended amount can result in toxicity. Massive doses of vitamins A, E, or K are needed before the body reaches toxic levels. The chart that follows can alert you to the symptoms of a nutrient toxicity.

Single-dose supplements can create the most problems. For example, prolonged megadoses of vitamin A can damage the liver. An overload of zinc interferes with the body's ability to absorb copper. When you upset the delicate nutrient balance of the body by mixing and matching supplements and foods fortified with nutrients, these products could end up doing more harm than good.

Vitamin Doses and Toxicity Levels

Vitamin	RDA	Suggested Dose for Disease Prevention	Signs of Toxicity
Fat soluble			
Vitamin A	5,000 IU	*	Nose bleeds, abdominal cramps, nausea, loss of appetite
Vitamin D	400 IU	400 IU	Constipation, nausea, kidney stones, weight loss
Vitamin E	15 IU	100–400 IU	Interferes with anticlotting medications
Vitamin K	No RDA	None	Interferes with anticlotting medications
Water Soluble			
Vitamin D	60 mg	100–500 mg	Nausea, diarrhea, abdominal cramps
Biotin	300 mcg	300 mcg	None reported
Folate	200 mcg	400 mcg	Insomnia, diarrhea, excess can mask B_{12} deficiency
Niacin	20 mg	20 mg	Flushing, heartburn, headaches, liver problems, low blood pressure
Pantothenic acid	10 mg	10 mg	Diarrhea
Riboflavin	1.8 mg	1.8 mg	None reported

Thiamin	1.5 mg	1.5 mg		Insomnia, rapid pulse, headache
Vitamin B$_6$	2 mg	1-2 mg		Depression, damage to nerves, difficulty walking
Vitamin B$_{12}$	2mcg	1-2 mcg		None reported

*It is safer to take your vitamin A as beta-carotene. Six milligrams of beta-carotene provides 100 percent of the RDA for vitamin A without any toxic side effects. The body converts beta-carotene into vitamin A as needed. Studies hint that the protective dose of beta-carotene may be as high as 15 to 30 milligrams.

Shopping for Supplements

If the doctor advises you to take a supplement or you've decided that your erratic eating habits could use some help, keep these tips in mind.

- Review nutrient amounts. A good rule of thumb is to keep within 100 to 150% of the RDA for a nutrient; higher levels can be toxic.
- Look carefully at the mix of nutrients offered. Some preparations are heavy on minerals; others have mostly vitamins.
- Forget special stress formulas. Vitamins can't ease tension or psychological stress.
- Steer clear of unproven preparations. Vitamin B$_{15}$, promoted as treatment from everything from allergies to aging, has no proven benefits. This is also true for laetrile, choline, and bioflavinoids.
- Note the expiration date. All vitamins lose potency over time.
- Test product quality by dropping the tablet in a glass with plain vinegar. It should begin to dissolve or be digested by the vinegar (which creates an acidic environment that mimics the one in your stomach) within fifteen to thirty minutes.
- Don't overlap supplements and fortified foods. Eating a breakfast cereal with 100 percent of the RDA for 8 different nutrients and taking a multivitamin preparation with 100 percent of the RDA for those same substances is redundant.
- Finally, make sure you realize that a vitamin pill can't make up for dietary indiscretions. Nor can it counteract bad lifestyle habits like smoking or eating too much fat. Clean up your diet if it needs fixing; use supplements to cover what's missing.

Reference List

Chandra, R.D. "Effect of vitamin and trace-element supplementation on immune responses and infection in elderly subjects." *Lancet;* 340: 1124–27, 1992.

Russell, R.M., et al. "Vitamin requirements of elderly people: an update." *American Journal of Clinical Nutrition;* 58: 4–14, 1993.

Rimm, E., et al. "Vitamin E consumption and the risk of coronary heart disease in men." *The New England Journal of Medicine;* 328: 1450–59, 1993.

Stampher, M., et al. "Vitamin E consumption and the risk of coronary heart disease in women." *The New England Journal of Medicine;* 328: 1450–59, 1993.

Barone, J., et al. "Vitamin supplement use and risk for oral and esophageal cancer." *Nutrition and Cancer;* 18: 31–41, 1992.

Subar, A.F. and Block, G. "Use of vitamin and mineral supplements: Demographics and amounts of nutrients consumed." *American Journal of Epidemiology;* 132 (6): 1091–1100, 1990.

Robertson, J.M., et al. "Vitamin E intake and risk of cataract in humans." *Annals of the New York Academy of Sciences;* 570: 372–82, 1989.

American Dietetic Association. "Position of the American Dietetic Association: Vegetarian Diets." *Journal of the American Dietetic Association;* 88: 351–55, 1988.

Bowerman, S.J.A. and Harrill, I. "Nutrient consumption of individuals taking or not taking nutrient supplements." *Journal of the American Dietetic Association;* 1983: 83: 298–305, 1983.

Willett, W., et al. "Vitamin supplement use among registered nurses. *American Journal of Clinical Nutrition;* 34: 1121–5, 1981.

Koplan, J.P., et al. "Nutrient intake and supplementation in the United States." *Journal of the American Dietetic Association;* 12: 1585–90, 1985.

Recommended Dietary Allowances, 10th edition. Washington D.C.: National Academy Press, 1989.

TEENAGERS AND NUTRITION

The teenage years present some special nutritional problems. At the same time that boys and girls are going through their largest growth spurt (elevating calorie demands to unusually high levels) they are exerting their independence in many areas, including food choices. Concerns about body image and staying thin can inspire the use of fad diets or lead to eating disorders. Habits such as meal skipping and snacking on empty-calorie foods become more common. Couple poor food choices with higher calorie demands and the situation can spell big nutritional problems.

There's not much parents can do to influence choices at this stage of the game, particularly since many teens are eating and sometimes working away from home. If you've discussed god nutrition and set a good example, chances are your teen will have developed some healthful eating habits. If lines of communication stay open, you can always offer suggestions based on what you've learned.

Meeting Growing Needs The Right Way

The average teenage boy sprouts up a full twelve inches or more and adds fifty to seventy pounds to his weight between the ages of twelve through sixteen. Girls between the ages of ten and fourteen add nine to ten inches in height and forty to fifty pounds. Fueling this huge growth spurt takes careful planning. (Active boys need as much as 3,000 to 4,000 calories per day; active girls 2,000 to 3,000 calories.)

Still, the same basic principles of healthy eating (see the Food Pyramid section in the Introduction, page 7) apply to teens that apply to adults. The only difference is that teenagers need extra servings from the milk and dairy group to help build growing bones. Studies show that teenage girls, probably because they eat fewer calories, have poorer diets than teenage boys. However, surveys find that both groups of teens have the same set of problem nutrients, nutrients that they typically fall short of in their everyday diets: calcium, iron, vitamin A, and vitamin C.

Calcium   Everyone knows that calcium is good for building strong bones, but a new study from Indiana finds that children who eat more calcium than is currently recommended end up having stronger, denser bones. The RDA for calcium for teens is 1,200 milligrams or the amount of calcium found in about four cups of milk. Food sources include low-fat milk, 1 percent chocolate milk, yogurt, ice milk, low-fat cheeses, leafy green vegetables such as kale and broccoli, canned salmon with the bones.

Vitamin A—Teens don't need more vitamin A than adults, but surveys show that they typically fall short of meeting their needs. Since the vitamin is critical for growth, vision, and immune health, teens need to stock up on vitamin-A-rich foods. Food sources include fortified milk and eggs. Beta-carotene-rich foods—orange vegetables (carrots, winter squash, sweet potatoes) and leafy green vegetables such as spinach and kale—can be converted to vitamin A by the body.

Iron—Iron deficiency anemia (see the chapter on Anemia, page 31) is common during teen years. An increase in muscle mass and blood volume creates a need for more iron in boys. Girls need extra iron to replace that lost through menstruation. Food sources include lean meats, chicken, fish, eggs, legumes (dried beans), whole grains, enriched breads and cereals, leafy green vegetables.

Vitamin C—Skipping breakfast and eating a lot of fast food may be two reasons why some teens don't eat enough vitamin C. Considering that this nutrient may play a role in warding off heart disease (see the chapter on Heart Health, page 85) and fighting infections (see Immunity, page 100) teens would do well to find some enjoyable sources of the vitamin. Food sources include citrus fruits and juices, strawberries, kiwifruit, broccoli, tomatoes, potatoes.

The Great American Snack Habit

Surveys show that teenagers obtain nearly one-quarter of their calories from snacks. While the extra calorie demands of a growing body can allow for some indulgence in potato chips, candy bars, and cola, healthier snacks are a better option. You can't stop a teen from eating candy bars and corn chips outside the home, but you can stock the cupboard and refrigerator with low-fat snacks, preferably the nutrient-dense variety.

Refrigerator: Fruit juices, skim or 1 percent milk, 1 percent chocolate milk, frozen fruit juice bars, frozen-yogurt bars, fudgesicles, ice milk. Low-fat cheese and lean deli meats (turkey, ham) for sandwiches.

Bread box: Bagels, English muffins, bran muffins, cinnamon raisin loaf, french rolls, whole-wheat bread.

Cupboard: Animal crackers, fig bars, vanilla wafers, graham crackers, angel-food cake, popcorn, pretzels.

Munching at the Mall

Teenagers do a lot of their snacking and eating away from home, buying food from vending machines, fast-food outlets, and shopping-mall food courts. Armed with the right information they can easily select and be satisfied with high-carb rather than high-fat snacks. (See the section on Fast Foods page 77 for more tips on low-fat snacking away from home.)

Choose	Instead of
Hot pretzel with mustard	Nachos with cheese
Frozen yogurt with fruit	Hot fudge sundae
Unbuttered popcorn	Potato chips or fries
Cinnamon raisin bagel	Donut
Vegetable pizza slice	Pepperoni pizza
Fresh fruit salad	Fried pie
Fruit juice spritzer	Soda or soft drinks
Oatmeal raisin cookie	Chocolate chip
Ham or turkey sandwich	Bologna sandwich

The Damaging Diet Mentality

Just as worrisome as teens who are haphazard snackers are teenagers who jump on the wrong kind of diet bandwagon. Worrying about shapes and physiques is natural, but trying to lose weight fast is unhealthy. Many teens ignore the hazards of strict diets and see only the appeal of a slimmer or more muscular silhouette. A recent Cleveland State University study finds that four out of ten teenage boys diet; nearly eighty percent of high-school girls are trying to lose weight.

Problems set in when teens resort to harmful weight-loss methods like purging (vomiting or laxatives) to shed unwanted pounds. In an alarming new report, researchers show that purging, diet pills, and fasting are common diet strategies in many Cleveland, Ohio high schools. Of girls who diet, 33 percent admit to putting themselves on a twenty-four-hour fast at least once per week. This is also true for one out of every four dieting boys.

Nutritionists worry that these drastic weight-loss measures will interfere with growth. Adolescent boys can require as much as 3,000 to 4,000 calories per day just to fuel growth.

Girls need high levels of calories too. However, if your teenager truly does have a weight problem, make sure they go about losing weight in the right way. (See the chapter on Weight Control, page 203.) Teenage girls shouldn't be eating fewer than 1,300 calories per day while dieting. Boys should drop no lower than 1,500 per day.

Is It an Eating Disorder?

When dieting or food becomes an obsession, teens can lose control over their relationship to food and eating disorders can develop. Teenage girls are more likely to fall victim to an eating disorder (anorexia or bulimia) than teenage boys. But be aware that eating disorders are more than a problem with food. Binging, purging, chronic fasting—these abnormal eating behaviors are typically tied to psychological issues.

Most experts define an eating disorder as a two-part illness, one with eating disturbances intertwined with underlying emotional problems. Since these disorders are complex, successful treatment must look not only at food intake but the emotional issues that are creating the abnormal response to food. If you suspect your teenager might have an eating disorder, seek help.

Eating to Ward off Acne

Estimates are that roughly 85 percent of teens experience some degree of acne. Experts speculate that lack of sleep, anxiety, and, for girls, the hormonal fluctuations that come with menstruation may be at least partly responsible for acne breakouts. However, the foods often fingered as culprits—chocolate, nuts, cola, french fries, and greasy burgers—probably don't cause acne. Research shows that when these foods are avoided, acne doesn't improve. However, alcohol is one diet item that can aggravate acne. Studies show that drinking large amounts of alcohol can cause acne to get worse. Luckily, whether treated or not, acne is one problem that teens eventually outgrow.

Reference List

Nutrition and Your Health: Dietary Guidelines for Americans. Hyattsville, MD: U.S. Department of Health and Human Services, 1992.
Ikeda, J. *Winning Weight Loss for Teens.* Palo Alto, CA: Bull Publishing, 1987.
Satter, E.M. "Childhood eating disorders." *Journal of the American Dietetic Association;* 86: 357–361, 1986.

Heilbrun, A.B. and Harris A. "Psychological defenses in females at risk for anorexia nervosa." *International Journal of Eating Disorders;* 5: 503–16, 1986.

Story, M. and Resnick, M.D. "Adolescents' views on foods and nutrition." *Journal of Nutrition Education;* 18: 188–92, 1986.

Human Nutrition Information Service. *CSF-II: Nationwide Food Consumption Survey—continuing survey of food intakes by individuals.* United States Department of Agriculture, 1985.

Pugliese, M.E., et al. "Fear of obesity: A cause of short stature and delayed puberty." *The New England Journal of Medicine;* 309: 513–18, 1983.

Michaelsson, G. "Diet and acne." *Nutrition Reviews;* 39(2): 104–106, 1981.

Greger, J.L., et al. "Nutritional status of adolescent girls in regard to zinc, copper and iron." *American Journal of Clinical Nutrition;* 31: 269–75, 1978.

VEGETARIANISM

Vegetarian diets encompass a wide variety of eating styles. Strict plans call for avoidance of all animal products; more liberal (semivegetarian) regimens allow for small quantities of meat or fish on a less-frequent basis. Regardless of the approach you decide to take, experts conclude that a diet focusing on fruits, vegetables, and whole grains can net you numerous health rewards. Studies confirm that vegetarians, as a group, tend to have lower blood-cholesterol levels, lower blood pressures and weigh less than their nonvegetarian counterparts. When you consider that most fruits, vegetables, and whole grains are low in fat and high in fiber, that doesn't seem at all surprising.

Yet the health benefits of a vegetarian eating style seem to go beyond simple good nutrition. Current scientific evidence indicates that fruits and vegetables and grains contain key ingredients that may offer protection against illnesses like heart disease and cancer. For example, a recent report in the medical journal *Lancet* suggests that isoflavonoids, compounds that tofu and rice contain in abundant amounts, may act to protect against prostate cancer. Japanese men, who have a lower death rate from prostate cancer, eat more tofu and rice than Westerners.

In another new study, German researchers are documenting lower death rates for heart disease and cancer among both strict and moderate vegetarians. Other reports suggest a role for fruits and vegetables in protecting against everything from lung cancer to osteoporosis. However, the health benefits you reap may depend on how you construct your vegetarian diet.

Practicing Vegetarianism by Degree

The term *vegetarianism* means different things to different people. Experts say it's not so much the vegetarian style you choose as what you do to make it nutritionally adequate. In fact, if you like meat, milk, and cheese you might find comfort in studies that suggest eating smaller quantities of these foods along with larger quantities of vegetables and grains may be just as protective to health as a strict vegetarian diet.

- *Semivegetarian*—Strict vegetarians don't like this term, but health experts say that a gradual shift toward eating more fruits, vegetables, and whole grains and less meat is not only healthy but realistic. As long as you eat a wide variety of foods and enough calories to maintain your weight, this kind of plan easily fulfills protein and nutrient requirements.

- *Lacto-ovovegetarian*—A moderate approach to vegetarian, this style of eating calls for milk, eggs, and dairy products to complement vegetables. Meats are avoided. Since milk and cheese provide high quality protein, you shouldn't experience nutritional problems as long as you eat at least two servings from the dairy group each day.
- *Vegan*—The strictest of vegetarian regimens, vegans avoid all animal products. Careful diet planning is necessary to ensure adequate amounts of key nutrients (calcium, iron, zinc, vitamin B_{12}) found mainly in animal foods.

Pitfalls of Vegetarian Diets

Before you crowd your plate with only vegetables, keep in mind that making a vegetarian diet healthful does take some careful planning. Three important strategies come to mind.

Beware the Fat Trap—Many vegetable-based recipes call for liberal use of nuts, cheese, and dairy products. Relying on these high-fat foods for protein could end up negating the health benefits of a vegetarian eating style. To keep fat intake low, follow these guidelines.

- Use fat-free and reduced-fat milk products. Some of the reduced-fat sour creams, milks, and cheeses are quite acceptable. Use evaporated skim milk as a replacement for whipping cream.
- Cut the amount of butter or oil in most recipes in half. (Replace the fat in baked goods with low-fat yogurt or mashed fruits such as bananas or prunes.) Rely on nonstick pans and vegetable-oil cooking sprays in order to keep added fats to a minimum.
- Thicken gravies or sauces by adding pureed vegetables such as potatoes or carrots, or rice instead of fat and flour.
- Use nuts sparingly. Sprinkle small amounts of chopped or slivered nuts onto a finished dish rather than mixing large amounts into a recipe.
- Add fresh herbs and acidic seasonings (flavored vinegars, citrus juices) to casseroles, stir-fries, and sauces to enhance flavor.
- Replace pastry in recipes with phyllo dough, a Greek pastry product found in the supermarket freezer case. Instead of coating with butter or margarine, spray the thin sheets lightly with vegetable-oil cooking spray.

Highlight Missing Nutrients—Another trouble spot in vegetarian diets is the high potential for nutrient deficiencies. Strict vegetarians or vegans need to be most concerned about these deficiencies. Without animal products in the diet it can be difficult to obtain adequate quantities of key nutrients such as iron, calcium, zinc, and vitamins D and B_{12}. Contrary to popular belief, obtaining adequate protein is usually not that difficult.

Iron: Meat contains an excellent and easily absorbable form of iron. Fortunately, dried beans, lentils, leafy green vegetables, and grains (enriched breads and cereals) are good food sources of the mineral, too. The hitch is that you will need to eat vitamin C-rich foods such as tomato juice, potatoes, and broccoli to help the body absorb the iron from vegetables more efficiently.

Food Sources of Iron

Item	Milligrams of Iron
Tofu, soft, 4 oz	6.7
Spinach, 1 cup cooked	6.4
Kidney beans, 1 cup cooked	5.2
Lima beans, 1 cup cooked	5.2
Hamburger, 4 oz with bun	4.9
Prune juice, 1 cup	3
Potato, baked with skin, 1 medium	2.8
Green peas, 1 cup cooked	2.5
Roast beef, 3 oz cooked	2.5
Broccoli, 1 cup cooked	1.8
Oatmeal, 1 cup cooked	1.6
Whole-wheat bread, 1 slice	.9

Calcium: If you don't include dairy products in your vegetarian diet, look to leafy green vegetables such as kale, broccoli, collard greens and Chinese cabbage (bok choy) to provide small quantities of the mineral. Since vegetables are not as high in calcium as dairy foods, you might want to consider calcium-fortified soy milk.

Food Sources of Calcium

Item	Milligrams calcium
Romano cheese, 1 oz	302
Skim milk, 8 oz	302
Cheddar cheese, 1 oz	204
Canned salmon with bones, 3 oz	203
Sardines with bones, 3 oz	199
Turnip greens, 1 cup cooked	198
Broccoli, 1 cup cooked	178

Bok choy, 1 cup cooked	158
Low-fat cottage cheese, 1 cup	138
Tofu, ½ cup	130
Orange, navel, 1 medium	56
Kidney beans, 1 cup cooked	50

Zinc: Look to everything from seafood to peanut butter to dried beans to provide generous amounts of this mineral that is crucial to wound healing and immunity. Until recently, scientists didn't realize the critical role zinc plays in keeping immune system cells (T-lymphocytes and neutrophils) tuned up and responsive to infections and foreign invaders.

Vitamin B_{12}:   Since this vitamin is only found in animal foods, strict vegetarians need to either drink soy milk fortified with B_{12} or take a B_{12} supplement.

Vitamin D: Sunlight helps the body to make vitamin D. Another source for the nutrient is fortified milks. If you don't drink milk or you live in a northern climate, supplements may be in order.

Protein: Most healthy adults need somewhere between fifty and sixty-three grams of protein per day. A cup of kidney beans provides fifteen grams of protein, or about one-fourth that requirement. Serve it with a cup of pasta or rice to add another four grams of protein. Add vegetables, breads, and other grains throughout the course of the day and you can easily meet or exceed your protein needs. Experts say that if you eat the variety and quantity of foods you need to maintain your weight, chances are good that protein intake will be adequate. However, the quality of that protein is another issue.

Select Complementary Proteins   If you eat small quantities of meat or include dairy products and eggs in your diet, protein quality will be high. However, if you decide to go the strict vegetarian route, keep in mind that plant proteins are not as high in quality as animal proteins. You'll need to mix and match vegetables and grains to mimic the high quality protein of meat. The chart below offers general guidelines.

High Quality Plant-Protein Combinations   Even though plant proteins are not as high in quality as animal proteins, what one plant protein lacks another can supply. (You don't necessarily have to eat vegetable protein complements at the same meal. Red beans at lunchtime can be complemented by rice at dinner.)

Combine	With	For Example
Barley	Lentils	Lentil soup
Cornmeal	Pinto beans	Bean burrito
Rice	Dried Beans	Red beans & rice
Whole grain bread	Peanuts	Peanut butter sandwich
Rye bread	Split peas	Pea soup & toast
Pasta	White beans	Pasta e fagoli
Pasta	Soybeans	Tofu casserole
Garbanzo beans	Sesame seeds	Hummus
Lentils	Cashews	Lentil nut loaf
Peanuts	Sunflower seeds	Trail mix

Should Kids Become Vegetarians?

Studies show that children can thrive and grow on vegetarian diets, as long as dietary plans are not too stringent. When researchers in Tennessee followed the growth patterns of a group of 404 vegetarian children they noticed only modestly slower gains in height and weight when these children were compared to the norm. Moreover, the differences tended to be made up in later years. Other new reports find that lower stature among preadolescent lacto-ovovegetarian girls tends to be temporary and that these girls continue to grow and eventually catch up to their nonvegetarian counterparts as they become older.

Of course, health professionals warn that strict vegetarian plans can be a problem, particularly for toddlers and preschool aged children. One of the main reasons is that it's hard to have a child this young eat the large volume of food needed to supply all the nutrients required for growth. Little stomachs can't always hold large amounts. In fact, if you plan to switch the whole family to a vegetarian eating style, experts favor using the lacto-ovovegetarian approach for children. That way kids will be assured of adequate amounts of protein, calcium, and other key nutrients needed in growing. One caveat: For children are under the age of two, make sure to use whole milk and regular cheese rather than reduced-fat varieties. At this age, youngsters need the fat, cholesterol, and calories whole-milk dairy products provide.

Reference List

Pennington, J.A.T. *Bowes & Church's Food Values of Portions Commonly Used,* 16th edition. Philadelphia: J.B. Lippincott Company, 1994.

Beilen, L.J. "Vegetarian diets, alcohol consumption, and hypertension." *Annals of the New York Academy of Sciences;* 676: 83–91, 1993.

Draper, A., et al. "The energy and nutrient intakes of different types of vegetarians: a case for supplements?" *British Journal of Nutrition;* 69(1):3–19, 1993.

Sabate, J., et al. "Lower height of lacto-ovovegetarian girls at preadolescence: an indication of physical maturation delay." *Journal of the American Dietetic Association;* 92(10): 1263–64, 1992.

Tesar, R., et al. "Axial and peripheral bone density and nutrient intakes of postmenopausal vegetarian and omnivorous women." *American Journal of Clinical Nutrition;* 56(4) 699–704, 1992.

Chang-Claude J., et al. "Mortality pattern of German vegetarians after 11 years of follow-up." *Epidemiology;* 3(5): 395–401, 1992.

Srikumar, T.S., et al. "Trace element status in healthy subjects switching from a mixed to a lactovegetarian diet for 12 months." *American Journal of Clinical Nutrition;* 55(4): 885–90, 1992.

Kjeldsen-Kragh, J., et al. "Controlled trial of fasting and one-year vegetarian diet in rheumatoid arthritis." *Lancet;* 338(8772): 899–902, 1991.

Dwyer, J.T. "Nutritional consequences of vegetarianism." *Annals of Reviews in Nutrition;* 11: 61–91, 1991.

Fraser, G.E., et al. "Diet and lung cancer in California Seventh-day Adventists." *American Journal of Epidemiology;* 133(7): 683–93, 1991.

Richter, E.A., et al. "Immune parameters in male athletes after a lacto-ovo vegetarian diet and a mixed Western diet." *Medicine and Science in Sports & Exercise;* 23(5): 517–21, 1991.

Resnicow, K., et al. "Diet and serum lipids in vegan vegetarians: a model for risk reduction." *Journal of the American Dietetic Association;* 91(4): 447–53, 1991.

Johansson, G.K., et al. "Shift from a mixed diet to a lactovegetarian diet: influence of some cancer-associated intestinal bacterial enzyme activities." *Nutrition and Cancer;* 14(3–4): 239–46, 1990.

Kestin, M., et al. "Cardiovascular disease risk factors in free-living men: comparison of two prudent diets, one based on lactoovovegetarianism and the other allowing lean meat." *American Journal of Clinical Nutrition;* 50(2): 280–7, 1989.

O'Connell, J.M., et al. "Growth of vegetarian children: The farm study." *Pediatrics;* 84: 475–84, 1989.

American Dietetic Association. "Position of The American Dietetic Association: Vegetarian Diets." *Journal of the American Dietetic Association;* 88: 351–55, 1988.

WEIGHT CONTROL

If you're like most weight-conscious Americans, you've tried to shed your excess pounds—all ten, twenty, or forty of them—at least three different times in the past year. Maybe you were successful at first. But chances are the weight came back. So, in absolute disgust, you have either decided to get off the dieting merry-go-round or planned to bide your time until you at least find a diet with a better success rate. Wherever you stand, don't despair. Very few people go through life without escaping the frustrations that come with trying to manage weight.

Fortunately, the factors that predispose some people to weight gain are becoming much clearer. Interesting new research sheds light on the roles that everything from heredity to musical tastes to television-watching habits play in determining body weight. Before you delve into the latest findings, however, there are two important points to consider. One, if you have any health conditions—pregnancy, diabetes—that might be negatively influenced by dieting, talk to your doctor before changing your style of eating. In the same vein, don't put growing children on a diet without a doctor's supervision. Well-intentioned parents have created serious health problems for their children by putting them on unneeded diets during their growing years. (See the chapter on Childhood Nutrition, page 53.)

Second, ask yourself if you really need to lose weight. That is, are excess pounds creating an undue health risk in your life? Or could your desire to lose weight stem from societal pressures or unrealistic expectations that would have you believing that the ideal figure is one that's model thin? Be aware that experts feel that it's more realistic to base ideal body weight on health rather than appearance. That's why your first step toward successful weight control is to figure out what is a healthy weight for you.

Are You Too Fat?

The mirror is probably the simplest, and definitely one of the most truthful, weight assessment tool. Shed your clothes and take a close look. If you are carrying around too much fat anywhere on your frame, the mirror will show it. You can also step on a bathroom scale and compare the resulting number to a weight table or chart. Although no weight table is perfect (figures are just estimates), the new weight tables published as part of the U.S. Dietary

Guidelines offer the most up-to-date guidelines on healthy weights.

Since numerous studies confirm it's not unhealthy to put on some weight as you age, you'll notice higher weight ranges for people over thirty-five. Bear in mind, however, that the upper end of the weight range is meant for larger-boned, muscular men (muscle weighs more than fat). If you are a petite 5'4" woman over the age of thirty-five, the weight range listed as healthy is 122 to 157 pounds. While that is quite a generous spread, the top end of the range—157 pounds—is definitely too much to carry if your frame is petite or even average. In other words, it's probably more realistic for most women to consider a healthy weight to be closer to the lower end of the weight range. And many men, unless they are unusually large framed or muscular, probably fit more in the middle of the range than on the upper end.

Height	Weight (lbs)	
	Ages 19-34	*Ages 35+*
5'0	97-128	108-138
5'1	101-132	111-143
5'2	104-137	115-148
5'3	107-141	119-152
5'4	111-146	122-157
5'5	114-150	126-162
5'6	118-155	130-167
5'7	121-160	134-172
5'8	125-164	138-178
5'9	129-169	142-183
5'10	132-174	146-188
5'11	136-179	151-194
6'0	140-184	155-199
6'1	144-189	159-205
6'2	148-195	164-210
6'3	152-200	168-216
6'4	156-205	173-222
6'5	160-211	177-228
6'6	164-216	182-234

Note: Measurements are without clothes and shoes.

*Put yourself into the high end of a weight range if you have higher muscle mass and heavier bones (most men fit into this category). Lower ranges are for people with less muscle mass.

Source: Nutrition and Your Health: Dietary Guidelines for Americans, 1990.

Location is Everything

The next step in assessing weight goes beyond the number on a scale. You'll need to address two other important issues: weight distribution and percentage of body fat. A muscular man may weigh more than the weight charts deem desirable. If the bulk of that weight is muscle (muscle weighs more than fat), however, the extra pounds won't create a health risk. A high body fat percentage, on the other hand, can be risky. So too can excess weight stored around the middle. While fat stored in the hips and thighs, or a pear-shaped fat distribution, appears to create no health risk, studies show that fat stored in a spare tire or apple shape increases the risk for diabetes and heart disease.

Taking a belly-to-hip measurement is another way of determining if you are an apple or pear. Start by placing a measuring tape around your waist (near your navel) and at the widest portion of your hips. Divide that waist measure by the total hip measurement. For women, a healthy belly to hip ratio is one that falls below 0.80. For men, a ratio below 0.95 is best.

Taking the Right Approach

Even though there is no doubt that extra pounds do spell trouble, (in the National Research Council's landmark report on *Diet and Health,* scientists cite obesity as a risk factor for everything from cancer to high blood pressure to diabetes) don't be in too much of a rush to shed body fat. In order to be successful, weight control requires changes in eating habits that are made for the long term. Indeed, at the crux of most weight problems are poor eating and exercise habits.

You must gradually learn to change an eating and activity style that promotes weight gain to one that helps you to lose weight. Cutting back on fat in your diet is the first and most effective step. Adding activity is the next step. To make the transition to lower-fat foods more pleasant, make changes in eating habits gradually. For instance, start by cooking one low-fat meal per week. Then, increase to two low-fat meals, three low-fat meals and so on. Follow the same system with your exercise regimen. Try taking a walk before work a few mornings a week (or a walk after dinner). Build up the time spent walking or exercising until you reach a goal of 45 minutes, three times per week.

At first these goals may seem overwhelming, but take your time. It's not necessary to change your eating and exercise behaviors overnight. Any weight-loss expert will tell you that behavior modification takes time. Moreover, different strategies work for different people. Here are a few behavior modification tips that might help you to modify your diet and exercise habits.

Forging New Eating Habits
- Eat slowly and savor each bite. (Conversing with others during the meal can help you to slow down.)
- Put down your fork between bites.
- Serve food on smaller plates or in smaller bowls.
- Eat in one designated place (preferably not in front of the TV or while standing up in the kitchen).
- Clear the cabinets of tempting, high-fat foods. Stock the pantry with low-fat snacks and ingredients.
- Plan an eating strategy for parties or special occasions; plan daily meals, too.

Forging New Exercise Habits
- Take a walk around the block when the urge to snack strikes.
- Schedule exercise as you do important appointments. That way you will make time for activity.
- Take the stairs instead of the elevator; park your car far enough away from your destination so that you'll need to take a short walk.
- Emphasize social activities that focus on exercise. Meet a friend for tennis instead of lunch; walk with a neighbor in the morning; jog with a coworker at lunch. Go out dancing, bowling, or play a round of golf with friends.

Counting Calories versus Counting Fat

After you begin to change general eating attitudes and behaviors, you'll want to get down to dieting specifics. One pound of stored body fat contains roughly 3,500 calories. If you want to lose a pound of fat a week, simple math dictates that you need to cut out 500 calories a day (or burn up 500 calories with activity). In reality, however, the rate at which weight is lost can vary. Experts advocate a slow, steady weight loss of one-half to one pound per week. You can achieve that goal by keeping active and either counting calories or counting fat.

Becoming a Calorie Counter   Estimates are that it takes ten calories per pound to maintain a desired body weight. If you currently weigh 140 pounds, multiply 140 x 10 = 1,400 calories. This calorie level will satisfy the routine or basal energy requirements needed to keep the lungs working, the heart beating, and all body processes going. Activities—jogging, house cleaning, stair climbing—create energy demands in addition to this basal level. Calculate the amount of calories spent on activity by using these formulas.

If you are sedentary:
Multiply desired body weight × 3.

If you are moderately active:
Multiply desired body weight × 5.

If you are very active (strenuous work)
Multiply desired body weight × 10.

If you want to lose weight, follow the rule of ten mentioned above but use your target weight (instead of current weight) in the formula. If you weigh 160 pounds but would like to weigh 145 pounds, multiply 145 × 10 = 1450 calories. Then, add the calories needed for activity. If you are sedentary or only do light activity multiply 145 × 3 = 435. Then add, 1,450 + 435 = 1,885 calories. This is the calorie level you would need to follow to lose weight gradually. Cutting calories below 1,200 calories per day makes it difficult to ensure that the diet contains needed quantities of most vitamins and minerals.

Becoming a Fat Counter   Since fat has about nine calories per gram and carbohydrate and protein have only four, it makes sense that cutting back on fat will automatically result in a cutback in calories. In fact, many weight-control experts feel that cutting back on fat (see the chapter on Low-Fat Eating, page 131) is a much easier way to achieve weight loss than counting calories. However, you will need to think about calories for just a moment, since fat budgets are set up based on the number of calories you eat each day. (Use the guidelines in the section above if you need to determine the number of calories you need to maintain weight or lose weight.)

You'll notice that there are three different fat budgets—30 percent, 25 percent, 20 percent—offered for each calorie level listed below. You can lose weight with any budget level as long as you select the number of calories needed for weight loss and then eat the corresponding number of fat grams listed. The reason for the choice in fat levels has to do with the fact that many experts feel that drawing closer to a goal of 20 percent or 25 percent of the calories from fat may be healthier for the heart and the rest of the body as well. However, if you haven't restricted fat in the past, the 30 percent level may be a more realistic place to start. Later, when you begin to adjust to a lower fat intake, you may want to drop down to 25 percent of the calories from fat or less.

If you eat	Limit fat grams to		
	30%	*25%*	*20%*
1,200 calories	40 grams	33 grams	27 grams
1,500 calories	50 grams	42 grams	33 grams
1,800 calories	60 grams	50 grams	40 grams
2,100 calories	70 grams	58 grams	47 grams
2,400 calories	80 grams	67 grams	53 grams

Learn the fat content of the foods you routinely eat (see the Encyclopedia of Daily Values starting on page 217 or look closely at food labels). Then examine the quantities of foods that you eat. Keep in mind that research shows that fat calories are more fattening than calories that come from carbohydrate or protein. Let's say you indulge in an extra 300 fat calories with a snack like potato chips or chocolate. The body processes those extra fat calories efficiently so that 297 of those calories get stored as body fat; only three calories are needed for the processing. Eat the same amount of extra carbohydrate calories, an oversized bagel, a couple of slices of toast with jam, and 25 percent of the energy—75 calories—will be lost to processing. The net number of calories stored as body fat is only 225.

Five More Steps to Success

People gain weight for a lot of different reasons, and research shows that people fight different battles when it comes to weight loss. Some of us inherit sluggish metabolisms. Others sabotage weight loss efforts with negative attitudes. Yet, in the end, managing weight is not an impossible task, particularly if you work to change the eating and exercise habits that caused you to gain weight in the first place. These five tips offer a good place to start.

1. Think Gradual.
   If you want to lose weight, chances are you will need to make a number of different changes in the way you eat and live. Rather than quit current eating habits cold turkey try to make one or two small changes at a time. Switch to mustard on your sandwich. Try one meatless meal a week. Increase your activity level. If you make changes gradually, you'll be more likely to stick with them long term.
2. Eat Something for Breakfast.
   Studies have long documented the fact that skipping a meal increases the chances that you will overeat at the next one, and in a new report from Vanderbilt University, scientists show that breakfast eaters experience fewer impulses to snack during the day and end up eating less total fat than those who forgo the morning meal. In fact, the best way to keep appetite under control is to establish a regular meal schedule.
3. Measure Portions.
   Even if you don't want to count calories or fat on a day-in-day-out basis, be sure to measure the amounts of foods that you eat in the beginning stages of weight control efforts. Intriguing new results from a study looking at perpetually unsuccessful dieters finds that most of these overweight people are dramatically underestimating how much they really eat.
4. Learn to Reward Yourself.

Weight control is difficult. Pat yourself on the back for any success, no matter how small. Losing one-quarter of a pound seems minuscule until you think of it as peeling one whole stick of margarine (one quarter pound of fat) from somewhere on your body. Why not treat yourself to a movie, a new paperback, or some little trinket to reinforce success? Conversely, rather than dwell on one diet slip-up, forgive yourself and review all your successes. New research finds that dieters who build themselves up with a positive attitude or mind-set are more likely to succeed.

5. Build a Support Network.
Recent research finds that dieters who have the support of a spouse are more likely to be successful at weight loss. If family members don't support your weight-control efforts look for a sympathetic friend or weight-loss support group.

Merits of Exercise

While changing eating habits, gaining family support, and other strategies help with weight loss, many dieters forget that exercise also plays a pivotal role. The reasons are twofold. First, aerobic exercise—brisk walking, jogging, bicycling—helps to rev up your metabolism. In fact, your resting metabolic rate is elevated not only during aerobic activity but continues to remain elevated for a short period after you stop. Just how long metabolic rate stays elevated is a hotly debated issue. Conservative estimates say that the rise lasts up to forty minutes after exercise has stopped. No matter how long it lasts, the fact remains that you are burning more calories while you exercise and for some time afterward.

Second, exercise helps to build muscle. Since muscle requires more calories to maintain than fat tissue, you will end up burning more calories when your body becomes a muscular body. Even without these extra benefits, exercise offers numerous other health benefits such as improved cardiovascular strength, improved mental attitude, lower blood-cholesterol levels, and lower blood pressure readings.

Intriguing New Diet Research

In a recent study, California researchers found that two out of every three dieters who are successful at controlling weight set up their own diet regimens rather than rely on commercial programs or diets planned by others. These dieters gradually change eating and exercise habits that caused them to put on weight in the first place, each finding the kind of eating style that works for them. Here are some current findings that offer new insight as to what helps and hinders weight loss regimens.

- *Television trouble*—A new report finds that people who spend four or more hours a day watching television are more than twice as likely to be obese as those who watch less than an hour of television each day. Experts speculate that the combination of snacking and sitting sets the stage for weight gain.
- *Late-night munching*—A new report finds that snacking late at night can actually slow metabolism. It seems that the body produces less heat and burns fewer calories to digest a food eaten after midnight than when that same food is eaten earlier in the day. Considering these findings, it's probably not such a good idea to eat dinner late either.
- *Blaming the genes*—Some people are predisposed to weight gain because of genetic influences. Yet, there's no reason to use "bad" genes as an excuse to give up on weight control. It may be harder to lose weight if you have a family history of obesity. But studies confirm it is not impossible.
- *Color coordinated*—Bright colors like orange, red, and yellow stimulate the appetite, according to studies from the Weight, Health and Stress Clinic at Johns Hopkins Medical Institute. Cool pastels and dark shades (black, brown, gun-metal gray) tend to douse hunger pangs. Keep these findings in mind when choosing tablecloths and dishware and when it's time to repaint dining-room walls.
- *Diet foods*—A recent study of foods with diet and health food labels finds that calorie counts can be underreported by as much as 85 percent. It seems that smaller companies and local brands are not as accurate at measuring calories as major brands—then again, you don't need any special foods to help you lose weight. Eat foods that are naturally low in fat: fruits, vegetables, whole grains, lean meats, low-fat dairy products. In fact, you can even eat your favorite foods—simply learn to eat high-calorie indulgences less often and in smaller quantities.
- *Spot-reducing scams*—Research confirms that it's useless to target a specific body areas for weight loss (hips, thighs, stomach) by using special exercises. Exercise can tone muscle in a particular area but it can't get rid of fat. In fact, the only way to lose "beer bellies" and "thunder thighs" is to cut back on fat, and do some kind of aerobic exercise such as brisk walking or jogging. As you create a demand for energy, the body relies on fat stores (the areas that contain the biggest fat stores go first) to supply needed fuel.
- *Musical pounds*—Researchers at Johns Hopkins Medical Institute in Baltimore find that playing soft classical music during meals can keep dieters from eating too fast and too much. Conversely, studies show that a pulsating rock 'n' roll rhythm causes diners to eat nearly twice as fast. More important, faster eaters end up eating much more.
- *Diet readiness*—New research suggests that major life changes—a divorce, a new job, a death in the family—can diminish weight-control efforts. It might be better to wait until you can give weight-loss efforts your full attention before starting a diet.
- *Fat tricks*—When scientists from Cornell University covertly cut the fat content of

foods served to the participants in one research study, volunteers ended up losing more than six pounds in just twelve weeks. Happily, participants were satisfied with the foods; no one noticed that fat had been trimmed.

References

National Institutes of Health Technology Assessment Conference Statement: Methods for Voluntary Weight Loss and Control. April, 1992.

Kuczmarski, R.J. "Prevalence of overweight and weight gain in the United States." *American Journal of Clinical Nutrition;* 55: 4955–59, 1992.

Ravussin, E., et al. "A brief overview of human energy metabolism and its relationship to essential obesity." *American Journal of Clinical Nutrition;* 55: 242S–245S, 1992.

Brownell, K.D., et al. "The heterogeneity of obesity. Fitting treatments to individuals." *Behavior Therapy;* 22:152–77, 1991.

Goodrick, G.K., et al. "Why treatments for obesity don't last." *Journal of the American Dietetic Association;* 91: 1255–57, 1991.

Lissner, L., et al. "Variability of body weight and health outcomes in the Framingham population." *The New England Journal of Medicine;* 324: 1839–44, 1991.

Pi-Synyer, X. "Health implications of obesity." *American Journal of Clinical Nutrition;* 53(Suppl): 1595–1603, 1991.

Wooley, S.C., et al. "Obesity treatment: the high cost of false hope." *Journal of the American Dietetic Association;* 91: 1248–51, 1991.

The American Dietetic Association. *The Healthy Weigh: a practical food guide.* 1991.

Hart, J., et al. "The importance of family support in a behavior modification weight loss program." *Journal of the American Dietetic Association;* 90(9): 1270–71, 1990.

Bouchard, C., et al. "The response to longterm overfeeding in identical twins. *The New England Journal of Medicine;* 322: 1477–82, 1990.

Rodin, J., et al. "Weight cycling and fat distribution." *International Journal of Obesity;* 14: 303–10, 1990.

Wadden, T.A., et al. "Long-term effects of dieting on resting metabolic rate in obese patients." *Journal of the American Medical Association;* 264: 707–711, 1990.

Stunkard, A.J., et al. "The body mass index of twins who have been reared apart." *The New England Journal of Medicine;* 322: 1483–87, 1990.

Ravussin, E., et al. "Reduced rate of energy expenditure as a risk factor for body weight gain." *The New England Journal of Medicine;* 318: 467–72, 1988.

Roberts, S.B., et al. "Energy expenditure and intake in infants born to lean and overweight mothers." *The New England Journal of Medicine;* 318 461–66, 1988.

Brownell, K.D., et al. "Improving long-term weight loss: pushing the limits of treatment." *Behavior Therapy;* 18: 353–374, 1987.

Callaway, C.W. *The Callaway Diet: Successful Permanent Weight Control for Starvers, Stuffers and Skippers.* New York: Bantam Books, 1990.

Foreyt, J.P. and Goodrick, K.G. *Living Without Dieting.* Houston: Harrison Publishing Company, 1992.

Nash, J.D. *Now That You've Lost It.* Palo Alto: Bull Publishing Company, 1992.

GLOSSARY

Amino acids—the building blocks of protein; made up of nitrogen-containing compounds attached to acids. The body can manufacture amino acids except for these nine essential building blocks: tryptophan, valine, threonine, isoleucine, leucine, lysine, phenylalanine, methionine, histidine. Essential amino acids must be supplied by diet.

Anemia—a condition in which there is a shortage of red blood cells or hemoglobin or both. Nutritional deficiencies can cause anemia, or it can be caused by other factors such as prolonged blood loss.

Antibody—a protein produced by the body in response to foreign invaders (antigens). Antibodies destroy and deactivate antigens by attaching to them and rendering them harmless.

Antigen—foreign substances (including proteins in foods) that provoke an immune response.

Antioxidant—a compound that reacts with oxygen in an effort to protect other substances from oxidation. Antioxidants added to processed foods keep oils and fats from spoiling. Antioxidants (vitamin C, vitamin E, beta-carotene) already in foods may protect against cancer, cataracts, and heart disease.

Arteries—vessels that carry blood away from the heart.

Atherosclerosis—The gradual build-up of plaque on artery and blood vessel walls that can interfere with blood flow. As blood vessels narrow due to plaque build-up, blood flow can be shut off leading to heart attack or stroke.

Basal metabolic rate—the rate at which the body burns or uses energy to support life-sustaining activities such as digestion and respiration.

Beta-carotene—the orange pigment found in many fruits and vegetables. It is not a nutrient, but the body can easily convert beta-carotene into vitamin A. Because it can act as an antioxidant, beta-carotene shows promise as a protector against heart disease and certain types of cancer.

Calories—term for kilocalories or units of energy. One kilocalorie is the amount of heat required to raise the temperature of one kilogram of water one degree celsius.

Carcinogen—an environmental substance or substance in food that influences the development of cancer.

Cholesterol—a crystalline fatlike substance found in the tissues of both animals and people.

(Plants do not contain cholesterol.) Cholesterol is necessary for growth, but excessive amounts of cholesterol in the blood increase the risk for heart disease.

Colostrum—a watery solution secreted in the first few days of breastfeeding that is rich in substances that help prevent infection.

Cruciferous vegetables—a group of plants that are members of the mustard family and have cross-shaped blossoms: cauliflower, cabbage, broccoli, collard greens, mustard greens, bok choy, brussel sprouts, radishes, rutabagas, and turnips. Studies conducted on animals found these vegetables may help protect against cancer.

Electrolytes—chemical substances that carry electrical charges when dissolved in water. Sodium and potassium are two electrolytes that help regulate fluid balance.

Estrogen—a female hormone that plays a role in maintaining the body's calcium balance and possibly helps protect women from heart disease in the premenopausal years. Estrogen levels begin to decline after menopause.

Fatty acids—building blocks of fat made up of carbon, oxygen, and hydrogen. The number of hydrogen atoms influences the degree of saturation. Unsaturated fats have fewer hydrogen atoms; saturated fats have more hydrogen.

Fiber—indigestible substances found in food. Most fibers are carbohydrates such as cellulose, hemicellulose, pectin, and gum. But lignin, a noncarbohydrate woody material that makes up the stems and bark of many plants, is sometimes classified as fiber. While the body lacks enzymes necessary to digest fiber, the substance is critical to health. Fibers can help lower blood cholesterol levels, prevent constipation, and possibly protect against certain types of cancer.

Glucose—a simple sugar used by the body for quick energy.

Gram—metric unit of weight measurement. Thirty grams is roughly equivalent to one ounce.

High-density lipoproteins (HDL)—one of several transport compounds made of protein and various amounts and types of fat. HDL packages carry cholesterol away from the arteries and blood vessels to the liver where it can be processed. High levels of HDL are associated with a decreased risk for heart disease.

Hormone—several of a group of powerful substances secreted by different body glands and tissues to help regulate different body functions. Insulin regulates blood sugar; thyroid hormones regulate metabolism. Glands that produce hormones include the adrenal glands, gonads (ovaries and testes), pancreas, parathyroid glands, pituitary gland, and the thyroid gland. Other tissues such as the kidneys, intestines, and the brain can also secrete hormones.

Hydrogenation—the chemical process of adding hydrogen to unsaturated fats (vegetable oils) to make them more solid. The solid fats produced contain more saturated fatty acids than the liquids from which they were made.

Immunity—ability to resist infection; largely the result of substances in the immune system (antibodies) that recognize and fight off foreign invaders that cause disease.

Insulin—a hormone secreted by the pancreas in response to an elevation in blood sugar. Insulin is the key that unlocks body cells so that glucose can enter. Without insulin or sufficient amounts of insulin, glucose would concentrate in the blood.

Irradiation—a food-processing procedure using gamma rays to destroy microorganisms and prolong shelf life of foods. Currently approved for use on spices, pork, poultry, and some fruit but not used extensively due to lack of widespread public acceptance.

Lactose—a disaccharide (double sugar) found in milk products; composed of galactose and glucose. Also called milk sugar.

Lactose intolerance—An inherited disorder characterized by lack of the enzyme needed to digest milk sugar. Without the enzyme, drinking milk can bring on abdominal pain, nausea, and diarrhea.

Legume—part of a large plant family of herbs, shrubs and trees, the pods or seeds of legumes are higher in protein than most plant foods: kidney bean, soybean, peanuts, black-eyed peas, lentils.

Low-density lipoproteins (LDL)—one of several transport compounds made of protein and various amounts and types of fat. LDL carry cholesterol from the liver to body tissues for storage. High levels of LDL are associated with an increased risk for heart disease.

Megadose—A dose that is ten times the level recommended as safe and adequate. The term is typically used when referring to vitamin supplements that offer excessive amounts of a nutrient, amounts that make the nutrient more like a drug, and thus bring on druglike side effects.

Menopause—The cessation of menstruation and the fluctuating hormone levels and biological changes that accompany it. Women enter menopause at around the age of forty-five to fifty.

Milligram—Metric unit of weight measurement that is frequently used to relate micronutrient needs. One milligram is equivalent to one-thousandth of a gram. (Approximately thirty grams make up one ounce.)

Minerals—inorganic elements, some of which are known to be vital to health in small or trace quantities.

Neurotransmitter—a chemical in the body that transmits a nerve impulse from one cell to the next. Serotonin, a compound that may help improve mood, is an example of one of these chemical messengers.

Nutrient density—the amount of nutrients in a serving of food in relation to that food's total energy contribution. If a food delivers a large amount of nutrients and has very few calories it is considered nutrient-dense.

Nutrients—substances obtained from food that promote growth, maintenance or repair of worn or injured body tissues. There are six classes of nutrients: carbohydrate, protein, fat, vitamins, minerals, and water.

Omega-3 fatty acids—a type of polyunsaturated fat that may help reduce the risk of heart disease. Omega-3 fats are found mainly in fatty fish such as salmon and mackerel.

Organic—substances that contain carbon. Organic compounds can come from nature or be created by scientists.

Osteoporosis—A bone disease of old age, osteoporosis is characterized by brittle, porous bones. Problems result when these bones fracture and crack with little stress.

Placebo—a pill or compound that is similar in appearance to an agent being tested in a clinical trial but has no effect. Often referred to as a *sugar pill,* but can contain other harmless but inactive substances.

Risk factors—characteristics, behaviors or traits that are linked with the development of chronic lifestyle illnesses such as heart disease, cancer, and osteoporosis.

RDA—the Recommended Dietary Allowances, set by the Food and Nutrition Board of the National Academy of Sciences, are the amount of a nutrient needed by normal, healthy people.

Serotonin—a neurotransmitter made within the brain from the amino acid tryptophan. It is believed to promote sleepiness and have a calming effect on mood.

Trans-fatty acids—the altered fat compounds produced when polyunsaturated vegetable oils are hydrogenated into solid fats like margarine. Studies suggest that trans-fats can raise blood-cholesterol levels.

Triglycerides—the chemical name for a major class of fats that contain one unit of glycerol attached to three fatty acids. Triglycerides are the major fats found in foods, and are also present in the blood.

Vegan—this type of vegetarian eats only plant foods, and they must plan their diets carefully.

Vitamins—complex organic substances, small quantities of which are vital to health.

Whole grains—the seeds of cereals (oats, wheat, barley) that are milled intact with only the inedible outer coating or husk peeled away during processing.

Part II

ENCYCLOPEDIA

OF DAILY VALUES

FOR BRAND NAME

AND BASIC FOODS

*Including Calories, Protein,
Fat, Saturated Fat, Cholesterol,
Carbohydrates, Fiber, Sodium,
Potassium, Calcium, Iron, Zinc,
Magnesium, Vitamin A, Vitamin C,
Thiamine, Riboflavin, Niacin,
Vitamin B_{12}, Folic Acid*

	Calories	Protein	Fat	Sat. Fat	Cholesterol	Carbohydrates	Fiber	Sodium	Potassium	Calcium	Iron	Zinc	Magnesium	Vitamin A	Vitamin C	Thiamin	Riboflavin	Niacin	Vitamin B12	Folic acid
ABALONE																				
raw 3 oz	89	24	*	*	24	2	*	11	6	3	15	5	10	*	3	11	5	6	10	*
fried 3 oz	161	28	9	7	27	3	*	21	7	3	18	5	12	*	3	12	6	8	10	*
ACEROLA, RAW																				
1/2 cup	31	*	*	*	*	2	4	*	4	*	*	—	4	15	2739	*	3	2	*	—
1 fruit	2	*	*	*	*	*	*	*	*	*	*	—	*	*	134	*	*	*	*	—
ACEROLA JUICE																				
8 fl oz	51	2	*			4	4		7	2	7	—	7	25	6451	3	9	5	*	—
ACORN																				
raw 1 oz	105	3	10	5	*	4	—	*	4	*	*	*	4	*	*	2	2	3	*	6
dried 1 oz	145	4	14	6	*	5	—	*	6	2	2	*	6	*	*	3	3	3	*	8
ACORN FLOUR																				
1 oz	142	4	13	6	*	5	—	*	6	*	2	*	8	*	*	3	3	3	*	8
ACORN SQUASH see SQUASH																				
ADZUKI BEAN																				
cooked 1/2 cup	147	14	*	*	*	9	—	*	17	3	13	14	15	*	*	9	4	4	*	35
cooked, salted 1/2 cup	147	14	*	*	*	9	—	12	17	3	13	14	15	*	*	9	4	4	*	35
ADZUKI BEAN, CANNED																				
sweetened 1/2 cup	351	9	*	*	*	27	—	13	5	3	9	15	11	*	*	10	5	5	*	40
ALFALFA SPROUTS																				
raw 1 cup	10	2	*	*	*	*	4	*	*	*	2	2	2	*	5	2	2	*	*	3
ALFREDO SAUCE see PASTA SAUCE																				
ALLSPICE, GROUND																				
1 tbsp	16	*	*	*	*	*	4	*	2	4	2	*	2	*	4	*	*	*	*	—
ALMOND																				
barbecue (Blue Diamond) 1 oz	160	10	25	5	*	2	12	9	3	10	6	2	20	*	*	2	15	6	—	—
blanched slivered (Blue Diamond) 1 oz	150	10	20	5	*	2	12	*	6	8	6	8	25	*	*	*	10	4	—	—
whole (Blue Diamond) 1 oz	150	10	20	5	*	2	12	*	4	8	8	8	25	*	*	*	8	4	—	—
chili w/ lemon (Blue Diamond) 1 oz	160	10	20	5	*	2	12	7	3	10	6	6	20	*	*	*	15	6	—	—
dried (generic) 1 oz	167	9	23	7	*	2	12	*	6	8	6	6	21	*	*	4	13	5	*	4
blanched (generic) 1 oz	166	10	23	7	*	2	8	*	6	7	6	6	20	*	*	3	11	4	*	3
dry roasted (generic) 1 oz	167	8	23	7	*	2	16	*	6	8	6	9	22	*	*	2	10	4	*	5
unsalted (Blue Diamond) 1 oz	150	10	20	5	*	2	16	*	5	10	8	8	25	*	*	*	25	*	—	—
w/ salt (generic) 1 oz	167	8	23	7	*	2	16	9	6	8	6	9	22	*	*	2	10	4	*	5
honey roasted (Blue Diamond) 1 oz	140	10	18	5	*	3	12	2	5	8	4	4	15	*	*	2	15	4	—	—
(generic) 1 oz	168	9	22	7	*	3	—	2	5	7	4	5	17	*	*	2	16	4	*	2
natural chopped (Blue Diamond) 1 oz	150	10	20	5	*	2	12	*	5	10	8	8	25	*	*	*	10	4	—	—
sliced (Blue Diamond) 1 oz	150	10	20	5	*	2	12	*	5	10	8	8	25	*	*	*	10	4	—	—

	Calories	Protein	Fat	Sat. Fat	Cholesterol	Carbohydrates	Fiber	Sodium	Potassium	Calcium	Iron	Zinc	Magnesium	Vitamin A	Vitamin C	Thiamin	Riboflavin	Niacin	Vitamin B₁₂	Folic acid
ALMOND (continued)																				
whole (Blue Diamond) 1 oz	150	10	20	5	*	2	16	*	5	10	8	8	25	*	*	*	15	4	—	—
oil roasted (generic) 1 oz	176	10	25	8	*	*	12	*	6	7	6	9	22	*	*	2	17	5	*	5
blanched (generic) 1 oz	174	9	25	8	*	2	12	*	6	6	8	3	21	*	*	*	5	6	*	5
w/salt (generic) 1 oz	174	9	25	8	*	2	12	9	6	6	8	3	21	*	*	*	5	6	*	5
unblanched w/ salt (generic) 1 oz	176	10	25	8	*	*	12	9	6	7	6	9	22	*	*	2	17	5	*	5
salted (Blue Diamond) 1 oz	150	10	20	5	*	*	12	6	3	6	4	6	20	*	*	2	15	4	—	—
smokehouse (Blue Diamond) 1 oz	150	10	22	5	*	*	12	7	3	4	8	2	20	*	*	2	20	4	—	—
sour cream & onion (Blue Diamond) 1 oz	150	10	22	5	*	*	12	6	3	6	4	6	20	*	*	2	15	4	—	—
toasted (generic) 1 oz	167	10	22	7	*	2	12	*	6	8	8	9	22	*	*	2	10	4	*	5
unsalted (Blue Diamond) 1 oz	150	10	20	5	*	2	16	*	5	10	8	8	25	*	*	*	25	*	—	—
ALMOND BUTTER																				
plain salted 1 tbsp	101	4	15	5	*	*	4	3	3	4	3	3	12	*	*	*	6	2	*	3
w/ honey & cinnamon salted 1 tbsp	96	4	13	4	*	*	4	*	3	4	3	3	12	*	*	*	6	2	*	3
unsalted 1 tbsp	96	4	13	4	*	*	—	*	3	4	3	3	12	*	*	*	6	2	*	3
ALMOND MEAL																				
partially defatted 1 oz	116	19	8	3	*	3	—	*	11	12	13	5	20	*	*	6	28	9	*	4
salted 1 oz	116	19	8	3	*	3	—	9	11	12	13	5	20	*	*	6	28	9	*	4
ALMOND OIL 1 tbsp	120	*	20	6	*	*	*	*	*	*	*	*	*	*	*	*	*	*	*	*
ALMOND PASTE 1 oz	127	6	12	4	*	4	16	*	5	7	5	5	18	*	*	4	12	4	*	4
ALMOND POWDER																				
partially defatted 1 oz	112	18	7	2	*	3	—	*	6	7	5	6	19	*	*	3	11	4	*	3
regular 1 oz	168	9	23	7	*	2	—	*	6	6	4	*	22	*	*	4	20	3	*	4
AMARANTH																				
raw 1/2 cup	4	*	*	*	*	*	*	*	2	3	2	*	2	8	10	*	*	*	*	3
boiled 1/2 cup	14	2	*	*	*	*	—	*	12	14	8	4	9	37	45	*	5	2	*	9
boiled w/ salt 1/2 cup	14	2	*	*	*	*	—	7	12	14	8	4	9	37	45	*	5	2	*	9
ANCHOVY																				
raw 3 oz	111	29	6	6	17	*	*	4	9	12	15	10	9	*	*	3	13	60	9	*
canned in oil 1/2 can	47	5	2	*	3	*	*	17	2	3	3	2	2	*	*	*	2	11	3	*
ANISE SEED 1 tbsp	23	2	2	—	*	*	4	*	3	4	14	2	3	*	*	2	2	*	*	*
ANTELOPE																				
roasted 4 oz	170	55	5	6	47	*	*	3	12	*	26	13	8	*	*	20	49	—	—	—

	Calories	Protein	Fat	Sat. Fat	Cholesterol	Carbohydrates	Fiber	Sodium	Potassium	Calcium	Iron	Zinc	Magnesium	Vitamin A	Vitamin C	Thiamin	Riboflavin	Niacin	Vitamin B₁₂	Folic acid
APPLE																				
raw																				
w/ out skin																				
1 fruit	73	*	*	*	*	6	8	*	4	*	*	*	*	*	9	*	*	*	—	*
w/ skin																				
1 fruit	81	*	*	*	*	7	16	*	5	*	*	*	2	*	13	2	*	*	—	*
boiled																				
1/2 cup slices	46	*	*	*	*	4	8	*	2	*	*	*	*	*	*	*	*	*	—	*
microwaved																				
1/2 cup slices	48	*	*	*	*	4	8	*	2	*	*	*	*	*	*	*	*	*	—	*
APPLE, CANNED																				
sweetened																				
1/2 cup slices	68	*	*	*	*	6	8	*	2	*	*	*	*	*	*	*	*	*	—	*
APPLE, DEHYDRATED, SULFURED																				
raw																				
1/2 cup	104	*	*	*	*	9	16	2	5	*	3	*	2	*	*	*	2	*	—	*
cooked																				
1/2 cup	72	*	*	*	*	6	—	*	4	*	2	*	*	*	*	*	2	*	—	*
APPLE, DRIED																				
1/4 cup	45	*	*	*	*	5	11	7	—	*	*	—	—	*	*	—	—	—	—	*
(generic) 1/2 cup halves	104	*	*	*	*	9	16	2	6	*	3	*	2	*	3	*	4	2	—	—
cooked																				
w/ out sugar																				
1/2 cup	73	*	*	*	*	7	12	*	4	*	2	*	*	*	2	*	*	*	—	—
w/ sugar																				
1/2 cup	116	*	*	*	*	10	12	*	4	*	2	*	*	*	2	*	*	*	—	—
APPLE, FROZEN																				
unsweetened																				
1/2 cup slices	41	*	*	*	*	4	4	*	2	*	*	*	*	*	*	*	*	*	*	*
heated																				
1/2 cup slices	48	*	*	*	*	4	—	*	2	*	*	*	*	*	*	*	*	*	*	*
APPLE BUTTER																				
(generic) 1 tbsp	33	*	*	*	*	3	*	*	*	*	*	*	*	*	*	*	*	*	*	*
(Smucker's Autumn Harvest)																				
1 tbsp	12	*	*	*	*	*	*	*	*	*	*	*	*	*	*	*	*	*	*	*
(Smucker's Natural) 1 tbsp	12	*	*	*	*	*	*	*	*	*	*	*	*	*	*	*	*	*	*	*
(Smucker's Simply Fruit) 1 tbsp	12	*	*	*	*	*	*	*	*	*	*	*	*	*	*	*	*	*	*	*
APPLE CHIPS																				
(Weight Watchers) 1 bag (3/4 oz)	70	*	*	*	*	6	12	5	—	*	*	—	—	*	*	—	—	—	—	—
APPLE CIDER																				
sparkling																				
(Welch's) 6 fl oz	100	*	*	*	*	8	*	*	—	*	*	*	*	*	*	*	*	*	*	*
spiced																				
(Knudsen Apple Blend) 8 fl oz	120	*	*	*	*	10	*	*	5	*	2	—	—	*	6	—	—	*	*	*
APPLE CRISP																				
(homemade) 1/2 cup	230	4	8	5	*	15	—	11	4	4	6	2	2	4	5	8	6	5	—	2
APPLE DISH, FROZEN																				
escalloped apples																				
(Stouffer's Side Dishes) 12 oz	180	*	5	—	—	12	12	3	3	*	*	—	—	*	80	2	*	*	—	—
APPLE DRINK																				
from concentrate																				
(Mott's Fruit Basket) 8 fl oz	120	*	*	*	*	10	*	*	9	2	6	—	—	*	25	*	*	*	—	—
APPLE DUMPLING																				
(Pepperidge Farm) 1 dumpling	260	4	20	—	—	11	—	10	—	*	4	—	—	*	*	2	2	2	—	—
APPLE FRITTERS																				
frozen																				
(Mrs. Paul's) 4 oz	240	8	14	10	2	12	—	21	—	2	2	—	—	*	15	10	8	*	—	—
APPLE FRUIT SQUARE																				
(Pepperidge Farm) 2 1/2 oz	220	2	18	—	—	9	—	7	—	*	4	—	—	*	*	*	*	*	—	—

	Calories	Protein	Fat	Sat. Fat	Cholesterol	Carbohydrates	Fiber	Sodium	Potassium	Calcium	Iron	Zinc	Magnesium	Vitamin A	Vitamin C	Thiamin	Riboflavin	Niacin	Vitamin B$_{12}$	Folic acid
APPLE JUICE, BOTTLED/CANNED																				
clear																				
(generic) 8 fl oz	117	*	*	*	*	10	*	*	8	2	5	*	2	*	4	3	2	*	*	*
(Knudsen) 8 fl oz	110	*	*	*	*	9	*	*	6	*	*	—	—	*	4	—	—	—	—	—
(Mott's) 8 fl oz	120	*	*	*	*	10	*	*	7	*	4	—	—	*	4	*	*	*	—	—
(Ocean Spray) 8 fl oz	110	—	*	*	*	9	*	*	7	*	*	—	—	*	*	—	—	—	—	—
gravenstein																				
(Heinke's) 8 fl oz	120	*	*	*	*	10	*	*	5	*	2	—	—	*	6	—	—	—	—	—
organic																				
(Knudsen) 8 fl oz	120	*	*	*	*	10	*	*	5	*	2	—	—	*	6	—	—	—	—	—
natural																				
(Heinke's) 8 fl oz	120	*	*	*	*	10	*	*	5	*	2	—	—	*	6	—	—	—	—	—
(Knudsen) 8 fl oz	120	*	*	*	*	10	*	*	5	*	2	—	—	*	6	—	—	—	—	—
(Mott's) 8 fl oz	120	*	*	*	*	10	*	*	7	*	4	—	—	*	4	*	*	*	—	—
(Red Cheek) 8 fl oz	120	*	*	*	*	10	*	*	7	*	4	—	—	*	4	—	—	—	—	—
from concentrate																				
(Knudsen) 8 fl oz	120	*	*	*	*	10	*	*	5	*	2	—	—	*	6	—	—	—	—	—
organic																				
(Heinke's) 8 fl oz	120	*	*	*	*	10	*	*	5	*	2	—	—	*	6	—	—	—	—	—
(Knudsen) 8 fl oz	120	*	*	*	*	10	*	*	5	*	2	—	—	*	6	—	—	—	—	—
(Santa Cruz Natural) 8 fl oz	120	*	*	*	*	10	*	*	5	*	2	—	—	*	6	—	—	—	—	—
vitamin C added																				
(generic) 8 fl oz	117	*	*	*	*	10	—	*	8	2	5	*	2	*	172	3	2	—	*	*
APPLE JUICE, FROM CONCENTRATE																				
(generic) 6 fl oz	350	2	*	*	*	29	4	2	27	4	11	2	9	*	7	2	7	*	*	*
(Red Cheek) 8 fl oz	120	*	*	*	*	10	*	*	7	*	4	—	—	*	4	*	*	*	—	—
vitamin C added																				
(generic) 6 fl oz	350	2	*	*	*	29	—	2	27	4	11	2	9	*	313	2	7	*	*	*
APPLE-APRICOT JUICE																				
(Knudsen Apple Blend) 8 fl oz	120	*	*	*	*	10	*	*	4	2	2	—	—	10	2	—	—	—	—	—
APPLE-BANANA JUICE																				
(Knudsen Apple Blend) 8 fl oz	120	*	*	*	*	10	*	*	5	*	2	—	—	*	6	—	—	—	—	—
APPLE-BOYSENBERRY CIDER																				
(Heinke's) 8 fl oz	120	*	*	*	*	10	*	*	5	*	2	—	—	*	6	—	—	—	—	—
APPLE-BOYSENBERRY JUICE																				
(Heinke's) 8 fl oz	120	*	*	*	*	10	*	*	5	*	2	—	—	*	6	—	—	—	—	—
(Knudsen Apple Blend) 8 fl oz	120	*	*	*	*	10	*	*	5	*	2	—	—	*	6	—	—	—	—	—
APPLE-CHERRY CIDER																				
(Heinke's) 8 fl oz	115	*	*	*	*	9	*	*	6	2	4	—	—	*	2	—	—	—	—	—
(Knudsen Apple Blend) 8 fl oz	130	*	*	*	*	11	*	*	7	2	4	—	—	*	2	—	—	—	—	—
from concentrate																				
(Knudsen) 8 fl oz	130	*	*	*	*	11	*	*	7	2	4	—	—	*	2	—	—	—	—	—
APPLE-CRANBERRY DRINK																				
(Mott's) 10 fl oz	180	*	*	*	*	15	*	*	2	*	*	—	—	*	*	*	*	*	—	—
(Ocean Spray Cranapple) 8 fl oz	160	—	*	*	*	14	2	*	—	*	*	—	—	*	100	—	—	—	—	—
(Tropicana) 6 fl oz	110	*	*	*	—	9	—	*	—	2	2	—	—	*	2	6	4	*	—	—
reduced calorie																				
(Ocean Spray Cranapple) 8 fl oz	50	—	*	*	*	4	*	*	4	*	*	—	—	*	100	—	—	—	—	—
APPLE-CRANBERRY JUICE																				
(Knudsen Apple Blend) 8 fl oz	120	*	*	*	*	10	*	*	5	*	2	—	—	*	6	—	—	—	—	—
(Mott's) 8 fl oz	120	*	*	*	*	10	*	*	9	2	4	—	—	*	4	*	*	*	—	—
(Smucker's) 8 fl. oz.	120	*	*	*	*	11	*	*	8	*	2	*	*	*	6	2	4	2	*	*
organic																				
(Santa Cruz Natural) 8 fl oz	120	*	*	*	*	10	*	*	5	*	2	—	—	*	6	—	—	—	—	—
APPLE-GRAPE JUICE																				
(Mott's) 8 fl oz	120	*	*	*	*	10	*	*	7	*	2	—	—	*	2	*	*	*	—	—

	Calories	Protein	Fat	Sat. Fat	Cholesterol	Carbohydrates	Fiber	Sodium	Potassium	Calcium	Iron	Zinc	Magnesium	Vitamin A	Vitamin C	Thiamin	Riboflavin	Niacin	Vitamin B₁₂	Folic acid
APPLE-GRAPE-CHERRY DRINK																				
aseptic pack (Welch's) 8 1/2 oz (1 box)	150	*	*	*	*	12	*	*	3	*	*	—	—	*	*	*	*	*	—	—
(Welch's Orchard) 8 1/2 oz (1 box)	150	*	*	*	*	12	*	*	3	*	*	*	*	*	*	*	*	*	*	*
from concentrate (Welch's) 6 fl oz	100	*	*	*	*	9	*	*	3	*	*	—	—	*	*	*	*	*	*	*
APPLE-GRAPE-RASPBERRY DRINK																				
(Welch's Orchard) 8 1/2 oz (1 box)	150	*	*	*	*	12	*	*	4	*	*	*	*	*	*	*	*	*	*	*
aseptic pack (Welch's) 8 1/2 oz (1 box)	150	*	*	*	*	12	*	*	4	*	*	—	—	*	*	*	*	*	—	—
from concentrate (Welch's) 6 fl oz	—	*	*	*	*	—	*	*	*	*	*	*	*	*	*	*	*	*	*	*
APPLE-PEACH JUICE																				
(Knudsen Apple Blend) 8 fl oz	120	*	*	*	*	10	*	*	5	*	2	—	—	*	6	—	—	—	—	—
APPLE-RASPBERRY DRINK																				
(Mott's) 10 fl oz	140	*	*	*	*	11	*	*	2	*	2			*	6	—	—	—	—	—
from concentrate (Mott's Fruit Basket) 8 fl oz	130	*	*	*	*	10	*	*	4	2	4			*	25	*	*	*	*	*
APPLE-RASPBERRY JUICE																				
(Heinke's) 8 fl oz	120	*	*	*	*	10	*	*	5	*	2	—	—	*	6	—	—	—	—	—
(Knudsen Apple Blend) 8 fl oz	120	*	*	*	*	10	*	*	5	*	2	—	—	*	6	—	—	—	—	—
(Mott's) 8 1/2 fl oz	120	*	*	*	*	10	*	*	8	*	4	—	—	*	10	*	*	*	—	—
organic (Santa Cruz Natural) 8 fl oz	120	*	*	*	*	10	*	*	5	*	2	—	—	*	6	—	—	—	—	—
APPLE-STRAWBERRY JUICE																				
(Knudsen Apple Blend) 8 fl oz	120	*	*	*	*	10	*	*	5	*	2	—	—	*	6	—	—	—	—	—
organic (Santa Cruz Natural) 8 fl oz	120	*	*	*	*	10	*	*	5	*	2	—	—	*	6	—	—	—	—	—
APPLE PIE see PIE																				
APPLESAUCE																				
chunky (Mott's) 5 oz	110	*	*	*	*	9	8	*	3	*	*	—	—	*	2	—	—	—	—	—
(Mussleman's) 1/2 cup	100	*	*	*	*	8	8	*	—	*	*	—	—	*	*	—	—	—	—	—
cinnamon (Mott's) 5 oz	120	*	*	*	*	10	4	*	2	*	*	—	—	*	4	—	—	—	—	—
sweetened (generic) 1/2 cup	97	*	*	*	*	8	8	*	2	*	2	*	*	*	4	*	2	*	—	*
(Mott's) 5 oz	110	*	*	*	*	9	4	*	2	*	*	—	—	*	4	—	—	—	—	—
vitamin C added (generic) 1/2 cup	97	*	*	*	*	8	—	*	2	*	2	*	*	*	4	*	2	*	—	—
unsweetened (generic) 1/2 cup	52	*	*	*	*	5	4	*	3	*	*	*	*	*	2	*	2	*	—	—
unsweetened vitamin C added (generic) 1/2 cup	52	*	*	*	*	5	—	*	3	*	*	*	*	*	43	*	2	*	—	—
APRICOT																				
1/2 cup halves	37	2	*	*	*	3	8	*	7	*	2	*	2	41	13	2	2	2	—	2
1 fruit	17	*	*	*	*	*	4	*	3	*	*	*	*	18	6	*	*	*	—	*
APRICOT, CANNED																				
in extra heavy syrup w/ out skin 1/2 cup	118	*	*	*	*	10	—	*	4	*	4	*	2	36	5	*	2	2	—	*
in extra light syrup w/ skin 1/2 cup halves	61	*	*	*	*	5	—	*	5	*	2	*	2	32	8	2	*	4	—	*
in heavy syrup w/ out skin 1/2 cup	107	*	*	*	*	9	—	*	5	*	3	*	3	32	6	2	2	3	—	*

	Calories	Protein	Fat	Sat. Fat	Cholesterol	Carbohydrates	Fiber	Sodium	Potassium	Calcium	Iron	Zinc	Magnesium	Vitamin A	Vitamin C	Thiamin	Riboflavin	Niacin	Vitamin B$_{12}$	Folic acid
APRICOT, CANNED (continued)																				
w/ skin																				
1/2 cup halves	107	*	*	*	*	9	8	*	5	*	2	*	2	32	7	2	2	2	—	*
(Del Monte) 1/2 cup	100	*	*	*	*	9	4	*	—	*	2	—	—	40	8	—	—	—	—	—
in juice																				
w/ skin																				
1/2 cup halves	60	*	*	*	*	5	8	*	6	*	2	*	3	42	10	*	*	2	—	*
in light syrup																				
w/ skin																				
1/2 cup halves	80	*	*	*	*	7	8	*	5	*	3	*	3	34	6	*	*	2	—	*
in water																				
w/ out skin																				
1/2 cup	25	*	*	*	*	2	—	*	5	*	3	*	3	41	3	2	2	2	—	*
w/ skin																				
1/2 cup halves	33	*	*	*	*	3	8	*	7	*	2	*	2	32	7	2	2	2	—	*
lite																				
w/ skin																				
(Del Monte) 1/2 cup	60	*	*	*	*	5	4	*	—	*	2	—	—	40	8	—	—	—	—	—
APRICOT, DEHYDRATED																				
raw																				
1/2 cup	192	5	*	*	*	17	—	*	32	4	21	4	9	152	9	2	5	11	—	*
cooked																				
1/2 cup	156	4	*	*	*	13	—	*	26	3	17	3	8	109	15	*	5	10	—	—
APRICOT, DRIED																				
(Del Monte Snap-E-Tom) 1/4 cup	45	3	*	*	*	5	14	*	—	*	—	—	—	51	5					
cooked																				
1/2 cup halves	106	3	*	*	*	9	16	*	17	2	12	2	5	59	3	*	2	6	—	—
cooked w/ sugar																				
1/2 cup halves	153	3	*	*	*	13	16	*	17	2	11	2	5	58	3	*	2	6	—	—
sulfured																				
1/2 cup halves	155	4	*	*	*	13	24	*	26	3	17	3	8	94	3	*	6	10	—	2
APRICOT, FROZEN																				
sweetened																				
1/2 cup	119	*	*	*	*	10	8	*	8	*	6	*	3	41	18	*	2	3	—	*
APRICOT KERNEL OIL																				
1 tbsp	120	*	22	5	*	*	*	*	*	*	*	*	*	*	*	*	*	*	*	*
APRICOT NECTAR																				
(Del Monte) 8 fl oz	140	2	*	*	*	12	4	*	—	*	2	—	—	50	50	—	—	—	—	—
(generic) 6 fl oz	105	*	*	*	*	9	4	*	6	*	4	*	2	49	2	*	2	2	*	*
(Knudsen Exotic Blends) 8 fl oz	120	*	*	*	*	10	*	*	4	2	2	—	—	10	2	—	—	—	—	—
vitamin C added																				
(generic) 8 fl oz	141	2	*	*	*	12	—	*	8	2	5	2	3	66	227	2	2	3	*	*
ARROWHEAD																				
raw																				
1 large corm	25	2	*	*	*	2	—	*	7	*	4	*	3	*	*	3	*	2	*	*
boiled																				
3 oz	66	6	*	*	*	5	—	*	21	*	6	*	10	*	*	8	3	5	*	2
boiled w/ salt																				
1 medium corm	9	*	*	*	*	*	—	*	3	*	*	*	*	*	*	*	*	*	*	*
ARTICHOKE																				
raw																				
1 medium artichoke	60	7	*	*	*	4	28	5	14	6	9	4	19	5	25	6	5	7	*	22
boiled																				
1 medium artichoke	60	7	*	*	*	4	24	5	12	5	9	4	18	4	20	5	5	6	*	15
boiled w/ salt																				
1 medium artichoke	60	7	*	*	*	4	24	17	12	5	9	4	18	4	20	5	5	6	*	15
ARTICHOKE, FROZEN																				
boiled																				
3 oz	36	4	*	*	*	2	—	2	6	2	2	2	6	3	7	3	7	4	*	24

	Calories	Protein	Fat	Sat. Fat	Cholesterol	Carbohydrates	Fiber	Sodium	Potassium	Calcium	Iron	Zinc	Magnesium	Vitamin A	Vitamin C	Thiamin	Riboflavin	Niacin	Vitamin B12	Folic acid
ARTICHOKE, FROZEN (continued)																				
boiled w/ salt																				
3 oz	36	4	*	*	*	2	—	10	6	2	2	2	6	3	7	3	7	4	*	24
ARTICHOKE HEART																				
boiled																				
1/2 cup	42	5	*	*	*	3	20	3	8	4	6	3	13	3	14	4	3	4	*	11
boiled w/ salt																				
1/2 cup	42	5	*	*	*	3	20	12	8	4	6	3	13	3	14	4	3	4	*	11
bottled																				
(Progresso) 1/2 cup	16	3	*	*	*	*	12	12	4	*	2	—	—	*	*	*	*	2	—	—
marinated																				
(Progresso) 1/2 cup	190	2	23	10	*	5	8	19	4	*	2	—	—	*	45	*	2	2	—	—
ARUGULA																				
raw																				
1/2 cup	3	*	*	*	*	*	—	*	*	2	*	*	*	5	2	*	*	*	*	2
1 leaf	1	*	*	*	*	*	—	*	*	*	*	*	*	*	*	*	*	*	*	*
ASPARAGUS																				
boiled																				
4 spears	14	3	*	*	*	*	4	*	3	*	2	2	*	6	11	5	4	3	*	22
1/2 cup	22	4	*	*	*	*	8	*	4	2	4	3	2	10	16	7	7	5	*	33
boiled w/ salt																				
1/2 cup	22	4	*	*	*	*	8	9	4	2	4	3	2	10	16	7	7	5	*	33
4 spears	14	3	*	*	*	*	4	6	3	*	2	2	*	6	11	5	4	3	*	22
ASPARAGUS, CANNED																				
low salt																				
(generic) 1/2 cup	17	4	*	*	*	*	8	*	5	2	4	4	3	12	33	4	6	5	*	26
salad tips																				
(Del Monte) 1/2 cup	20	3	*	*	*	*	4	17	—	*	2	—	—	8	30	—	—	—	—	—
spears																				
(Del Monte) 1/2 cup	20	3	*	*	*	*	4	17	—	*	2	—	—	8	30	—	—	—	—	—
(generic) 1/2 cup	23	4	*	*	*	*	8	20	6	2	12	3	3	13	37	5	7	6	*	29
(Green Giant) 1/2 cup	18	3	*	*	*	*	4	17	5	*	2	—	—	6	20	2	6	2	—	—
extra long																				
(Del Monte) 1/2 cup	20	3	*	*	*	*	4	17	—	*	2	—	—	8	30	—	—	—	—	—
spears, cut																				
(Bush Bros) 1/2 cup	25	5	*	*	*	*	4	16	—	*	10	—	—	8	15	—	—	—	—	—
(Del Monte) 1/2 cup	20	3	*	*	*	*	4	17	—	*	2	—	—	8	30	—	—	—	—	—
(Green Giant) 1/2 cup	18	3	*	*	*	*	4	17	5	*	2	—	—	6	20	2	6	2	—	—
50% less salt																				
(Green Giant) 1/2 cup	18	3	*	*	*	*	4	9	5	*	2	—	—	6	20	2	6	2	—	—
spears, white																				
(Green Giant) 1/2 cup	16	3	*	*	*	*	4	17	6	*	2	—	—	10	30	4	4	4	—	—
tips																				
(Del Monte) 1/2 cup	20	3	*	*	*	*	4	17	—	*	2	—	—	8	30	—	—	—	—	—
ASPARAGUS, FROZEN																				
cuts																				
(Green Giant Harvest Fresh) 1/2 cup	25	5	*	*	*	*	8	4	8	2	4	—	—	10	20	4	4	4	—	—
spears																				
boiled																				
(generic) 4 spears	17	3	*	*	*	*	8	*	4	*	2	2	2	10	24	3	4	3	*	20
boiled w/ salt																				
(generic) 4 spears	17	3	*	*	*	*	8	6	4	*	2	2	2	10	24	3	4	3	*	20
ASPARAGUS COMBINATION, FROZEN																				
asparagus pilaf																				
(Green Giant Garden Gourmet)																				
1 pkg (9 1/2 oz)	190	8	6	10	3	12	12	25	6	4	25	—	—	60	20	60	10	30	—	—

	Calories	Protein	Fat	Sat. Fat	Cholesterol	Carbohydrates	Fiber	Sodium	Potassium	Calcium	Iron	Zinc	Magnesium	Vitamin A	Vitamin C	Thiamin	Riboflavin	Niacin	Vitamin B12	Folic acid
AU JUS GRAVY																				
canned																				
(Franco-American) 1/4 cup	10	*	*	*	—	*	—	14	—	*	*	—	—	*	*	*	*	2	—	—
(generic) 1/4 cup	12	2	*	*	—	*	—	3	2	*	3	5	*	*	2	*	3	4	2	*
from mix																				
(generic) 1/4 cup	14	*	2	—	—	*	—	35	2	2	*	*	*	*	*	*	*	2	3	*	*
(Knorr) 1/4 cup	18	*	2	—	—	*	—	18	—	*	*	*	*	*	*	*	*	*	*	*
AVOCADO																				
all types																				
1 fruit	324	7	47	—	*	5	48	*	34	2	11	6	20	25	26	14	14	19	—	31
1/2 cup puree	185	4	27	—	*	3	28	*	20	*	7	3	11	14	15	8	8	11	—	18
California																				
1 fruit	306	6	46	—	*	4	—	*	31	2	11	5	18	21	23	12	12	17	—	28
Florida																				
1 fruit	340	8	42	—	*	9	72	*	42	3	9	9	26	37	40	22	22	29	—	41
AVOCADO OIL																				
1 tbsp	124	*	20	8	*	*	*	*	*	*	*	*	*	*	*	*	*	*	*	*
BABASSU OIL																				
1 tbsp	120	*	22	55	*	*	*	*	*	*	*	*	*	*	*	*	*	*	*	*
BABY FOOD, INFANT																				
apple juice																				
(Beech-Nut Stage 1) 4 oz jar	60	0	0	0	0	15	—	10	—	*	2	—	—	*	120	*	*	*	—	—
(Gerber 1st) 4 fl oz jar	60	0	0	0	0	14	—	—	89	*	*	—	—	*	120	*	*	*	—	—
applesauce																				
(Beech-Nut Stage 1) 4 oz jar	70	0	0	0	0	16	—	0	—	*	*	—	—	*	45	2	2	*	—	—
applesauce (Beech-Nut Baby's First)																				
2 1/2 oz jar	50	0	0	0	0	11	—	0	—	*	*	—	—	*	35	*	2	*	—	—
(Gerber 1st) 2 1/2 oz jar	35	0	0	0	0	9	—	—	102	*	*	—	—	*	45	*	2	*	—	—
bananas (Beech-Nut Baby's First)																				
2 1/2 oz jar	70	2	0	0	0	16	—	0	—	*	*	—	—	2	45	2	4	2	—	—
(Beech-Nut Stage 1) 4 oz jar	110	2	0	0	0	25	—	0	—	*	2	—	—	4	45	4	6	4	—	—
(Gerber 1st) 2 1/2 oz jar	70	2	0	0	0	17	—	—	312	*	*	—	—	*	45	2	6	4	—	—
barley cereal (Beech-Nut Stage 1)																				
1/2 oz dry + 2 1/2 oz formula	120	8	4	—	—	18	—	25	—	20	50	—	—	6	4	50	50	50	—	—
(Gerber 1st) 1/2 oz + 2 1/2 oz formula	110	10	4	—	—	16	—	—	—	20	80	—	—	10	10	50	50	30	—	—
beef & broth																				
(Beech-Nut Stage 1) 2 1/2 oz jar	80	35	5	—	—	0	—	40	—	*	6	—	—	*	*	2	15	20	—	—
butternut squash (Beech-Nut Baby's First)																				
2 1/2 oz jar	30	2	0	0	0	7	—	0	—	*	*	—	—	150	*	4	2	4	—	—
(Beech-Nut Stage 1) 4 oz jar	50	4	0	0	0	10	—	0	—	2	2	—	—	150	4	8	6	8	—	—
carrots (Beech-Nut Baby's First)																				
2 1/2 oz jar	25	0	0	0	0	6	—	80	—	2	*	—	—	460	*	2	4	2	—	—
(Beech-Nut Stage 1) 4 oz jar	40	2	0	0	0	9	—	65	—	4	*	—	—	700	*	4	6	6	—	—
(Gerber 1st) 2 1/2 oz jar	25	2	0	0	0	5	—	—	234	2	*	—	—	250	*	2	4	2	—	—
chicken & broth																				
(Beech-Nut Stage 1) 2 1/2 oz jar	70	35	4	—	—	0	—	55	—	2	6	—	—	*	*	4	15	20	—	—
grape juice																				
(Beech-Nut Stage 1) 4 oz jar	100	0	0	0	0	23	—	10	—	2	*	—	—	*	120	*	4	4	—	—
red																				
(Gerber 1st) 4 fl oz jar	80	0	0	0	0	20	—	—	52	2	*	—	—	*	120	*	*	*	—	—
white																				
(Gerber 1st) 4 fl oz jar	80	0	0	0	0	19	—	—	41	2	*	—	—	*	120	*	*	*	—	—

	Calories	Protein	Fat	Sat. Fat	Cholesterol	Carbohydrates	Fiber	Sodium	Potassium	Calcium	Iron	Zinc	Magnesium	Vitamin A	Vitamin C	Thiamin	Riboflavin	Niacin	Vitamin B₁₂	Folic acid

BABY FOOD, INFANT (continued)

green beans

	Calories	Protein	Fat	Sat. Fat	Cholesterol	Carbohydrates	Fiber	Sodium	Potassium	Calcium	Iron	Zinc	Magnesium	Vitamin A	Vitamin C	Thiamin	Riboflavin	Niacin	Vitamin B₁₂	Folic acid
(Beech-Nut Stage 1) 4 oz jar	35	4	0	0	0	7	—	0	—	8	6	—	—	30	*	4	10	4	—	—
(Gerber 1st) 2 1/2 oz jar	25	2	0	0	0	5	—	—	182	2	2	—	—	4	*	2	6	2	—	—
lamb & broth																				
(Beech-Nut Stage 1) 2 1/2 oz jar	60	35	3	—	—	0	—	50	—	*	6	—	—	*	*	4	20	25	—	—
oatmeal (Gerber 1st) 1/2 oz + 2 1/2 oz formula	100	15	4	—	—	14	—	—	—	20	80	—	—	10	10	50	50	30	—	—
oatmeal cereal (Beech-Nut Stage 1) 1/2 oz dry + 2 1/2 oz formula	120	10	5	—	—	16	—	25	—	20	50	—	—	6	4	50	50	50	—	—
peaches (Beech-Nut Baby's First) 2 1/2 oz jar	50	2	0	0	0	10	—	0	—	*	*	—	—	20	45	*	4	6	—	—
(Beech-Nut Stage 1) 4 oz jar	60	2	0	0	0	14	—	0	—	*	*	—	—	35	45	2	6	10	—	—
(Gerber 1st) 2 1/2 oz jar	30	0	0	0	0	7	—	—	157	*	*	—	—	6	45	*	2	4	—	—
pear juice (Beech-Nut Stage 1) 4 oz jar	60	0	0	0	0	15	—	5	—	*	*	—	—	*	120	*	6	2	—	—
(Gerber 1st) 4 fl oz jar	60	0	0	0	0	14	—	—	127	*	*	—	—	*	120	*	*	*	—	—
pears (Beech-Nut Baby's First) 2 1/2 oz jar	50	0	0	0	0	12	—	0	—	*	*	—	—	*	45	*	2	*	—	—
(Beech-Nut Stage 1) 4 oz jar	70	0	0	0	0	17	—	0	—	2	*	—	—	*	45	6	6	4	—	—
(Gerber 1st) 2 1/2 oz jar	40	0	0	0	0	10	—	—	121	*	*	—	—	*	45	*	2	*	—	—
peas (Beech-Nut Baby's First) 2 1/2 oz jar	40	8	0	0	0	7	—	0	—	*	4	—	—	15	8	8	6	8	—	—
(Beech-Nut Stage 1) 4 oz jar	70	10	0	0	0	12	—	0	—	2	4	—	—	30	4	15	10	10	—	—
(Gerber 1st) 2 1/2 oz jar	30	8	0	0	0	6	—	—	87	2	4	—	—	6	*	6	6	6	—	—
prunes (Gerber 1st) 2 1/2 oz jar	70	2	0	0	0	17	—	—	306	2	*	—	—	*	*	*	10	6	—	—
rice cereal (Beech-Nut Stage 1) 1/2 oz dry + 2 1/2 oz formula	120	8	4	—	—	18	—	20	—	20	50	—	—	6	4	50	50	50	—	—
(Gerber 1st) 1/2 oz + 2 1/2 oz formula	110	10	4	—	—	16	—	—	—	20	80	—	—	10	10	50	50	30	—	—
squash (Gerber 1st) 2 1/2 oz jar	25	2	0	0	0	5	—	—	192	2	*	—	—	15	*	*	4	2	—	—
sweet potatoes (Beech-Nut Baby's First) 2 1/2 oz jar	50	2	0	0	0	11	—	10	—	*	*	—	—	230	*	2	4	2	—	—
(Beech-Nut Stage 1) 4 oz jar	80	4	0	0	0	18	—	40	—	2	*	—	—	400	4	4	6	4	—	—
(Gerber 1st) 2 1/2 oz jar	45	2	0	0	0	10	—	—	254	*	*	—	—	130	*	2	2	2	—	—
turkey & broth (Beech-Nut Stage 1) 2 1/2 oz jar	90	30	6	—	—	0	—	40	—	6	4	—	—	*	*	2	20	20	—	—
veal & broth (Beech-Nut Stage 1) 2 1/2 oz jar	70	40	3	—	—	0	—	50	—	*	4	—	—	*	*	2	20	30	—	—
BABY FOOD, JUNIOR																				
apple banana juice (Gerber 2nd) 4 oz jar	60	0	0	0	0	15	—	—	123	*	*	—	—	*	120	*	*	*	—	—
apple-banana juice (Beech-Nut Stage 2) 4 oz jar	70	0	0	0	0	16	—	0	—	*	*	—	—	*	120	*	2	2	—	—
apple cherry juice (Gerber 2nd) 4 oz jar	60	0	0	0	0	14	—	—	115	*	*	—	—	*	120	*	2	*	—	—
apple-cherry juice (Beech-Nut Stage 2) 4 oz jar	70	0	0	0	0	17	—	10	—	*	2	—	—	*	120	*	2	*	—	—
apple & chicken dinner (Gerber 2nd) 4 oz jar	70	0	2	—	—	12	—	—	0	4	2	—	—	*	*	2	10	6	—	—

PERCENTAGE DAILY VALUE

	Calories	Protein	Fat	Sat. Fat	Cholesterol	Carbohydrates	Fiber	Sodium	Potassium	Calcium	Iron	Zinc	Magnesium	Vitamin A	Vitamin C	Thiamin	Riboflavin	Niacin	Vitamin B12	Folic acid
BABY FOOD, JUNIOR (continued)																				
apple grape juice (Gerber 2nd) 4 oz jar	60	0	0	0	0	15	—	—	97	*	*	—	—	*	120	*	2	*	—	—
apple & ham dinner (Gerber 2nd) 4 oz jar	70	0	1	—	—	14	—	—	0	*	2	—	—	*	*	8	8	6	—	—
apple juice w/ yogurt (Gerber 2nd) 4 oz jar	100	10	2	—	—	18	—	—	143	15	*	—	—	*	120	4	10	*	—	—
apple peach juice (Gerber 2nd) 4 oz jar	60	0	0	0	0	14	—	—	117	*	*	—	—	*	120	*	*	2	—	—
apple, peach & strawberry dessert (Beech-Nut Stage 2) 4 oz jar	100	0	0	0	0	23	—	0	—	*	*	—	—	8	45	2	6	4	—	—
apple plum juice (Gerber 2nd) 4 oz jar	60	0	0	0	0	15	—	—	110	*	*	—	—	*	120	*	*	2	—	—
apple prune juice (Gerber 2nd) 4 oz jar	60	0	0	0	0	16	—	—	139	*	2	—	—	*	120	*	10	2	—	—
apple & strawberry dessert (Beech-Nut Stage 2) 4 oz jar	100	0	2	—	—	22	—	0	—	*	*	—	—	6	45	2	6	*	—	—
apple & turkey dinner (Gerber 2nd) 4 oz jar	80	0	2	—	—	13	—	—	0	*	4	—	—	*	*	4	10	6	—	—
apple yogurt dessert (Beech-Nut Stage 2) 4 oz jar	110	4	0	0	0	24	—	25	—	6	*	—	—	*	45	2	10	*	—	—
apple-cranberry juice (Beech-Nut Stage 2) 4 oz jar	60	0	0	0	0	15	—	10	—	*	2	—	—	*	120	*	*	*	—	—
apple-grape juice (Beech-Nut Stage 2) 4 oz jar	70	0	0	0	0	18	—	15	—	*	2	—	—	*	120	*	2	*	—	—
apples & apricots (Beech-Nut Stage 2) 4 oz jar	70	0	0	0	0	16	—	0	—	2	*	—	—	40	45	2	4	2	—	—
apples & bananas (Beech-Nut Stage 2) 4 oz jar	70	0	0	0	0	26	—	0	—	*	*	—	—	*	45	2	2	*	—	—
apples & blueberries (Beech-Nut Stage 2) 4 oz jar	80	0	0	0	0	20	—	0	—	2	2	—	—	*	45	15	15	2	—	—
(Gerber 2nd) 4 oz jar	50	0	0	0	0	13	—	—	77	*	*	—	—	*	45	*	4	*	—	—
apples & cherries (Beech-Nut Stage 2) 4 oz jar	80	0	0	0	0	18	—	0	—	*	2	—	—	2	45	2	4	*	—	—
apples & pears (Beech-Nut Stage 2) 4 oz jar	80	0	0	0	0	20	—	0	—	*	2	—	—	*	45	4	4	2	—	—
apples, pears, & bananas (Beech-Nut Stage 2) 4 oz jar	90	0	0	0	0	22	—	0	—	2	*	—	—	*	45	4	8	2	—	—
applesauce (Gerber 2nd) 4 oz jar	60	0	0	0	0	14	—	—	77	*	*	—	—	*	45	2	2	*	—	—
applesauce w/ apricot (Gerber 2nd) 4 oz jar	60	0	0	0	0	14	—	—	119	*	*	—	—	15	45	2	2	*	—	—
apricots, pears & apples (Beech-Nut Stage 2) 4 oz jar	90	2	0	0	0	20	—	0	—	4	2	—	—	70	45	2	6	4	—	—
apricots w/ tapioca (Gerber 2nd) 4 oz jar	80	0	0	0	0	19	—	—	108	*	*	—	—	35	45	*	*	2	—	—
banana apple dessert (Gerber 2nd) 4 oz jar	80	0	0	0	0	19	—	—	69	*	*	—	—	*	45	*	*	*	—	—
banana flan dessert (Beech-Nut Stage 2) 4 oz jar	110	0	0	0	0	26	—	0	—	*	*	—	—	2	45	2	2	*	—	—
banana juice w/ yogurt (Gerber 2nd) 4 oz jar	110	15	2	—	—	21	—	—	173	15	*	—	—	*	120	4	10	2	—	—
bananas, pears & apples (Beech-Nut Stage 2) 4 oz jar	100	2	0	0	0	23	—	0	—	4	*	—	—	2	45	4	10	4	—	—
bananas w/ pineapple & tapioca (Gerber 2nd) 4 oz jar	60	0	0	0	0	14	—	—	98	*	*	—	—	*	45	*	2	2	—	—
banana pineapple dessert (Beech-Nut Stage 2) 4 oz jar	110	2	0	0	0	26	—	15	—	*	*	—	—	2	45	2	4	2	—	—

BABY FOOD, JUNIOR (continued)

	Calories	Protein	Fat	Sat. Fat	Cholesterol	Carbohydrates	Fiber	Sodium	Potassium	Calcium	Iron	Zinc	Magnesium	Vitamin A	Vitamin C	Thiamin	Riboflavin	Niacin	Vitamin B₁₂	Folic acid
banana pudding (Beech-Nut Stage 2) 4 oz jar	110	0	2	—	—	26	—	0	—	*	*	—	—	2	45	2	2	*	—	—
banana vanilla dessert (Gerber Tropical) 4 oz jar	100	2	1	—	0	21	—	—	90	2	*	—	—	*	45	2	8	2	—	—
bananas w/ tapioca (Gerber 2nd) 4 oz jar	90	2	0	0	0	21	—	—	149	*	*	—	—	*	45	2	6	2	—	—
banana yogurt dessert (Beech-Nut Stage 2) 4 oz jar	130	6	0	0	0	26	—	30	—	6	*	—	—	*	45	2	15	2	—	—
(Gerber 2nd) 4 oz jar	90	4	0	0	—	21	—	—	114	6	*	—	—	*	45	*	6	2	—	—
beans & rice dinner (Gerber Tropical) 4 oz jar	60	8	2	—	0	9	—	—	118	2	6	—	—	*	*	4	2	2	—	—
beef (Gerber 2nd) 2 1/2 oz jar	80	50	4	—	—	0	—	—	212	*	4	—	—	*	*	*	10	20	—	—
beef dinner (Beech-Nut Stage 2) 4 oz jar	130	8	9	—	—	10	—	45	—	4	2	—	—	220	*	6	10	8	—	—
beef & egg noodle dinner (Beech-Nut Stage 2) 4 oz jar	100	4	7	—	—	8	—	50	—	4	2	—	—	250	*	6	10	10	—	—
(Gerber 2nd) 4 oz jar	80	10	3	—	—	10	—	—	73	*	2	—	—	25	*	4	4	8	—	—
beets (Gerber 2nd) 4 oz jar	45	4	0	0	0	10	—	—	219	2	2	—	—	*	*	*	4	*	—	—
broccoli & chicken dinner (Gerber 2nd) 4 oz jar	50	15	2	—	—	4	—	—	175	6	4	—	—	8	20	2	10	6	—	—
carrot & beef dinner (Gerber 2nd) 4 oz jar	70	10	3	—	—	7	—	—	209	2	2	—	—	180	*	2	8	8	—	—
carrots (Gerber 2nd) 4 oz jar	30	2	0	0	0	7	—	—	191	4	*	—	—	380	*	2	4	2	—	—
carrots & peas (Beech-Nut Stage 2) 4 oz jar	60	8	0	0	0	9	—	25	—	2	4	—	—	310	*	10	15	8	—	—
cherry vanilla pudding (Gerber 2nd) 4 oz jar	80	0	0	0	—	19	—	—	43	*	*	—	—	*	*	*	*	*	—	—
chicken (Gerber 2nd) 2 1/2 oz jar	90	50	6	—	—	0	—	—	175	4	4	—	—	*	*	*	8	25	—	—
chicken noodle dinner (Beech-Nut Stage 2) 4 oz jar	70	4	4	—	—	8	—	45	—	8	2	—	—	310	*	4	10	10	—	—
(Gerber 2nd) 4 oz jar	70	10	2	—	—	11	—	—	79	4	2	—	—	2	*	4	6	8	—	—
chicken & rice dinner (Beech-Nut Stage 2) 4 oz jar	80	4	3	—	—	11	—	70	—	10	4	—	—	420	*	4	8	6	—	—
(Gerber Tropical) 4 oz jar	60	10	2	—	0	8	—	—	59	2	2	—	—	*	*	2	4	4	—	—
chicken soup (Beech-Nut Stage 2) 4 oz jar	80	4	4	—	—	10	—	50	—	8	4	—	—	320	*	4	10	10	—	—
corn cereal (Gerber Tropical) 1/2 oz + 2 1/2 oz milk	110	10	4	—	—	12	—	—	—	30	80	—	—	6	2	50	70	25	—	—
cottage cheese dessert w/ pine-apple juice (Beech-Nut Stage 2) 4 oz jar	120	8	0	0	0	25	—	15	—	2	*	—	—	2	45	6	8	*	—	—
creamed corn (Beech-Nut Stage 2) 4 oz jar	90	6	0	0	0	18	—	20	—	2	*	—	—	6	*	*	10	4	—	—
(Gerber 2nd) 4 oz jar	80	8	1	—	—	15	—	—	101	4	*	—	—	*	*	*	4	6	—	—
creamed spinach (Gerber 2nd) 4 oz jar	50	10	1	—	—	8	—	—	202	10	4	—	—	100	2	2	15	2	—	—
Dutch apple dessert (Beech-Nut Stage 2) 4 oz jar	100	0	0	0	0	24	—	15	—	2	*	—	—	*	45	2	4	*	—	—
(Gerber 2nd) 4 oz jar	100	0	2	—	0	20	—	—	36	*	*	—	—	*	45	*	*	*	—	—
egg yolks (Gerber 2nd) 2 1/2 oz jar	130	35	11	—	—	1	—	—	70	8	8	—	—	10	*	4	15	*	—	—

BABY FOOD, JUNIOR (continued)

	Calories	Protein	Fat	Sat. Fat	Cholesterol	Carbohydrates	Fiber	Sodium	Potassium	Calcium	Iron	Zinc	Magnesium	Vitamin A	Vitamin C	Thiamin	Riboflavin	Niacin	Vitamin B12	Folic acid
fruit dessert (Beech-Nut Stage 2) 4 oz jar	80	0	0	0	0	20	—	0	—	*	*	—	—	4	45	4	4	*	—	—
(Gerber 2nd) 4 oz jar	90	2	0	0	0	23	—	—	99	*	*	—	—	2	45	2	2	4	—	—
garden vegetables (Beech-Nut Stage 2) 4 oz jar	60	8	0	0	0	11	—	10	—	4	4	—	—	140	2	8	10	8	—	—
(Gerber 2nd) 4 oz jar	45	10	1	—	0	7	—	—	169	4	4	—	—	140	*	6	8	6	—	—
grape juice fortified w/ iron (Beech-Nut Stage 2) 4 oz jar	100	0	0	0	0	23	—	10	—	*	15	—	—	*	120	2	*	*	—	—
green bean & turkey dinner (Gerber 2nd) 4 oz jar	70	15	2	—	—	9	—	—	188	4	4	—	—	8	*	4	15	10	—	—
green beans (Gerber 2nd) 4 oz jar	35	6	0	0	0	7	—	—	155	6	2	—	—	10	*	2	8	2	—	—
guava dessert (Beech-Nut Stage 2) 4 oz jar	110	2	0	0	0	25	—	10	—	*	*	—	—	10	45	4	8	6	—	—
guava w/ mixed fruit juice (Gerber Tropical) 4 oz jar	70	0	0	0	0	18	—	—	121	2	*	—	—	2	120	2	6	6	—	—
guava w/ tapioca dessert (Gerber Tropical) 4 oz jar	80	0	0	0	0	21	—	—	70	*	*	—	—	6	45	*	*	2	—	—
ham (Gerber 2nd) 2 1/2 oz jar	90	50	6	—	—	0	—	—	232	*	4	—	—	*	*	8	10	20	—	—
Hawaiian delight dessert (Gerber 2nd) 4 oz jar	90	6	0	0	0	22	—	—	82	8	*	—	—	*	45	4	2	*	—	—
high protein cereal (Gerber 2nd) 1/2 oz + 2 1/2 oz apple juice	90	20	1	—	—	15	—	—	—	15	80	—	—	*	70	45	45	25	—	
island fruit dessert (Beech-Nut Stage 2) 4 oz jar	100	0	0	0	0	24	—	15	—	*	*	—	—	15	45	4	4	2	—	—
lamb (Gerber 2nd) 2 1/2 oz jar	80	60	4	—	—	0	—	—	202	*	6	—	—	*	*	*	10	20	—	—
macaroni & beef dinner (Beech-Nut Stage 2) 4 oz jar	110	8	6	—	—	11	—	45	—	4	2	—	—	260	*	6	10	10	—	—
macaroni & cheese dinner (Gerber 2nd) 4 oz jar	80	10	3	—	—	10	—	—	54	10	*	—	—	*	*	4	4	6	—	—
macaroni tomato beef dinner (Gerber 2nd) 4 oz jar	70	10	2	—	—	11	—	—	123	2	2	—	—	25	*	4	4	8	—	—
mango, banana, & passionfruit dessert (Gerber Tropical) 4 oz jar	80	0	0	0	0	20	—	—	87	*	*	—	—	6	45	*	2	2	—	—
mango dessert (Beech-Nut Stage 2) 4 oz jar	110	2	0	0	0	26	—	10	—	*	*	—	—	50	45	4	8	4	—	—
mango w/ mixed fruit juice (Gerber Tropical) 4 oz jar	70	0	0	0	0	18	—	—	102	2	2	—	—	2	120	2	4	4	—	—
mango nectar (Beech-Nut Stage 2) 4 oz jar	80	0	0	0	0	18	—	0	—	*	*	—	—	20	120	*	*	*	—	—
mango w/ tapioca (Gerber Tropical) 4 oz jar	80	0	0	0	0	21	—	—	64	*	*	—	—	25	45	*	*	2	—	—
mixed cereal (Beech-Nut Stage 2) 1/2 oz dry + 2 1/2 oz formula	120	10	4	—	—	17	—	25	—	20	50	—	—	6	4	50	50	50	—	—
plain (Gerber 2nd) 1/2 oz + 2 1/2 oz apple juice	90	6	1	—	—	20	—	—	—	15	80	—	—	*	70	45	45	25	—	
w/ applesauce & bananas (Gerber 2nd) 4 oz jar	90	4	1	—	—	20	—	—	51	*	45	—	—	*	45	45	45	45	—	—
w/ banana (Gerber 2nd) 1/2 oz + 2 1/2 oz apple juice	90	4	1	—	—	20	—	—	—	15	80	—	—	*	70	45	45	25	—	

BABY FOOD, JUNIOR (continued)

	Calories	Protein	Fat	Sat. Fat	Cholesterol	Carbohydrates	Fiber	Sodium	Potassium	Calcium	Iron	Zinc	Magnesium	Vitamin A	Vitamin C	Thiamin	Riboflavin	Niacin	Vitamin B12	Folic acid
mixed cereal & apples (Beech-Nut Stage 2) 4 oz jar	70	2	0	0	0	14	—	0	—	*	35	—	—	4	45	45	45	45	—	—
mixed fruit juice (Beech-Nut Stage 2) 4 oz jar	70	0	0	0	0	16	—	10	—	*	2	—	—	10	120	2	4	*	—	—
(Gerber 2nd) 4 oz jar	60	0	0	0	0	14	—	—	120	*	*	—	—	*	120	4	*	*	—	—
w/ yogurt (Gerber 2nd) 4 oz jar	100	15	2	—	—	18	—	—	152	15	*	—	—	*	120	6	15	*	—	—
mixed fruit yogurt dessert (Beech-Nut Stage 2) 4 oz jar	120	4	2	—	—	27	—	15	—	6	*	—	—	*	45	6	8	*	—	—
(Gerber 2nd) 4 oz jar	90	4	0	0	—	21	—	—	131	6	*	—	—	2	45	2	6	2	—	—
mixed vegetables (Beech-Nut Stage 2) 4 oz jar	45	4	0	0	0	9	—	10	—	4	2	—	—	410	*	8	15	4	—	—
(Gerber 2nd) 4 oz jar	50	6	1	—	0	9	—	—	120	2	2	—	—	130	*	2	*	2	—	—
oatmeal w/ applesauce & bananas (Gerber 2nd) 4 oz jar	90	6	1	—	—	20	—	—	65	*	45	—	—	*	45	45	45	45	—	—
w/ banana (Gerber 2nd) 1/2 oz + 2 1/2 oz apple juice	90	8	1	—	—	19	—	—	—	15	80	—	—	*	70	45	45	25	—	—
oatmeal & apples (Beech-Nut Stage 2) 4 oz jar	70	2	0	0	0	14	—	0	—	*	35	—	—	2	45	45	45	45	—	—
oatmeal & bananas (Beech-Nut Stage 2) 1/2 oz dry + 2 1/2 oz formula	120	8	4	—	—	18	—	20	—	20	40	—	—	6	4	40	40	40	—	—
orange juice (Gerber 2nd) 4 oz jar	60	2	0	0	0	13	—	—	168	2	*	—	—	*	120	10	2	2	—	—
papaya w/ mixed fruit juice (Gerber Tropical) 4 oz jar	70	0	0	0	0	18	—	—	106	2	*	—	—	*	120	*	4	2	—	—
papaya nectar (Beech-Nut Stage 2) 4 oz jar	80	0	0	0	0	20	—	10	—	*	*	—	—	45	120	2	2	*	—	—
papaya & pineapple dessert (Gerber Tropical) 4 oz jar	90	0	0	0	0	22	—	—	96	*	2	—	—	2	45	2	4	*	—	—
papaya w/ tapioca (Gerber Tropical) 4 oz jar	70	0	0	0	0	17	—	—	64	*	*	—	—	2	45	*	*	*	—	—
peach cobbler (Gerber 2nd) 4 oz jar	90	2	0	0	0	21	—	—	67	*	*	—	—	4	45	*	*	4	—	—
peach & mango dessert (Gerber Tropical) 4 oz jar	80	0	0	0	0	19	—	—	57	*	*	—	—	10	45	*	*	2	—	—
peach nectar (Beech-Nut Stage 2) 4 oz jar	70	0	0	0	0	17	—	0	—	4	*	—	—	40	120	2	6	4	—	—
peach yogurt dessert (Beech-Nut Stage 2) 4 oz jar	130	6	0	0	0	27	—	30	—	6	*	—	—	15	45	10	8	4	—	—
(Gerber 2nd) 4 oz jar	90	4	0	0	—	21	—	—	121	4	*	—	—	2	45	*	6	4	—	—
peaches (Gerber 2nd) 4 oz jar	70	2	0	0	0	17	—	—	148	*	*	—	—	8	45	*	2	6	—	—
peaches & bananas (Beech-Nut Stage 2) 4 oz jar	70	2	0	0	0	16	—	10	—	10	4	—	—	20	45	2	2	10	—	—
pear-peach juice w/ yogurt (Gerber 2nd) 4 oz jar	90	15	1	—	—	18	—	—	171	15	*	—	—	4	120	4	15	4	—	—
pear yogurt dessert (Beech-Nut Stage 2) 4 oz jar	130	4	3	—	—	28	—	30	—	8	*	—	—	*	45	2	10	*	—	—
pears (Gerber 2nd) 4 oz jar	60	0	0	0	0	15	—	—	103	*	*	—	—	*	45	2	2	2	—	—
pears & pineapple (Beech-Nut Stage 2) 4 oz jar	80	0	0	0	0	20	—	0	—	2	*	—	—	*	45	6	6	2	—	—
(Gerber 2nd) 4 oz jar	60	0	0	0	0	15	—	—	102	*	*	—	—	*	45	2	4	2	—	—
peas (Gerber 2nd) 4 oz jar	60	15	1	—	0	9	—	—	102	2	6	—	—	8	6	8	6	10	—	—

	Calories	Protein	Fat	Sat. Fat	Cholesterol	Carbohydrates	Fiber	Sodium	Potassium	Calcium	Iron	Zinc	Magnesium	Vitamin A	Vitamin C	Thiamin	Riboflavin	Niacin	Vitamin B₁₂	Folic acid
BABY FOOD, JUNIOR (continued)																				
pineapple & banana dessert (Gerber Tropical) 4 oz jar	90	0	0	0	0	22	—	—	80	*	*	—	—	*	45	4	6	*	—	—
plums, apples & rice (Beech-Nut Stage 2) 4 oz jar	110	0	0	0	0	25	—	10	—	2	*	—	—	8	45	2	4	2	—	—
plums w/tapioca (Gerber 2nd) 4 oz jar	80	0	0	0	0	20	—	—	81	*	*	—	—	4	*	*	4	2	—	—
prunes & pears (Beech-Nut Stage 2) 4 oz jar	110	2	0	0	0	26	—	10	—	6	2	—	—	35	*	4	6	6	—	—
prunes w/tapioca (Gerber 2nd) 4 oz jar	90	2	0	0	0	21	—	—	167	*	*	—	—	10	*	2	8	4	—	—
rice & apples (Beech-Nut Stage 2) 1/2 oz dry + 2 1/2 oz formula	120	6	4	—	—	19	—	20	—	20	40	—	—	6	4	40	40	40	—	—
(Beech-Nut Stage 2) 4 oz jar	60	2	0	0	0	13	—	0	—	*	35	—	—	2	45	45	45	45	—	—
rice & bananas (Beech-Nut Stage 2) 1/2 oz dry + 2 1/2 oz formula	120	6	4	—	—	19	—	20	—	20	40	—	—	6	4	40	40	40	—	—
rice cereal w/ applesauce & bananas (Gerber 2nd) 4 oz jar	90	4	0	0	—	21	—	—	48	2	45	—	—	*	45	45	45	45	—	—
w/ banana (Gerber 2nd) 1/2 oz + 2 1/2 oz apple juice	90	4	1	—	—	20	—	—	—	15	80	—	—	*	70	45	45	25	—	—
rice cereal w/mango (Gerber Tropical) 1/2 oz + 2 1/2 oz milk	100	10	3	—	—	12	—	—	—	30	80	—	—	6	2	50	70	25	—	—
squash (Gerber 2nd) 4 oz jar	35	2	0	0	0	8	—	—	166	4	*	—	—	35	4	2	4	*	—	—
sweet potatoes (Gerber 2nd) 4 oz jar	70	4	0	0	0	16	—	—	236	2	2	—	—	160	2	2	4	4	—	—
tropical blend juice (Beech-Nut Stage 2) 4 oz jar	90	0	0	0	0	21	—	0	—	2	*	—	—	2	120	2	2	2	—	—
tropical fruit medley (Gerber Tropical) 4 oz jar	70	0	0	0	0	18	—	—	39	*	*	—	—	2	45	2	*	*	—	—
turkey (Gerber 2nd) 2 1/2 oz jar	80	50	5	—	—	0	—	—	209	*	2	—	—	*	*	*	10	20	—	—
turkey dinner (Beech-Nut Stage 2) 4 oz jar	90	10	4	—	—	10	—	40	—	15	6	—	—	220	*	6	15	10	—	—
turkey rice dinner (Gerber 2nd) 4 oz jar	70	10	3	—	—	9	—	—	91	*	2	—	—	40	*	2	4	8	—	—
turkey & rice dinner (Beech-Nut Stage 2) 4 oz jar	70	4	3	—	—	10	—	50	—	6	4	—	—	290	*	4	10	8	—	—
vanilla custard pudding (Gerber 3rd) 4 oz jar	100	10	1	—	—	21	—	—	64	10	*	—	—	*	*	*	6	*	—	—
(Beech-Nut Stage 2) 4 oz jar	130	8	0	0	0	22	—	55	—	10	*	—	—	2	*	4	20	*	—	—
veal (Gerber 2nd) 2 1/2 oz jar	70	50	4	—	—	0	—	—	224	*	2	—	—	*	*	*	10	25	—	—
vegetable bacon dinner (Gerber 2nd) 4 oz jar	90	8	5	—	—	10	—	—	125	2	2	—	—	70	*	4	2	6	—	—
vegetable beef dinner (Beech-Nut Stage 2) 4 oz jar	90	4	5	—	—	11	—	35	—	4	2	—	—	260	*	6	10	8	—	—
(Gerber 2nd) 4 oz jar	70	10	3	—	—	10	—	—	98	*	2	—	—	50	*	2	2	6	—	—
vegetable chicken dinner (Beech-Nut Stage 2) 4 oz jar	80	8	4	—	—	10	—	40	—	6	2	—	—	260	*	4	10	10	—	—
(Gerber 2nd) 4 oz jar	70	10	2	—	—	11	—	—	78	2	2	—	—	35	*	2	2	6	—	—
vegetable ham dinner (Beech-Nut Stage 2) 4 oz jar	80	8	3	—	—	10	—	30	—	4	4	—	—	220	*	10	10	10	—	—
(Gerber 2nd) 4 oz jar	70	8	3	—	—	10	—	—	77	*	*	—	—	30	*	2	2	4	—	—

	Calories	Protein	Fat	Sat. Fat	Cholesterol	Carbohydrates	Fiber	Sodium	Potassium	Calcium	Iron	Zinc	Magnesium	Vitamin A	Vitamin C	Thiamin	Riboflavin	Niacin	Vitamin B₁₂	Folic acid
BABY FOOD, JUNIOR (continued)																				
vegetable lamb dinner (Beech-Nut Stage 2) 4 oz jar	80	4	0	0	0	11	—	55	—	8	4	—	—	370	*	6	10	8	—	—
vegetable turkey dinner (Gerber 2nd) 4 oz jar	60	10	2	—	—	9	—	—	74	*	*	—	—	25	*	2	2	6	—	—
BABY FOOD, TODDLER																				
apple-carrot juice (Gerber 3rd) 4 oz jar	50	0	0	0	0	12	—	—	81	2	2	—	—	45	120	*	4	*	—	—
apple-sweet potato juice (Gerber 3rd) 4 oz jar	60	0	0	0	0	14	—	—	137	4	2	—	—	45	120	2	4	*	—	—
apples & bananas (Beech-Nut Stage 3) 6 oz jar	100	0	0	0	0	25	—	0	—	*	*	—	—	*	45	2	2	*	—	—
apples & blueberries (Gerber 3rd) 6 oz jar	80	0	0	0	0	20	—	—	91	*	*	—	—	*	45	2	6	*	—	—
apples & cherries (Beech-Nut Stage 3) 6 oz jar	100	0	0	0	0	24	—	0	—	*	2	—	—	2	45	4	4	*	—	—
applesauce (Beech-Nut Stage 3) 6 oz jar	90	0	0	0	0	22	—	0	—	*	*	—	—	*	45	4	4	*	—	—
(Gerber 3rd) 6 oz jar	80	0	0	0	0	21	—	—	93	*	*	—	—	*	45	2	4	*	—	—
apricots, pears & apples (Beech-Nut Stage 3) 6 oz jar	120	4	0	0	0	27	—	0	—	2	2	—	—	90	45	4	6	6	—	—
apricots w/ tapioca (Gerber 3rd) 6 oz jar	120	2	0	0	0	29	—	—	134	*	2	—	—	35	45	2	*	2	—	—
bananas, pears, & apples (Beech-Nut Stage 3) 6 oz jar	130	2	0	0	0	31	—	0	—	*	2	—	—	6	45	6	6	4	—	—
bananas, pineapple, & tapioca (Gerber 3rd) 6 oz jar	90	2	0	0	0	21	—	—	110	*	*	—	—	*	45	2	4	2	—	—
bananas w/ tapioca (Gerber 3rd) 6 oz jar	130	2	0	0	0	32	—	—	142	*	*	—	—	*	45	4	6	4	—	—
beef (Gerber 3rd) 2 1/2 oz jar	80	60	4	—	—	0	—	—	216	*	8	—	—	*	*	*	10	15	—	—
beef egg noodle dinner (Beech-Nut Stage 3) 6 oz jar	120	15	5	—	—	14	—	50	—	4	4	—	—	280	*	8	10	10	—	—
(Gerber 3rd) 6 oz jar	110	20	4	—	—	15	—	—	94	2	4	—	—	90	*	6	6	10	—	—
broccoli, carrots & cheese (Gerber 3rd) 6 oz jar	80	10	2	—	—	12	—	—	98	8	2	—	—	110	10	4	4	4	—	—
carrots (Beech-Nut Stage 3) 6 oz jar	60	4	0	0	0	13	—	170	—	4	2	—	—	900	*	4	8	8	—	—
(Gerber 3rd) 6 oz jar	50	4	0	0	0	11	—	—	176	6	*	—	—	550	*	2	6	4	—	—
chicken (Gerber 3rd) 2 1/2 oz jar	90	60	6	—	—	0	—	—	168	2	4	—	—	*	*	*	6	25	—	—
chicken noodle dinner (Beech-Nut Stage 3) 6 oz jar	100	15	3	—	—	14	—	55	—	6	4	—	—	170	*	6	10	10	—	—
(Gerber 3rd) 6 oz jar	100	15	3	—	—	15	—	—	84	2	4	—	—	40	*	4	6	15	—	—
chicken & stars microwave (Beech-Nut Stage 3) 6 oz tub	130	25	3	—	—	17	—	240	—	6	8	—	—	80	*	10	15	25	—	—
cottage cheese dessert w/ pineapple juice (Beech-Nut Stage 3) 6 oz jar	170	10	2	—	—	36	—	20	—	*	*	—	—	*	45	6	10	*	—	—
cream of broccoli soup (Gerber 3rd) 6 oz jar	45	10	2	—	—	5	—	—	38	15	2	—	—	*	*	*	6	2	—	—
cream of potato soup (Gerber 3rd) 6 oz jar	70	8	2	—	—	10	—	—	122	15	2	—	—	*	*	4	10	8	—	—
cream of tomato soup (Gerber 3rd) 6 oz jar	80	10	2	—	—	13	—	—	296	15	4	—	—	6	*	6	15	10	—	—
cream of vegetable soup (Gerber 3rd) 6 oz jar	60	8	2	—	—	8	—	—	78	15	2	—	—	10	*	4	10	4	—	—
creamed green beans (Gerber 3rd) 6 oz jar	80	10	1	—	—	16	—	—	114	8	2	—	—	6	*	2	8	4	—	—

	Calories	Protein	Fat	Sat. Fat	Cholesterol	Carbohydrates	Fiber	Sodium	Potassium	Calcium	Iron	Zinc	Magnesium	Vitamin A	Vitamin C	Thiamin	Riboflavin	Niacin	Vitamin B₁₂	Folic acid
BABY FOOD, TODDLER (continued)																				
Dutch apple dessert (Gerber 3rd) 6 oz jar	130	0	2	—	0	29	—	—	40	*	*	—	—	*	45	*	2	*	—	—
fruit dessert (Beech-Nut Stage 3) 6 oz jar	120	2	0	0	0	28	—	5	—	*	*	—	—	8	45	4	8	4	—	—
(Gerber 3rd) 6 oz jar	120	0	0	0	0	30	—	—	79	2	*	—	—	15	*	2	*	2	—	—
green beans (Beech-Nut Stage 3) 6 oz jar	45	6	0	0	0	10	—	0	—	8	8	—	—	30	*	6	20	4	—	—
ham (Gerber 3rd) 2 1/2 oz jar	90	60	6	—	—	0	—	—	237	*	4	—	—	*	*	8	10	20	—	—
Hawaiian delight dessert (Gerber 3rd) 6 oz jar	150	8	0	0	0	35	—	—	76	10	*	—	—	*	45	6	10	*	—	—
macaroni & beef dinner (Beech-Nut Stage 3) 6 oz jar	130	15	6	—	—	16	—	70	—	6	4	—	—	400	*	8	20	15	—	—
mixed cereal w/ applesauce & bananas (Gerber 3rd) 6 oz jar	140	6	1	—	—	31	—	—	58	*	45	—	—	*	45	45	45	45	—	—
mixed fruit yogurt dessert (Beech-Nut Stage 3) 6 oz jar	160	6	2	—	—	36	—	30	—	8	*	—	—	4	45	8	15	2	—	—
mixed vegetables (Gerber 3rd) 6 oz jar	70	8	0	0	0	15	—	—	144	4	6	—	—	120	*	8	8	8	—	—
oatmeal w/ applesauce & bananas (Gerber 3rd) 6 oz jar	140	6	2	—	—	28	—	—	64	*	45	—	—	*	45	45	45	45	—	—
orange juice (Beech-Nut Stage 3) 6 oz jar	60	0	0	0	0	14	—	0	—	2	*	—	—	6	120	8	4	2	—	—
orange-carrot juice (Gerber 3rd) 4 oz jar	50	2	0	0	0	12	—	—	174	2	*	—	—	45	120	8	8	2	—	—
papaya dessert (Beech-Nut Stage 3) 6 oz jar	110	0	3	—	—	25	—	10	—	*	*	—	—	35	45	2	4	2	—	—
peach cobbler (Gerber 3rd) 6 oz jar	130	2	0	—	0	31	—	—	85	*	*	—	—	4	45	2	2	4	—	—
peaches (Beech-Nut Stage 3) 6 oz jar	90	4	0	0	0	22	—	0	—	*	*	—	—	40	45	2	6	15	—	—
(Gerber 3rd) 6 oz jar	110	4	1	—	0	25	—	—	164	*	*	—	—	10	45	*	4	10	—	—
pears (Beech-Nut Stage 3) 6 oz jar	100	2	0	0	0	24	—	0	—	*	*	—	—	*	45	4	4	4	—	—
(Gerber 3rd) 6 oz jar	100	2	1	—	0	22	—	—	121	2	*	—	—	*	45	2	4	2	—	—
pears & pineapples (Gerber 3rd) 6 oz jar	100	2	1	—	0	22	—	—	116	2	*	—	—	*	45	6	4	2	—	—
peas (Gerber 3rd) 6 oz jar	80	20	1	—	0	14	—	—	91	4	10	—	—	15	2	10	8	15	—	—
pineapple-carrot juice (Gerber 3rd) 4 oz jar	60	2	0	0	0	13	—	—	115	2	*	—	—	40	120	10	6	2	—	—
plums w/ tapioca (Gerber 3rd) 6 oz jar	130	2	0	0	0	31	—	—	102	2	*	—	—	6	*	*	6	4	—	—
rice w/ mixed fruit cereal (Gerber 3rd) 6 oz jar	130	6	0	0	—	31	—	—	50	4	45	—	—	*	45	45	45	45	—	—
seashells in tomato sauce microwave (Beech-Nut Stage 3) 6 oz tub	140	15	4	—	—	25	—	260	—	4	8	—	—	210	*	6	8	10	—	—
spaghetti & beef dinner (Beech-Nut Stage 3) 6 oz jar	130	15	6	—	—	16	—	65	—	4	4	—	—	320	*	6	20	15	—	—
spaghetti rings in meat sauce microwave (Beech-Nut Stage 3) 6 oz tub	160	25	5	—	—	22	—	300	—	6	6	—	—	210	*	15	20	20	—	—
spaghetti w/ tomato sauce & beef (Gerber 3rd) 6 oz jar	120	20	3	—	—	19	—	—	128	4	4	—	—	35	*	10	10	15	—	—
squash (Gerber 3rd) 6 oz jar	60	4	1	—	0	12	—	—	167	4	2	—	—	60	4	2	8	6	—	—
sweet potatoes (Beech-Nut Stage 3) 6 oz jar	110	6	0	0	0	26	—	80	—	4	2	—	—	600	2	6	8	4	—	—
(Gerber 3rd) 6 oz jar	100	6	0	0	0	24	—	—	255	4	2	—	—	260	*	4	6	4	—	—

	Calories	Protein	Fat	Sat. Fat	Cholesterol	Carbohydrates	Fiber	Sodium	Potassium	Calcium	Iron	Zinc	Magnesium	Vitamin A	Vitamin C	Thiamin	Riboflavin	Niacin	Vitamin B₁₂	Folic acid

BABY FOOD, TODDLER (continued)

	Calories	Protein	Fat	Sat. Fat	Cholesterol	Carbohydrates	Fiber	Sodium	Potassium	Calcium	Iron	Zinc	Magnesium	Vitamin A	Vitamin C	Thiamin	Riboflavin	Niacin	Vitamin B12	Folic acid
tomato macaroni beef dinner (Gerber 3rd) 6 oz jar	110	15	2	—	—	19	—	—	117	2	4	—	—	45	*	2	8	10	—	—
turkey (Gerber 3rd) 2 1/2 oz jar	90	60	5	—	—	0	—	—	203	*	2	—	—	*	*	*	10	20	—	—
turkey & rice dinner (Beech-Nut Stage 3) 6 oz jar	100	10	3	—	—	14	—	60	—	6	2	—	—	250	*	4	8	10	—	—
(Gerber 3rd) 6 oz jar	100	20	3	—	—	14	—	—	112	2	2	—	—	60	*	2	8	15	—	—
vanilla custard pudding (Beech-Nut Stage 3) 6 oz jar	180	10	5	—	—	30	—	80	—	15	2	—	—	2	*	4	20	*	—	—
(Gerber 3rd) 6 oz jar	150	15	2	—	—	31	—	—	67	15	2	—	—	*	*	2	8	*	—	—
vanilla flan (Beech-Nut Stage 3) 6 oz jar	130	8	0	0	0	22	—	70	—	10	*	—	—	2	*	8	25	*	—	—
veal (Gerber 3rd) 2 1/2 oz jar	80	60	4	—	—	0	—	—	224	*	2	—	—	*	*	*	10	25	—	—
vegetable bacon dinner (Gerber 3rd) 6 oz jar	130	15	6	—	—	17	—	—	92	2	2	—	—	130	*	6	6	6	—	—
vegetable beef dinner (Beech-Nut Stage 3) 6 oz jar	120	10	5	—	—	16	—	60	—	2	4	—	—	350	*	6	8	10	—	—
(Gerber 3rd) 6 oz jar	120	15	4	—	—	16	—	—	144	2	4	—	—	110	*	4	4	10	—	—
vegetable chicken dinner (Beech-Nut Stage 3) 6 oz jar	110	15	4	—	—	14	—	75	—	8	4	—	—	320	*	6	15	15	—	—
(Gerber 3rd) 6 oz jar	100	15	3	—	—	15	—	—	86	4	2	—	—	70	*	2	2	10	—	—
vegetable ham dinner (Gerber 3rd) 6 oz jar	110	15	4	—	—	16	—	—	102	2	2	—	—	80	*	4	4	8	—	—
vegetable stew w/ beef microwave (Beech-Nut Stage 3) 6 oz tub	110	15	4	—	—	13	—	270	—	*	8	—	—	80	*	6	8	15	—	—
vegetable turkey dinner (Gerber 3rd) 6 oz jar	100	15	3	—	—	15	—	—	78	2	2	—	—	45	*	2	6	8	—	—
BACON																				
(Armour) 2 slices	80	8	11	13	5	*	*	14	25	*	—	—	*	*	—	—	—	—	—	—
(Bryan) 2 slices	73	7	9	—	4	*	*	8	25	*	—	—	*	*	—	—	—	—	—	—
(Oscar Mayer) 2 slices	64	6	8	10	4	*	*	12	*	*	*	*	*	*	*	3	*	2	*	*
(Thorn Apple Valley) 2 slices	70	7	9	—	4	*	*	11	25	—	—	—	*	*	—	—	—	—	—	—
black pepper (Bryan) 2 slices	73	7	9	—	4	*	*	8	25	*	—	—	*	*	—	—	—	—	—	—
Canadian (Oscar Mayer) 2 slices	54	14	*?	4	8	*	*	26	4	*	*	6	*	*	*	—	—	—	—	—
center cut (Oscar Mayer) 2 slices	50	6	6	8	4	· *	*	10	2	*	*	*	*	*	*	3	*	3	2	*
low salt (Bryan) 2 slices	73	7	9	—	4	*	*	6	—	*	—	—	*	*	—	—	—	—	—	—
(Oscar Mayer) 2 slices	78	8	10	12	4	*	*	10	6	*	*	4	*	*	—	—	—	—	—	—
(Thorn Apple Valley) 2 slices	10	10	14	—	—	*	*	9	—	—	—	—	*	*	—	—	—	—	—	—
maple (Armour) 2 slices	80	8	11	14	4	*	*	10	—	*	—	2	—	*	—	—	—	—	—	—
meatless (generic) 1 strip	25	*	4	2	*	*	*	5	*	*	*	*	*	*	*	23	2	3	*	*
smoky hollow (Bryan) 2 slices	73	7	9	—	4	*	*	8	—	*	—	—	*	*	—	—	—	—	—	—
thick slice (Range) 1 oz	152	3	25	30	6	*	*	8	*	*	*	2	*	*	10	5	2	4	—	—
(Thorn Apple Valley) 2 slices	93	8	12	—	—	*	*	15	—	—	—	—	*	*	—	—	—	—	—	—
turkey (Oscar Mayer) 2 slices	64	6	8	8	8	*	*	16	2	*	*	4	*	*	*	—	—	—	—	—
BACON BITS																				
(Hormel Bacon Bits) 1 oz	117	20	11	15	5	*	—	42	10	1	4	9	3	*	*	2	9	15	—	—

	Calories	Protein	Fat	Sat. Fat	Cholesterol	Carbohydrates	Fiber	Sodium	Potassium	Calcium	Iron	Zinc	Magnesium	Vitamin A	Vitamin C	Thiamin	Riboflavin	Niacin	Vitamin B₁₂	Folic acid
(Hormel Bacon Pieces) 1 oz	94	20	8	10	9	*	—	27	6	1	4	11	2	*	*	18	8	13	—	—
(Libby's Crumbles) 1 tbsp	25	2	2	—	—	*	*	—	—	*	*	*	*	*	*	*	*	*	—	—
(Oscar Mayer) 1 tbsp	21	4	2	2	2	*	*	8	*	*	*	2	*	*	*	3	2	3	2	—
BACON & HORSERADISH DIP																				
(Kraft) 2 tbsp	60	2	8	15	*	*	*	8	*	*	*	—	—	*	*	*	*	*	*	—
premium *(Kraft)* 2 tbsp	50	2	8	15	5	*	*	11	*	2	*	—	—	2	*	*	2	*	*	—
BACON & ONION DIP																				
(Kraft) 2 tbsp	60	2	8	15	5	*	*	7	*	2	*	—	—	2	*	4	4	*	*	—
BAGEL																				
cinnamon raisin *(Thomas')* 1 bagel	160	10	2	5	*	12	4	7	—	6	10	—	—	*	*	15	8	8	—	—
egg *(Lender's)* 1 bagel	160	10	2	*	3	10	6	13	—	*	10	—	—	4	*	10	10	10	—	—
egg *(Thomas')* 1 bagel	180	15	2	5	12	11	4	8	—	6	10	—	—	*	*	15	10	8	—	—
onion *(Lender's)* 1 bagel	160	10	2	*	*	10	6	13	—	*	10	—	—	*	*	15	10	10	—	—
onion *(Thomas')* 1 bagel	180	15	2	5	*	12	4	8	4	6	10	—	—	*	*	15	10	8	—	—
plain *(Lender's)* 1 bagel	160	10	2	*	*	10	6	13	—	*	10	—	—	*	*	15	10	10	—	—
plain *(Thomas')* 1 bagel	170	15	2	5	*	11	4	8	—	6	10	—	—	*	*	15	10	8	—	—
BAGEL CHIPS																				
onion & garlic *(Pepperidge Farm)* 1 oz	140	4	6	*	*	6	*	7	*	*	*	—	—	*	*	12	4	12	—	—
three cheese *(Pepperidge Farm)* 1 oz	140	8	9	*	*	5	*	7	*	*	*	—	—	*	*	12	4	12	—	—
BAKING POWDER																				
(Davis) 1/4 tsp	0	*	*	*	*	*	*	4	*	*	*	*	*	*	*	*	*	*	*	*
BAKING SODA																				
(Arm & Hammer) 1/4 tsp	0	*	*	*	*	*	*	10	*	*	*	*	*	*	*	*	*	*	*	*
BALSAM-PEAR LEAF																				
raw 1/2 cup	7	2	*	*	*	*	*	4	*	4	2	3	*	5	8	35	3	5	*	8
boiled 1/2 cup	10	2	*	*	*	*	*	4	*	5	*	2	*	7	10	27	3	5	*	6
boiled w/ salt 1/2 cup	10	2	*	*	*	*	*	4	3	5	*	2	*	7	10	27	3	5	*	6
BALSAM-PEAR POD																				
raw 1/2 cup	8	*	*	*	*	*	*	4	*	4	*	3	2	4	66	*	*	*	*	8
boiled 1/2 cup	12	*	*	*	*	*	*	4	*	6	*	3	2	*	34	2	2	*	*	8
BAMBOO SHOOT																				
raw 1/2 cup	21	3	*	*	*	*	*	8	*	12	*	2	6	*	*	5	8	3	2	*
boiled 1/2 cup	7	2	*	*	*	*	*	8	*	9	*	*	2	*	*	*	*	2	*	*
boiled w/ salt 1/2 cup	7	2	*	*	*	*	*	8	6	9	*	*	2	*	*	*	*	2	*	*
BAMBOO SHOOT, CANNED																				
(generic) 1/2 cup	12	2	*	*	*	*	*	8	*	*	*	*	3	*	*	*	*	*	*	*
(La Choy) 1/2 cup	12	2	*	*	*	*	*	4	*	*	*	*	—	—	*	*	*	*	—	—
BANANA																				
1 fruit	105	2	*	*	*	9	12	*	13	*	2	*	8	2	17	3	7	3	—	5
BANANA CHIPS																				
3 oz	441	3	44	123	*	17	28	*	13	2	6	4	16	*	9	5	*	3	*	3
BANANA, COOKING see PLANTAIN																				

	Calories	Protein	Fat	Sat. Fat	Cholesterol	Carbohydrates	Fiber	Sodium	Potassium	Calcium	Iron	Zinc	Magnesium	Vitamin A	Vitamin C	Thiamin	Riboflavin	Niacin	Vitamin B12	Folic acid
BANANA TOPPING																				
creamy glaze for bananas (Marie's) 2 1/4 oz	120	*	8	—	—	6	*	4	—	*	*	—	—	*	*	*	*	*	—	—
BARBECUE LOAF																				
pork & beef 1 oz	49	7	4	5	3	*	*	16	3	2	2	5	*	*	9	7	4	3	8	*
BARBECUE SAUCE																				
(Hunt's) 2 tbsp	40	*	*	*	*	4	*	14	2	6	2	—	—	*	4	*	*	*	*	*
(Kraft) 2 tbsp	45	*	2	*	*	3	*	19	2	*	*	—	—	4	*	*	*	*	*	*
(Kraft Thick & Spicy) 2 tbsp	50	*	2	*	*	4	*	18	2	*	2	—	—	4	*	*	*	*	*	*
chunky (Kraft Thick & Spicy) 2 tbsp	60	*	2	*	*	4	*	17	2	*	2	—	—	4	*	*	*	*	*	*
country style (Hunt's) 2 tbsp	40	*	*	*	*	4	*	12	2	6	2	—	—	*	4	*	*	*	*	*
fat free hickory (Heinz) 2 tbsp	40	*	*	*	*	3	4	20	—	2	*	—	—	15	*	*	*	*	*	*
original (Heinz) 2 tbsp	40	*	*	*	*	3	4	20	—	2	*	—	—	15	*	*	*	*	*	*
garlic (Kraft) 2 tbsp	40	*	*	*	*	3	*	17	2	*	*	—	—	4	*	*	*	*	*	*
hickory (Hunt's) 2 tbsp	40	*	*	*	*	4	*	14	2	6	2	—	—	*	4	*	*	*	*	*
(Kraft) 2 tbsp	45	*	2	*	*	3	*	18	2	*	*	—	—	4	*	*	*	*	*	*
(Kraft Thick & Spicy) 2 tbsp	50	*	2	*	*	4	*	18	2	*	2	—	—	6	*	*	*	*	*	*
homestyle (Hunt's) 2 tbsp	40	*	*	*	*	4	*	14	2	6	4	—	—	*	4	*	*	*	*	*
honey (Hain) 1 tbsp	28	*	2	—	*	*	*	5	—	*	*	*	*	*	*	*	*	*	*	*
(Kraft Thick & Spicy) 2 tbsp	60	*	2	*	*	4	*	14	3	2	2	—	—	4	*	*	*	*	*	*
hot (Kraft) 2 tbsp	45	*	2	*	*	3	*	22	2	*	*	—	—	4	*	*	*	*	*	*
Italian style (Kraft) 2 tbsp	50	*	2	*	*	3	*	12	2	*	*	—	—	4	*	*	*	*	*	*
Kansas City style (Hunt's) 2 tbsp	40	*	*	*	*	4	*	8	3	8	2	—	—	*	4	*	*	*	*	*
(Kraft) 2 tbsp	50	*	2	*	*	4	*	11	3	2	4	—	—	2	*	*	*	*	*	*
(Kraft Thick & Spicy) 2 tbsp	60	*	2	*	*	4	*	11	4	2	2	—	—	2	*	*	*	*	*	*
mesquite (Kraft) 2 tbsp	45	*	2	*	*	3	*	17	2	*	*	—	—	6	*	*	*	*	*	*
(Kraft Thick & Spicy) 2 tbsp	50	*	2	*	*	4	*	18	2	*	2	—	—	4	*	*	*	*	*	*
New Orleans style (Hunt's) 2 tbsp	40	*	*	*	*	4	*	12	2	6	2	—	—	*	4	*	*	*	*	*
onion (Kraft) 2 tbsp	50	*	2	*	*	4	*	14	2	*	*	—	—	4	*	*	*	*	*	*
southern style (Hunt's) 2 tbsp	40	*	*	*	*	4	*	14	2	6	2	—	—	*	4	*	*	*	*	*
Texas style (Hunt's) 2 tbsp	50	*	*	*	*	4	*	12	2	8	4	—	—	4	4	*	*	*	*	*
western style (Hunt's) 2 tbsp	40	*	*	*	*	4	*	14	2	10	2	—	—	*	4	*	*	*	*	*
BASIL																				
fresh 1 tbsp	1	*	*	*	*	*	*	*	*	*	*	*	*	4	2	*	*	*	*	*
ground 1 tbsp	11	*	*	*	*	*	4	*	4	10	10	2	5	8	5	*	*	2	*	—

	Calories	Protein	Fat	Sat. Fat	Cholesterol	Carbohydrates	Fiber	Sodium	Potassium	Calcium	Iron	Zinc	Magnesium	Vitamin A	Vitamin C	Thiamin	Riboflavin	Niacin	Vitamin B₁₂	Folic acid

BASS

freshwater
raw
1 fillet: 90, 25, 4, 3, 18, *, *, 2, 8, 6, 7, 3, 6, 2, 3, 4, 3, 5, 26, *

sea
raw
1 fillet: 125, 40, 4, 4, 18, *, *, 4, 9, *, 2, 3, 13, 5, *, 9, 9, 10, 6, *

sea
baked/broiled
1 fillet: 125, 40, 4, 4, 18, *, *, 4, 9, *, 2, 3, 13, 4, *, 9, 9, 10, 5, *

striped
raw
1 fillet: 154, 47, 6, 4, 42, *, *, 5, 12, 2, 7, 4, 16, 3, *, 11, 3, 17, 101, *

striped
broiled/baked
1 fillet: 154, 47, 6, 4, 43, *, *, 5, 12, 2, 7, 4, 16, 3, *, 9, 3, 16, 91, *

all varieties
broiled/baked
1 fillet: 91, 25, 4, 3, 18, *, *, 2, 8, 6, 7, 3, 6, *, 2, 4, 3, 5, 24, *

BAY LEAF, CRUMBLED
1 tbsp: 6, *, *, *, *, *, *, *, *, *, 2, 4, *, *, 2, *, *, *, *, *

BEAN SPROUT
kidney
raw
1/2 cup: 27, 6, *, *, *, *, —, *, 5, 2, 4, 2, 5, *, 59, 23, 14, 13, *, 14

BEAN
See also specific listings

BEAN, BAKED

	Calories	Protein	Fat	Sat. Fat	Cholesterol	Carbohydrates	Fiber	Sodium	Potassium	Calcium	Iron	Zinc	Magnesium	Vitamin A	Vitamin C	Thiamin	Riboflavin	Niacin	Vitamin B₁₂	Folic acid
(B & M) 1/2 cup	150	12	3	3	*	9	—	14	12	6	20	—	—	*	*	15	4	4	—	—
(Bush Bros) 1/2 cup	150	12	2	3	—	10	28	23	—	6	10	—	—	*	*	—	—	—	—	—
(generic) 1/2 cup	118	10	*	*	*	9	24	21	11	6	2	12	10	4	7	13	4	3	*	8
(Green Giant) 1/2 cup	130	10	*	*	*	5	12	12	3	3	5	—	—	*	2	4	*	*	—	—
(homemade) 1/2 cup	190	12	10	13	2	9	28	22	13	8	14	6	14	*	2	11	4	3	*	15
(Joan of Arc) 1/2 cup	130	10	*	*	*	5	12	12	3	3	5	—	—	*	2	4	*	*	—	—
barbecue (B & M) 1/2 cup	150	10	3	3	*	9	20	17	13	6	15	—	—	*	*	*	4	2	—	—
(Campbell's) 1/2 cup	130	8	3	—	*	11	24	18	—	4	8	—	—	6	4	2	2	2	—	—
Boston w/ honey (Health Valley) 1/2 cup	100	12	*	*	*	3	19	4	5	3	8	—	—	19	11	5	2	3	—	—
no salt added (Health Valley) 1/2 cup	212	7	*	*	*	7	11	—	11	4	11	—	—	27	13	8	3	4	—	—
brown sugar & bacon (Campbell's) 1/2 cup	150	8	5	—	*	12	—	18	—	6	10	—	—	*	*	4	2	2	—	—
w/ beef (generic) 1/2 cup	161	14	7	11	10	7	—	26	12	6	12	11	8	6	4	5	4	6	*	14
w/ franks (generic) 1/2 cup	182	14	13	15	3	7	36	23	9	6	12	16	9	4	5	5	4	6	*	10
(Libby's) 1/2 cup	330	12	*	*	7	6	19	19	—	5	8	—	—	13	*	—	—	—	—	—
microwave (Hormel Kid's Kitchen) 1/2 cup	310	12	*	*	8	6	—	17	11	5	9	7	8	3	8	5	4	6	—	—
homestyle (Campbell's) 1/2 cup	130	10	3	—	*	11	52	18	—	6	10	—	—	4	4	2	2	2	—	—
honey (B & M) 1/2 cup	120	12	*	*	*	9	22	19	12	5	18	—	—	*	*	*	3	2	—	—
maple (B & M) 1/2 cup	120	12	*	5	*	9	22	19	13	5	20	—	—	*	*	2	3	3	—	—
(Friends) 1/2 cup	120	12	*	—	*	9	22	19	13	5	20	—	—	*	*	2	3	3	—	—
New England (Campbell's) 1/2 cup	150	8	5	—	*	7	—	14	—	10	10	—	—	*	*	2	2	2	—	—

	Calories	Protein	Fat	Sat. Fat	Cholesterol	Carbohydrates	Fiber	Sodium	Potassium	Calcium	Iron	Zinc	Magnesium	Vitamin A	Vitamin C	Thiamin	Riboflavin	Niacin	Vitamin B12	Folic acid
BEAN, BAKED (continued)																				
old fashioned																				
in brown sugar & molasses																				
(Campbell's) 1/2 cup	150	8	5	—	*	9	24	14	—	10	10	—		*	*	2	2	2	—	—
w/ onions																				
(Bush Bros) 1/2 cup	150	12	2	3	*	9	24	21	—	4	10	—		*	*	—	—	—	—	—
w/ pork																				
(Bush Bros) 1/2 cup	120	10	2	3	—	7	24	23	—	4	10	—		2	*	—	—	—	—	—
(Campbell's) 1/2 cup	120	8	3	—	*	7	20	15	—	4	8	—		4	*	4	*	*	—	—
(generic) 1/2 cup	134	11	3	4	3	8	28	22	11	7	12	12	11	4	4	4	3	3	*	11
(Hunt's) 1/2 cup	135	10	2	*	*	9	32	18	10	4	11	—		*	2	10	4	4	—	—
deluxe																				
(Bush Bros) 1/2 cup	160	7	2	3	2	9	32	20	—	4	8	—		16	*	—	—	—	—	—
fanci pak																				
(Bush Bros) 1/2 cup	160	12	2	3	—	9	28	15	—	4	8	—		8	*	—	—	—	—	—
vegetarian																				
(B & M) 1/2 cup	160	—	*	*	9	10	29	20	—	6	20	—		*	*	—	—	—	—	—
(Bush Bros) 1/2 cup	140	10	2	*	*	8	24	23	—	4	8	—		10	*	—	—	—	—	—
(Campbell's) 1/2 cup	110	10	2	—	*	7	20	17	—	6	10	—		6	*	2	2	4	—	—
(Heinz) 1/2 cup	115	12	*	*	*	7	—	18	—	5	13	—		*	*	15	4	4	—	—
low sodium																				
(B & M) 1/2 cup	150	12	2	3	*	9	24	5	18	6	20	—		*	*	*	4	2	—	—
w/ miso																				
(Health Valley) 1/2 cup	180	7	*	*	*	7	12	1	10	3	8	—		27	13	8	4	4	—	—
in sweet sauce																				
(generic) 1/2 cup	140	11	3	4	3	9	28	18	10	8	12	13	11	3	6	4	5	2	*	12
in tomato sauce																				
(generic) 1/2 cup	123	11	2	3	3	8	24	23	11	7	23	49	11	3	7	4	3	3	*	7
(Green Giant/Joan of Arc) 1/2 cup	90	9	*	*	*	4	10	9	3	2	3	—		*	*	*	*	*	—	—
BEAN, CANNED																				
beans 'n fixn's																				
(Hunt's Big John's) 1/2 cup	170	8	9	11	2	9	24	20	12	4	11	—		*	9	12	5	6	—	—
mexe-beans																				
(Old El Paso) 1/2 cup	163	17	2	*	*	10	52	26	17	4	15	—		15	—	15	6	2	—	—
mixed																				
(Bush Bros) 1/2 cup	110	12	*	*	*	6	24	21	—	4	8	—		*	*	—	—	—	—	—
BEAN, CHILI																				
(Gebhardt) 1/2 cup	115	12	2	*	*	7	20	24	13	5	11	—		*	4	12	5	4	—	—
(Hunt's) 1/2 cup	100	10	*	*	*	6	24	20	11	3	11	—		*	3	11	4	3	—	—
50% less salt																				
(Green Giant/Joan of Arc) 1/2 cup	100	12	*	*	*	4	14	7	6	2	8	—		2	*	2	3	2	—	—
extra spicy																				
(Green Giant/Joan of Arc) 1/2 cup	100	12	*	*	*	4	12	12	4	2	4	—		6	*	2	2	2	—	—
hot																				
(Bush Bros) 1/2 cup	120	3	2	3	*	7	24	20	—	2	8	—		10	*	—	—	—	—	—
(Campbell's) 1/2 cup	110	8	3	—	*	6	20	18	—	4	10	—		6	2	2	2	*	—	—
spicy																				
(Green Giant/Joan of Arc) 1/2 cup	100	12	*	*	*	4	14	13	6	2	8	—		2	*	2	3	2	—	—
BEAN DIP																				
fiesta																				
(Chi-Chi's) 1 oz	30	2	2	*	*	*	—	5	3	*	2	1	2	*	*	*	*	*	*	*
hot																				
(Frito-Lay) 2 tbsp	35	3	2	*	*	2	8	9	—	—	—	—		—	—	—	—	—	—	—
(Hain) 2 tbsp	40	3	2	—	*	2	*	5	4	*	6	*	*	*	*	*	*	*	*	*
jalapeño																				
(Frito-Lay) 2 tbsp	40	3	2	3	*	2	*	6	—	—	—	—		—	—	—	—	—	—	—
(Old El Paso) 2 tbsp	28	6	*	*	*	*	8	4	3	*	*	—		*	*	*	*	*	—	—

	Calories	Protein	Fat	Sat. Fat	Cholesterol	Carbohydrates	Fiber	Sodium	Potassium	Calcium	Iron	Zinc	Magnesium	Vitamin A	Vitamin C	Thiamin	Riboflavin	Niacin	Vitamin B$_{12}$	Folic acid
BEAN DIP (continued)																				
Mexican (Hain) 2 tbsp	35	3	2	—	*	2	*	5	4	*	4	*	*	*	*	*	*	*	*	*
onion (Hain) 2 tbsp	35	3	2	—	*	2	*	5	4	*	4	*	*	*	*	*	*	*	*	*
BEAN, GARBANZO																				
(Bush Bros) 1/2 cup	130	10	3	3	*	7	36	21	—	6	8	—	—	*	*	—	—	—	—	—
BEAN, REFRIED																				
(Chi-Chi's) 1/2 cup	250	8	*	*	*	5	—	21	11	3	8	5	8	5	3	*	3	*	—	—
(Gebhardt) 1/2 cup	100	12	3	4	*	7	27	20	12	4	11	—	—	*	2	13	4	3	—	—
(Old El Paso) 1/2 cup	80	10	3	—	*	5	20	18	9	4	12	—	—	*	*	2	2	2	—	—
(Rosarita) 1/2 cup	100	12	3	4	*	6	24	20	12	4	10	—	—	*	*	4	2	4	—	—
w/ bacon (Rosarita) 1/2 cup	110	12	3	5	5	7	24	23	13	5	15	—	—	*	1	5	6	3	—	—
canned (generic) 1/2 cup	118	12	2	3	3	7	28	16	10	4	12	10	10	*	13	2	*	2	*	3
w/ cheese (Old El Paso) 1/2 cup	260	46	9	15	3	11	40	39	21	*	16	—	—	—	—	—	—	—	—	—
fat free (Old El Paso) 1/2 cup	90	10	*	*	*	6	—	15	11	2	8	—	—	*	*	2	8	2	—	—
w/ green chiles (Old El Paso) 1/2 cup	98	20	2	x	x	5	20	21	10	4	12	—	—	x	x	x	x	x	—	—
(Rosarita) 1/2 cup	90	10	3	4	*	6	24	19	12	4	11	—	—	*	5	4	2	4	—	—
w/ jalapeño (Gebhardt) 1/2 cup	115	10	3	4	*	6	27	11	11	4	11	—	—	*	2	12	4	3	—	—
w/ nacho cheese (Rosarita) 1/2 cup	110	12	3	5	*	7	24	20	13	4	15	—	—	*	1	4	4	4	—	—
w/ onions (Rosarita) 1/2 cup	110	12	3	4	*	7	24	20	13	5	15	—	—	*	1	2	2	4	—	—
w/ sausage (Old El Paso) 1/2 cup	360	40	25	*	*	5	*	25	7	8	20	—	—	*	*	*	4	8	—	—
spicy (Rosarita) 1/2 cup	100	12	3	4	*	6	24	21	13	5	11	—	—	*	*	4	2	3	—	—
vegetarian (Hain) 1/2 cup	70	10	2	*	*	5	8	12	9	2	15	—	—	*	*	10	2	*	—	—
(Old El Paso) 1/2 cup	70	10	2	*	*	5	20	25	9	2	15	—	—	*	*	10	2	*	—	—
(Rosarita) 1/2 cup	100	12	3	3	*	6	24	20	12	4	10	—	—	*	*	4	2	4	—	—
BEAN SALAD, CANNED																				
3 bean (Green Giant) 1/2 cup	70	3	*	*	*	6	12	20	5	4	8	—	—	2	*	*	2	2	—	—
BEAN SPROUT																				
mung boiled 1/2 cup	13	2	*	*	*	*	*	*	2	*	2	2	2	*	12	2	4	3	*	5
boiled, salted 1/2 cup	13	2	*	*	*	*	*	6	2	*	2	2	2	*	12	2	4	3	*	5
stir-fried 1/2 cup	31	4	*	*	*	2	—	*	4	*	7	4	5	*	17	6	7	4	*	11
raw 1/2 cup	16	3	*	*	*	*	4	*	2	*	3	*	3	*	11	3	4	2	*	8
kidney boiled 3 oz	28	7	*	*	*	*	—	*	5	2	4	2	5	*	50	20	14	13	*	10
boiled, salted 3 oz	28	7	*	*	*	*	—	9	5	2	4	2	5	*	50	20	14	13	*	10
navy boiled 3 oz	66	10	*	*	*	4	—	*	8	*	10	5	24	*	24	22	12	5	*	23
boiled, salted 3 oz	66	10	*	*	*	4	—	9	8	*	10	5	24	*	24	22	12	5	*	23

	Calories	Protein	Fat	Sat. Fat	Cholesterol	Carbohydrates	Fiber	Sodium	Potassium	Calcium	Iron	Zinc	Magnesium	Vitamin A	Vitamin C	Thiamin	Riboflavin	Niacin	Vitamin B12	Folic acid
BEAN SPROUT (continued)																				
raw 1/2 cup	35	5	*	*	*	2	—	*	5	*	6	3	13	*	16	14	7	3	*	17
boiled 3 oz	19	3	*	*	*	*	—	2	2	*	3	*	4	*	9	4	3	3	*	6
boiled, salted 3 oz	19	3	*	*	*	*	—	10	2	*	3	*	4	*	9	4	3	3	*	6
pinto raw 3 oz	53	7	*	*	*	3	—	5	7	4	9	3	11	*	31	13	9	10	*	25
BEAN SPROUT, CANNED																				
(La Choy) 1/2 cup	8	*	*	*	*	*	2	*	*	*	2	—	—	*	15	*	*	*	—	—
mung (generic) 1/2 cup	7	*	*	*	*	*	*	4	*	*	*	*	*	*	*	*	3	*	*	2
BEAR																				
simmered 4 oz	293	61	23	—	*	*	—	—	*	*	67	—	—	*	*	8	—	—	—	—
BEARNAISE SAUCE																				
from mix (generic) 1/4 cup	225	15	9	—		12	—	88	5	10	2	3	5	*	2	5	8	2	5	2
mix (Knorr) 1/4 oz	170	2	26	—	2	2	—	15	—	4	*	*	*	10	*	*	2	*	*	*
BEAVER																				
roasted 4 oz	240	66	12	—	46	*	*	3	13	2	63	—	8	*	—	4	21	12	156	3
BEECHNUT																				
dried (generic) 1 oz	164	3	22	8	*	3	—	*	8	*	4	*	*	*	7	6	6	*	*	8
BEEF, BLADE																				
prime lean & fat braised 3 oz	354	36	45	61	29	*	*	2	5	*	14	44	4	*	*	4	12	10	31	*
lean only braised 3 oz	270	44	27	36	30	*	*	2	6	*	17	58	5	*	*	5	14	11	35	*
BEEF, BOTTOM ROUND																				
all types lean & fat braised 3 oz	234	41	22	27	27	*	*	2	7	*	15	28	5	*	*	4	12	16	33	2
roasted 3 oz	222	42	19	24	27	*	*	2	7	*	15	29	5	*	*	4	12	16	34	2
lean only braised 3 oz	189	45	13	15	27	*	*	2	7	*	16	31	5	*	*	4	13	17	35	2
roasted 3 oz	156	41	9	10	22	*	*	2	9	*	15	26	6	*	*	5	12	17	38	3
choice lean & fat braised 3 oz	224	42	20	25	27	*	*	2	7	*	15	29	5	*	*	4	12	16	34	2
roasted 3 oz	173	40	12	14	22	*	*	2	9	*	15	26	6	*	*	5	12	17	38	3
lean only braised 3 oz	191	45	13	15	27	*	*	2	7	*	16	31	5	*	*	4	13	17	35	2
roasted 3 oz	164	41	10	11	22	*	*	2	9	*	15	26	6	*	*	5	12	17	38	3

	Calories	Protein	Fat	Sat. Fat	Cholesterol	Carbohydrates	Fiber	Sodium	Potassium	Calcium	Iron	Zinc	Magnesium	Vitamin A	Vitamin C	Thiamin	Riboflavin	Niacin	Vitamin B$_{12}$	Folic acid
BEEF, BOTTOM ROUND (continued)																				
prime																				
lean & fat																				
braised																				
3 oz	252	41	25	31	27	*	*	2	7	*	15	28	5	*	*	4	12	16	33	2
lean only																				
braised																				
3 oz	212	45	17	19	27	*	*	2	7	*	16	31	5	*	*	4	13	17	35	2
select																				
lean & fat																				
braised																				
3 oz	215	42	18	23	27	*	*	2	7	*	15	29	5	*	*	4	12	16	34	2
roasted																				
3 oz	150	40	8	9	22	*	*	2	9	*	15	26	6	*	*	5	12	17	38	3
lean only																				
braised																				
3 oz	182	45	12	13	27	*	*	2	7	*	16	31	5	*	*	4	13	17	35	2
roasted																				
3 oz	145	41	7	8	22	*	*	2	9	*	15	26	6	*	*	5	12	17	38	3
BEEF, BRAIN																				
pan-fried																				
3 oz	167	18	21	16	565	*	*	6	9	*	10	8	3	*	5	7	13	16	214	*
simmered																				
3 oz	136	16	16	13	581	*	*	4	6	*	10	7	3	*	*	5	8	9	121	2
BEEF, BRISKET																				
all types																				
lean & fat																				
braised																				
3 oz	332	33	42	56	26	*	*	2	6	*	10	28	4	*	*	3	9	13	31	*
lean only																				
braised																				
3 oz	205	42	17	20	26	*	*	3	7	*	13	39	5	*	*	4	11	16	36	2
flat half																				
lean & fat																				
braised																				
3 oz	311	35	38	51	27	*	*	2	6	*	11	27	4	*	*	3	9	13	32	*
lean only																				
braised																				
3 oz	180	45	11	13	27	*	*	2	7	*	13	36	5	*	*	4	11	16	37	2
point half																				
lean & fat																				
braised																				
3 oz	347	31	46	62	26	*	*	2	5	*	10	30	3	*	*	3	9	12	32	*
lean only																				
braised																				
3 oz	224	40	21	27	26	*	*	3	7	*	13	42	5	*	*	4	11	15	36	2
BEEF, EYE ROUND																				
all types																				
lean & fat																				
roasted																				
3 oz	207	38	19	25	21	*	*	2	9	*	9	25	5	*	*	4	8	15	30	2
lean only																				
roasted																				
3 oz	156	41	8	11	20	*	*	2	10	*	9	27	6	*	*	5	9	16	31	2
choice																				
lean & fat																				
roasted																				
3 oz	207	38	19	25	21	*	*	2	9	*	9	25	5	*	*	4	8	15	30	2
lean only																				
roasted																				
3 oz	156	41	9	11	20	*	*	2	10	*	9	27	6	*	*	5	9	16	31	2

	Calories	Protein	Fat	Sat. Fat	Cholesterol	Carbohydrates	Fiber	Sodium	Potassium	Calcium	Iron	Zinc	Magnesium	Vitamin A	Vitamin C	Thiamin	Riboflavin	Niacin	Vitamin B12	Folic acid
BEEF, EYE ROUND (continued)																				
prime																				
lean & fat																				
roasted																				
3 oz	213	38	20	26	20	*	*	2	9	*	9	25	5	*	*	5	8	15	30	2
lean only																				
roasted																				
3 oz	168	41	11	14	20	*	*	2	10	*	9	27	6	*	*	5	9	16	31	2
select																				
lean & fat																				
roasted																				
3 oz	201	38	18	24	20	*	*	2	9	*	9	25	5	*	*	4	8	15	30	2
lean only																				
roasted																				
3 oz	151	41	8	10	20	*	*	2	10	*	9	27	6	*	*	5	9	16	31	2
BEEF, FLANK																				
choice																				
lean & fat																				
braised																				
3 oz	224	38	22	30	20	*	*	2	8	*	16	33	5	*	*	8	9	19	47	2
broiled																				
3 oz	192	37	16	23	19	*	*	3	10	*	12	26	5	*	*	6	9	21	45	2
lean only																				
braised																				
3 oz	201	40	17	24	20	*	*	3	8	*	16	34	5	*	*	8	9	20	48	2
broiled																				
3 oz	176	38	13	19	19	*	*	3	10	*	12	27	5	*	*	6	9	21	46	2
BEEF, GROUND																				
all types																				
lean & fat																				
braised																				
3 oz	326	36	40	54	29	*	*	2	5	*	14	44	4	*	*	4	11	10	31	*
lean only																				
braised																				
3 oz	213	44	17	22	30	*	*	2	6	*	17	58	5	*	*	5	14	11	35	*
braised																				
3 oz	230	44	20	27	30	*	*	2	6	*	17	58	5	*	*	5	14	11	35	*
choice																				
lean & fat																				
braised																				
3 oz	330	36	41	55	29	*	*	2	5	*	14	44	4	*	*	4	11	10	31	*
lean only																				
braised																				
3 oz	234	44	21	28	30	*	*	2	6	*	17	58	5	*	*	5	14	11	35	*
extra lean																				
baked																				
medium																				
3 oz	213	35	21	27	23	*	*	2	5	*	11	30	4	*	*	2	12	18	24	2
well-done																				
3 oz	233	43	21	27	30	*	*	2	7	*	14	39	5	*	*	3	15	23	26	2
broiled																				
medium																				
3 oz	218	36	21	28	24	*	*	2	8	*	11	31	4	*	*	3	13	21	31	2
well-done																				
3 oz	225	40	21	27	28	*	*	3	9	*	13	36	5	*	*	4	16	25	36	2
fried																				
medium																				
3 oz	217	35	22	28	23	*	*	2	8	*	11	31	4	*	*	3	13	20	28	2
well-done																				
3 oz	224	40	21	27	26	*	*	3	9	*	13	35	5	*	*	4	15	23	33	2

	Calories	Protein	Fat	Sat. Fat	Cholesterol	Carbohydrates	Fiber	Sodium	Potassium	Calcium	Iron	Zinc	Magnesium	Vitamin A	Vitamin C	Thiamin	Riboflavin	Niacin	Vitamin B₁₂	Folic acid

BEEF, GROUND (continued)

frozen
broiled
medium

	Calories	Protein	Fat	Sat. Fat	Cholesterol	Carbohydrates	Fiber	Sodium	Potassium	Calcium	Iron	Zinc	Magnesium	Vitamin A	Vitamin C	Thiamin	Riboflavin	Niacin	Vitamin B₁₂	Folic acid
BEEF, GROUND (continued)																				
frozen broiled medium 3 oz	240	35	26	33	27	*	*	3	7	*	10	31	4	*	*	3	10	22	35	2
lean only baked medium 3 oz	228	34	24	31	22	*	*	2	5	*	10	29	4	*	*	3	9	18	25	2
well-done 3 oz	248	42	24	31	28	*	*	2	7	*	13	37	4	*	*	4	12	23	32	3
broiled medium 3 oz	231	35	24	31	25	*	*	3	7	*	10	30	4	*	*	3	10	22	33	2
well-done 3 oz	238	40	23	30	29	*	*	3	8	*	12	35	5	*	*	3	12	25	38	2
fried medium 3 oz	234	34	25	32	24	*	*	3	7	*	10	29	4	*	*	3	11	20	32	2
well-done 3 oz	235	39	23	30	27	*	*	3	8	*	12	33	5	*	*	3	12	23	36	2
regular baked medium 3 oz	244	33	27	35	25	*	*	2	5	*	11	28	3	*	*	2	8	20	33	2
well-done 3 oz	269	41	28	36	31	*	*	3	7	*	14	34	4	*	*	2	10	25	41	2
broiled medium 3 oz	246	34	27	35	25	*	*	3	7	*	12	29	4	*	*	2	9	25	41	2
well-done 3 oz	248	39	25	33	29	*	*	3	8	*	13	33	5	*	*	2	10	27	46	2
fried medium 3 oz	260	34	30	38	25	*	*	3	7	*	12	29	4	*	*	2	10	25	38	2
well-done 3 oz	243	38	25	32	28	*	*	3	8	*	13	32	5	*	*	2	10	27	42	2
select lean & fat braised 3 oz	311	36	37	51	29	*	*	2	5	*	14	45	4	*	*	4	12	10	32	*
lean only braised 3 oz	218	44	18	24	30	*	*	2	6	*	17	58	5	*	*	5	14	11	35	*
BEEF, HEART *simmered* 3 oz	149	41	7	7	55	*	*	2	6	*	35	18	5	*	2	8	77	17	202	*
BEEF, KIDNEY *simmered* 3 oz	122	36	4	5	110	*	*	5	4	*	34	24	4	21	*	11	203	26	724	21
BEEF, LIVER *braised* 3 oz	137	35	6	8	110	*	*	2	6	*	32	34	4	607	33	11	205	46	1002	46
pan-fried 3 oz	184	38	10	12	136	2	*	4	9	*	30	31	5	614	33	12	207	61	1577	47
BEEF, PORTERHOUSE *choice* lean & fat broiled 3 oz	254	36	28	38	24	*	*	2	9	*	13	27	5	*	*	5	11	17	30	2
lean only broiled 3 oz	185	40	14	19	23	*	*	2	10	*	14	31	6	*	*	6	12	20	32	2

	Calories	Protein	Fat	Sat. Fat	Cholesterol	Carbohydrates	Fiber	Sodium	Potassium	Calcium	Iron	Zinc	Magnesium	Vitamin A	Vitamin C	Thiamin	Riboflavin	Niacin	Vitamin B12	Folic acid
BEEF, RIB																				
all types																				
lean & fat broiled 3 oz	308	30	39	54	24	*	*	2	7	*	10	28	4	*	*	4	9	13	39	*
roasted 3 oz	324	31	42	57	24	*	*	2	7	*	10	29	4	*	*	4	9	14	35	2
choice																				
lean & fat broiled 3 oz	313	30	40	55	24	*	*	2	7	*	10	28	4	*	*	4	9	13	39	*
roasted 3 oz	328	31	42	59	24	*	*	2	7	*	10	29	4	*	*	4	9	14	35	2
prime																				
lean & fat broiled 3 oz	347	30	46	64	24	*	*	2	7	*	10	28	4	*	*	4	8	13	39	*
roasted 3 oz	361	30	48	67	24	*	*	2	7	*	10	29	4	*	*	4	8	14	35	2
select																				
lean & fat broiled 3 oz	289	31	36	50	24	*	*	2	7	*	10	29	4	*	*	4	9	13	40	*
roasted 3 oz	306	32	38	53	24	*	*	2	7	*	10	30	4	*	*	4	9	14	36	2
whole																				
all types lean only broiled 3 oz	194	37	17	24	23	*	*	2	9	*	12	37	5	*	*	5	10	16	46	2
lean only roasted 3 oz	204	39	18	25	23	*	*	3	9	*	12	39	5	*	*	5	10	17	41	2
choice lean only broiled 3 oz	198	37	18	24	23	*	*	2	9	*	12	37	5	*	*	5	10	16	46	2
lean only roasted 3 oz	209	39	19	26	23	*	*	3	9	*	12	39	5	*	*	5	10	17	41	2
prime lean only broiled 3 oz	238	37	24	34	23	*	*	2	9	*	12	37	5	*	*	5	10	16	46	2
lean only roasted 3 oz	248	39	25	35	23	*	*	3	9	*	12	39	5	*	*	5	10	17	41	2
select lean only broiled 3 oz	181	37	15	21	23	*	*	2	9	*	12	37	5	*	*	5	10	16	46	2
lean only roasted 3 oz	191	39	16	22	23	*	*	3	9	*	12	39	5	*	*	5	10	17	41	2
BEEF, RIB EYE																				
choice																				
lean & fat broiled 3 oz	261	35	29	39	24	*	*	2	8	*	11	34	5	*	*	5	9	18	42	2
lean only broiled 3 oz	191	40	15	20	23	*	*	2	10	*	12	40	6	*	*	6	11	20	47	2

	Calories	Protein	Fat	Sat. Fat	Cholesterol	Carbohydrates	Fiber	Sodium	Potassium	Calcium	Iron	Zinc	Magnesium	Vitamin A	Vitamin C	Thiamin	Riboflavin	Niacin	Vitamin B$_{12}$	Folic acid
BEEF, ROUND																				
choice																				
lean & fat broiled 3 oz	233	36	24	31	24	*	*	2	9	*	11	23	5	*	*	5	10	16	39	2
lean only broiled 3 oz	165	40	10	13	23	*	*	2	10	*	13	26	6	*	*	6	11	18	42	2
select																				
lean & fat broiled 3 oz	223	36	22	29	24	*	*	2	9	*	11	24	5	*	*	5	10	16	39	2
lean only broiled 3 oz	156	40	9	11	23	*	*	2	10	*	13	26	6	*	*	6	11	18	42	2
BEEF, SHANK																				
choice																				
lean & fat simmered 3 oz	207	45	16	20	22	*	*	2	10	3	17	55	6	*	*	7	10	23	51	2
lean only 3 oz	171	48	8	10	22	*	*	2	11	3	18	59	6	*	*	8	11	25	53	2
BEEF, SHORT RIB																				
choice																				
lean & fat braised 3 oz	400	31	55	76	27	*	*	2	5	*	11	28	3	*	*	3	7	10	37	*
lean only braised 3 oz	251	44	24	33	26	*	*	2	8	*	16	44	5	*	*	4	10	14	49	2
BEEF, SIRLOIN																				
all types																				
lean & fat broiled 3 oz	238	39	24	32	25	*	*	2	9	*	14	33	6	*	*	6	13	16	38	2
lean only broiled 3 oz	177	43	11	15	25	*	*	2	10	*	16	37	7	*	*	7	15	18	40	2
choice																				
lean & fat broiled 3 oz	241	39	24	33	25	*	*	2	9	*	14	32	6	*	*	6	13	16	38	2
pan-fried 3 oz	288	39	32	43	28	*	*	2	9	*	15	30	6	*	*	7	14	16	45	2
lean only broiled 3 oz	179	43	12	16	25	*	*	2	10	*	16	37	7	*	*	7	15	18	40	2
fried 3 oz	202	46	14	18	28	*	*	3	11	*	18	36	7	*	*	8	16	18	52	2
prime																				
lean & fat broiled 3 oz	271	38	30	41	25	*	*	2	8	*	14	31	6	*	*	6	13	16	37	2
lean only broiled 3 oz	201	43	16	21	25	*	*	2	10	*	16	37	7	*	*	7	15	18	40	2
select																				
lean & fat broiled 3 oz	232	39	23	31	25	*	*	2	9	*	14	32	6	*	*	6	13	16	38	2
lean only broiled 3 oz	170	43	10	14	25	*	*	2	10	*	16	37	7	*	*	7	15	18	40	2

	Calories	Protein	Fat	Sat. Fat	Cholesterol	Carbohydrates	Fiber	Sodium	Potassium	Calcium	Iron	Zinc	Magnesium	Vitamin A	Vitamin C	Thiamin	Riboflavin	Niacin	Vitamin B₁₂	Folic acid
BEEF, SWEETBREADS																				
braised																				
3 oz	271	31	33	37	83	*	*	4	10	*	7	12	2	*	43	5	11	8	21	*
BEEF, T-BONE																				
choice																				
lean & fat																				
broiled																				
3 oz	275	34	32	44	24	*	*	2	8	*	12	25	5	*	*	5	10	17	30	2
lean only																				
broiled																				
3 oz	182	40	14	18	23	*	*	2	10	*	14	31	6	*	*	6	12	20	32	2
BEEF, TENDERLOIN																				
all types																				
lean & fat																				
broiled																				
3 oz	226	37	22	30	24	*	*	2	9	*	15	29	6	*	*	7	13	15	35	*
roasted																				
3 oz	258	35	29	39	25	*	*	2	8	*	15	25	5	*	*	5	14	13	36	2
lean only																				
broiled																				
3 oz	173	40	12	16	24	*	*	2	10	*	17	32	6	*	*	7	15	17	36	2
roasted																				
3 oz	186	39	15	19	24	*	*	2	10	*	17	29	6	*	*	6	16	14	39	2
choice																				
lean & fat																				
broiled																				
3 oz	230	37	23	31	24	*	*	2	9	*	15	28	6	*	*	7	13	15	34	2
roasted																				
3 oz	262	35	30	40	25	*	*	2	8	*	15	25	5	*	*	5	14	13	36	2
lean only																				
broiled																				
3 oz	176	40	13	16	24	*	*	2	10	*	17	32	6	*	*	7	15	17	36	2
roasted																				
3 oz	190	39	15	20	24	*	*	2	10	*	17	29	6	*	*	6	16	14	39	2
prime																				
lean & fat																				
broiled																				
3 oz	270	35	31	41	24	*	*	2	9	*	15	27	6	*	*	6	13	15	34	2
roasted																				
3 oz	304	33	38	50	25	*	*	2	8	*	14	24	5	*	*	5	13	13	35	2
lean only																				
broiled																				
3 oz	197	40	16	21	24	*	*	2	10	*	17	32	6	*	*	7	15	17	36	2
roasted																				
3 oz	217	39	20	26	24	*	*	2	10	*	17	29	6	*	*	6	16	14	39	2
select																				
lean & fat																				
broiled																				
3 oz	216	37	21	27	24	*	*	2	9	*	15	29	6	*	*	7	14	15	35	2
roasted																				
3 oz	245	35	27	36	25	*	*	2	8	*	15	26	5	*	*	5	14	13	36	2
lean only																				
broiled																				
3 oz	167	40	11	14	24	*	*	2	10	*	17	32	6	*	*	7	15	17	36	2
roasted																				
3 oz	177	39	13	17	24	*	*	2	10	*	17	29	6	*	*	6	16	14	39	2
BEEF, TIP ROUND																				
all types																				
lean & fat																				
roasted																				
3 oz	213	37	20	26	24	*	*	2	9	*	13	36	5	*	*	5	12	15	39	2

	Calories	Protein	Fat	Sat. Fat	Cholesterol	Carbohydrates	Fiber	Sodium	Potassium	Calcium	Iron	Zinc	Magnesium	Vitamin A	Vitamin C	Thiamin	Riboflavin	Niacin	Vitamin B_{12}	Folic acid
BEEF, TIP ROUND (continued)																				
lean only roasted 3 oz	162	41	10	12	23	*	*	2	9	*	14	40	6	*	*	6	13	16	41	2
choice																				
lean & fat roasted 3 oz	216	37	20	27	24	*	*	2	9	*	13	36	5	*	*	5	12	15	39	2
lean only roasted 3 oz	164	41	10	12	23	*	*	2	9	*	14	40	6	*	*	6	13	16	41	2
prime																				
lean & fat roasted 3 oz	241	37	25	33	24	*	*	2	8	*	13	35	5	*	*	5	12	14	38	2
lean only roasted 3 oz	181	41	13	16	23	*	*	2	9	*	14	40	6	*	*	6	13	16	41	2
select																				
lean & fat roasted 3 oz	205	38	18	24	24	*	*	2	9	*	13	36	5	*	*	5	12	15	39	2
lean only roasted 3 oz	156	41	9	11	23	*	*	2	9	*	14	40	6	*	*	6	13	16	41	2
BEEF, TONGUE																				
simmered 3 oz	241	31	27	38	30	*	*	2	4	*	16	27	4	*	*	2	17	9	83	*
BEEF, TOP LOIN																				
all types																				
lean & fat broiled 3 oz	238	36	25	33	22	*	*	2	8	*	11	26	5	*	*	5	9	20	27	2
lean only broiled 1 steak	396	93	27	35	49	*	*	6	22	2	27	68	13	*	*	12	23	52	65	4
choice																				
lean & fat broiled 3 oz	243	36	26	35	22	*	*	2	8	*	11	26	5	*	*	5	9	20	27	2
lean only broiled 1 steak	406	93	28	37	50	*	*	6	22	2	27	68	13	*	*	12	23	52	65	4
prime																				
lean & fat broiled 3 oz	288	35	34	46	23	*	*	2	8	*	10	25	5	*	*	4	9	19	27	2
lean only broiled 1 steak	439	85	38	49	45	*	*	5	20	*	25	62	12	*	*	11	21	48	59	4
select																				
lean & fat broiled 3 oz	223	37	22	30	22	*	*	2	9	*	11	26	5	*	*	5	9	20	27	2
lean only broiled 1 steak	372	93	23	30	50	*	*	6	22	2	27	68	13	*	*	12	23	52	65	4
BEEF, TOP ROUND																				
all types																				
lean & fat braised 3 oz	178	50	8	10	25	*	*	2	8	*	15	25	5	*	*	4	12	16	38	2

	Calories	Protein	Fat	Sat. Fat	Cholesterol	Carbohydrates	Fiber	Sodium	Potassium	Calcium	Iron	Zinc	Magnesium	Vitamin A	Vitamin C	Thiamin	Riboflavin	Niacin	Vitamin B₁₂	Folic acid

BEEF, TOP ROUND (continued)

	Calories	Protein	Fat	Sat. Fat	Cholesterol	Carbohydrates	Fiber	Sodium	Potassium	Calcium	Iron	Zinc	Magnesium	Vitamin A	Vitamin C	Thiamin	Riboflavin	Niacin	Vitamin B₁₂	Folic acid
broiled 3 oz	179	44	12	14	24	*	*	2	10	*	13	31	6	*	*	6	13	25	34	3
lean only braised 3 oz	169	51	7	8	25	*	*	2	8	*	16	26	6	*	*	4	12	16	38	2
broiled 3 oz	162	45	8	9	24	*	*	2	11	*	14	32	7	*	*	7	13	26	35	3
choice lean & fat braised 3 oz	184	50	9	11	25	*	*	2	8	*	15	25	5	*	*	4	12	16	38	2
broiled 3 oz	181	44	12	15	24	*	*	2	10	*	13	31	6	*	*	6	13	25	34	3
fried 3 oz	247	45	22	28	27	*	*	2	11	*	13	24	7	*	*	6	13	21	45	2
lean only braised 3 oz	176	51	8	9	25	*	*	2	8	*	16	26	6	*	*	4	12	16	38	2
broiled 3 oz	165	45	8	10	24	*	*	2	11	*	14	32	7	*	*	7	13	26	35	3
fried 3 oz	193	50	11	12	27	*	*	2	12	*	15	26	7	*	*	6	14	23	48	3
prime lean & fat broiled 3 oz	201	44	15	19	24	*	*	2	10	*	13	30	6	*	*	6	13	25	34	2
lean only broiled 3 oz	183	45	12	13	24	*	*	2	11	*	14	32	7	*	*	7	13	26	35	3
select lean & fat braised 3 oz	170	50	7	8	25	*	*	2	8	*	15	25	5	*	*	4	12	16	38	2
broiled 3 oz	176	44	11	14	24	*	*	2	10	*	13	30	6	*	*	6	13	25	34	2
lean only braised 3 oz	162	51	5	6	25	*	*	2	8	*	16	26	6	*	*	4	12	16	38	2
broiled 3 oz	156	45	7	8	24	*	*	2	11	*	14	32	7	*	*	7	13	26	35	3

BEEF, CORNED see CORNED BEEF

BEEF, COLD CUTS

	Calories	Protein	Fat	Sat. Fat	Cholesterol	Carbohydrates	Fiber	Sodium	Potassium	Calcium	Iron	Zinc	Magnesium	Vitamin A	Vitamin C	Thiamin	Riboflavin	Niacin	Vitamin B₁₂	Folic acid
cured thin sliced (generic) 5 slices	37	10	*	*	3	*	*	13	3	*	3	6	*	*	5	*	2	6	9	*
luncheon meat dried (Hormel) 1 oz	45	13	2	3	7	*	—	47	*	*	6	15	2	*	8	1	6	7	—	*
roast (Oscar Mayer) 1 slice	59	17	2	4	9	*	*	22	5	*	5	12	2	*	*	—	—	—	—	—
smoked, chopped cured (generic) 2 slices	70	19	4	5	9	*	*	30	6	*	9	15	3	*	20	3	6	13	16	*

BEEF DINNER, FROZEN

	Calories	Protein	Fat	Sat. Fat	Cholesterol	Carbohydrates	Fiber	Sodium	Potassium	Calcium	Iron	Zinc	Magnesium	Vitamin A	Vitamin C	Thiamin	Riboflavin	Niacin	Vitamin B₁₂	Folic acid
(Banquet Extra Helping) 15 1/2 oz	430	60	20	—	33	14	—	51	21	4	30	—	—	40	15	10	15	20	—	—
w/ barbecue sauce (Swanson) 11 oz	460	60	23	—	—	17	—	35	—	8	25	—	—	25	8	10	20	20	—	—
marinated slow-cooked (Le Menu) 11 oz	310	32	22	—	—	9	—	30	—	8	20	—	—	40	90	25	20	15	—	—

	Calories	Protein	Fat	Sat. Fat	Cholesterol	Carbohydrates	Fiber	Sodium	Potassium	Calcium	Iron	Zinc	Magnesium	Vitamin A	Vitamin C	Thiamin	Riboflavin	Niacin	Vitamin B$_{12}$	Folic acid
BEEF DINNER, FROZEN (continued)																				
pepper steak																				
(Healthy Choice) 11 oz	260	33	8	10	13	13	—	21	7	2	6	—	—	20	50	10	4	4	—	—
pot roast																				
(Budget Gourmet Light & Healthy) 10 1/2 oz	230	40	11	15	20	6	—	21	17	2	10	—	—	100	20	15	20	35	—	—
old fashioned																				
(Le Menu) 7 2/3 oz	250	40	11	—	—	7	—	25	—	4	20	—	—	210	15	6	15	25	—	—
yankee																				
(Healthy Choice) 11 oz	260	32	6	10	18	12	—	17	10	4	10	—	—	10	15	10	10	8	—	—
(Swanson) 11 1/2 oz	270	35	11	—	—	12	—	28	—	6	15	—	—	45	8	8	20	30	—	—
(Swanson Hungry-Man) 16 oz	420	60	17	—	—	16	—	38	—	8	30	—	—	35	8	10	25	35	—	—
ribs w/ barbecue sauce																				
(Healthy Choice Homestyle) 11 oz	330	47	9	10	23	13	—	22	19	6	10	—	—	6	8	15	15	15	—	—
roast																				
(Top Shelf) 10 oz	240	47	9	10	20	6	—	37	27	2	15	30	12	40	4	50	25	30	—	—
salisbury steak																				
(Armour Classics) 11 1/4 oz	350	37	26	—	18	9	—	59	15	10	25	—	—	6	40	15	20	10	—	—
(Armour Classics Lite) 11 1/2 oz	300	35	17	—	13	10	—	41	19	8	25	—	—	6	20	25	15	15	—	—
(Banquet Extra Helping) 16 1/4 oz	590	55	43	—	28	19	—	115	29	10	20	—	—	*	2	15	20	35	—	—
(Healthy Choice) 11 1/2 oz	280	32	11	15	17	15	—	23	17	6	15	—	—	8	8	20	20	20	—	—
(Le Menu) 10 1/2 oz	360	35	26	—	—	10	—	28	—	10	20	—	—	15	40	8	20	15	—	—
(Swanson) 10 1/2 oz	390	35	26	—	—	14	—	37	—	6	15	—	—	4	2	8	10	20	—	—
(Swanson Hungry-Man) 16 1/4 oz	630	70	49	—	—	17	—	67	—	20	30	—	—	6	6	10	20	20	—	—
(Top Shelf) 10 oz	320	42	23	35	23	7	—	38	23	2	15	38	10	*	6	2	15	25	—	—
old fashioned																				
(Le Menu Healthy) 10 1/4 oz	270	40	8	10	8	12	—	20	—	10	15	—	—	35	60	10	25	25	—	—
parmigiana																				
(Armour Classics) 11 1/2 oz	410	37	32	—	20	11	—	47	15	10	25	—	—	6	10	20	15	15	—	—
w/ mushroom gravy																				
(Healthy Choice Homestyle) 11 oz	280	35	9	15	18	12	—	21	18	6	15	—	—	2	*	15	20	15	—	—
sirloin																				
chopped																				
(Swanson) 10 1/2 oz	340	40	26	—	—	10	—	31	—	6	20	—	—	100	8	6	10	20	—	—
in wine sauce																				
(Budget Gourmet Light & Healthy) 11 oz	280	30	12	10	8	12	—	23	13	4	10	—	—	100	15	20	20	35	—	—
salisbury steak																				
(Budget Gourmet Light & Healthy) 11 oz	280	30	14	20	13	10	—	22	18	10	10	—	—	60	35	15	25	35	—	—
special recipe																				
(Budget Gourmet Light & Healthy) 11 oz	250	30	14	15	20	10	—	23	13	6	10	—	—	100	10	20	25	30	—	—
w/ barbecue sauce																				
(Healthy Choice) 11 oz	280	28	6	10	8	15	—	10	18	4	10	—	—	15	45	15	10	10	—	—
sirloin tips																				
(Healthy Choice) 11 1/4 oz	280	37	11	15	22	10	—	15	15	2	10	—	—	70	70	10	10	15	—	—
(Le Menu) 7 2/3 oz	290	38	17	—	—	8	—	31	—	10	20	—	—	210	45	10	25	20	—	—
(Swanson) 7 oz	190	30	11	—	—	6	—	18	—	4	10	—	—	30	8	6	10	10	—	—
(Swanson Hungry-Man) 15 3/4 oz	450	60	22	—	—	17	—	52	—	8	35	—	—	35	15	15	25	20	—	—
sliced																				
(Swanson) 11 1/4 oz	330	60	12	—	—	12	—	29	—	4	25	—	—	10	10	10	15	25	—	—

	Calories	Protein	Fat	Sat. Fat	Cholesterol	Carbohydrates	Fiber	Sodium	Potassium	Calcium	Iron	Zinc	Magnesium	Vitamin A	Vitamin C	Thiamin	Riboflavin	Niacin	Vitamin B₁₂	Folic acid
BEEF DINNER, FROZEN (continued)																				
steak, chopped (Swanson Hungry-Man) 16 3/4 oz	640	70	57	—	—	14	—	67	—	6	30	—	—	8	15	10	20	40	—	—
stroganoff (Armour Classics Lite) 11 1/4 oz	250	30	9	—	18	11	—	21	9	4	15	—	—	50	70	15	10	8	—	—
teriyaki (Budget Gourmet Light & Healthy) 10 3/4 oz	260	30	11	10	10	12	—	22	11	4	6	—	—	50	35	15	15	25	—	—
vegetable w/ beef pot pie (Banquet) 7 oz	510	20	51	—	8	13	—	36	5	2	10	—	—	10	2	20	15	20	—	—
BEEF ENTREE																				
brunswick stew (homemade) 1 cup	231	44	10	—	—	6	—	18	14	4	11	14	11	9	23	9	12	33	3	5
stew (homemade) 1 cup	222	38	8	—	—	7	—	19	15	3	17	38	10	133	24	12	14	18	26	6
BEEF ENTREE, CANNED																				
corned beef hash (Libby's) 1 cup	490	37	55	85	32	9	36	52	—	2	10	—	—	*	*	—	—	—	—	—
(Mary Kitchen) 7 1/2 oz	47	37	5	5	3	*	—	5	2	1	2	3	1	*	*	—	1	2	—	—
pepper oriental (La Choy) 3/4 cup	100	12	6	8	3	4	8	56	5	2	10	—	—	*	9	2	6	8	—	—
pepper steak (La Choy Classics) 3/4 cup	180	28	14	17	20	3	4	32	14	2	10	—	—	*	*	10	10	25	—	—
roast beef hash (Libby's) 1 cup	460	32	51	65	27	8	12	58	—	2	10	—	—	*	*	—	—	—	—	—
(Mary Kitchen) 7 1/2 oz	46	37	5	5	3	*	—	4	2	1	2	3	1	*	*	7	1	2	—	—
roast beef w/ gravy (Libby's) 2/3 cup	140	60	5	8	23	*	*	33	—	*	8	—	—	*	2	—	—	—	—	—
stew (Dinty Moore) 8 oz	220	18	20	30	10	5	—	36	15	3	9	17	6	73	4	2	7	12	—	—
(Healthy Choice) 7 1/2 oz	140	25	3	—	12	5	—	22	12	2	10	—	—	30	6	6	8	10	—	—
(Libby's) 7 3/4 oz	290	20	31	25	13	6	20	35	—	2	8	—	—	25	*	—	—	—	—	—
(Weight Watchers) 7 1/2 oz	120	23	3	5	7	5	16	19	9	2	10	—	—	40	*	—	—	—	—	—
microwave (Healthy Choice) 7 1/2 oz	140	25	3	—	12	5	—	10	12	2	10	—	—	30	6	6	8	10	—	—
sweet & sour (La Choy Dinner Classics) 3/4 cup	310	53	9	6	17	10	2	36	10	4	15	—	—	*	3	6	15	70	—	—
w/ pepper bi-pack (La Choy) 3/4 cup	80	12	3	3	6	3	8	40	5	2	10	—	—	*	24	27	4	8	—	—
BEEF ENTREE, FROZEN																				
cantonese (Budget Gourmet) 9 oz	270	25	14	—	13	10	—	37	13	2	6	—	—	45	50	25	15	25	—	—
chimichanga (Old El Paso) 1 chimichanga	310	15	31	25	3	12	—	20	6	4	20	—	—	*	*	15	20	15	—	—
creamed, chipped (Stouffer's) 9 oz	150	15	17	15	13	2	4	29	7	10	6	—	—	*	*	4	15	10	—	—
(Swanson) 9 oz	410	30	34	—	—	13	—	42	—	6	10	—	—	35	6	15	15	25	—	—
over biscuit (Stouffer's) 9 oz	460	—	43	35	23	13	12	69	12	15	20	—	—	*	*	—	—	—	—	—
london broil (Weight Watchers) 7 1/2 oz	110	28	5	5	8	*	8	13	12	4	10	—	—	8	6	—	—	—	—	—
oriental style (Budget Gourmet Light & Healthy) 10 oz	290	30	12	15	10	12	—	35	14	4	6	—	—	25	25	10	15	35	—	—

	Calories	Protein	Fat	Sat. Fat	Cholesterol	Carbohydrates	Fiber	Sodium	Potassium	Calcium	Iron	Zinc	Magnesium	Vitamin A	Vitamin C	Thiamin	Riboflavin	Niacin	Vitamin B₁₂	Folic acid
BEEF ENTREE, FROZEN (continued)																				
(Stouffer's Lean Cuisine) 8 5/8 oz	290	33	14	10	13	10	—	25	11	2	10	—	—	15	2	6	10	15	—	—
(Stouffer's Lunch Express) 9 5/8 oz	80	—	12	8	7	11	16	51	11	4	10	—	—	40	20					
pepper oriental (Chun King) 13 oz	310	28	5	—	13	18	—	54	11	2	20	—	—	30	30	10	15	10	—	
pepper steak (Armour Classics Lite) 11 1/4 oz	220	28	6	—	12	10	—	40	9	4	10	—	—	10	25	10	15	8	—	
(Healthy Choice) 9 1/2 oz	250	30	6	10	13	12	—	23	7	2	10	—	—	4	45	10	10	8	—	—
pepper steak w/ rice (Budget Gourmet) 10 oz	300	25	12	—	12	13	—	30	9	2	6	—	—	25	20	10	10	25	—	
(Stouffer's) 10 1/2 oz	330	33	14	13	12	15	12	27	18	2	6	—	—	4	20	10	10	20	—	
pot pie (Stouffer's) 10 oz	450	30	40	45	22	12	12	47	7	4	15	—	—	40	2	20	25	20	—	—
(Swanson) 7 oz	370	20	29	—	—	—	—	30	—	2	15	—	—	25	*	15	10	15		
(Swanson Hungry-Man) 14 oz	600	60	45	—	—	10	—	54	—	6	25	—	—	170	10	30	30	35	—	—
pot roast homestyle (Stouffer's) 8 7/8 oz	270	33	15	15	13	8	16	27	20	4	10	—	—	30	1	20	15	25	—	
reuben sandwich (Weight Watchers) 5 oz	250	20	9	10	7	14	20	17	11	8	10	—	—	8	15					
roast beef sandwich (Swanson) 10 1/4 oz	340	25	15	—	—	17	—	29	—	6	10	—	—	*	20	20	15	10	—	
romanoff supreme (Weight Watchers) 9 1/2 oz	240	20	12	15	8	13	24	24	12	15	10	—	—	6	6					
salisbury steak (Light & Elegant) 9 oz	200	30	12	—	18	5	—	42	19	6	20	—	—	10	4	10	15	15	—	
(Weight Watchers) 8 1/2 oz	250	32	14	15	10	8	16	25	13	10	15	—	—	6	*					
w/ macaroni & cheese (Stouffer's) 9 5/8 oz	370	42	29	30	17	9	—	51	10	20	15	—	—	2	*	10	25	15	—	
(Stouffer's Lean Cuisine) 9 1/2 oz	270	45	12	15	17	7	—	21	16	15	20	—	—	*	*	15	20	15	—	
w/ mashed potatoes (Swanson) 9 oz	340	35	29	—	—	8	—	40	—	6	15	—	—	*	4	6	10	15	—	
salisbury steak w/gravy (Morton) 9 oz	270	18	25	—	12	7	—	53	11	4	10	—	—	60	6	8	8	6	—	
sandwich, barbecue (Hormel Quickmeal) 4 1/4 oz	370	25	26	25	18	13	—	25	9	4	15	15	8	*	*	25	15	20	—	
sirloin cheddar melt (Budget Gourmet) 9 1/2 oz	380	30	32	—	28	10	—	40	23	15	8	—	—	10	20	15	20	30	—	—
in herb sauce (Budget Gourmet Light & Healthy) 9 1/2 oz	250	30	14	15	10	7	—	36	19	4	10	—	—	8	6	15	20	40	—	—
salisbury steak (Budget Gourmet Light & Healthy) 9 oz	220	25	12	15	8	8	—	30	15	6	10	—	—	40	15	15	20	30	—	—
supreme (Budget Gourmet) 9 oz	320	30	23	—	28	9	—	26	7	4	10	—	—	4	8	15	20	30	—	—
sirloin tips (Swanson) 7 oz	190	30	11	—	—	6	—	18	—	4	10	—	—	30	8	6	10	10	—	
(Weight Watchers) 7 1/2 oz	200	33	9	15	10	7	8	23	5	*	8	—	—	6	4	—	—	—	—	
w/ country vegetables (Budget Gourmet) 10 oz	290	25	26	—	13	6	—	34	12	6	10	—	—	35	25	20	15	25	—	
w/ mushroom gravy (Healthy Choice) 9 1/2 oz	260	33	9	10	12	11	—	24	4	4	10	—	—	6	10	20	20	10	—	—

	Calories	Protein	Fat	Sat. Fat	Cholesterol	Carbohydrates	Fiber	Sodium	Potassium	Calcium	Iron	Zinc	Magnesium	Vitamin A	Vitamin C	Thiamin	Riboflavin	Niacin	Vitamin B₁₂	Folic acid
BEEF ENTREE, FROZEN (continued)																				
steak biscuit sandwich *(Hormel Quickmeal)* 1 (4 1/4 oz)	330	22	23	—	18	12	—	35	9	6	10	11	6	*	*	15	15	15	—	—
steak & mushroom pie *(Mrs. Paterson's)* 1 pie (5 1/2 oz)	410	27	40	50	32	14	—	33	8	8	11	12	5	17	5	17	21	19	—	—
stew microwave *(Hormel Micro Cup)* 7 1/2 oz	230	22	23	25	15	4	—	47	14	2	9	16	6	32	4	3	6	12	—	—
stroganoff *(Budget Gourmet Light & Healthy)* 8 3/4 oz	260	30	15	25	17	9	—	20	7	6	15	—	—	10	6	20	20	25	—	—
(Stouffer's) 9 3/4 oz	380	38	31	35	28	10	8	46	11	4	10	—	—	2	*	8	20	15	—	—
Swiss steak *(Swanson)* 10 oz	350	60	17	—	—	12	—	29	—	4	20	—	—	15	20	10	10	20	—	—
w/ potatoes *(Stouffer's)* 8 1/8 oz	270	—	15	15	15	8	8	37	21	2	10	—	—	*	10	—	—	—	—	—
western style *(Swanson)* 11 1/2 oz	430	45	29	—	—	14	—	44	—	8	20	—	—	10	25	8	10	30	—	—
BEEF GRAVY																				
canned *(Franco-American)* 1/4 cup	35	*	3	—	—	*	*	12	—	*	—	—	—	*	*	*	*	*	—	—
hearty *(Pepperidge Farm)* 1/4 cup	25	2	2	—	—	*	—	10	—	*	—	—	—	*	*	*	*	6	*	—
from dry mix *(generic)* 1/4 cup	31	4	2	—	—	*	*	14	*	*	2	4	*	*	*	*	*	2	*	*
BEEF JERKY																				
smoked *(generic)* 1 stick	109	7	15	21	9	*	—	12	*	*	4	3	*	6	2	2	5	4	3	*
BEEF SPREAD																				
(Underwood) 2 1/8 oz	140	15	17	25	15	*	*	15	4	*	8	—	—	*	*	*	4	10	—	—
BEEF SUET																				
1 oz	242	44	—	74	*	*	*	*	*	*	*	*	*	*	*	*	*	*	*	*
BEEF TALLOW																				
1 tbsp	115	*	6	32	*	*	*	*	*	*	*	*	*	*	*	*	*	*	*	*
BEEFALO																				
roasted 4 oz	212	58	11	15	22	*	*	4	—	3	19	48	—	*	—	2	7	28	48	5
BEER																				
light 12 fl oz	99	*	*	*	*	2	*	*	2	2	*	*	4	*	*	2	6	7	*	4
regular 12 fl oz	146	2	*	*	*	4	4	*	3	2	*	*	5	*	*	*	5	8	*	5
BEERWURST																				
beef 1 1 oz slice	93	6	13	19	6	*	*	12	*	*	2	5	*	*	8	*	2	5	9	*
pork 1 1 oz slice	67	7	8	9	6	*	*	15	2	*	*	3	*	*	14	10	3	5	4	*
BEET																				
raw 2 beets	70	4	*	*	*	5	20	5	15	3	7	4	9	*	13	3	4	3	*	45
boiled 1/2 cup slices	37	2	*	*	*	3	4	3	7	*	4	2	5	*	5	2	2	*	*	17
2 beets	44	3	*	*	*	3	8	3	9	2	4	2	6	*	6	2	2	2	*	20
boiled w/ salt 1/2 cup slices	37	2	*	*	*	3	4	10	7	*	4	2	5	*	5	2	2	*	*	17
BEET, CANNED																				
(Bush Bros) 1/2 cup slices	40	3	*	*	*	3	8	15	—	2	4	—	—	*	*	—	—	—	—	—
(Del Monte) 1/2 cup slices	35	2	*	*	*	3	8	12	—	*	2	—	—	*	4	—	—	—	—	—

	Calories	Protein	Fat	Sat. Fat	Cholesterol	Carbohydrates	Fiber	Sodium	Potassium	Calcium	Iron	Zinc	Magnesium	Vitamin A	Vitamin C	Thiamin	Riboflavin	Niacin	Vitamin B₁₂	Folic acid
BEET, CANNED (continued)																				
(generic) 1/2 cup slices	26	*	*	*	*	2	8	10	4	*	9	*	4	*	6	*	2	*	*	6
Harvard solid & liquid (generic) 1/2 cup slices	90	2	*	*	*	7	—	8	6	*	2	2	6	*	5	*	4	*	*	9
low salt solid & liquid (generic) 1/2 cup slices	36	2	*	*	*	3	4	2	5	2	5	2	5	*	8	*	3	*	*	9
pickled (Del Monte) 1/2 cup slices	80	2	*	*	*	6	8	16	—	*	2			*	6					
solid & liquid (generic) 1/2 cup slices	74	2	*	*	*	6	—	13	5	*	3	2	4	*	4	*	3	*	*	8
whole (Del Monte) 1/2 cup	35	2	*	*	*	3	8	12	—	*	2			*	4					
solid & liquid (generic) 1/2 cup slices	36	2	*	*	*	3	4	13	5	2	5	2	5	*	8	*	3	*	*	9
whole, tiny (Del Monte) 1/2 cup	35	2	*	*	*	3	8	12	—	*	2			*	4					
BEET GREENS																				
raw 1/2 cup	4	*	*	*	*	*	4	2	3	2	3	*	3	23	9	*	2	*	*	*
boiled 1/2 cup	19	3	*	*	*	*	8	7	19	8	8	2	12	73	30	6	12	2	*	3
boiled w/ salt 1/2 cup	19	3	*	*	*	—		14	19	8	8	2	12	73	30	6	12	2	*	3
BERLINER																				
pork & beef 1 1 oz slice	65	7	8	9	4	*	*	15	2	*	2	5	*	*	3	7	4	4	13	*
BERRY DRINK																				
berry nectar, organic (Heinke's) 8 fl oz	120	3	*	*	*	10	*	*	5	*	*			*	6					
(Santa Cruz Natural) 8 fl oz	110	*	*	*	*	9	*	*	2	4	4	—	—	*	2	—	—	—	—	—
(Tang) 8 1/2 fl oz	140	*	*	*	*	12	*	*	*	*	*	—	—	*	100	*	10	10	*	20
(Tropicana) 6 fl oz	90	*	*	*	—	8	—	*	—	*	—			*	2	6	4	*	—	—
BISCUIT																				
from mix (Robin Hood) 1 biscuit	90	3	5	5	*	5	—	2	—	2	4			*	*	6	2	4	—	—
from refrigerated dough (Pillsbury Heat 'n Eat) 1 biscuit	280	8	23	15	*	11	—	25	2	2	8			*	*	10	20	8	—	—
baking powder (1869 Brand) 1 biscuit	100	3	8	5	*	4	—	13	*	*	4			*	*	6	4	4	—	—
butter (Pillsbury) 1 biscuit	50	2	*	*	*	3	—	7	3	*	2			*	*	4	2	2	—	—
butter tastin' (Big Country) 1 biscuit	100	3	6	5	*	4	—	13	3	*	4			*	*	6	4	4	—	—
(1869 Brand) 1 biscuit	100	3	8	5	*	4	—	12	*	*	4			*	*	6	4	4	—	—
(Grands!) 1 biscuit	190	7	14	10	*	7	—	23	2	2	6			*	*	10	8	6	—	—
country (Pillsbury) 1 biscuit	50	2	2	*	*	3	—	7	3	*	2			*	*	4	2	2	—	—
flaky (Hungry Jack) 1 biscuit	100	3	6	3	*	4	—	12	*	*	2			*	*	6	2	2	—	—
buttermilk (Big Country) 1 biscuit	100	3	6	3	*	5	—	13	3	*	4			*	*	8	4	4	—	—
(Pillsbury) 1 biscuit	50	2	2	*	*	3	—	7	3	*	2			*	*	4	2	2	—	—
(Pillsbury Heat 'n Eat) 1 biscuit	170	7	8	5	*	9	—	22	2	2	6			*	*	10	8	8	—	—
cinnamon raisin (Grands!) 1 biscuit	190	5	11	10	*	9	—	22	3	2	6			*	*	10	6	6	—	—
extra lights (Ballard Ovenready) 1 biscuit	50	2	*	*	*	3	—	7	3	*	2			*	*	4	2	2	—	—

	Calories	Protein	Fat	Sat. Fat	Cholesterol	Carbohydrates	Fiber	Sodium	Potassium	Calcium	Iron	Zinc	Magnesium	Vitamin A	Vitamin C	Thiamin	Riboflavin	Niacin	Vitamin B₁₂	Folic acid
BISCUIT (continued)																				
extra rich (Hungry Jack) 1 biscuit	150	2	2	*	*	3	—	7	3	*	2	—	—	*	*	4	2	2	—	—
flaky (Hungry Jack) 1 biscuit	90	3	6	3	*	4	—	12	*	*	2	—	—	*	*	6	2	4	—	—
fluffy (Hungry Jack) 1 biscuit	90	3	6	5	*	4	—	12	*	*	2	—	—	*	*	6	2	4	—	—
honey tastin' flaky (Hungry Jack) 1 biscuit	90	3	6	3	*	4	—	12	*	*	4	—	—	*	*	6	2	4	—	—
regular (1869 Brand) 1 biscuit	100	3	8	5	*	4	—	13	*	*	4	—	—	*	*	6	4	4	—	—
southern style (Big Country) 1 biscuit	100	3	6	3	*	5	—	13	3	*	4	*	—	*	*	8	4	4	—	*
tender layer (Pillsbury) 1 biscuit	50	2	2	*	*	3	—	7	3	*	2	—	—	*	*	4	2	2	—	—
flaky (Hungry Jack) 1 biscuit	80	2	6	3	*	4	—	12	*	*	2	—	—	*	*	6	2	4	—	—
ready to eat old fashioned (Arnold) 1 biscuit	60	3	5	—	'	3	—	4	—	2	4	—	—	*	*	8	2	4	—	—
BISON																				
roasted 4 oz	162	54	4	5	31	*	*	3	12	*	21	28	7	*	*	—	—	—	—	—
BLACK BEAN																				
cooked (generic) 1/2 cup	114	13	*	*	*	7	28	*	9	2	10	6	15	*	*	14	3	2	*	32
cooked, salted (generic) 1/2 cup	114	13	*	*	*	7	28	8	9	2	10	6	15	*	*	14	3	2	*	32
BLACK BEAN, CANNED																				
(Progresso) 1/2 cup	90	15	2	*	*	6	26	15	8	4	10	*	*	*	*	8	2	*	*	—
dry, canned in brine (Green Giant) 1/2 cup	90	12	*	*	*	7	24	24	11	4	8	—	—	*	*	10	2	2	*	—
(Joan of Arc) 1/2 cup	90	12	*	*	*	7	24	24	11	4	8	—	—	*	*	10	2	2	*	—
w/ garden vegetables (Health Valley) 7 1/2 oz	213	23	*	*	*	4	58	7	8	15	23	—	—	150	*	15	15	6	—	—
w/ tofu weiners (Health Valley) 1/2 cup	240	20	7	—	*	4	44	9	6	12	20	—	—	80	2	12	12	5	—	—
BLACK TURTLE BEAN																				
cooked (generic) 1/2 cup	120	13	*	*	*	7	20	*	11	5	15	5	11	*	*	14	3	2	*	20
cooked, salted (generic) 1/2 cup	120	13	*	*	*	7	20	9	11	5	15	5	11	*	*	14	3	2	*	20
BLACK TURTLE BEAN, CANNED																				
(generic) 1/2 cup	109	12	*	*	*	7	—	19	11	4	13	4	11	*	5	11	8	4	*	18
(Hain) 1/2 cup	70	10	2	*	*	5	24	13	11	4	10	—	—	*	*	6	*	2	*	—
BLACK CHERRY DRINK																				
from mix unsweetened (Kool-Aid) 8 fl oz prep. w/ out sugar	2	*	*	*	*	*	*	*	*	*	*	*	*	*	10	*	*	*	*	*
(Kool-Aid) 8 fl oz prep. w/ sugar	100	*	*	*	*	8	*	*	*	*	*	*	*	*	10	*	*	*	*	*
BLACK CHERRY JUICE																				
(Heinke's) 8 fl oz	180	*	*	*	*	14	*	2	8	2	*	*	*	*	*	—	—	—	*	*
(Knudsen) 8 fl oz	180	3	*	*	*	14	*	2	8	2	*	*	*	*	*	—	—	—	*	*
(Smucker's) 8 fl. oz.	130	*	*	*	*	10	*	*	10	2	4	*	*	2	6	2	4	2	*	*
from concentrate (Knudsen Exotic Blends) 8 fl oz	130	*	*	*	*	11	*	*	10	2	6	*	*	*	*	—	—	—	*	*

	Calories	Protein	Fat	Sat. Fat	Cholesterol	Carbohydrates	Fiber	Sodium	Potassium	Calcium	Iron	Zinc	Magnesium	Vitamin A	Vitamin C	Thiamin	Riboflavin	Niacin	Vitamin B₁₂	Folic acid
BLACKBERRY 1/2 cup	37	*	*	*	*	3	16	*	4	2	2	*	4	2	25	*	2	*	*	6
BLACKBERRY, CANNED in heavy syrup 1/2 cup	118	3	*	*	*	10	16	*	4	3	5	2	5	6	6	2	3	2	*	8
BLACKBERRY, FROZEN unsweetened 1 cup	97	3	*	*	*	8	32	*	6	4	7	3	8	3	8	3	4	9	*	13
BLACKEYE PEA, CANNED from fresh (Bush Bros) 1/2 cup	110	12	2	*	*	6	20	21	—	2	8	—	—	*	*	—	—	—	—	—
from dry (Bush Bros) 1/2 cup	100	8	*	*	*	6	16	17	—	2	8	—	—	*	*	—	—	—	—	—
w/bacon (Bush Bros) 1/2 cup	110	10	2	3	—	6	20	26	—	*	8	—	—	*	*	—	—	—	—	—
w/bacon & jalapeño (Bush Bros) 1/2 cup	120	10	4	5	—	5	20	27	—	*	10	—	—	*	*	—	—	—	—	—
BLACKEYE PEA COMBINATION CANNED w/snap beans (Bush Bros) 1/2 cup	110	12	*	*	*	6	20	23	—	2	8	—	—	*	*	—	—	—	—	—
BLOOD SAUSAGE 1 1 oz slice	107	7	15	19	11	*	*	8	*	*	10	2	*	*	*	*	2	2	5	*
BLOODY MARY 1 cocktail (5 fl oz)	115	*	*	*	*	*	—	14	6	*	3	*	3	10	*	3	2	3	*	5
BLUEBERRY raw 1/2 cup	81	2	*	*	*	7	16	*	4	*	*	*	2	3	31	5	4	3	—	2
BLUEBERRY, CANNED in heavy syrup 1/2 cup	113	*	*	*	*	9	8	*	*	2	*	*	2	2	3	4	*	—		*
BLUEBERRY, FROZEN sweetened 1 cup	186	2	*	*	*	17	20	*	4	*	5	*	2	4	3	7	3	—		3
unsweetened 1 cup	79	*	2	*	*	6	16	*	2	*	2	*	2	3	6	3	3	4	—	3
BLUEBERRY GLAZE (Marie's) 2 1/3 oz	90	*	*	*	*	7	*	3	—	*	*	*	*	*	*	*				
BLUEBERRY NECTAR (Knudsen Exotic Blends) 8 fl oz	130	*	*	*	*	11	*	*	*	7	2	4	—	*	2					
BLUEBERRY-CRANBERRY DRINK (Ocean Spray) 8 fl oz	160	*	*	*	*	14	*	*	*	*	*	*	—	*	100					
BLUEFISH raw 1 fillet	186	50	10	7	29	*	*	4	16	*	4	8	12	12	*	6	7	45	134	*
broiled/baked 1 fillet	186	50	10	7	30	*	*	4	16	*	4	8	12	11	*	5	7	42	121	*
BOAR, WILD roasted 4 oz	181	53	8	8	—	*	*	—			2	—	—	*	*	23	9	—	—	—
BOCKWURST pork & veal (generic) 1 1 oz slice	87	6	12	15	6	*	*	13	2	*	3	*	*	*	*	8	3	6	4	*
BOK CHOY see CABBAGE																				
BOLOGNA beef (Bryan) 1 oz	90	5	12	—	5	*	*	12	—	—	—									
(generic) 1 1 oz slice	88	6	12	17	5	*	*	12	*	*	3	4	*	*	10	*	2	3	7	*
(Oscar Mayer) 1 slice	90	5	13	18	6	*	*	12	*	*	2	4	*	*	*	*	2	3	7	*
light (Oscar Mayer) 1 slice	54	5	6	8	4	*	*	13	*	*	2	4	*	*	*	*	—	—	—	—

Encyclopedia of Daily Values

	Calories	Protein	Fat	Sat. Fat	Cholesterol	Carbohydrates	Fiber	Sodium	Potassium	Calcium	Iron	Zinc	Magnesium	Vitamin A	Vitamin C	Thiamin	Riboflavin	Niacin	Vitamin B₁₂	Folic acid
BOLOGNA (continued)																				
beef & pork																				
(Bryan) 1 oz	90	55	12	—	5	*	*	12	—				*	*		—	—	—	—	
(generic) 1 1 oz slice	90	6	12	15	5	*	*	12	*	*	2	4	*	*	10	3	2	4	6	*
(Oscar Mayer) 1 slice	89	5	13	16	6	*	*	13	*	*	2	3	*	*	*	5	2	3	5	*
(Oscar Mayer Healthy) 1 slice	20	5	*	*	2	*	*	10	*	*	2	2	*	*	*	—	—	—	—	—
light (Oscar Mayer) 1 slice	55	5	6	7	4	*	*	13	*	*	2	3	*	*	*	—	—	—	—	—
skinless (Oscar Mayer) 1 slice	86	5	12	15	7	*	*	11	*	*	2	3	*	*	*	—	—	—	—	—
garlic (Oscar Mayer) 1 slice	131	8	18	22	8	*	*	20	2	*	3	4	2	*	*	—	—	—	—	—
Lebanon (generic) 1 1 oz slice	60	9	6	9	7	*	*	16	2	*	4	8	*	*	10	*	3	6	12	*
pork (generic) 1 1 oz slice	70	7	9	10	6	*	*	14	2	*	4	*	*	*	17	10	3	6	4	*
ring (Oscar Mayer) 1 slice	86	5	12	15	6	*	*	10	*	*	2	3	*	*	*	5	2	4	6	—
BOLOGNA, TURKEY see TURKEY, COLD CUTS																				
BOLOGNESE SAUCE																				
mix (Knorr) 1/2 oz	60	2	3	—	2	3	*	34	—		2	*	*	10	45	4	6	4	*	*
BORAGE																				
raw 1/2 cup	9	*	*	*	*	*	—	*	6	4	8	*	6	37	26	2	4	2	*	2
boiled 3 oz	21	3	*	*	*	*	—	3	12	9	17	*	12	75	46	3	8	4	*	2
boiled w/ salt 3 oz	21	3	*	*	*	*	—	11	12	9	17	*	12	75	46	3	8	4	*	2
BOULLION see SOUP, FROM MIX																				
BOYSENBERRY, CANNED																				
in heavy syrup 1/2 cup	113	2	*	*	*	10	12	*	3	2	3	2	4	*	13	2	2	*	*	11
BOYSENBERRY, FROZEN																				
unsweetened 1/2 cup	33	*	*	*	*	2	10	*	3	2	3	*	2	*	4	3	*	3	*	21
BOYSENBERRY JUICE																				
(Farmer's Market) 8 fl oz	120	*	*	*	*	10	*	*	2	*	—	—	*		4	—	—	—	*	—
(Smucker's) 8 fl oz	120	*	*	*	*	10	*	*	9	2	4	*	*	*	2	2	4	2	*	*
BOYSENBERRY NECTAR																				
(Knudsen Exotic Blends) 8 fl oz	130	*	*	*	*	11	*	*	7	2	4	*	*	*	2	—	—	—	*	*
BRAINS see specific meat																				
BRATWURST																				
pork 1 1 oz slice	85	7	11	13	6	*	*	7	2	*	2	4	*	*	*	10	3	5	4	*
BRAUNSCHWEIGER (see also LIVERWURST)																				
(Oscar Mayer) 1 slice	95	6	13	15	16	*	*	13	2	*	15	6	*	88	5	4	26	13	87	3
German brand (Oscar Mayer) 1 slice	97	6	14	15	15	*	*	13	2	*	15	6	*	102	5	4	28	12	83	7
pork (generic) 1 1 oz slice	102	6	14	16	15	*	*	13	2	*	15	5	*	80	5	5	25	12	95	3
tube (Oscar Mayer) 1 oz	95	6	13	15	16	*	*	13	*	*	15	6	*	93	5	4	25	12	86	4
BRAZIL NUT																				
dried 1 oz	186	7	29	23	*	*	8	*		5	5	9	16	*	*	19	2	2	*	*
BREAD, APPLE CINNAMON																				
from mix (Pillsbury) 1 slice (1/12 recipe)	180	3	9	5	7	10	—	7	*	2	4	—	—	*	*	6	6	4	—	—

	Calories	Protein	Fat	Sat. Fat	Cholesterol	Carbohydrates	Fiber	Sodium	Potassium	Calcium	Iron	Zinc	Magnesium	Vitamin A	Vitamin C	Thiamin	Riboflavin	Niacin	Vitamin B₁₂	Folic acid
BREAD, APPLE CINNAMON (continued)																				
no cholesterol recipe																				
(Pillsbury) 1 slice (1/12 recipe)	190	3	9	5	*	10	—	7	*	2	4	—	—	*	*	8	4	4	—	—
BREAD, APPLE WALNUT																				
(Pepperidge Farm Swirl) 1 oz	80	6	2	*	*	5	8	5	—	2	4	—	—	*	*	6	4	6	—	—
BREAD, BANANA																				
from mix																				
(Pillsbury) 1 slice (1/12 recipe)	170	5	9	3	*	9	—	9	*	*	4	—	—	2	*	6	6	4	—	—
BREAD, BLUEBERRY																				
from mix																				
no cholesterol recipe																				
(Pillsbury) 1 slice (1/12 recipe)	180	3	9	5	*	10	—	7	*	2	4	—	—	*	*	8	6	4	—	—
BREAD, BRAN																				
country																				
light																				
(Brownberry) 1 slice	40	4	*	*	*	3	12	3	—	*	2	—	—	*	*	4	2	2	—	—
light																				
(Arnold Bakery) 1 slice	40	4	*	*	*	3	12	3	—	*	2	—	—	*	*	4	2	2	—	—
natural																				
(Brownberry) 1 slice	60	2	2	*	*	3	8	7	—	*	6	—	—	*	*	8	6	6	—	—
BREAD, BROWN																				
plain																				
(B & M) 1/2" slice	92	3	*	*	*	7	8	14	4	4	4	—	—	*	*	4	4	2	—	—
(Friends) 1/2" slice	92	3	*	*	*	7	8	14	4	4	4	—	—	*	*	4	4	2	—	—
raisin																				
(B & M) 1/2" slice	94	3	*	*	*	7	8	13	5	4	4	—	—	*	*	4	4	2	—	—
(Friends) 1/2" slice	94	3	*	*	*	7	8	13	5	4	4	—	—	*	*	4	4	2	—	—
BREAD, CINNAMON																				
(Arnold) 1 slice	70	2	2	*	*	4	4	4	—	4	—	—	—	*	*	*	4	4	—	—
(Pepperidge Farm Swirl) 1 oz	90	4	5	*	*	5	8	5	—	*	4	—	—	*	*	8	4	4	—	—
cinnamon chip																				
(Arnold) 1 slice	80	4	3	—	*	4	4	4	—	*	2	—	—	*	*	4	2	2	—	—
w/ raisins																				
(Pepperidge Farm Swirl) 1 oz	90	2	3	*	*	5	4	4	—	2	4	—	—	*	*	6	4	4	—	—
(Wonder) 1 slice	60	5	2	3	*	4	4	4	2	2	6	—	—	*	*	6	4	4	—	—
BREAD, CORN																				
from mix																				
(Ballard) 1/16 mix	150	7	5	3	10	8	—	24	3	4	6	—	—	2	*	15	10	8	—	—
twists																				
from refrigerated dough																				
(Pillsbury) 1 twist	70	2	5	3	*	3	—	6	*	*	2	—	—	*	*	2	2	2	—	—
BREAD, CRACKED WHEAT TWIST																				
from mix																				
(Hearty Grains) 1 twist	80	3	3	*	*	5	4	5	4	*	4	—	—	*	*	4	2	4	—	—
BREAD, CRANBERRY																				
from mix																				
(Pillsbury) 1 slice (1/12 recipe)	160	3	6	3	7	10	—	6	*	*	4	—	—	*	*	8	6	4	—	—
no cholesterol recipe																				
(Pillsbury) 1 slice (1/12 recipe)	170	5	6	3	*	10	—	7	*	*	4	—	—	*	*	8	6	4	—	—
BREAD, DATE																				
date-nut loaf																				
(Thomas') 1 oz	90	2	3	—	2	6	4	7	—	*	4	—	—	*	*	4	2	2	—	—
from mix																				
(Pillsbury) 1 slice (1/12 recipe)	160	3	5	3	7	10	—	6	2	*	4	—	—	*	*	6	6	4	—	—
(Pillsbury) 1 slice (1/12 recipe)	160	3	5	3	*	11	—	6	2	*	4	—	—	*	*	6	4	4	—	—
BREAD, FRENCH																				
(Bread du Jour) 1 slice	70	5	2	3	*	4	3	6	*	4	6	—	—	*	*	10	6	6	—	—
(Wonder) 1 slice	70	5	2	3	*	4	3	6	*	4	6	—	—	*	*	4	6	6	—	—
from refrigerated dough																				
(Pillsbury) 1 slice	60	3	*	*	*	4	—	5	*	*	4	—	—	*	*	6	4	4	—	—

	Calories	Protein	Fat	Sat. Fat	Cholesterol	Carbohydrates	Fiber	Sodium	Potassium	Calcium	Iron	Zinc	Magnesium	Vitamin A	Vitamin C	Thiamin	Riboflavin	Niacin	Vitamin B₁₂	Folic acid
BREAD, FRENCH (continued)																				
Parisan																				
(DiCarlo's) 1 slice	70	3	2	3	*	4	3	7	*	4	4	—	—		*	*	6	4	6	—	—
petite loaves																				
(Bread du Jour) 1 loaf	230	17	3	3	*	15	10	22	3	15	20	—	—		*	*	35	20	20	—	—
stick																				
(Arnold Francisco) 1 oz	70	4	2	—	*	4	4	6	—	2	6	—	—		*	*	6	4	4	—	—
(Savoni) 1 oz	80	4	2	—	*	5	4	—	—	2	4	—	—		*	*	6	4	4	—	—
twin																				
(Pepperidge Farm) 1 oz	80	4	2	*	*	5	*	7	—	2	4	—	—		*	*	8	6	6	—	—
BREAD, HONEY BRAN																				
honey																				
(Pepperidge Farm Old Fashioned) 1 slice	90	4	2	—	*	6	4	7	—	*	6	—	—		*	*	10	6	6	—	—
BREAD, HONEY WHEATBERRY																				
(Pepperidge Farm Hearty) 1 slice	100	5	2	*	*	6	8	8	—	2	4	—	—		*	*	8	4	4	—	—
BREAD, ITALIAN																				
(Wonder) 1 slice	70	5	2	3	*	4	3	7	*	4	4	—	—		*	*	8	4	6	—	—
brown & serve																				
(Pepperidge Farm) 1 oz	80	4	2	*	*	5	*	6	—	2	4	—	—		*	*	10	6	6	—	—
light																				
(Arnold Bakery) 1 slice	40	4	*	*	*	2	12	3	—	*	2	—	—		*	*	4	2	2	—	—
(Brownberry) 1 slice	40	2	2	*	*	3	8	4	—	*	4	—	—		*	*	4	4	4	—	—
(Wonder) 1 slice	40	3	*	*	*	2	12	5	*	4	4	—	—		*	*	6	4	4	—	—
sliced																				
(Arnold Francisco) 1 slice	70	4	2	—	—	4	—	5	—	2	2	—	—		*	*	6	4	4	—	—
stick																				
(Arnold Francisco) 1 oz	90	4	2	—	—	6	—	5	—	2	4	—	—		*	*	6	4	6	—	—
BREAD, MULTI-GRAIN																				
from mix																				
(Hearty Grains) 1 slice	80	3	3	*	*	5	4	10	5	*	4	—	—		*	*	6	2	4	—	—
BREAD, NINE GRAIN																				
(Pepperidge Farm Wholesome Choice) 1 slice	90	7	2	*	*	5	8	7	—	2	4	—	—		*	*	6	4	4	—	—
BREAD, NUT																				
from mix																				
(Pillsbury) 1 slice (1/12 recipe)	170	5	9	3	7	9	—	8	*	2	4	—	—		*	*	8	6	4	—	—
no cholesterol recipe																				
(Pillsbury) 1 slice (1/12 recipe)	170	5	9	3	*	9	—	8	2	2	4	—	—		*	*	8	6	4	—	—
BREAD, OATMEAL																				
(Arnold) 1 slice	60	2	2	*	*	4	8	4	—	*	2	—	—		*	*	4	2	2	—	—
(Pepperidge Farm Light) 1 slice	40	2	*	*	*	3	8	4	—	*	4	—	—		*	*	6	2	4	—	—
(Pepperidge Farm Old Fashioned) 1 slice	90	4	2	—	*	6	4	8	—	2	6	—	—		*	*	10	4	6	—	—
thin sliced																				
(Pepperidge Farm) 1 slice	70	4	2	—	*	4	4	7	—	*	4	—	—		*	*	6	4	4	—	—
w/ bran																				
(Oatmeal Goodness) 1 slice	80	7	2	3	*	5	5	6	2	6	6	—	—		*	*	8	6	6	—	—
w/ sunflower seeds																				
(Oatmeal Goodness) 1 slice	80	7	2	3	*	5	5	6	2	6	6	—	—		*	*	8	6	6	—	—
crunchy																				
(Pepperidge Farm Hearty) 1 slice	100	7	3	*	*	6	8	7	—	2	4	—	—		*	*	10	6	6	—	—
light																				
(Arnold Bakery) 1 slice	40	4	*	*	*	3	8	2	—	*	2	—	—		*	*	4	2	2	—	—
(Brownberry) 1 slice	40	2	2	*	*	3	8	4	—	*	4	—	—		*	*	6	4	4	—	—
w/ bran																				
(Oatmeal Goodness) 1 slice	40	3	*	*	*	2	11	4	*	6	4	—	—		*	*	4	2	4	—	—

	Calories	Protein	Fat	Sat. Fat	Cholesterol	Carbohydrates	Fiber	Sodium	Potassium	Calcium	Iron	Zinc	Magnesium	Vitamin A	Vitamin C	Thiamin	Riboflavin	Niacin	Vitamin B₁₂	Folic acid
						PERCENTAGE DAILY VALUE														

BREAD, OATMEAL (continued)

	Calories	Protein	Fat	Sat. Fat	Cholesterol	Carbohydrates	Fiber	Sodium	Potassium	Calcium	Iron	Zinc	Magnesium	Vitamin A	Vitamin C	Thiamin	Riboflavin	Niacin	Vitamin B₁₂	Folic acid
w/ wheat (Oatmeal Goodness) 1 slice	40	3	*	*	*	2	11	4	*	6	*	—	—	*	*	4	2	4	—	—
natural (Brownberry) 1 slice	60	2	2	*	*	4	4	6	—	*	6	—	—	*	*	8	6	6	—	—
sandwich natural (Brownberry) 1 slice	70	2	3	5	*	4	8	5	—	2	4	—	—	*	*	4	2	2	—	—
soft (Brownberry) 1 slice	60	2	2	*	*	4	8	4	—	*	4	—	—	*	*	4	4	4	—	—
(Pepperidge Farm) 1 slice	60	2	*	*	*	4	—	4	—	4	10	—	—	*	*	10	6	8	—	—

BREAD, OATMEAL RAISIN

	Calories	Protein	Fat	Sat. Fat	Cholesterol	Carbohydrates	Fiber	Sodium	Potassium	Calcium	Iron	Zinc	Magnesium	Vitamin A	Vitamin C	Thiamin	Riboflavin	Niacin	Vitamin B₁₂	Folic acid
(Arnold) 1 slice	60	2	2	*	*	4	8	4	—	*	4	—	—	*	*	4	4	4	—	—
(Brownberry) 1 slice	60	2	2	*	*	4	8	4	—	*	4	—	—	*	*	4	4	4	—	—
from mix (Hearty Grains) 1 slice	90	3	3	3	*	5	4	9	4	*	4	—	—	*	*	6	2	2	—	—
no cholesterol recipe (Pillsbury) 1 slice (1/12 recipe)	190	5	11	5	*	10	—	7	3	2	6	—	—	*	*	10	4	4	—	—

BREAD, OATMEAL TWIST

	Calories	Protein	Fat	Sat. Fat	Cholesterol	Carbohydrates	Fiber	Sodium	Potassium	Calcium	Iron	Zinc	Magnesium	Vitamin A	Vitamin C	Thiamin	Riboflavin	Niacin	Vitamin B₁₂	Folic acid
from mix (Hearty Grains) 1 twist	80	3	3	3	*	5	4	5	4	*	4	—	—	*	*	6	2	2	—	—

BREAD, ORANGE RAISIN

	Calories	Protein	Fat	Sat. Fat	Cholesterol	Carbohydrates	Fiber	Sodium	Potassium	Calcium	Iron	Zinc	Magnesium	Vitamin A	Vitamin C	Thiamin	Riboflavin	Niacin	Vitamin B₁₂	Folic acid
(Brownberry) 1 slice	70	2	2	*	*	4	4	4	—	*	4	—	—	*	*	4	4	4	—	—

BREAD, PAN CUBANO

	Calories	Protein	Fat	Sat. Fat	Cholesterol	Carbohydrates	Fiber	Sodium	Potassium	Calcium	Iron	Zinc	Magnesium	Vitamin A	Vitamin C	Thiamin	Riboflavin	Niacin	Vitamin B₁₂	Folic acid
(Arnold August Bros.) 1 roll	230	10	5	—	*	14	8	21	—	8	15	—	—	*	*	20	10	10	—	—

BREAD PAN DE AQUA

	Calories	Protein	Fat	Sat. Fat	Cholesterol	Carbohydrates	Fiber	Sodium	Potassium	Calcium	Iron	Zinc	Magnesium	Vitamin A	Vitamin C	Thiamin	Riboflavin	Niacin	Vitamin B₁₂	Folic acid
(Arnold August Bros.) 1 oz	80	4	2	—	*	5	4	6	—	2	4	—	—	*	*	6	4	4	—	—

BREAD, PITA

	Calories	Protein	Fat	Sat. Fat	Cholesterol	Carbohydrates	Fiber	Sodium	Potassium	Calcium	Iron	Zinc	Magnesium	Vitamin A	Vitamin C	Thiamin	Riboflavin	Niacin	Vitamin B₁₂	Folic acid
oat bran (Thomas') 1/2 pita	80	4	2	*	*	5	8	7	—	4	2	—	—	*	*	6	2	4	—	—
wheat (Arnold) 1/2 pita	71	6	*	*	—	5	—	—	—	7	4	—	—	*	*	6	4	4	—	—
white (Arnold) 1/2 pita	71	6	*	*	—	5	—	—	—	7	4	—	—	*	*	6	4	4	—	—
large (Thomas') 1 pita	150	8	*	*	*	10	8	12	—	10	10	—	—	*	*	15	8	8	—	—
mini (Pepperidge Farm Wholesome Choice) 1 pita	70	4	6	*	*	5	4	4	—	4	4	—	—	*	*	8	8	6	—	—
regular (Pepperidge Farm Wholesome Choice) 1 pita	70	4	*	*	*	5	4	4	—	4	6	—	—	*	*	8	8	6	—	—
(Thomas') 1 pita	80	4	2	*	*	5	4	6	—	4	2	—	—	*	*	10	4	6	—	—
whole wheat (Thomas') 1/2 pita	70	4	2	*	*	4	8	6	—	4	4	—	—	*	*	10	2	6	—	—

BREAD, PUMPERNICKEL

	Calories	Protein	Fat	Sat. Fat	Cholesterol	Carbohydrates	Fiber	Sodium	Potassium	Calcium	Iron	Zinc	Magnesium	Vitamin A	Vitamin C	Thiamin	Riboflavin	Niacin	Vitamin B₁₂	Folic acid
(Arnold) 1 slice	70	4	2	*	*	4	4	7	—	2	6	—	—	*	*	8	4	4	—	—
(Arnold August Bros.) 1 slice	80	4	2	—	*	5	4	9	—	2	6	—	—	*	*	8	4	4	—	—
(Pepperidge Farm) 1 slice	80	4	2	*	*	5	8	10	—	2	6	—	—	*	*	8	4	6	—	—
natural (Brownberry) 1 slice	70	4	2	*	*	4	4	6	—	2	4	—	—	*	*	8	4	4	—	—
party (Pepperidge Farm) 4 slices	60	4	2	*	*	4	4	7	—	2	4	—	—	*	*	6	4	4	—	—

BREAD, RAISIN

	Calories	Protein	Fat	Sat. Fat	Cholesterol	Carbohydrates	Fiber	Sodium	Potassium	Calcium	Iron	Zinc	Magnesium	Vitamin A	Vitamin C	Thiamin	Riboflavin	Niacin	Vitamin B₁₂	Folic acid
(Arnold) 1 slice	70	2	2	*	*	4	4	4	—	4	—	—	—	*	*	*	4	4	—	—
(Sun Maid) 1 slice	70	2	2	5	*	4	4	4	—	*	4	—	—	*	*	4	4	4	—	—
w/ walnuts (Brownberry) 1 slice	70	2	2	*	*	4	4	4	—	*	4	—	—	*	*	4	4	4	—	—
(Brownberry) 1 slice	70	2	5	5	*	3	8	4	—	*	6	—	—	*	*	6	4	4	—	—

Encyclopedia of Daily Values

	Calories	Protein	Fat	Sat. Fat	Cholesterol	Carbohydrates	Fiber	Sodium	Potassium	Calcium	Iron	Zinc	Magnesium	Vitamin A	Vitamin C	Thiamin	Riboflavin	Niacin	Vitamin B12	Folic acid
BREAD, RYE																				
caraway																				
(Brownberry) 1 slice	70	4	2	*	*	5	4	7	—	*	6	—	—	*	*	8	6	4	—	—
deli style																				
(Arnold) 1 slice	50	4	2	*	*	3	4	5	—	4	4	—	—	*	*	4	2	2	—	—
dijon																				
(Pepperidge Farm) 1 slice	50	4	2	*	*	3	4	7	—	2	4	—	—	*	*	4	4	4	—	—
dill																				
(Brownberry) 2 slices	150	6	3	5	*	9	4	7	—	*	10	—	—	*	*	10	8	10	—	—
hearty																				
(Beefsteak) 1 slice	60	3	2	3	*	4	3	7	*	*	4	—	—	*	*	6	4	4	—	—
Jewish																				
dijon																				
(Arnold) 1 slice	70	4	2	—	*	5	4	9	—	2	4	—	—	*	*	8	4	4	—	—
melba thin																				
(Arnold) 1 slice	40	2	2	*	*	3	4	4	—	*	4	—	—	*	*	6	4	8	—	—
seeded																				
(Arnold) 1 slice	70	4	2	*	*	4	4	6	—	2	6	—	—	*	*	8	6	4	—	—
(Pepperidge Farm) 1 slice	80	4	2	*	*	5	8	9	—	2	6	—	—	*	*	10	6	6	—	—
unseeded																				
(Arnold) 1 slice	70	4	2	*	*	5	4	6	—	2	6	—	—	*	*	8	6	4	—	—
mild																				
(Beefsteak) 1 slice	70	5	2	3	*	4	4	7	*	2	4	—	—	*	*	8	4	4	—	—
onion																				
(Arnold August Bros.) 1 slice	80	4	2	—	*	5	4	9	—	2	6	—	—	*	*	8	4	4	—	—
(Beefsteak) 1 slice	60	3	2	3	*	4	3	7	*	*	4	—	—	*	*	6	4	4	—	—
party																				
(Pepperidge Farm) 4 slices	60	4	2	*	*	4	4	10	—	2	4	—	—	*	*	8	4	6	—	—
seeded																				
(Arnold) 1 slice	80	4	2	*	*	5	4	7	—	2	6	—	—	*	*	8	4	4	—	—
(Arnold August Bros.) 1 slice	80	4	2	—	*	5	4	9	—	2	6	—	—	*	*	8	4	4	—	—
soft																				
(Beefsteak) 1 slice	60	3	2	3	*	4	3	7	*	*	4	—	—	*	*	6	4	4	—	—
(Brownberry) 1 slice	40	4	*	*	*	3	8	3	—	2	2	—	—	*	*	4	2	2	—	—
light																				
(Arnold Bakery) 1 slice	40	4	*	*	*	3	8	3	*	2	2	—	—	*	*	4	2	2	—	—
seeded																				
(Arnold Bakery) 1 slice	70	4	2	*	*	4	4	7	—	2	4	—	—	*	*	4	4	4	—	—
unseeded																				
(Arnold Bakery) 1 slice	70	4	2	*	*	4	4	7	—	2	4	—	—	*	*	4	4	4	—	—
thin sliced																				
(Arnold August Bros.) 1 slice	40	2	3	—	*	3	4	5	—	*	4	—	—	*	*	6	2	2	—	—
natural																				
(Brownberry) 1 slice	50	2	2	*	*	3	4	7	—	*	2	—	—	*	*	4	2	2	—	—
unseeded																				
(Arnold) 1 slice	80	4	2	—	*	5	4	7	—	2	6	—	—	*	*	8	4	4	—	—
(Arnold August Bros.) 1 slice	80	4	2	—	*	5	4	9	—	2	6	—	—	*	*	8	4	4	—	—
(Pepperidge Farm) 1 slice	80	4	2	*	*	5	8	9	—	2	6	—	—	*	*	10	6	6	—	—
natural																				
(Brownberry) 1 slice	150	6	3	*	*	9	4	7	—	4	10	—	—	*	*	10	8	10	—	—
BREAD, SEVEN GRAIN																				
(Pepperidge Farm Hearty) 1 slice	100	5	2	*	*	6	8	7	—	*	4	—	—	*	*	8	4	6	—	—
(Pepperidge Farm Light) 1 slice	40	4	*	*	*	3	8	6	—	4	6	—	—	*	*	6	2	4	—	—
buttertop																				
(Home Pride) 1 slice	70	5	2	3	*	4	5	6	2	2	6	—	—	*	*	8	6	8	—	—
BREAD, SOURDOUGH																				
(Arnold Francisco) 1 slice	90	4	2	—	*	6	4	10	—	2	6	—	—	*	*	8	4	6	—	—

	Calories	Protein	Fat	Sat. Fat	Cholesterol	Carbohydrates	Fiber	Sodium	Potassium	Calcium	Iron	Zinc	Magnesium	Vitamin A	Vitamin C	Thiamin	Riboflavin	Niacin	Vitamin B12	Folic acid
BREAD, SOURDOUGH (continued)																				
light																				
(Arnold Bakery) 1 slice	40	4	*	*	*	2	8	2	—	*	2	—	—	*	*	4	2	2	—	—
(Wonder) 1 slice	40	3	*	*	*	2	12	5	*	4	4	—	—	*	*	6	4	6	—	—
BREAD, SPROUTED WHEAT																				
(Pepperidge Farm) 1 slice	70	4	3	—	*	4	8	4	—	*	4	—	—	*	*	6	2	4	—	—
BREAD, TWELVE GRAIN																				
natural																				
(Arnold) 1 slice	60	4	2	*	*	3	4	4	—	*	4	—	—	*	*	4	4	2	—	—
(Brownberry) 1 slice	60	4	2	*	*	4	4	5	—	*	4	—	—	*	*	4	4	2	—	—
BREAD, VIENNA																				
(Pepperidge Farm Light) 1 slice	40	2	*	*	*	3	8	4	—	*	2	6	—	*	*	8	2	*	—	—
thick sliced																				
(Pepperidge Farm) 1 oz	70	4	2	*	*	4	*	5	—	*	2	4	—	*	*	6	4	6	—	—
BREAD, WHEATBERRY																				
(Arnold) 1 slice	80	4	2	*	*	5	12	6	—	*	4	—	—	*	*	6	2	2	—	—
BREAD, WHITE																				
(Arnold Brick Oven) 1 slice	60	2	2	*	*	4	4	5	—	*	4	—	—	*	*	4	2	2	—	—
(Wonder) 1 slice	70	3	2	3	*	4	3	6	*	4	4	—	—	*	*	8	4	6	—	—
buttermilk																				
(Wonder) 1 slice	70	3	2	3	*	4	3	6	*	4	4	—	—	*	*	8	6	6	—	—
buttertop																				
(Home Pride) 1 slice	70	5	2	3	*	4	6	7	2	4	6	—	—	*	*	8	6	6	—	—
country																				
(Arnold) 1 slice	100	4	3	5	2	6	4	8	—	*	4	—	—	*	*	8	6	6	—	—
(Brownberry) 1 slice	100	4	3	5	*	6	4	8	—	*	6	—	—	*	*	8	6	4	—	—
(Pepperidge Farm Hearty) 1 slice	90	5	2	*	*	6	8	8	—	*	6	4	—	*	*	10	6	6	—	—
extra fiber																				
(Arnold Brick Oven) 1 slice	50	—	2	*	*	3	8	4	—	—	—	—	—	—	—	—	—	—	—	—
light																				
(Arnold Bakery) 1 slice	40	4	*	*	*	3	8	3	—	*	2	—	—	*	*	4	2	2	—	—
(Arnold Brick Oven) 1 slice	40	2	*	*	*	2	8	3	—	6	2	—	—	*	*	4	4	2	—	—
(Home Pride) 1 slice	40	3	*	*	*	2	10	5	*	8	4	—	—	*	*	6	4	4	—	—
(Wonder) 1 slice	40	3	*	*	*	2	8	5	*	8	4	—	—	*	*	8	4	4	—	—
from mix																				
(Pillsbury) 1 slice (1/12 recipe)	170	5	8	5	12	9	—	8	*	*	4	—	—	*	*	6	6	4	—	—
natural																				
(Arnold) 1 slice	80	4	2	*	*	5	8	7	—	*	4	—	—	*	*	6	4	6	—	—
(Brownberry) 1 slice	60	2	2	*	*	4	4	6	—	*	4	—	—	*	*	6	6	6	—	—
from refrigerated dough																				
(Pillsbury Pipin' Hot) 1 slice	70	5	3	*	*	4	—	7	*	*	4	—	—	*	*	40	4	4	—	—
robust																				
(Beefsteak) 1 slice	70	5	2	3	*	4	3	6	*	4	6	—	—	*	*	15	6	6	—	—
sandwich																				
(Brownberry) 1 slice	60	2	2	*	*	4	4	5	—	*	4	—	—	*	*	4	4	4	—	—
(Pepperidge Farm) 1 slice	65	3	2	*	*	4	*	5	—	2	4	—	—	*	*	8	4	4	—	—
sliced																				
(Pepperidge Farm) 1 slice	80	2	3	*	*	5	*	3	—	2	4	—	—	*	*	6	4	4	—	—
soft																				
(Arnold Brick Oven) 1 slice	80	—	3	*	*	5	4	5	—	*	4	—	—	*	*	—	—	—	—	—
(Brownberry) 1 slice	80	4	3	—	*	4	4	5	—	*	4	—	—	*	*	6	4	4	—	—
country																				
(Arnold) 1 slice	70	4	2	*	*	4	4	6	—	2	4	—	—	*	*	6	2	2	—	—
thin sliced																				
(Arnold Brick Oven) 1 slice	40	2	2	—	*	4	4	3	—	*	2	—	—	*	*	2	2	2	—	—
(Pepperidge Farm) 1 slice	40	2	*	*	*	3	*	3	—	*	2	—	—	*	*	4	2	2	—	—

PERCENTAGE DAILY VALUE

	Calories	Protein	Fat	Sat. Fat	Cholesterol	Carbohydrates	Fiber	Sodium	Potassium	Calcium	Iron	Zinc	Magnesium	Vitamin A	Vitamin C	Thiamin	Riboflavin	Niacin	Vitamin B12	Folic acid
BREAD, WHITE (continued)																				
toasting																				
(Pepperidge Farm) 1 slice	90	4	2	*	*	6	4	4	—	2	6	—	—	*	*	10	6	6	—	—
BREAD, WHOLE WHEAT																				
100% light																				
(Arnold Brick Oven) 1 slice	40	4	2	—	*	2	12	4	—	*	2	—	—	*	*	4	2	2	—	—
stoneground																				
(Arnold) 1 slice	50	4	2	*	*	3	8	4	—	*	2	—	—	*	*	4	2	2	—	—
BREAD, WHOLE WHEAT, PARTIAL																				
(Arnold Brick Oven) 1 slice	60	2	3	*	*	3	8	4	—	2	4	—	—	*	*	4	2	4	—	—
(Fresh & Natural) 1 slice	70	7	2	3	*	4	6	5	2	2	4	—	—	*	*	6	4	6	—	—
(Oatmeal Goodness) 1 slice	80	7	2	3	*	5	5	6	2	6	6	—	—	*	*	8	6	6	—	—
(Pepperidge Farm Light) 1 slice	40	4	*	*	*	3	8	4	—	2	4	—	—	*	*	6	2	4	—	—
(Pepperidge Farm Old Fashioned) 1 slice	90	4	3	—	*	6	8	8	—	2	6	—	—	*	*	8	4	6	—	—
100% (Wonder) 1 slice	60	7	2	3	*	3	7	5	2	4	6	—	—	*	*	6	4	6	—	—
100%, soft (Wonder) 1 slice	60	7	2	3	*	3	7	5	2	4	6	—	—	*	*	6	4	6	—	—
apple honey (Brownberry) 1 slice	60	2	2	5	*	4	8	5	—	*	6	—	—	*	*	6	6	4	—	—
Austrian (Bread du Jour) 1 slice	70	5	2	3	*	4	5	6	*	4	6	—	—	*	*	8	6	6	—	—
bran'nola country oat																				
(Arnold) 1 slice	90	4	5	*	*	5	12	5	—	2	6	—	—	*	*	6	4	4	—	—
(Brownberry) 1 slice	90	4	5	*	*	5	12	5	—	2	6	—	—	*	*	6	4	4	—	—
bran'nola dark wheat																				
(Arnold) 1 slice	90	6	5	*	*	5	12	6	—	2	4	—	—	*	*	6	4	4	—	—
(Brownberry) 1 slice	90	6	5	*	*	5	12	6	—	2	4	—	—	*	*	6	4	4	—	—
bran'nola hearty wheat																				
(Arnold) 1 slice	100	4	5	*	*	5	12	7	—	2	6	—	—	*	*	6	4	4	—	—
(Brownberry) 1 slice	100	4	5	*	*	5	12	7	—	2	6	—	—	*	*	6	4	4	—	—
bran'nola nutty grains																				
(Arnold) 1 slice	90	6	3	*	*	5	12	5	—	2	6	—	—	*	*	6	4	4	—	—
(Brownberry) 1 slice	90	6	3	*	*	5	12	5	—	2	6	—	—	*	*	6	4	4	—	—
bran'nola original																				
(Arnold) 1 slice	90	4	3	*	*	5	12	6	—	2	6	—	—	*	*	6	4	4	—	—
(Brownberry) 1 slice	90	4	3	*	*	5	12	6	—	2	6	—	—	*	*	6	4	4	—	—
buttertop (Home Pride) 1 slice	70	5	2	3	*	4	6	7	2	4	6	—	—	*	*	8	6	6	—	—
country style (Wonder) 1 slice	70	5	2	3	*	4	4	7	*	4	6	—	—	*	*	8	6	6	—	—
cracked (Wonder) 1 slice	70	5	2	3	*	4	3	7	—	4	4	—	—	*	*	10	6	8	—	—
thin sliced (Pepperidge Farm) 1 slice	70	4	2	—	*	4	4	6	—	*	4	—	—	*	*	6	4	4	—	—
family (Wonder) 1 slice	70	3	2	3	*	4	4	6	*	4	6	—	—	*	*	10	6	6	—	—
golden (Wonder) 1 slice	70	5	2	3	*	4	4	7	*	4	6	—	—	*	*	8	6	6	—	—
light (Arnold Bakery) 1 slice	40	4	*	*	*	*	8	3	—	*	2	—	—	*	*	4	2	2	—	—
health nut																				
natural (Brownberry) 1 slice	70	2	3	5	*	4	8	7	—	*	4	—	—	*	*	6	2	6	—	—
hearth (Brownberry) 1 slice	70	3	2	*	*	4	8	6	—	*	4	—	—	*	*	6	4	6	—	—
hearty (Beefsteak) 1 slice	70	5	2	3	*	4	6	7	2	6	6	—	—	*	*	8	6	6	—	—

	Calories	Protein	Fat	Sat. Fat	Cholesterol	Carbohydrates	Fiber	Sodium	Potassium	Calcium	Iron	Zinc	Magnesium	Vitamin A	Vitamin C	Thiamin	Riboflavin	Niacin	Vitamin B$_{12}$	Folic acid
BREAD, WHOLE WHEAT, PARTIAL (continued)																				
honey buttertop																				
(Home Pride) 1 slice	100	5	3	3	*	6	7	9	2	6	8	—	—	*	*	10	8	8	—	—
light																				
(Brownberry) 1 slice	40	2	2	*	*	3	8	3	—	*	2	—	—	*	*	4	2	2	—	—
(Home Pride) 1 slice	40	3	*	*	*	2	10	5	*	8	4	—	—	*	*	6	4	4	—	—
(Thomas') 1 slice	40	2	2	5	*	2	8	3	—	10	2	—	—	*	*	4	2	2	—	—
(Wonder) 1 slice	40	3	*	*	*	2	8	5	*	8	4	—	—	*	*	8	4	4	—	—
natural																				
(Brownberry) 1 slice	60	2	2	*	*	4	8	7	—	*	4	—	—	*	*	4	4	4	—	—
(Brownberry) 1 slice	80	4	2	*	*	5	8	8	—	*	6	—	—	*	*	8	6	4	—	—
from refrigerated dough																				
(Pillsbury Pipin' Hot) 1 slice	70	3	3	*	*	4	—	7	*	*	*	—	—	*	*	40	4	4	—	—
sesame																				
(Pepperidge Farm Hearty) 1 slice	100	7	2	*	*	6	8	8	—	2	6	—	—	*	*	8	4	6	—	—
soft																				
(Arnold) 1 slice	100	6	3	*	*	6	8	7	—	*	4	—	—	*	*	8	4	4	—	—
(Arnold Brick Oven) 1 slice	80	4	3	*	*	5	4	5	—	*	4	—	—	*	*	—	—	—	—	—
(Brownberry) 1 slice	70	6	2	5	*	5	4	5	—	*	2	—	—	*	*	4	2	2	—	—
(Pepperidge Farm) 1 slice	50	4	*	*	*	4	—	4	—	2	2	—	—	*	*	6	2	4	—	—
stoneground																				
(Pepperidge Farm Wholesome Choice) 1 slice	90	7	2	*	*	6	8	7	—	2	2			*	*	10	6	6		
(Wonder) 1 slice	80	7	2	3	*	4	9	7	3	4	6	—	—	*	*	8	4	6	—	—
thin sliced																				
(Pepperidge Farm) 1 slice	60	4	2	—	*	4	8	5	—	2	4	—	—	*	*	6	2	4	—	—
very thin sliced																				
(Pepperidge Farm) 1 slice	40	2	2	*	*	2	*	3	—	*	2	—	—	*	*	2	*	2	—	—
BREADCRUMBS																				
Italian																				
(Arnold) 1/2 oz	50	2	2	*	*	3	4	8	—	*	2	—	—	*	*	4	2	2	—	—
Italian																				
(Progresso) 1/4 cup	110	7	3	*	*	7	—	18	2	6	10	—	—	*	*	10	8	10	—	—
plain																				
(Arnold) 1/2 oz	50	2	2	*	*	3	4	3	—	*	4	—	—	*	*	4	2	2	—	—
(Progresso) 1/4 cup	110	7	3	*	*	7	—	10	2	4	8	—	—	*	*	10	6	10	—	—
seasoned																				
(Contadina) 1/4 cup	76	8	*	*	*	4	3	20	—	4	6	—	—	*	*	—	—	—	—	—
BREADSTICK																				
cheddar cheese																				
(Pepperidge Farm) 1 oz	120	8	6	10	2	6	8	10	*	*	2	—	—	*	*	8	4	4	—	—
garlic																				
(Stella d'Oro) 2 breadsticks	80	3	3	—	*	5	—	5	—	—	—	—	—	—	—	—	—	—	—	—
onion																				
(Pepperidge Farm) 1 oz	120	8	3	*	*	7	8	6	*	*	2	—	—	*	*	12	4	12	—	—
(Stella d'Oro) 2 breadsticks	80	3	3	—	*	4	—	3	—	—	—	—	—	—	—	—	—	—	—	—
pesto																				
(Pepperidge Farm) 1 oz	120	8	3	10	*	6	8	10	*	*	2	—	—	*	*	8	4	4	—	—
plain																				
(Stella d'Oro) 2 breadsticks	80	3	3	—	*	5	—	3	—	—	—	—	—	—	—	—	—	—	—	—
regular																				
(Stella d'Oro) 2 breadsticks	80	3	3	—	*	5	—	3	—	—	—	—	—	—	—	—	—	—	—	—
sesame																				
(Pepperidge Farm) 1 oz	120	4	6	*	*	7	*	7	*	4	12	—	—	*	*	12	4	12	—	—
(Stella d'Oro) 1 breadstick	50	2	4	—	*	2	—	2	—	—	—	—	—	—	—	—	—	—	—	—

	Calories	Protein	Fat	Sat. Fat	Cholesterol	Carbohydrates	Fiber	Sodium	Potassium	Calcium	Iron	Zinc	Magnesium	Vitamin A	Vitamin C	Thiamin	Riboflavin	Niacin	Vitamin B12	Folic acid
BREADSTICK (continued)																				
soft																				
from refrigerated dough																				
(Pillsbury) 1 stick	100	5	3	3	*	6	—	10	*	*	6	—	—	*	*	80	6	6	—	—
wheat																				
(Stella d'Oro) 2 breadsticks	80	3	4	—	*	4	—	2												
BREADFRUIT																				
1/4 fruit	99	2	*	*	*	9	20	*	13	2	3	*	6	*	46	7	2	4	—	*
1/2 cup	113	2	*	*	*	10	20	*	15	2	3	*	7	*	53	8	2	5	—	*
BREADFRUIT SEED																				
raw																				
1 oz	54	4	2	2	*	3	—	*	8	*	6	2	4	*	3	9	5	*	*	4
boiled																				
1 oz	48	3	*	*	*	3	—	*	7	2	*	2	4	*	3	5	3	8	*	3
roasted																				
1 oz	59	3	*	*	*	4	—	*	9	2	*	2	4	2	4	8	4	11	*	4
BREADNUT TREE SEED																				
raw																				
1 oz	62	3	*	*	*	4	—	*	10	3	3	2	5	*	13	*	*	*	*	5
dried																				
1 oz	104	4	*	*	*	7	16	*	16	3	7	4	8	*	22	*	2	3	—	8
BREAKFAST BAR																				
chocolate chip																				
(Carnation) 1 bar	200	10	17	21	*	7	—	7	3	2	25	20	15	35	45	20	2	25	10	25
chocolate crunch																				
(Carnation) 1 bar	190	10	15	20	*	7	—	6	4	2	25	20	15	35	45	20	2	25	10	25
peanut butter w/ chocolate chips																				
(Carnation) 1 bar	200	10	17	15	*	7	—	7	3	2	25	20	15	35	45	20	2	25	10	25
peanut butter crunch																				
(Carnation) 1 bar	190	10	15	14	*	7	—	7	3	2	25	20	15	35	45	20	2	25	10	25
BREAKFAST, FROZEN																				
bagel sandwich																				
ham & cheese																				
(Weight Watchers) 3 oz	200	20	8	10	5	9	4	20	6	6	6	—	—	*	4	—	—	—	—	—
biscuit																				
sausage																				
(Weight Watchers) 3 oz	230	18	17	18	8	7	16	23	4	2	6	—	—	*	4	—	—	—	—	—
w/ sausage, egg, & cheese																				
(Swanson Breakfast Sandwich) 5 1/2 oz	470	30	45	—	—	12	—	52	—	15	15	—	—	4	*	20	10	10	—	—
biscuit sandwich																				
bacon patty																				
(Swanson Breakfast Sandwich) 3 1/4 oz	340	20	35	—	—	7	—	41	—	6	10	—	—	*	*	10	8	8	—	—
egg, cheese & bacon																				
(Swanson Breakfast Sandwich) 4 1/4 oz	360	20	29	—	—	12	—	40	—	15	15	—	—	*	*	15	15	10	—	—
sausage																				
(Hormel Quickmeal) 1 (3 3/4 oz)	350	17	34	—	13	10	—	36	7	6	8	8	5	*	*	30	15	15	—	—
(Swanson Breakfast Sandwich) 3 1/4 oz	300	25	29	—	—	8	—	49	—	6	10	—	—	*	20	10	15	15	—	—
sausage & cheese																				
(Hormel Quickmeal) 1 (4 1/4 oz)	420	22	42	50	20	10	—	44	9	15	10	11	6	4	*	25	20	10	—	—
sausage & egg																				
(Hormel Quickmeal) 1 (4 1/2 oz)	350	18	32	—	37	10	—	32	8	8	10	9	5	2	*	25	20	10	—	—
burrito																				
bacon																				
(Swanson Breakfast Sandwich) 3 1/2 oz	250	20	17	—	—	9	—	22	—	8	10	—	—	2	2	6	6	4	—	—

	Calories	Protein	Fat	Sat. Fat	Cholesterol	Carbohydrates	Fiber	Sodium	Potassium	Calcium	Iron	Zinc	Magnesium	Vitamin A	Vitamin C	Thiamin	Riboflavin	Niacin	Vitamin B12	Folic acid
BREAKFAST, FROZEN (continued)																				
w/ home fried potatoes *(Swanson Fiesta Breakfast)* 5 3/4 oz	330	20	28	—	—	10	—	25	—	8	10	—	—	2	*	10	10	8	—	—
original *(Swanson Breakfast Sandwich)* 3 1/2 oz	200	15	11	—	—	8	—	21	—	10	10	—	—	2	6	2	2	2	—	—
sausage *(Swanson Breakfast Sandwich)* 3 oz	250	20	20	—	—	8	—	21	—	8	8	—	—	2	2	6	4	4	—	—
egg, Canadian bacon & cheese on muffin *(Swanson Breakfast Sandwich)* 4 oz	290	30	23	—	—	8	—	31	—	15	10	—	—	2	*	15	15	10	—	—
eggs, Canadian bacon, & cheese w/ green chiles on muffin *(Swanson Fiesta Breakfast)* 4 3/4 oz	280	25	22	—	—	9	—	28	—	15	10	—	—	4	*	20	15	*	—	—
flapsticks (pancake & sausage) blueberry *(Jimmy Dean)* 1 flapstick	170	7	15	—	5	5	—	12	—	*	4	—	—	*	*	20	10	10	—	—
plain *(Jimmy Dean)* 1 flapstick	170	7	18	—	5	4	—	12	—	4	4	—	—	*	*	20	10	10	—	—
French toast cinnamon swirl w/ sausage *(Swanson Breakfast Entree)* 5 1/2 oz	440	25	42	—	—	13	—	24	—	10	15	—	—	4	*	25	20	15	—	—
mini *(Swanson Breakfast Blast)* 3 oz	180	8	8	—	—	10	—	8	—	8	8	—	—	2	4	10	8	*	—	—
French toast w/ sausage *(Swanson Breakfast Entree)* 5 1/2 oz	410	20	35	—	—	12	—	25	—	10	15	—	—	2	*	30	20	15	—	—
sticks *(Swanson Breakfast Blast)* 3 3/4 oz	280	10	14	—	—	15	—	9	—	8	4	—	—	8	*	2	4	2	—	—
muffin sandwich Canadian bacon & egg w/ cheese *(Hormel Quickmeal)* 1 4 1/2 oz	250	27	12	20	38	10	—	28	8	20	10	3	7	4	2	25	20	10	—	—
English *(Healthy Choice)* 4 1/4 oz	200	27	5	5	7	10	—	21	6	15	20	—	—	6	6	30	25	15	—	—
(Weight Watchers) 4 oz	220	20	8	10	5	10	4	15	9	6	6	—	—	4	6	—	—	—	—	—
omelet w/ turkey sausage *(Healthy Choice)* 4 3/4 oz	210	27	6	10	7	10	—	20	17	20	20	—	—	6	*	25	30	15	—	—
sausage & egg w/ cheese *(Hormel Quickmeal)* 1 (5 oz)	76	5	6	—	9	2	—	6	2	4	2	3	1	1	*	7	5	3	—	—
omelet ham & cheese *(Weight Watchers)* 4 oz	220	23	9	10	10	9	12	19	6	10	6	—	—	6	8	—	—	—	—	—
omelet western, on English muffin *(Healthy Choice)* 4 3/4 oz	200	27	5	10	5	10	—	20	6	20	20	—	—	10	6	30	30	10	—	—
omelet sandwich *(Weight Watchers)* 3 3/4 oz	220	23	8	5	10	9	4	17	5	20	10	—	—	8	*	—	—	—	—	—
garden *(Weight Watchers)* 3 2/3 oz	210	15	9	10	5	9	8	20	5	15	4	—	—	8	4	—	—	—	—	—
pancakes w/ bacon *(Swanson Breakfast Entree)* 4 1/2 oz	400	20	31	—	—	14	—	43	—	6	10	—	—	*	*	20	15	8	—	—

	Calories	Protein	Fat	Sat. Fat	Cholesterol	Carbohydrates	Fiber	Sodium	Potassium	Calcium	Iron	Zinc	Magnesium	Vitamin A	Vitamin C	Thiamin	Riboflavin	Niacin	Vitamin B12	Folic acid
BREAKFAST, FROZEN (continued)																				
mini (Swanson Breakfast Blast) 4 1/4 oz	300	10	12	—	—	17	—	24	—	6	4	—	—	*	4	4	6	10		
w/sausage (Swanson Breakfast Entree) 6 oz	470	25	35	—	—	18	—	39	—	8	15	—	—	*	*	30	20	15	—	—
silver dollar, w/sausage (Swanson Breakfast Entree) 3 3/4 oz	320	15	25	—	—	12	—	28	—	6	10	—	—	*	*	20	15	8	—	—
silver dollar, w/scrambled eggs (Swanson Breakfast Entree) 4 1/4 oz	290	15	31	—	—	7	—	23	—	2	2	—	—	*	*	10	10	6	—	—
scrambled eggs, Canadian bacon & cheese (Swanson Fiesta Breakfast) 6 1/2 oz	390	25	45	—	—	6	—	29	—	10	10	—	—	2	*	15	25	*	—	—
scrambled eggs & home fries (Swanson Breakfast Entree) 4 1/3 oz	260	15	29	—	—	5	—	16	—	6	8	—	—	*	2	15	4	4	—	—
scrambled eggs, home fries, & bacon (Swanson Breakfast Entree) 5 1/4 oz	350	25	42	—	—	5	—	29	—	6	10	—	—	*	2	10	15	6	—	—
scrambled eggs & sausage w/hash browns (Swanson Breakfast Entree) 6 1/4 oz	430	25	52	—	—	6	—	31	—	6	10	—	—	*	*	10	20	8	—	—
waffles & sausage (Swanson Breakfast Entree) 2 1/4 oz	230	10	22	—	—	7	—	13	—	4	4	—	—	*	*	15	10	6	—	—
BREAKFAST, INSTANT																				
chocolate (Carnation) 1 envelope prep. w/ 8 fl oz low fat milk	250	25	5	20	7	13	*	10	21	40	25	25	25	45	50	25	30	25	25	25
diet (Carnation) 1 envelope prep. w/ 8 fl oz low fat milk	190	25	9	15	7	8	*	9	20	40	25	25	25	45	50	25	30	25	25	25
made w/ whole milk (Pillsbury) 8 fl oz	250	25	8	15	7	13	*	9	17	25	25	—	25	30	30	25	25	25	25	25
chocolate malt (Carnation) 1 envelope prep. w/ 8 fl oz low fat milk	250	25	9	20	7	13	*	10	17	40	25	25	25	45	50	25	30	25	25	25
diet (Carnation) 1 envelope prep. w/ 8 fl oz low fat milk	190	25	9	20	7	7	*	10	17	40	25	25	25	45	50	25	30	25	25	25
made w/ whole milk (Pillsbury) 8 fl oz	250	23	8	15	7	12	*	10	16	25	25	—	25	30	30	25	25	25	25	25
coffee (Carnation) 1 envelope prep. w/ 8 fl oz low fat milk	280	25	8	15	7	13	*	9	19	40	25	25	25	45	50	25	30	25	25	25
original (Carnation) 1 cup	240	25	9	15	7	12	*	8	17	35	25	25	25	25	*	25	25	25	25	25
strawberry (Carnation) 1 envelope prep. w/ 8 fl oz low fat milk	280	25	8	15	7	14	*	12	17	40	25	25	25	45	50	25	30	25	25	25
diet (Carnation) 1 envelope prep. w/ 8 fl oz low fat milk	190	25	8	15	7	8	*	9	17	40	25	25	25	45	50	25	30	25	25	25
made w/ whole milk (Pillsbury) 8 fl oz	250	23	8	10	7	13	*	9	11	25	25	—	25	30	30	25	25	25	25	25
vanilla (Carnation) 1 envelope prep. w/ 8 fl oz low fat milk	250	25	8	15	7	13	*	9	17	40	25	25	25	45	50	25	30	25	25	25

	Calories	Protein	Fat	Sat. Fat	Cholesterol	Carbohydrates	Fiber	Sodium	Potassium	Calcium	Iron	Zinc	Magnesium	Vitamin A	Vitamin C	Thiamin	Riboflavin	Niacin	Vitamin B$_{12}$	Folic acid
						PERCENTAGE DAILY VALUE														
BREAKFAST, INSTANT (continued)																				
diet (Carnation) 1 envelope prep. w/ 8 fl oz low fat milk	190	25	8	15	7	8	*	9	17	40	25	25	25	45	50	25	30	25	25	25
BREAKFAST STRIP																				
(generic) 3 slices	153	18	18	25	13	*	*	32	4	*	6	14	2	*	20	2	5	11	19	*
turkey w/ pork (Oscar Mayer Healthy Favorites) 1 slice	18	3	2	2	3	*	*	6	*	*	*	2	*	*	*				—	—
BROADBEAN																				
raw 1/2 cup	40	5	*	*	*	2	8	*	4	*	6	2	5	4	30	6	4	4	*	13
cooked 1/2 cup	94	11	*	*	*	6	—	9	6	3	7	6	9	*	*	5	4	3	*	22
cooked w/ salt 1/2 cup	94	11	*	*	*	6	20	*	6	3	7	6	9	*	*	5	4	3	*	22
BROADBEAN, CANNED																				
1/2 cup	91	12	*	*	*	5	—	24	9	3	7	5	10	*	4	2	4	6	*	10
BROCCOLI																				
flower raw 1/2 cup chopped	12	2	*	*	*	*	—	*	4	2	2	*	3	26	68	2	3	*	*	8
leaf raw 1/2 cup chopped	12	2	*	*	*	*	—	*	4	2	2	*	3	141	68	2	3	*	*	8
spear boiled 1 head	50	9	*	*	*	3	20	2	15	8	8	5	11	50	224	7	12	5	*	22
raw 1 head	42	7	*	*	*	3	20	2	14	7	7	4	9	47	234	7	11	5	*	27
stalks raw 1/2 cup chopped	12	2	*	*	*	*	—	*	4	2	2	*	3	4	68	2	3	*	*	8
whole boiled 1/2 cup chopped	22	4	*	*	*	*	8	*	6	4	4	2	5	22	97	3	5	2	*	10
boiled, salted 1/2 cup chopped	22	4	*	*	*	*	—	8	6	4	4	2	5	22	97	3	5	2	*	10
raw 1/2 cup chopped	12	2	*	*	*	*	4	*	4	2	2	*	3	14	68	2	3	*	*	8
BROCCOLI, FROZEN																				
chopped (Bird's Eye) 3 1/3 oz	25	5	*	*	*	2	12	*	—	4	2	*	2	45	90	4	4	*	—	15
boiled (generic) 1/2 cup	26	5	*	*	*	2	12	*	5	5	3	2	5	35	61	3	4	2	*	13
boiled, salted (generic) 1/2 cup	26	5	*	*	*	2	—	10	5	5	3	2	5	35	61	3	4	2	*	13
cuts (Green Giant) 1/2 cup	18	3	*	*	*	2	16	*	6	2	*	—	—	15	80	2	4	*	—	—
(Green Giant Harvest Fresh) 1/2 cup	16	3	*	*	*	*	8	4	4	2	*	—	—	10	60	*	4	*	—	—
cuts in butter sauce (Green Giant One Serving) 4 1/2 oz	45	5	3	3	2	2	12	17	6	4	2	—	—	10	90	2	6	2	—	—
cuts in cheese flavored sauce (Green Giant One Serving) 5 oz	80	7	3	3	2	4	8	29	9	8	4	—	—	40	50	*	10	2	—	—
spears (Bird's Eye Deluxe) 3 1/3 oz	30	5	*	*	*	2	—	*	—	4	4	2	4	25	120	6	8	2	*	25
(Green Giant Harvest Fresh) 1/2 cup	20	3	*	*	*	*	8	5	4	4	2	—	—	10	90	*	4	2	—	—

	Calories	Protein	Fat	Sat. Fat	Cholesterol	Carbohydrates	Fiber	Sodium	Potassium	Calcium	Iron	Zinc	Magnesium	Vitamin A	Vitamin C	Thiamin	Riboflavin	Niacin	Vitamin B₁₂	Folic acid

BROCCOLI, FROZEN (continued)

	Calories	Protein	Fat	Sat. Fat	Cholesterol	Carbohydrates	Fiber	Sodium	Potassium	Calcium	Iron	Zinc	Magnesium	Vitamin A	Vitamin C	Thiamin	Riboflavin	Niacin	Vitamin B12	Folic acid
(Green Giant Select) 4–5 spears	18	3	*	*	*	2	12	*	6	2	4	—	—	10	70	*	4	2	—	—
boiled (generic) 1/2 cup	26	5	*	*	*	2	12	*	5	5	3	2	5	35	61	3	4	2	*	7
boiled, w/ salt (generic) 1/2 cup	26	5	*	*	*	2	—	10	5	5	3	2	5	35	61	3	4	2	*	7
spears in butter sauce (Green Giant) 1/2 cup	40	3	3	3	2	2	8	15	7	2	2	—	—	20	70	2	4	2	—	—
spears in cheese flavored sauce (Green Giant) 1/2 cup	60	5	3	3	*	3	8	22	7	6	2	—	—	20	60	2	10	2	—	—

BROCCOLI COMBINATION, FROZEN

	Calories	Protein	Fat	Sat. Fat	Cholesterol	Carbohydrates	Fiber	Sodium	Potassium	Calcium	Iron	Zinc	Magnesium	Vitamin A	Vitamin C	Thiamin	Riboflavin	Niacin	Vitamin B12	Folic acid
broccoli fanfare (Green Giant Valley Combinations) 1/2 cup	80	5	3	*	*	5	12	14	5	2	2	—	—	6	40	4	4	4	—	—
w/ carrots & rotini in cheese flavored sauce (Green Giant One Serving) 1 pkg (5 1/2 oz)	100	8	3	3	2	6	12	18	8	6	6	—	—	170	10	10	6	6	—	—
w/ cauliflower (Green Giant Valley Combinations) 1/2 cup	60	3	3	*	*	3	12	14	4	2	*	—	—	25	35	2	2	2	—	—
w/ cauliflower & carrots (Green Giant One Serving) 1/2 cup	30	5	*	*	*	2	12	2	7	4	4	—	—	70	50	*	4	2	—	—
in butter sauce (Green Giant) 1/2 cup	30	3	2	3	2	*	12	10	4	2	2	—	—	80	35	*	2	*	—	—
in cheese sauce (Green Giant) 1/2 cup	60	5	3	3	*	3	8	20	7	6	2	—	—	30	20	2	10	*	—	—
w/ cauliflower & carrots in cheese sauce (Green Giant One Serving) 1 pkg (5 oz)	80	5	3	3	2	4	8	27	9	8	2	—	—	70	30	*	10	2	—	—
w/ red peppers (Green Giant Select) 1/2 cup	25	3	*	*	*	*	8	*	5	4	2	—	—	20	35	*	*	2	—	—

BROTWURST

	Calories	Protein	Fat	Sat. Fat	Cholesterol	Carbohydrates	Fiber	Sodium	Potassium	Calcium	Iron	Zinc	Magnesium	Vitamin A	Vitamin C	Thiamin	Riboflavin	Niacin	Vitamin B12	Folic acid
pork & beef 1 1 oz slice	92	7	12	14	6	*	*	13	2	*	2	4	*	*	13	5	4	5	10	*

BROWN BREAD see BREAD

BROWN GRAVY

	Calories	Protein	Fat	Sat. Fat	Cholesterol	Carbohydrates	Fiber	Sodium	Potassium	Calcium	Iron	Zinc	Magnesium	Vitamin A	Vitamin C	Thiamin	Riboflavin	Niacin	Vitamin B12	Folic acid
canned (La Choy) 1 tsp	15	*	*	*	*	*	*	—	—	—	*	—	*	—	—	*	—	—	—	—
from mix (Hain) 1/4 pkg	16	*	*	*	*	*	*	25	2	10	*	*	*	*	*	*	*	*	*	*
(Knorr) 1/4 cup	13	*	*	—	*	*	—	6	—	*	*	*	*	*	*	6	*	*	*	*
(Pillsbury) 1/4 cup	16	*	*	*	*	*	*	7	*	*	*	*	*	*	*	*	*	*	*	*
(Weight Watchers) 1/4 cup	10	2	*	*	—	*	—	15	—	*	*	—	*	*	—	—	—	—	—	—
w/ mushrooms (Weight Watchers) 1/4 cup	10	2	*	*	—	*	—	11	—	*	*	—	*	*	—	—	—	—	—	—
w/ onions (Weight Watchers) 1/4 cup	10	2	*	*	—	*	—	13	—	*	*	—	*	*	—	—	—	—	—	—

BROWNIE see also CAKE

	Calories	Protein	Fat	Sat. Fat	Cholesterol	Carbohydrates	Fiber	Sodium	Potassium	Calcium	Iron	Zinc	Magnesium	Vitamin A	Vitamin C	Thiamin	Riboflavin	Niacin	Vitamin B12	Folic acid
frozen hot fudge (Pepperidge Farm) 3 oz	370	8	28	—	25	15	—	6	—	4	6	—	—	*	*	6	6	4	—	—
microwave frosted (Betty Crocker MicroRave) 1 brownie	180	3	11	10	*	9	—	5	5	*	4	—	—	*	*	2	2	2	—	—
(Duncan Hines) 1 brownie	210	5	12	8	*	12	*	8	—	*	8	—	—	*	*	—	—	—	—	—
from mix caramel supreme (Betty Crocker) 1 brownie	120	2	6	5	3	7	—	5	2	*	2	—	—	*	*	2	2	*	—	—

BROWNIE see also CAKE (continued)

	Calories	Protein	Fat	Sat. Fat	Cholesterol	Carbohydrates	Fiber	Sodium	Potassium	Calcium	Iron	Zinc	Magnesium	Vitamin A	Vitamin C	Thiamin	Riboflavin	Niacin	Vitamin B$_{12}$	Folic acid
chewy fudge basic recipe (Duncan Hines) 1 brownie	160	3	11	8	3	8	4	5	—	*	4	—	—	*	*	—	—	—	—	—
no cholesterol recipe (Duncan Hines) 1 brownie	160	3	11	5	*	8	4	5	—	*	4	—	—	*	*	—	—	—	—	—
chocolate chip supreme (Betty Crocker) 1 brownie	130	2	8	10	3	7	—	4	2	*	4	—	—	*	*	2	2	*	—	—
dark chocolate plain (Duncan Hines) 1 brownie	170	3	12	8	5	8	4	5	—	*	4	—	—	*	*	—	—	—	—	—
w/ milk chocolate chunks (Duncan Hines) 1 brownie	160	3	11	8	3	9	4	4	—	*	4	—	—	*	*	—	—	—	—	—
double chocolate basic recipe (Pillsbury Great Additions) 1 2" square	140	2	9	10	3	6	—	3	2	*	2	—	—	*	*	2	2	*	—	—
no cholesterol recipe (Pillsbury Great Additions) 1 2" square	130	2	9	10	*	6	—	3	2	*	2	—	—	*	*	2	2	*	—	—
double fudge basic recipe (Duncan Hines) 1 brownie	170	3	11	8	7	10	4	5	—	*	4	—	—	*	*	—	—	—	—	—
no cholesterol recipe (Duncan Hines) 1 brownie	170	3	9	5	*	10	4	5	—	*	4	—	—	*	*	—	—	—	—	—
fudge (Betty Crocker) 1 brownie	140	2	8	5	3	7	—	4	2	*	4	—	—	*	*	2	2	*	—	—
(Pillsbury) 1 2" square	140	3	9	5	5	7	—	4	2	*	2	—	—	*	*	2	2	2	—	—
from mix fudge (Robin Hood) 1 brownie	100	2	6	—	—	5	—	3	2	*	2	—	—	*	*	2	2	*	—	—
light (Betty Crocker) 1 brownie	100	2	2	—	*	7	—	4	2	*	2	—	—	*	*	2	2	*	—	—
no cholesterol recipe (Pillsbury) 1 2" square	140	2	9	5	*	7	—	4	2	*	2	—	—	*	*	2	2	2	—	—
funfetti frosted basic recipe (Pillsbury Great Additions) 1 2" square	160	2	11	5	3	8	—	4	2	*	4	—	—	*	*	2	2	2	—	—
no cholesterol recipe (Pillsbury Great Additions) 1 2" square	150	2	9	5	*	8	—	4	2	*	4	—	—	*	*	2	2	2	—	—
German chocolate supreme (Betty Crocker) 1 brownie	160	2	11	10	3	8	—	5	3	*	4	—	—	*	*	2	2	*	—	—
light fudge basic recipe (Pillsbury Lovin' Lites) 1 (1/24 recipe)	100	2	3	3	3	6	—	3	*	*	2	—	—	*	*	2	2	2	—	—
(Pillsbury) 1 (1/24 recipe)	100	2	3	3	*	6	—	4	*	*	2	—	—	*	*	2	2	2	—	—
milk chocolate chunk basic recipe (Duncan Hines) 1 brownie	170	3	11	5	7	9	4	5	—	*	4	—	—	*	*	—	—	—	—	—
no cholesterol recipe (Duncan Hines) 1 brownie	170	3	9	5	*	9	4	5	—	*	4	—	—	*	*	—	—	—	—	—
original supreme (Betty Crocker) 1 brownie	140	2	8	5	7	7	—	4	2	*	6	—	—	*	*	2	2	*	—	—
party supreme (Betty Crocker) 1 brownie	160	2	9	5	3	9	—	4	3	*	4	—	—	*	*	2	2	*	—	—
peanut butter basic recipe (Duncan Hines) 1 brownie	160	3	12	8	3	8	4	5	—	*	4	—	—	*	*	—	—	—	—	—

	Calories	Protein	Fat	Sat. Fat	Cholesterol	Carbohydrates	Fiber	Sodium	Potassium	Calcium	Iron	Zinc	Magnesium	Vitamin A	Vitamin C	Thiamin	Riboflavin	Niacin	Vitamin B$_{12}$	Folic acid
														PERCENTAGE DAILY VALUE						
BROWNIE see also CAKE (continued)																				
no cholesterol recipe (Duncan Hines) 1 brownie	160	3	12	8	*	8	4	5	—	*	4	—	—	*	*	—	—	—	—	—
turtle basic recipe (Duncan Hines) 1 brownie	160	3	9	8	7	9	4	5	—	*	4	—	—	*	*	—	—	—	—	—
no cholesterol recipe (Duncan Hines) 1 brownie	160	3	9	8	*	9	4	5	—	*	4	—	—	*	*	—	—	—	—	—
walnut basic recipe (Duncan Hines) 1 brownie	170	3	12	8	3	8	4	4	—	*	4	—	—	*	*	—	—	—	—	—
walnut basic recipe (Pillsbury Great Additions) 1 2" square	140	3	12	5	3	5	—	3	2	*	2	—	—	*	*	2	2	2	—	—
no cholesterol recipe (Duncan Hines) 1 brownie	170	3	12	5	*	8	4	4	—	*	4	—	—	*	*	—	—	—	—	—
walnut no cholesterol recipe (Pillsbury Great Additions) 1 2" square	130	3	11	5	*	5	—	3	2	*	2	—	—	*	*	2	2	2	—	—
walnut supreme (Betty Crocker) 1 brownie	130	2	9	5	3	6	—	4	2	*	4	—	—	*	*	2	*	*	—	—
from mix, microwave fudge (Pillsbury) 1 (1/9 recipe)	190	3	14	10	*	8	—	5	3	*	6	—	—	*	*	4	2	2	—	—
fudge w/ frosting (Pillsbury) 1 (1/9 recipe)	240	3	17	15	*	11	—	6	4	*	8	—	—	*	*	4	2	2	—	—
BRUSSELS SPROUTS																				
raw 1/2 cup	19	2	*	*	*	*	8	*	5	2	3	*	3	8	62	4	2	2	*	7
4 sprouts	33	4	*	*	*	2	12	*	8	3	6	2	4	13	108	7	4	3	*	12
boiled 1/2 cup	30	3	*	*	*	2	12	*	7	3	5	2	4	11	81	6	4	2	*	12
4 sprouts	33	4	*	*	*	2	16	*	8	3	6	2	4	12	87	6	4	3	*	13
boiled w/ salt 1/2 cup	30	3	*	*	*	2	—	8	7	3	5	2	4	11	81	6	4	2	*	12
BRUSSELS SPROUTS, FROZEN																				
boiled w/ salt 1/2 cup	33	5	*	*	*	2	—	8	7	2	3	2	5	9	59	5	5	2	*	20
in butter sauce (Green Giant) 1/2 cup	40	5	2	3	2	3	16	12	8	2	2	—	—	10	70	4	4	2	—	—
BURBOT																				
raw 1 fillet	104	37	*	*	23	*	*	5	13	6	6	6	9	*	*	29	10	9	15	*
broiled/baked 1 fillet	104	37	*	*	23	*	*	5	13	6	6	6	9	*	*	26	9	9	14	*
BURDOCK ROOT																				
raw 1/2 cup	42	2	*	*	*	3	8	*	5	2	3	*	6	*	3	*	*	*	*	3
1 root	112	4	*	*	*	9	20	*	14	6	7	3	15	*	8	*	3	2	*	9
boiled 1/2 cup	55	2	*	*	*	4	4	*	6	3	3	2	6	*	3	2	2	*	*	3
1 root	146	6	*	*	*	12	12	*	17	8	7	4	16	*	7	4	6	3	*	8
boiled w/ salt 1/2 cup	55	2	*	*	*	4	—	6	6	3	3	2	6	*	3	2	2	*	*	3
BURRITO, FROZEN																				
(Old El Paso) 1 burrito	299	25	20	20	8	12	16	18	6	4	10	—	—	*	2	15	10	15	—	—
bean & cheese (Old El Paso) 1 burrito	300	20	14	20	5	15	—	35	7	15	15	—	—	4	8	15	15	15	—	—
beef (Hormel) 4 oz	300	15	20	25	12	12	—	26	7	2	8	7	6	2	*	20	10	10	—	—

	Calories	Protein	Fat	Sat. Fat	Cholesterol	Carbohydrates	Fiber	Sodium	Potassium	Calcium	Iron	Zinc	Magnesium	Vitamin A	Vitamin C	Thiamin	Riboflavin	Niacin	Vitamin B₁₂	Folic acid
BURRITO, FROZEN (continued)																				
beef & bean																				
hot																				
(Old El Paso) 1 burrito	320	20	15	20	5	15	—	35	7	6	20	—	—	*	4	20	15	20	—	—
medium																				
(Healthy Choice Quick Meals) 5 1/3 oz	270	20	11	15	5	14	—	22	8	6	15	—	—	2	6	25	10	10	—	—
(Old El Paso) 1 burrito	320	20	15	20	5	15	—	33	8	6	20	—	—	*	*	20	10	15	—	—
(Patio) 5 oz	370	18	25	—	8	14	—	35	10	4	15	—	—	6	*	20	10	10	—	—
mild																				
(Healthy Choice Quick) 5 1/3 oz	270	20	11	15	5	14	—	22	8	6	15	—	—	2	6	25	10	10	—	—
(Old El Paso) 1 burrito	330	20	14	15	5	16	—	29	7	6	20	—	—	*	*	25	15	20	—	—
beef & bean green chili																				
mild																				
(Patio) 5 oz	330	20	18	—	10	14	—	32	11	4	20	—	—	*	*	30	10	15	—	—
beef & bean red chili																				
hot																				
(Patio) 5 oz	340	18	20	—	7	15	—	34	11	4	15	—	—	10	*	30	15	10	—	—
red hot																				
(Patio) 5 oz	360	20	23	—	8	14	—	33	10	4	15	—	—	10	*	30	15	2	—	—
brito																				
beef & bean																				
(Patio) 3 oz	210	7	14	—	5	9	—	12	5	*	6	—	—	10	*	6	2	2	—	—
chicken & cheese, spicy																				
(Patio) 3 oz	210	7	14	—	8	9	—	12	3	4	4	—	—	*	*	4	4	2	—	—
nacho beef																				
(Patio) 3 oz	220	12	17	—	8	8	—	15	4	2	4	—	—	2	*	4	4	2	—	—
nacho cheese																				
(Patio) 3 2/3 oz	250	12	15	—	7	11	—	14	6	10	4	—	—	2	*	4	6	4	—	—
cheese																				
(Hormel) 4 oz	250	15	8	10	10	14	—	28	10	6	8	6	8	2	*	15	8	8	—	—
chicken con queso																				
mild																				
(Healthy Choice Quick Meals) 5 1/3 oz	280	25	12	10	7	13	—	21	7	10	15	—	—	2	10	30	20	15	—	—
red chili																				
(Hormel) 4 oz	280	15	15	20	12	13	—	26	7	2	8	6	7	2	*	20	10	10	—	—
BURRITO SEASONING MIX																				
(Old El Paso) 1/8 pkg	17	2	*	*	*	*	4	11	2	*	*	—	—	8	25	*	*	*	—	—
BUTTER																				
stick																				
salted																				
(generic) 1 pat	36	*	20	13	4	*	*	2	*	*	*	*	*	3	*	*	*	*	*	*
(Land O'Lakes) 1 tbsp	100	*	17	35	10	*	*	4	—	*	*	*	*	8	*	*	*	*	*	*
salted, light																				
(Land O'Lakes) 1 tbsp	50	*	8	20	5	*	*	3	—	*	*	*	*	8	*	*	*	*	*	*
unsalted																				
(generic) 1 pat	36	*	18	13	4	*	*	*	*	*	*	*	*	3	*	*	*	*	*	*
(Land O'Lakes) 1 tbsp	100	*	17	35	10	*	*	*	—	*	*	*	*	8	*	*	*	*	*	*
unsalted, light																				
(Land O'Lakes) 1 tbsp	50	*	8	20	5	*	*	*	—	*	*	*	*	6	*	*	*	*	*	*
whipped																				
salted																				
(generic) 1 pat	27	*	5	10	3	*	*	*	*	*	*	*	*	2	*	*	*	*	*	*
salted																				
(Land O'Lakes) 1 tbsp	60	*	11	25	7	*	*	3	—	*	*	*	*	6	*	*	*	*	*	*
salted, light																				
(Land O'Lakes) 1 tbsp	34	*	5	15	3	*	*	2	—	*	*	*	*	8	*	*	*	*	*	*
unsalted																				
(Land O'Lakes) 1 tbsp	60	*	11	25	7	*	*	*	—	*	*	*	*	6	*	*	*	*	*	*

	Calories	Protein	Fat	Sat. Fat	Cholesterol	Carbohydrates	Fiber	Sodium	Potassium	Calcium	Iron	Zinc	Magnesium	Vitamin A	Vitamin C	Thiamin	Riboflavin	Niacin	Vitamin B12	Folic acid
BUTTER BEAN, CANNED																				
baby (Bush Bros) 1/2 cup	120	12	*	*	*	6	20	21	—	4	10	—	—	*	*	—	—	—	—	—
dry, canned in brine (Green Giant/Joan of Arc) 1/2 cup	35	10	*	*	*	2	8	10	4	2	4	—	—	*	*	*	*	*	—	—
green (Bush Bros) 1/2 cup	110	10	2	*	*	6	24	14	—	2	8	—	—	*	*	—	—	—	—	—
large (Bush Bros) 1/2 cup	100	10	*	*	*	6	20	19	—	2	8	—	—	*	*	—	—	—	—	—
speckled (Bush Bros) 1/2 cup	110	10	*	*	*	6	20	17	—	6	10	—	—	6	*	—	—	—	—	—
BUTTERBUR																				
raw 1/2 cup	7	*	*	*	*	*	—	*	9	5	*	*	2	*	25	*	*	*	*	*
boiled 3 oz	7	*	*	*	*	*	—	*	9	5	*	*	2	*	27	*	*	*	*	*
boiled w/ salt 3 oz	7	*	*	*	*	*	—	8	9	5	*	*	2	*	27	*	*	*	*	*
BUTTERBUR, CANNED																				
1/2 cup chopped	2	*	*	*	*	*	—	*	*	2	2	*	*	*	12	*	*	*	*	*
BUTTERFISH																				
raw 1 fillet	47	9	4	6	7	*	*	*	3	*	2	2	*	*	*	3	3	7	10	*
broiled/baked 1 fillet	47	9	4	—	7	*	*	*	3	*	2	2	*	*	*	2	3	7	8	*
BUTTERMILK																				
cultured 1 cup	99	14	3	7	3	4	*	11	11	29	*	7	7	2	4	6	*	*	9	3
dry, sweet 1 cup	464	69	11	22	28	20	*	26	54	142	2	32	33	5	11	31	*	5	76	14
BUTTERNUT																				
dried (generic) 1 oz	174	12	25	2	*	*	4	*	3	2	6	6	17	*	2	7	2	*	*	5
BUTTERNUT SQUASH see SQUASH																				
BUTTERSCOTCH CARAMEL																				
(generic) 2 tbsp	103	*	*	*	*	9	*	6	*	2	*	*	*	*	*	*	2	*	*	*
BUTTERSCOTCH MORSELS																				
(Nestlé) 1 tbsp	80	*	6	20	*	3	*	*	*	*	*	*	*	*	*	*	—	*	*	*
BUTTERSCOTCH TOPPING																				
(Kraft) 2 tbsp	240	*	8	*	*	16	*	12	*	2	*	*	*	*	*	*	*	*	*	*
(Smucker's) 2 tbsp	140	2	2	—	*	11	*	3	*	2	*	*	*	*	*	*	2	*	*	*
(Smucker's Special Recipe) 2 tbsp	160	2	5	—	*	11	*	2	*	2	*	*	*	*	*	*	2	*	*	*
CABBAGE, BOK-CHOY																				
raw 1/2 cup shredded	5	*	*	*	*	*	*	*	3	4	2	*	2	21	26	*	*	*	*	6
boiled w/ salt 1/2 cup shredded	10	2	*	*	*	*	—	10	9	8	5	*	2	44	37	2	3	2	*	9
CABBAGE, GREEN																				
raw 1/2 cup shredded	9	*	*	*	*	*	*	4	*	2	2	*	*	*	19	*	*	*	*	4
boiled 1/2 cup shredded	17	*	*	*	*	*	8	*	2	2	*	*	*	2	25	3	2	*	*	4
boiled w/ salt 1/2 cup shredded	17	*	*	*	*	*	8	8	2	2	*	*	*	2	25	3	2	*	*	4

PERCENTAGE DAILY VALUE

	Calories	Protein	Fat	Sat. Fat	Cholesterol	Carbohydrates	Fiber	Sodium	Potassium	Calcium	Iron	Zinc	Magnesium	Vitamin A	Vitamin C	Thiamin	Riboflavin	Niacin	Vitamin B12	Folic acid
CABBAGE, HARVEST																				
raw																				
1/2 cup shredded	8	*	*	*	*	*	—	*	2	2	*	*	*	*	30	*	*	*	*	5
CABBAGE, PE-TSAI																				
raw																				
1/2 cup shredded	6	*	*	*	*	*	*	*	3	3	*	*	*	9	17	*	*	*	*	8
boiled w/ salt																				
1/2 cup shredded	8	*	*	*	*	*	—	6	4	2	*	*	*	12	16	2	2	*	*	8
CABBAGE, RED																				
raw																				
1/2 cup shredded	9	*	*	*	*	*	4	*	2	2	*	*	*	*	33	*	*	*	*	2
boiled																				
1/2 cup shredded	16	*	*	*	*	*	8	*	3	3	*	*	2	*	43	2	*	*	*	2
boiled w/ salt																				
1/2 cup shredded	16	*	*	*	*	*	—	8	3	3	*	*	2	*	43	2	*	*	*	2
CABBAGE, SAVOY																				
raw																				
1/2 cup shredded	9	*	*	*	*	*	4	*	2	*	*	*	2	7	18	2	*	*	*	7
boiled																				
1/2 cup shredded	18	2	*	*	*	*	—	*	4	2	2	*	4	13	21	2	*	*	*	8
boiled w/ salt																				
1/2 cup shredded	18	2	*	*	*	*	—	8	4	2	2	*	4	13	21	2	*	*	*	8
CACCIATORE SAUCE																				
(General Mills Recipe Sauce)																				
1/6 jar (4 oz)	40	2	*			3	—	24	8	2	6	—	—	4	*	4	2	4	—	—
CAKE, FROZEN																				
apple crisp																				
(Pepperidge Farm Classic)																				
4 1/2 oz	240	*	12	—	13	14	4	5	—	4	6	—	—	*	*	4	4	*	—	—
(Weight Watchers) 1 crisp	190	2	8	5	*	13	16	4	*	*	4	—	—	*	*	—	—	—	—	—
black forest																				
(Pepperidge Farm Classic) 3 oz	220	8	15	10	3	11	—	5	—	*	6	—	—	*	*	*	2	*	—	—
Boston creme																				
(Pepperidge Farm Special Recipe) 2 oz	190	2	12	—	10	9	—	3	—	2	4	—	—	*	*	*	4	*	—	—
brownie																				
peanut butter fudge																				
(Weight Watchers) 1 1/4 oz	100	3	5	5	2	6	12	6	3	*	4	—	—	*	*	—	—	—	—	—
Swiss mocha fudge																				
(Weight Watchers) 1 1/4 oz	90	3	3	*	2	6	8	6	3	*	4	—	—	*	*	—	—	—	—	—
brownie a la mode																				
(Weight Watchers) 1 brownie	190	10	6	5	2	12	16	7	7	8	6	—	—	*	*	—	—	—	—	—
brownie cheesecake																				
(Weight Watchers) 1 brownie	200	15	8	5	3	11	16	11	5	8	6	—	—	2	2	—	—	—	—	—
brownie, mint frosted																				
(Weight Watchers) 1 1/4 oz	100	3	3	*	2	7	12	5	3	*	4	—	—	*	*	—	—	—	—	—
caramel fudge a la mode																				
(Weight Watchers) 1 small cake	180	7	5	5	2	11	*	7	5	8	4	—	—	*	*	—	—	—	—	—
cheesecake																				
almond amaretto																				
(Weight Watchers) 3 oz	170	13	8	13	2	8	12	7	3	8	2	—	—	4	*	—	—	—	—	—
chocolate																				
(Weight Watchers) 3 1/4 oz	190	13	6	10	2	10	12	9	5	8	6	—	—	2	*	—	—	—	—	—
strawberry																				
(Weight Watchers) 4 oz	180	12	8	10	5	9	8	10	3	8	2	—	—	4	4	—	—	—	—	—
chocolate frosted brownie																				
(Weight Watchers) 1 brownie	100	3	4	5	*	7	12	6	4	*	4	—	—	*	2	—	—	—	—	—
chocolate fudge																				
(Pepperidge Farm) 1 3/4 oz	180	2	15	—	7	8	—	6	—	*	4	—	—	—	—	*	2	*	—	—
chocolate fudge stripe																				
(Pepperidge Farm) 1 3/4 oz	170	2	14	—	7	7	—	6	—	*	4	—	—	*	*	*	2	*	—	—

	Calories	Protein	Fat	Sat. Fat	Cholesterol	Carbohydrates	Fiber	Sodium	Potassium	Calcium	Iron	Zinc	Magnesium	Vitamin A	Vitamin C	Thiamin	Riboflavin	Niacin	Vitamin B12	Folic acid
CAKE, FROZEN (continued)																				
chocolate mousse (Pepperidge Farm Special) 2 oz	190	4	14	—	7	8	—	4	—	*	4	—	—	*	*	*	2	—	—	—
(Sara Lee) 1/5 cake	400	—	38	100	10	12	8	8	—	*	10	—	—	4	6	—	—	—	—	—
coconut (Pepperidge Farm) 1 3/4 oz	180	2	12	—	7	8	—	5	—	2	2	—	—	*	*	2	2	*	—	—
coffee cake (Sara Lee) 1/8 cake	220	—	14	8	5	11	4	9	—	*	4	—	—	*	2	—	—	—	—	—
devil's food (Pepperidge Farm) 1 3/4 oz	180	2	14	—	7	8	—	6	—	*	2	—	—	*	*	*	2	*	—	—
double chocolate (Sara Lee) 1/8 cake	260	3	20	55	8	8	4	11	—	*	8	—	—	2	4	—	—	—	—	—
double fudge (Weight Watchers) 2 3/4 oz	190	7	7	5	2	11	8	6	6	6	8	—	—	*	*	—	—	—	—	—
fudge golden layer (Sara Lee) 1/8 cake	270	5	20	50	5	12	4	7	—	*	4	—	—	2	4	—	—	—	—	—
German chocolate (Pepperidge Farm) 1 3/4 oz	180	2	15	—	7	7	—	7	—	2	2	—	—	*	*	2	4	2	—	—
(Pepperidge Farm Classic) 3 oz	250	*	20	20	15	10	—	10	—	*	*	—	—	*	*	*	6	*	—	—
golden (Pepperidge Farm) 1 3/4 oz	180	2	14	—	7	8	—	5	—	2	2	—	—	*	*	*	2	2	—	—
Irish creme (Weight Watchers) 3 oz	170	7	8	5	3	9	12	10	3	10	8	—	—	22	*	—	—	—	—	—
lemon mousse (Pepperidge Farm Special) 1 1/2 oz	170	2	14	15	7	7	—	5	—	*	*	—	—	*	*	*	2	—	—	—
Mississippi mud pie (Pepperidge Farm Classic) 3 oz	260	2	26	15	2	9	—	*	—	*	6	—	—	*	*	*	2	*	—	—
pineapple cream (Pepperidge Farm Special) 2 oz	190	2	11	—	7	9	—	5	—	2	4	—	—	*	*	4	2	2	—	—
pound (generic) 2 oz slice	642	20	4	3	*	46	8	32	7	10	26	5	6	2	*	19	40	8	*	2
chocolate swirl (Sara Lee) 1/4 cake	330	8	22	30	22	15	4	13	—	2	10	—	—	4	6	—	—	—	—	—
fat free chocolate (Pepperidge Farm) 1 oz	70	*	2	—	*	5	*	4	—	*	2	—	—	*	*	*	2	*	—	—
golden (Pepperidge Farm) 1 oz	70	*	*	*	*	5	*	3	—	*	*	—	—	*	*	*	*	*	—	—
plain (Sara Lee) 1/4 cake	320	7	25	45	28	13	3	8	—	*	6	—	—	8	2	—	—	—	—	—
shortcake strawberry (Weight Watchers) 4 oz	180	7	2	3	2	11	44	7	4	8	*	—	—	2	8	—	—	—	—	—
strawberry cheesecake (Pepperidge Farm Classic) 4 oz	250	8	12	—	42	14	—	9	—	6	4	—	—	*	*	*	6	*	—	—
strawberry cream (Pepperidge Farm Special) 2 oz	190	2	11	—	7	10	—	5	—	2	4	—	—	*	*	1	2	2	—	—
strawberry stripe (Pepperidge Farm) 1 1/2 oz	160	2	12	—	7	7	—	5	—	*	2	—	—	*	*	2	2	*	—	—
vanilla (Pepperidge Farm) 1 3/4 oz	190	2	12	—	7	8	—	5	—	*	*	—	—	*	*	*	2	*	—	—
CAKE, FROM MIX																				
angel food (Duncan Hines) 1/12 cake	140	7	*	*	*	10	4	5	—	2	*	—	—	*	*	—	—	—	—	—
(Pillsbury Lovin' Loaf) 1/8 cake	90	3	*	*	*	7	—	9	*	2	*	—	—	*	*	*	2	*	—	—

CAKE, FROM MIX (continued)

	Calories	Protein	Fat	Sat. Fat	Cholesterol	Carbohydrates	Fiber	Sodium	Potassium	Calcium	Iron	Zinc	Magnesium	Vitamin A	Vitamin C	Thiamin	Riboflavin	Niacin	Vitamin B12	Folic acid
banana (Pillsbury Plus) 1/12 cake	250	5	17	15	18	12	—	12	*	4	4	—	—	*	*	6	8	4	—	—
no cholesterol recipe (Pillsbury Plus) 1/12 cake	190	5	6	5	*	12	—	12	*	2	2	—	—	*	*	6	6	4	—	—
banana supreme (Duncan Hines) 1/12 cake	250	5	17	10	15	12	2	11	—	8	6	—	—	*	*	—	—	—	—	—
no cholesterol recipe (Duncan Hines) 1/12 cake	240	3	15	8	*	12	2	11	—	8	6	—	—	*	*	—	—	—	—	—
black forest cherry (Pillsbury Bundt) 1/16 cake	270	5	18	10	13	14	—	13	5	2	8	—	—	*	*	6	8	4	—	—
no cholesterol recipe (Pillsbury Bundt) 1/16 cake	260	5	17	10	*	14	—	13	5	2	6	—	—	*	*	4	8	4	—	—
blueberry streusel (Pillsbury Streusel Swirl) 1/16 cake	260	5	17	10	13	13	—	8	*	2	4	—	—	*	*	6	6	4	—	—
no cholesterol recipe (Pillsbury Streusel Swirl) 1/16 cake	250	5	15	10	*	13	—	8	*	2	2	—	—	*	*	4	6	4	—	—
Boston creme (Pillsbury Bundt) 1/16 cake	260	5	15	10	13	14	—	12	2	4	4	—	—	*	*	6	6	4	—	—
no cholesterol recipe (Pillsbury Bundt) 1/16 cake	250	3	14	10	*	14	—	12	2	4	4	—	—	*	*	6	6	4	—	—
butter chocolate (Betty Crocker SuperMoist) 1/12 cake	280	7	22	35	25	12	—	17	5	4	8	—	—	6	*	6	6	4	—	—
butter pecan (Betty Crocker SuperMoist) 1/12 cake	250	5	17	15	18	12	—	13	*	8	4	—	—	*	*	6	8	4	—	—
no cholesterol recipe (Betty Crocker SuperMoist) 1/12 cake	220	5	11	10	*	12	—	13	*	8	6	—	—	*	*	6	6	4	—	—
butter recipe (Duncan Hines) 1/10 cake	320	5	25	35	27	14	8	8	—	6	4	—	—	*	*	—	—	—	—	—
(Pillsbury Plus) 1/12 cake	260	5	18	25	25	12	—	15	*	8	4	—	—	6	*	6	8	4	—	—
no cholesterol recipe (Pillsbury Plus) 1/12 cake	250	5	17	5	*	12	—	15	*	6	2	—	—	6	*	6	6	4	—	—
butter recipe chocolate (Pillsbury Plus) 1/12 cake	250	7	20	30	25	11	—	17	5	10	8	—	—	6	*	6	6	4	—	—
no cholesterol recipe (Pillsbury Plus) 1/12 cake	240	5	18	5	*	11	—	17	6	10	6	—	—	6	*	6	6	4	—	—
butter yellow (Betty Crocker SuperMoist) 1/12 cake	260	5	17	30	25	12	—	14	*	8	4	—	—	*	*	6	6	4	—	—
caramel (Duncan Hines) 1/12 cake	250	5	17	10	15	12	2	11	—	8	6	—	—	*	*	—	—	—	—	—
no cholesterol recipe (Duncan Hines) 1/12 cake	240	3	15	8	*	12	2	11	—	8	6	—	—	*	*	—	—	—	—	—
carrot (Betty Crocker SuperMoist) 1/12 cake	250	5	15	10	18	12	—	12	2	4	6	—	—	*	*	6	6	4	—	—
(Pillsbury Plus) 1/12 cake	260	5	18	15	18	11	—	12	2	4	4	—	—	50	*	8	8	4	—	—
no cholesterol recipe (Betty Crocker SuperMoist) 1/12 cake	210	5	5	10	*	12	—	12	2	4	6	—	—	*	*	8	4	4	—	—
(Pillsbury Plus) 1/12 cake	190	5	8	5	*	12	—	12	2	4	4	—	—	50	*	8	6	4	—	—
cherry chip (Betty Crocker SuperMoist) 1/12 cake	190	5	5	5	*	12	—	11	*	*	4	—	—	*	*	6	4	4	—	—

	Calories	Protein	Fat	Sat Fat	Cholesterol	Carbohydrates	Fiber	Sodium	Potassium	Calcium	Iron	Zinc	Magnesium	Vitamin A	Vitamin C	Thiamin	Riboflavin	Niacin	Vitamin B12	Folic acid
CAKE, FROM MIX (continued)																				
chocolate, dark (Pillsbury Plus) 1/12 cake	250	5	18	15	18	11	—	14	2	10	6	—	—	*	*	6	6	4	—	—
no cholesterol recipe (Pillsbury Plus) 1/12 cake	180	5	8	10	*	11	—	14	2	10	4	—	—	*	*	6	6	4	—	—
chocolate caramel (Pillsbury Bundt) 1/16 cake	290	5	20	10	15	14	—	15	5	2	8	—	—	*	*	6	8	2	—	—
reduced cholesterol recipe (Pillsbury Bundt) 1/16 cake	280	5	18	10	2	14	—	15	5	2	8	—	—	*	*	4	8	2	—	—
chocolate chip (Betty Crocker SuperMoist) 1/12 cake	290	5	23	15	18	11	—	12	2	8	4	—	—	*	*	6	8	4	—	—
(Pillsbury Plus) 1/12 cake	240	5	15	15	12	11	—	12	*	8	4	—	—	*	*	6	6	4	—	—
no cholesterol recipe (Betty Crocker SuperMoist) 1/12 cake	220	5	12	10	*	12	—	12	2	8	6	—	—	*	*	8	6	4	—	—
(Pillsbury Plus) 1/12 cake	190	5	8	10	*	12	—	12	*	6	4	—	—	*	*	6	6	4	—	—
chocolate chocolate chip (Betty Crocker SuperMoist) 1/12 cake	260	5	18	15	18	11	—	17	3	6	8	—	—	*	*	6	8	4	—	—
chocolate eclair (Pillsbury Bundt) 1/16 cake	260	5	15	10	13	14	—	12	2	4	4	—	—	*	*	6	6	4	—	—
no cholesterol recipe (Pillsbury Bundt) 1/16 cake	250	3	14	10	*	14	—	12	2	4	4	—	—	*	*	6	6	4	—	—
chocolate fudge (Betty Crocker SuperMoist) 1/12 cake	260	5	18	15	18	11	—	19	3	6	8	—	—	*	*	6	6	2	—	—
chocolate macaroon (Pillsbury Bundt) 1/16 cake	280	5	22	20	13	12	—	14	5	*	6	—	—	*	*	6	8	4	—	—
no cholesterol recipe (Pillsbury Bundt) 1/16 cake	270	5	22	20	*	12	—	14	5	*	8	—	—	*	*	6	8	4	—	—
chocolate mousse (Pillsbury Bundt) 1/16 cake	260	5	18	10	13	12	—	13	5	2	6	—	—	*	*	6	8	2	—	—
no cholesterol recipe (Pillsbury Bundt) 1/16 cake	250	5	17	10	*	12	—	13	5	2	6	—	—	*	*	6	8	2	—	—
chocolate pudding (Betty Crocker Classic) 1/6 cake	230	5	8	10	12	15	—	10	5	4	4	—	—	4	*	4	4	2	—	—
cinnamon crumb microwave (Duncan Hines) 1/8 cake	170	3	11	8	*	9	2	7	—	*	4	—	—	*	*	—	—	—	—	—
cinnamon streusel (Pillsbury Streusel Swirl) 1/16 cake	260	5	17	10	13	13	—	8	*	2	4	—	—	*	*	6	6	4	—	—
no cholesterol recipe (Pillsbury Streusel Swirl) 1/16 cake	250	3	15	10	*	13	—	8	*	2	4	—	—	*	*	4	4	4	—	—
dark fudge (Duncan Hines) 1/12 cake	290	7	23	15	15	11	4	16	—	6	6	—	—	*	*	—	—	—	—	—
no cholesterol recipe (Duncan Hines) 1/12 cake	280	7	23	10	*	11	4	16	—	6	6	—	—	*	*	—	—	—	—	—
devil's food (Betty Crocker SuperMoist) 1/12 cake	260	7	18	15	18	12	—	18	4	2	10	—	—	*	*	6	6	4	—	—
(Duncan Hines) 1/12 cake	290	7	23	15	15	11	4	16	—	6	6	—	—	*	*	—	—	4	—	—
(Duncan Hines DeLights) 1/12 cake	220	5	9	8	12	14	4	17	—	6	6	—	—	*	*	—	—	—	—	—
(Pillsbury Lovin'Lites) 1/12 cake	170	7	5	5	12	11	—	16	5	10	8	—	—	*	*	6	6	4	—	—
(Pillsbury Plus) 1/12 cake	270	7	22	15	18	11	—	15	5	10	8	—	—	*	*	6	6	4	—	—

CAKE, FROM MIX (continued)

	Calories	Protein	Fat	Sat. Fat	Cholesterol	Carbohydrates	Fiber	Sodium	Potassium	Calcium	Iron	Zinc	Magnesium	Vitamin A	Vitamin C	Thiamin	Riboflavin	Niacin	Vitamin B₁₂	Folic acid
light (Betty Crocker SuperMoist) 1/12 cake	200	7	6	10	18	12	—	14	5	6	8	—	—	*	*	6	4	2	—	—
no cholesterol recipe (Betty Crocker SuperMoist) 1/12 cake	220	5	11	10	*	12	—	18	4	2	10	—	—	*	*	8	6	4	—	—
(Betty Crocker SuperMoist) 1/12 cake	180	5	5	10	*	12	—	15	6	6	10	—	—	*	*	8	6	2	—	—
(Duncan Hines) 1/12 cake	280	7	23	10	*	11	4	16	—	6	6	—	—	*	*	—	—	—	—	—
(Pillsbury Lovin'Lites) 1/12 cake	160	7	3	3	*	11	—	16	5	10	6	—	—	*	*	6	6	4	—	—
devil's food w/ chocolate frosting (Betty Crocker MicroRave) 1/6 cake	310	5	26	25	12	12	—	10	4	4	6	—	—	2	*	4	4	2	—	—
no cholesterol recipe (Betty Crocker MicroRave) 1/6 cake	240	5	14	15	*	12	—	10	4	4	6	—	—	2	*	4	4	2	—	—
French vanilla (Duncan Hines) 1/12 cake	250	5	17	10	15	12	2	11	—	8	6	—	—	*	*	—	—	—	—	—
no cholesterol recipe (Duncan Hines) 1/12 cake	240	3	15	8	*	12	2	11	—	8	6	—	—	*	*	—	—	—	—	—
fudge (Duncan Hines) 1/10 cake	320	5	26	40	27	13	8	12	—	2	8	—	—	*	*	—	—	—	—	—
fudge marble (Betty Crocker SuperMoist) 1/12 cake	260	5	18	15	18	12	—	17	2	8	4	—	—	*	*	6	8	4	—	—
(Duncan Hines) 1/12 cake	250	5	17	10	15	12	2	11	—	8	6	—	—	*	*	—	—	—	—	—
(Duncan Hines DeLights) 1/12 cake	220	5	8	8	12	14	4	17	—	6	6	—	—	*	*	—	—	—	—	—
no cholesterol recipe (Betty Crocker SuperMoist) 1/12 cake	220	5	11	10	*	12	—	12	—	8	6	—	—	*	*	8	6	4	—	—
(Duncan Hines) 1/12 cake	240	3	15	8	*	12	2	11	—	8	6	—	—	*	*	—	—	—	—	—
fudge swirl (Pillsbury Plus) 1/12 cake	270	5	18	15	18	12	—	12	2	8	4	—	—	*	*	6	8	4	—	—
no cholesterol recipe (Pillsbury Plus) 1/12 cake	200	5	8	10	*	12	—	12	2	6	4	—	—	*	*	6	6	4	—	—
funfetti (Pillsbury Plus) 1/12 cake	230	5	14	15	*	12	—	12	*	2	2	—	—	*	*	6	6	4	—	—
no oil recipe (Pillsbury Plus) 1/12 cake	190	5	6	5	*	12	—	12	*	2	4	—	—	*	*	8	6	4	—	—
German chocolate (Betty Crocker SuperMoist) 1/12 cake	260	5	18	15	18	12	—	17	2	2	6	—	—	*	*	6	8	4	—	—
(Pillsbury Plus) 1/12 cake	250	5	17	15	18	11	—	12	2	2	4	—	—	*	*	6	8	4	—	—
no cholesterol recipe (Betty Crocker SuperMoist) 1/12 cake	220	5	12	10	*	12	—	17	2	2	6	—	—	*	*	8	6	4	—	—
(Pillsbury Plus) 1/12 cake	180	5	6	5	*	11	—	12	2	2	4	—	—	*	*	8	6	4	—	—
w/ coconut pecan frosting (Betty Crocker MicroRave) 1/6 cake	320	5	28	25	12	12	—	10	2	4	6	—	—	*	*	4	4	2	—	—
golden vanilla (Betty Crocker SuperMoist) 1/12 cake	280	5	22	15	18	12	—	11	*	6	6	—	—	*	*	6	6	4	—	—
no cholesterol recipe (Betty Crocker SuperMoist) 1/12 cake	220	5	11	10	*	12	—	11	*	6	6	—	—	*	*	6	4	4	—	—

CAKE, FROM MIX (continued)

	Calories	Protein	Fat	Sat. Fat	Cholesterol	Carbohydrates	Fiber	Sodium	Potassium	Calcium	Iron	Zinc	Magnesium	Vitamin A	Vitamin C	Thiamin	Riboflavin	Niacin	Vitamin B12	Folic acid
lemon (Betty Crocker SuperMoist) 1/12 cake	260	5	17	15	18	12	—	12	*	8	6	—	—	*	*	8	8	4	—	—
(Pillsbury Plus) 1/12 cake	240	5	15	10	18	11	—	12	*	6	4	—	—	*	*	6	8	4	—	—
no cholesterol recipe (Betty Crocker SuperMoist) 1/12 cake	220	5	11	10	*	12	—	12	*	8	6	—	—	*	*	8	6	4	—	—
(Pillsbury Plus) 1/12 cake	180	5	5	5	*	12	—	12	*	6	2	—	—	*	*	6	6	4	—	—
lemon chiffon (Betty Crocker Classic) 1/12 cake	200	7	8	5	12	12	—	8	2	2	4	—	—	*	*	6	8	4	—	—
lemon pudding (Betty Crocker SuperMoist) 1/6 cake	230	3	8	10	12	15	—	11	*	4	2	—	—	*	*	4	4	2	—	—
lemon supreme (Duncan Hines) 1/12 cake	250	5	17	10	15	12	2	11	—	8	6	—	—	*	*	—	—	—	—	—
(Pillsbury Streusel Swirl) 1/16 cake	260	5	17	10	13	12	—	12	*	4	4	—	—	*	*	6	6	4	—	—
no cholesterol recipe (Duncan Hines) 1/12 cake	240	3	15	8	*	12	2	11	—	8	6	—	—	*	*	—	—	—	—	—
(Pillsbury Streusel Swirl) 1/16 cake	250	5	15	10	*	12	—	12	*	4	2	—	—	*	*	4	4	4	—	—
milk chocolate (Betty Crocker SuperMoist) 1/12 cake	260	7	18	15	18	11	—	14	4	6	6	—	—	*	*	6	8	2	—	—
no cholesterol recipe (Betty Crocker SuperMoist) 1/12 cake	210	5	11	10	*	11	—	14	4	6	8	—	—	*	*	6	6	2	—	—
orange supreme (Duncan Hines) 1/12 cake	250	5	17	10	15	12	2	11	—	8	6	—	—	*	*	—	—	—	—	—
no cholesterol recipe (Duncan Hines) 1/12 cake	240	3	15	8	*	12	2	11	—	8	6	—	—	*	*	—	—	—	—	—
pineapple creme (Pillsbury Bundt) 1/16 cake	280	3	17	10	13	14	—	12	*	4	4	—	—	*	*	6	6	4	—	—
no cholesterol recipe (Pillsbury Bundt) 1/16 cake	270	3	15	10	*	14	—	12	*	4	2	—	—	*	*	6	6	4	—	—
pineapple supreme (Duncan Hines) 1/12 cake	250	5	17	10	15	12	2	11	—	8	6	—	—	*	*	—	—	—	—	—
no cholesterol recipe (Duncan Hines) 1/12 cake	240	3	15	8	*	12	2	11	—	8	6	—	—	*	*	—	—	—	—	—
pineapple upside down (Betty Crocker Classic) 1/9 cake	270	3	15	15	8	14	—	10	2	4	4	—	—	*	*	4	4	2	—	—
no cholesterol recipe (Betty Crocker SuperMoist) 1/9 cake	270	3	15	15	*	14	—	10	2	4	4	—	—	*	*	4	4	2	—	—
pound (Betty Crocker Classic) 1/12 cake	200	3	14	15	12	9	—	7	*	2	4	—	—	*	*	4	4	4	—	—
rainbow chip (Betty Crocker SuperMoist) 1/12 cake	250	5	17	15	18	12	—	13	*	10	4	—	—	*	*	6	8	4	—	—
raspberry (Duncan Hines) 1/12 cake	250	5	17	10	15	12	2	11	—	8	6	—	—	*	*	—	—	—	—	—
no cholesterol recipe (Duncan Hines) 1/12 cake	240	3	15	8	*	12	2	11	—	8	6	—	—	*	*	—	—	—	—	—
sour cream chocolate (Betty Crocker SuperMoist) 1/12 cake	260	5	18	15	18	12	—	18	3	2	8	—	—	*	*	6	6	4	—	—

CAKE, FROM MIX (continued)

	Calories	Protein	Fat	Sat. Fat	Cholesterol	Carbohydrates	Fiber	Sodium	Potassium	Calcium	Iron	Zinc	Magnesium	Vitamin A	Vitamin C	Thiamin	Riboflavin	Niacin	Vitamin B₁₂	Folic acid
no cholesterol recipe (Betty Crocker SuperMoist) 1/12 cake	220	5	12	10	*	12	—	18	3	2	8	—		—	*	*	6	6	4	—	—
sour cream white (Betty Crocker SuperMoist) 1/12 cake	180	5	5	5	*	12	—	12	*	*	4	—		—	*	*	6	6	4	—	—
spice (Betty Crocker SuperMoist) 1/12 cake	260	5	17	15	18	12	—	13	*	10	6	—		—	*	*	6	8	4	—	—
no cholesterol recipe (Betty Crocker SuperMoist) 1/12 cake	220	5	11	10	*	12	—	13	*	10	6	—		—	*	*	6	6	4	—	—
strawberry (Pillsbury Plus) 1/12 cake	250	5	17	15	18	12	—	13	*	6	4	—		—	*	*	6	8	4	—	—
no cholesterol recipe (Pillsbury Plus) 1/12 cake	190	5	6	5	*	12	—	13	*	6	2	—		—	*	*	6	6	4	—	—
strawberry supreme (Duncan Hines) 1/12 cake	250	5	17	10	15	12	2	11	—	8	6	—		—	*	—	—	—	—	—	—
no cholesterol recipe (Duncan Hines) 1/12 cake	240	3	15	8	*	12	2	11	—	8	6	—		—	*	*	—	—	—	—	—
sunshine vanilla (Pillsbury Plus) 1/12 cake	260	5	18	15	18	11	—	12	*	8	4	—		—	*	*	6	8	4	—	—
no cholesterol recipe (Pillsbury Plus) 1/12 cake	190	5	8	10	*	12	—	12	*	6	2	—		—	*	*	6	6	4	—	—
swirl (Betty Crocker SuperMoist) 1/12 cake	260	5	17	15	18	12	—	12	*	8	6	—		—	*	*	6	8	4	—	—
no cholesterol recipe (Betty Crocker SuperMoist) 1/12 cake	220	5	11	10	*	12	—	12	*	8	6	—		—	*	*	8	6	4	—	—
Swiss chocolate (Duncan Hines) 1/12 cake	290	7	23	15	15	11	4	16	—	6	6	—		—	*	*	—	—	—	—	—
no cholesterol recipe (Duncan Hines) 1/12 cake	280	7	23	10	*	11	4	16	—	6	6	—		—	*	*	—	—	—	—	—
tunnel of fudge (Pillsbury Bundt) 1/16 cake	310	5	25	15	13	14	—	14	6	*	8	—		—	*	*	4	8	2	—	—
no cholesterol recipe (Pillsbury Bundt) 1/16 cake	300	5	23	15	*	14	—	14	6	*	6	—		—	*	*	4	8	2	—	—
tunnel of lemon (Pillsbury Bundt) 1/16 cake	270	3	14	10	13	15	—	12	*	4	4	—		—	*	*	6	6	4	—	—
no cholesterol recipe (Pillsbury Bundt) 1/16 cake	260	3	12	10	*	15	—	12	*	4	2	—		—	*	*	6	6	4	—	—
white (Betty Crocker SuperMoist) 1/12 cake	230	3	15	10	*	11	—	13	*	6	4	—		—	*	*	8	6	4	—	—
(Pillsbury Lovin'Lites) 1/12 cake	180	5	5	3	12	12	—	13	*	8	4	—		—	*	*	6	6	4	—	—
(Pillsbury Plus) 1/12 cake	220	5	14	10	*	11	—	12	*	2	2	—		—	*	*	6	6	4	—	—
basic recipe (Duncan Hines) 1/12 cake	240	3	15	10	*	12	2	9	—	6	6	—		—	*	*	—	—	—	—	—
light (Betty Crocker SuperMoist) 1/12 cake	180	3	5	5	*	12	—	14	*	8	4	—		—	*	*	6	6	4	—	—
no cholesterol recipe (Pillsbury Lovin'Lites) 1/12 cake	170	5	3	3	*	12	—	13	*	8	2	—		—	*	*	6	6	4	—	—
no oil recipe (Pillsbury Plus) 1/12 cake	190	5	6	5	*	12	—	12	*	2	4	—		—	*	*	8	6	4	—	—
w/ 3 whole eggs (Duncan Hines) 1/12 cake	250	5	18	13	15	12	2	9	—	6	6	—		—	*	*	—	—	—	—	—

	Calories	Protein	Fat	Sat. Fat	Cholesterol	Carbohydrates	Fiber	Sodium	Potassium	Calcium	Iron	Zinc	Magnesium	Vitamin A	Vitamin C	Thiamin	Riboflavin	Niacin	Vitamin B$_{12}$	Folic acid
CAKE, FROM MIX (continued)																				
yellow																				
(Betty Crocker SuperMoist) 1/12 cake	260	5	17	15	18	12	—	12	*	8	6	—	—	*	*	6	8	4	—	—
(Duncan Hines) 1/12 cake	250	5	17	10	15	12	2	11	—	8	6	—	—	*	*	—	—	—	—	—
(Duncan Hines DeLights) 1/12 cake	220	5	7	8	12	15	2	13	—	4	4	—	—	*	*	—	—	—	—	—
(Pillsbury Lovin'Lites) 1/12 cake	180	5	5	3	12	12	—	12	*	8	4	—	—	*	*	6	6	4	—	—
(Pillsbury Plus) 1/12 cake	260	5	18	15	18	11	—	12	*	8	4	—	—	*	*	6	8	4	—	—
light																				
(Betty Crocker SuperMoist) 1/12 cake	200	5	6	10	18	12	—	13	*	6	4	—	—	*	*	8	8	4	—	—
no cholesterol recipe *(Betty Crocker)* 1/12 cake	190	5	5	5	*	12	—	14	*	6	6	—	—	*	*	8	6	4	—	—
(Betty Crocker SuperMoist) 1/12 cake	220	5	11	10	*	12	—	12	*	8	6	—	—	*	*	8	6	4	—	—
(Duncan Hines) 1/12 cake	240	3	15	8	*	12	2	11	—	8	6	—	—	*	—	—	—	—	—	—
(Pillsbury Lovin'Lites) 1/12 cake	170	5	3	3	*	12	—	13	*	8	2	—	—	*	*	6	6	4	—	—
(Pillsbury Plus) 1/12 cake	190	5	8	10	*	12	—	12	*	6	2	—	—	*	*	6	6	4	—	—
unfrosted *(generic)* 1/12 of 9 in. cake	195	6	6	8	18	12	4	12	*	7	4	2	*	2	*	4	8	3	2	2
yellow w/ chocolate frosting *(Betty Crocker MicroRave)* 1/6 cake	300	3	26	20	12	12	—	9	2	6	2	—	—	2	*	4	4	2	—	—
no cholesterol recipe *(Betty Crocker MicroRave)* 1/6 cake	230	3	14	15	*	12	—	10	2	6	4	—	—	2	*	6	4	2	—	—
CAKE, FROM REFRIGERATED DOUGH																				
cinnamon streusel *(Pillsbury)* 1/6 cake	230	5	17	10	*	10	—	10	*	*	6	—	—	*	*	80	4	6	—	—
pecan crumb *(Pillsbury)* 1/6 cake	230	5	18	10	*	10	—	10	*	*	6	—	—	*	*	80	4	6	—	—
CAKE, SNACK																				
apple spice *(Hostess)* 1 cake	130	3	2	3	*	10	2	6	*	2	2	—	—	*	*	2	4	2	—	—
banana w/ vanilla frosting from mix *(Pillsbury)* 1 cake	170	2	11	10	3	9	—	7	*	4	2	—	—	*	*	2	2	2	—	—
carrot w/ cream cheese frosting from mix *(Pillsbury)* 1 cake	170	2	11	10	3	8	—	8	*	4	2	—	—	25	*	2	2	2	—	—
Choco-bliss *(Hostess)* 1 cake	200	3	14	20	2	10	5	9	4	2	4	—	—	*	*	4	2	—	—	—
Choco-diles *(Hostess)* 1 cake	240	3	17	40	7	11	6	7	5	2	8	—	—	*	*	4	4	*	—	—
chocolate w/ chocolate fudge frosting from mix *(Pillsbury)* 1 cake	160	3	11	10	3	8	—	9	5	2	2	—	—	*	*	2	2	2	—	—
coffee cake apple & cinnamon *(Hostess Stroozls)* 1 cake	140	3	2	3	*	11	2	7	*	2	2	—	—	*	*	6	10	4	—	—
cinnamon streusel *(Weight Watchers)* 2 1/4 oz	160	5	6	5	2	9	8	8	2	4	2	—	—	*	*	—	—	—	—	—
raspberry *(Hostess Stroozls)* 1 cake	140	3	2	3	*	11	4	7	*	2	2	—	—	*	*	6	10	4	—	—
cookie cake, chocolate chip *(Hostess)* 1 cake	150	3	20	15	12	11	8	5	2	2	4	—	—	*	*	6	10	4	—	—

PERCENTAGE DAILY VALUE

	Calories	Protein	Fat	Sat. Fat	Cholesterol	Carbohydrates	Fiber	Sodium	Potassium	Calcium	Iron	Zinc	Magnesium	Vitamin A	Vitamin C	Thiamin	Riboflavin	Niacin	Vitamin B₁₂	Folic acid
CAKE, FROM MIX (continued)																				
corn																				
(generic) 2 cakes	70	2	*	*	*	5	*	4	*	*	*	2	5	*	*	3	*	5	*	*
(verylona) 2 cakes	70	2	*	*	*	5	—	*	*	*	*	2	5	*	*	3	*	5	*	*
crumb coffee																				
regular																				
(Hostess) 1 cake	120	2	8	10	3	6	3	3	*	2	4	—	—	*	*	4	4	4	—	—
w/ cinnamon, 97% fat free																				
(Hostess) 1 cake	80	2	2	3	*	6	2	4	*	2	2	—	—	*	*	2	2	2	—	—
dessert cup																				
(Hostess) 1 cake	90	3	3	3	5	6	2	4	*	2	4	—	—	*	*	4	4	2	—	—
Ding Dong																				
(Hostess) 1 cake	170	3	14	30	2	7	4	5	4	2	6	—	—	*	*	2	2	*	—	—
Doo Dads																				
1/2 cup	129	5	8	—	*	6	8	15	2	2	4	4	4	*	*	7	4	8	*	3
Ho Ho's																				
(Hostess) 1 cake	120	2	9	20	3	5	2	3	3	2	4	—	—	*	*	2	2	2	—	—
Lil' Angels																				
(Hostess) 1 cake	90	2	3	—	*	5	—	4	—	2	2	—	—	*	*	2	2	*	—	—
orange swirl																				
(Hostess) 1 cake	230	5	18	30	3	9	4	6	2	6	6	—	—	*	*	8	8	4	—	—
Sno Balls																				
(Hostess) 1 cake	150	2	6	10	*	9	4	7	2	*	2	—	—	*	*	*	*	2	—	—
Suzy q's																				
banana																				
(Hostess) 1 cake	240	3	14	—	7	13	—	8	—	4	4	—	—	*	*	6	6	4	—	—
regular																				
(Hostess) 1 cake	250	3	15	20	5	12	8	12	3	2	8	—	—	*	*	4	4	2	—	—
Tiger Tails																				
(Hostess) 1 cake	240	7	12	20	8	13	5	12	2	2	6	—	—	*	*	6	8	4	—	—
CALAMARI *see* **SQUID**																				
CANDY																				
butter mints																				
(Kraft) 1 piece	8	*	*	*	*	*	*	*	*	*	*	—	—	*	*	*	*	*	—	—
butter rum																				
(Pearson) 2 pieces	60	*	2	8	*	4	*	*	*	*	*	*	*	*	*	*	*	*	*	*
butterscotch																				
(generic) 1 oz	112	*	2	*	*	9	*	*	*	*	*	*	*	*	*	*	*	*	*	*
caramels																				
(generic) 1 package	271	5	9	24	2	18	4	7	4	10	*	2	3	*	*	*	8	*	*	*
(Kraft) 1 piece	60	*	2	*	*	2	*	*	*	*	*	—	—	*	*	*	*	*	—	—
(Pearson) 2 pieces	60	*	2	8	*	4	*	2	*	*	*	*	*	*	*	*	*	*	*	*
(Rolo) 1 package	261	5	18	—	4	13	*	4	4	7	2	3	4	*	2	2	8	*	6	*
caramels, chocolate flavored																				
(generic) 1 bar	230	2	2	2	*	19	4	*	2	2	*	2	5	*	*	*	2	*	*	*
Cherry Nibs																				
(Y & S) 1 oz	106	*	*	*	*	9	—	3	*	2	*	*	*	*	*	*	*	*	*	*
chewing gum																				
(generic) 1 stick	10	*	*	*	*	*	*	*	*	*	*	*	*	*	*	*	*	*	*	*
chocolate covered almonds																				
(Hershey's) 1 bag (1 1/2 oz)	564	9	57		4	15	—	2	14	36	8	12	30	*	—	4	29	6	—	—
chocolate covered peanuts																				
(Goobers) 1 1/3 oz	210	10	20	25	—	6	12	*	6	6	2	—	—	*	*	4	4	10	*	*
chocolate covered raisins																				
(Raisinets) 1 1/2 oz	200	4	12	20	—	10	8	*	—	4	2	—	—	*	*	2	4	*	*	*
chocolate fondant																				
(generic) 1 small patty	40	*	2	3	*	3	*	*	*	*	*	*	2	*	*	*	*	*	*	*
Chocolate Fudgies																				
(Kraft) 1 piece	65	*	2	*	*	2	*	*	*	*	*	—	—	*	*	*	*	*	—	—

	Calories	Protein	Fat	Sat. Fat	Cholesterol	Carbohydrates	Fiber	Sodium	Potassium	Calcium	Iron	Zinc	Magnesium	Vitamin A	Vitamin C	Thiamin	Riboflavin	Niacin	Vitamin B$_{12}$	Folic acid
CANDY (continued)																				
Chocolate Kisses																				
(Hershey's) 6 pieces	540	4	47	91	8	19	—	3	12	20	7	9	16	*	—	5	20	2	—	—
Chocolate Kisses w/ almonds																				
(Hershey's) 6 pieces	554	6	52	—	—	17	—	3	12	23	7	—	—	*	—	3	24	3	—	—
chocolate mint																				
(Pearson) 2 pieces	60	*	2	8	*	4	*	2	*	*	*	*	*	*	*	*	*	*	*	*
chocolate parfait																				
(Pearson) 2 pieces	60	*	3	10	*	4	*	*	*	*	*	*	*	*	*	*	*	*	*	*
coffee																				
(Pearson) 2 pieces	60	*	2	8	*	4	*	2	*	*	*	*	*	*	*	*	*	*	*	*
fruit chews																				
(Starburst) 1 package	234	*	8	—	*	17	—	*	*	*	*	*	*	*	52	*	*	*	*	*
fudge																				
brown sugar w/ nuts																				
(homemade) 1 piece	55	*	2	*	*	4	—	*	*	2	*	*	2	*	*	*	*	*	*	*
chocolate plain																				
(homemade) 1 piece	65	*	2	5	*	4	*	*	*	*	*	*	*	*	*	*	*	*	*	*
w/ nuts																				
(homemade) 1 piece	81	*	5	6	*	5	*	*	*	*	*	*	2	*	*	*	*	*	*	*
chocolate marshmallow w/ nuts																				
(homemade) 1 piece	96	*	7	11	2	5	*	*	*	*	*	*	2	*	*	*	*	*	*	*
peanut butter plain																				
(homemade) 1 piece	59	*	2	*	*	4	*	*	*	*	*	*	*	*	*	*	*	*	*	*
vanilla plain																				
(homemade) 1 piece	59	*	*	3	*	4	*	*	*	*	*	*	*	*	*	*	*	*	*	*
w/ nuts																				
(homemade) 1 piece	62	*	3	3	*	4	*	*	*	*	*	*	*	*	*	*	*	*	*	*
golden almond solitaires																				
(generic) 1 package	455	16	48	—	3	13	—	2	12	31	7	10	25	*	*	3	25	5	7	5
gumdrops																				
(generic) 10 small	135	*	*	*	*	12	*	*	*	*	*	*	*	*	*	*	*	*	*	*
hard candy																				
(generic) 2 large	22	*	*	*	*	2	*	*	*	*	*	*	*	*	*	*	*	*	*	*
jellies																				
(generic) 1 tbsp	51	*	*	*	*	4	*	*	*	*	*	*	*	*	*	*	*	*	*	*
jellybeans																				
(generic) 10 large	104	*	*	*	*	9	*	*	*	*	*	2	*	*	*	*	*	*	*	*
licorice																				
(Pearson) 2 pieces	60	*	2	8	*	4	*	2	*	*	*	*	*	*	*	*	*	*	*	*
lollipop																				
(generic) 1 lollipop	22	*	*	*	*	2	*	*	*	*	*	*	*	*	*	*	*	*	*	*
M & M's																				
peanut butter																				
1 bag	240	6	18	—	—	9		2	—	4	2	—	—	*	*	*	4	8	—	—
plain																				
1 bag	230	2	15	—	—	12		2	—	4	2	—	—	*	*	*	4	*	—	—
milk chocolate																				
plain chips																				
(generic) 1 cup	872	20	80	157	12	34	24	6	19	32	13	16	26	6	*	9	30	3	11	3
w/ peanuts																				
(generic) 10 pieces	208	9	21	29	*	7	8	*	6	4	3	5	9	*	*	3	4	8	3	*
w/ raisins																				
(generic) 10 pieces	39	*	2	5	*	2	*	*	*	*	*	*	*	*	*	*	*	*	*	*
mints																				
(After Eight) 2 mints	70	*	3	—	*	4	*	*	*	*	*	*	*	*	*	*	*	*	*	*
nonpareils																				
(Sno-Caps) 2 1/3 oz	300	*	20	40	*	16	12	*	2	*	2	*	*	*	*	*	*	*	*	*
party mints																				
(Kraft) 1 piece	8	*	*	*	*	*	*	*	*	*	*	*	—	*	*	*	*	*	—	—

	Calories	Protein	Fat	Sat. Fat	Cholesterol	Carbohydrates	Fiber	Sodium	Potassium	Calcium	Iron	Zinc	Magnesium	Vitamin A	Vitamin C	Thiamin	Riboflavin	Niacin	Vitamin B$_{12}$	Folic acid
CANDY (continued)																				
peanut brittle																				
(generic) 2 oz	257	7	17	14	2	13	4	11	3	2	4	4	7	2	*	7	2	10	*	10
(Kraft) 1 piece	130	6	8	5	*	7	*	6	2	*	*	—	—	*	*	*	*	6	—	—
peanut butter & chocolate																				
(Reese's Pieces) 1 package	258	12	18	—	*	11	8	3	7	7	5	4	11	*	*	2	8	16	3	8
peanut butter cup																				
(Reese's) 6 small cups	204	8	20	49	2	7	8	5	5	3	3	4	9	*	*	*	5	8	3	3
crunchy																				
(Reese's) 2 cups	554	11	54	—	2	16	—	10	12	9	9	12	24	*	—	19	9	29	—	—
peanut butter parfait																				
(Pearson) 2 pieces	60	*	3	10	*	4	*	2	*	*	*	*	*	*	*	*	*	*	*	*
pecan caramels																				
(Demet's Turtles) 2 pieces	180	*	15	—	*	3	*	*	3	4	*	*	*	*	*	*	4	*	*	*
praline																				
(homemade) 1 piece	177	2	15	4	*	8	—	*	2	*	3	5	5	*	*	8	*	*	*	*
Skittles																				
1 bag	270	*	3	—	—	20	—	*	*	*	*	—	*	*	50	*	*	*	—	—
1 package	255	*	3	—	*	21	*	*	*	*	*	*	*	*	*	*	*	*	*	*
taffy																				
(homemade) 1 piece	56	*	*	*	*	5	—	*	*	*	*	*	*	*	*	*	*	*	*	*
toffee																				
(homemade) 1 piece	65	*	6	13	4	3	—	*	*	*	*	*	*	3	*	*	*	*	*	*
truffle																				
(homemade) 1 piece	59	*	6	13	2	2	—	*	*	2	*	*	*	*	*	*	2	*	*	*
turtles																				
(Nestlé) 2 pieces	160	—	14	15	—	7	4	*	—	—	—	—	—	—	—	—	—	—	—	—
Twizzlers																				
1 package	263	4	2	—	*	22	*	8	*	2	2	*	*	*	*	*	2	*	*	*
CANDY BAR																				
100 Grand																				
1 bar	195	3	13	—	*	10	*	3	3	5	2	2	4	*	*	*	6	*	3	*
3 Musketeers																				
1 bar	250	3	12	20	*	15	4	5	2	2	2	2	4	*	*	*	5	*	2	*
5th Avenue																				
1 bar	280	8	20	—	*	14	—	5	6	4	3	4	9	*	*	*	8	10	2	8
Aero																				
(Nestlé) 1 3/8 oz	210	6	20	35	3	9	8	*	4	8	*	—	—	*	*	2	8	*	*	*
Almond Joy																				
1 bar	232	4	21	42	*	10	—	3	5	4	3	3	8	*	*	*	4	*	*	*
Alpine White																				
w/ almonds																				
1 bar	350	10	35	59	2	10	12	2	7	14	2	5	6	*	*	3	15	*	9	2
Baby Ruth																				
2 oz	280	8	18	35	*	13	8	6	4	2	2	2	8	*	*	*	4	10	*	*
Bar None																				
1 bar	224	6	22	—	2	7	4	2	5	6	3	4	8	*	*	2	7	3	3	3
Bit-o-Honey																				
1 bar	186	2	6	—	*	13	—	5	2	3	*	*	3	*	*	*	7	*	*	*
Bounty																				
dark																				
1 bar	280	*	25	—	—	11	—	2	—	*	4	—	—	*	*	*	*	*	—	—
milk																				
1 bar	280	*	22	—	—	11	—	2	—	4	*	—	—	*	*	*	*	*	—	—
Buncha Crunch																				
1 1/2 oz	200	—	15	25	2	9	—	4	—	—	—	—	—	—	—	—	—	—	—	—
Butterfinger																				
2 oz	280	6	17	30	*	14	4	5	4	*	2	2	8	*	*	*	*	10	*	*

CANDY BAR (continued)

	Calories	Protein	Fat	Sat. Fat	Cholesterol	Carbohydrates	Fiber	Sodium	Potassium	Calcium	Iron	Zinc	Magnesium	Vitamin A	Vitamin C	Thiamin	Riboflavin	Niacin	Vitamin B$_{12}$	Folic acid
Caramello 1 bar	220	5	18	—	4	10	—	2	4	9	3	3	5	3	*	*	11	3	5	*
chocolate, sweet (generic) 1 bar	207	3	22	41	*	8	8	*	3	*	6	4	12	*	*	*	6	*	*	*
Chunky 1 bar	198	6	18	47	*	8	8	*	6	6	3	5	7	*	*	2	9	4	2	2
dark chocolate (Hershey Special Dark) 1 bar	195	3	19	—	*	8	8	*	4	*	5	4	12	*	*	*	6	*	*	*
golden almond chocolate 1 bar	466	15	49	—	3	14	—	2	11	28	7	10	24	2	*	3	26	5	6	5
Golden III chocolate bar 1 bar	471	10	46	—	6	17	—	3	12	27	3	7	15	2	*	4	15	*	7	3
Kit Kat 1 pkg (2.8 oz)	405	9	35	67	5	16	—	3	7	14	4	5	9	—	2	3	12	—	8	*
Krackel 1 bar	236	5	20	28	3	10	—	3	5	8	2	4	6	*	*	2	8	*	5	*
Kudos 1 bar	200	4	18	—	—	6	—	3	—	2	2	—	—	*	*	2	2	6	—	—
Mars almond 1 bar	234	7	18	—	*	10	4	4	5	8	3	4	9	2	*	*	9	2	3	2
plain 1 bar	240	6	17	—	—	10	4	—	8	2	—	—	—	*	*	*	8	2	—	—
milk chocolate plain (generic) 1 bar	226	5	21	41	3	9	8	*	5	8	3	4	7	2	*	2	8	*	3	*
(Hershey) 1 bar	540	6	47	91	8	19	—	3	11	20	6	9	16	*	—	5	22	*	—	—
(Nestlé) 1 1/2 oz	220	4	20	35	3	8	8	*	5	6	2	—	—	*	*	2	10	*	*	*
(Symphony) 1 bar	209	5	20	—	4	8	—	*	4	9	2	3	6	*	*	2	9	*	3	*
w/ almonds (generic) 1 bar	216	6	22	35	3	7	12	*	5	9	4	4	9	*	*	2	10	2	4	*
(Hershey) 1 bar	559	8	54	80	9	16	—	5	13	26	9	11	23	2	—	*	17	2	—	—
(Nestlé) 1 1/2 oz	200	6	22	—	*	6	*	*	5	8	2	—	—	*	*	2	10	2	—	—
w/ crisped rice (generic) 1 bar	223	5	18	36	3	9	4	3	4	8	2	3	6	*	*	2	8	*	3	*
(Nestlé Crunch) 1 1/2 oz	230	4	18	35	2	9	4	2	3	6	*	—	—	*	*	2	8	*	*	*
Milky Way dark 1 bar	220	2	12	—	—	12	—	5	—	2	2	—	—	*	*	*	2	*	—	—
regular 1 bar	251	4	14	24	4	14	4	6	4	8	3	3	5	2	*	*	8	*	5	*
Mounds 1 package	195	3	18	31	*	10	8	3	3	*	11	4	9	*	*	*	2	*	*	*
Mr. Goodbar 1 bar	257	10	25	45	3	9	8	*	6	6	3	6	12	*	*	2	8	12	4	9
Munch 1 bar	220	8	22	—	—	6	—	5	—	2	2	—	—	*	*	2	2	10	—	—
Oh! Henry 1 bar	246	10	15	19	2	12	8	6	5	6	2	5	9	*	*	*	5	8	3	5
PB Max 1 bar	240	8	23	—	—	7	—	6	—	2	2	—	—	*	*	4	2	10	—	—
peanut (generic) 1 bar	235	12	23	10	*	7	4	4	5	4	2	4	8	5	*	3	4	18	*	7
Peppermint Patty (York) 1 patty	411	2	3	—	*	26	—	2	—	2	8	5	16	*	—	*	2	6	4	*
Skor 1 bar	211	3	21	—	8	7	—	4	3	4	*	2	3	2	*	*	8	*	2	*

PERCENTAGE DAILY VALUE

	Calories	Protein	Fat	Sat. Fat	Cholesterol	Carbohydrates	Fiber	Sodium	Potassium	Calcium	Iron	Zinc	Magnesium	Vitamin A	Vitamin C	Thiamin	Riboflavin	Niacin	Vitamin B₁₂	Folic acid
CANDY BAR (continued)																				
Snickers																				
1 bar	278	10	21	37	2	12	8	7	6	7	3	5	9	*	*	2	7	9	4	6
w/ peanut butter																				
1 bar	280	8	28	—	—	8	—	6	—	4	2	—	—	*	*	4	2	10	—	—
Twix																				
caramel																				
1 package	272	5	21	—	2	12	4	5	3	7	2	3	4	*	*	2	6	*	4	*
original																				
1 bar	280	4	22	—	—	13	—	5	—	4	*	—	—	*	*	*	4	*	—	—
peanut butter																				
1 package	253	9	22	—	2	9	8	6	5	6	6	5	10	*	*	4	5	9	2	3
Whatchamacallit																				
1 bar	257	8	20	—	4	10	8	5	5	6	3	4	7	*	*	21	8	5	3	*
CANOLA OIL																				
(generic) 1 tbsp	124	*	20	5	*	*	*	*	*	*	*	*	*	*	*	*	*	*	*	*
(Wesson) 1 tbsp	120	*	22	5	*	*	*	*	*	*	*	*	—	*	*	*	*	*	*	*
w/ added vitamin E																				
(Hollywood) 1 tbsp	120	*	22	5	*	*	*	*	*	*	*	*	*	*	*	*	*	*	*	*
CANOLA & CORN OIL BLEND																				
(Crisco) 1 tbsp	120	*	22	8	*	*	*	*	*	*	*	*	*	*	*	*	*	*	*	*
CANTALOUPE																				
1/2 fruit	93	4	*	*	*	7	8	*	24	3	3	3	7	172	188	6	3	8	*	11
1/2 cup cubed	28	*	*	*	*	2	4	*	7	*	*	*	2	52	56	2	*	2	*	3
CAPERS																				
bottled																				
(Progresso) 1 tbsp	10	*	*	*	*	*	*	6	*	*	*	*	—	—	*	*	*	*	*	—
CAPON *see* **CHICKEN**																				
CARAMBOLA																				
1 fruit	42	*	*	*	*	3	12	*	6	*	2	*	3	13	45	2	2	3	—	—
1/2 cup cubes	23	*	*	*	*	2	8	*	3	*	2	*	2	7	24	*	*	*	—	—
CARAMEL *see* **CANDY**																				
CARAWAY SEED																				
1 tbsp	22	2	2	*	*	*	12	*	3	5	6	2	4	*	2	2	*	*	*	—
CARDAMOM, GROUND																				
1 tbsp	18	*	*	*	*	*	—	*	2	2	4	3	3	*	—	*	*	*	*	—
CARAMEL ROLL																				
w/ nuts																				
from refrigerated dough																				
(Pillsbury) 1 piece (1 1/4 oz)	160	3	12	10	*	6	—	10	*	*	4	—	—	*	*	4	4	4	—	—
CARAMEL SAUCE																				
(Knorr) 2 tbsp	120	*	*	*	*	10	—	—	*	*	*	*	*	*	*	*	*	*	*	*
CARAMEL TOPPING																				
(Kraft) 2 tbsp	120	*	*	*	*	8	*	4	3	8	*	—	—	*	*	*	4	*	*	*
hot																				
(Smucker's Special Recipe) 2 tbsp	150	2	6	—	*	9	*	3	*	*	*	*	*	*	*	*	*	*	—	*
regular																				
(Smucker's) 2 tbsp	140	2	2	—	*	11	*	5	*	2	*	*	*	*	*	*	2	*	*	*
CARDOON																				
raw																				
3 oz	17	*	*	*	*	*	4	6	10	6	3	*	9	2	3	*	*	*	*	6
boiled																				
3 oz	19	*	*	*	*	*	—	6	9	6	3	*	9	2	2	*	2	*	*	5
boiled w/ salt																				
3 oz	19	*	*	*	*	*	—	15	9	6	3	*	9	2	2	*	2	*	*	5
CARIBOU																				
roasted																				
4 oz	189	56	8	10	41	*	*	3	10	2	39	40	8	*	6	19	60	33	125	*

	Calories	Protein	Fat	Sat. Fat	Cholesterol	Carbohydrates	Fiber	Sodium	Potassium	Calcium	Iron	Zinc	Magnesium	Vitamin A	Vitamin C	Thiamin	Riboflavin	Niacin	Vitamin B12	Folic acid
CARISSA																				
1 fruit	12	*	*	*	*	*	—	*	*	*	*	—	*	*	13	*	*	*	*	—
1/2 cup slices	47	*	2	—	*	3	—	*	6	*	5	—	3	*	47	2	3	*	*	*
CAROB																				
1 bar	464	19	44	37	*	14	24	5	22	40	7	8	10	*	3	*	32	5	14	7
CAROB FLOUR																				
1 cup	394	8	*	*	*	30	164	*	24	36	17	6	14	*	*	4	28	10	*	8
CAROB MILK																				
1 cup milk + 3 tsp powder	195	14	13	*	11	7	*	6	11	29	4	6	8	6	4	6	23	*	14	3
CARP																				
raw																				
1 fillet	277	65	19	12	48	*	*	4	21	9	15	21	16	*	6	17	7	18	55	*
baked/broiled																				
1 fillet	275	65	19	12	48	*	*	4	21	9	15	22	16	*	5	16	7	18	42	*
CARROT																				
raw																				
1/2 cup shredded	24	*	*	*	*	2	8	*	5	*	*	*	2	309	9	4	2	3	*	2
1 medium	31	*	*	*	*	2	8	*	7	2	*	*	3	405	11	5	2	3	*	3
baby																				
1 large	6	*	*	*	*	*	—	*	*	*	*	*	*	6	2	*	*	*	*	*
boiled																				
1/2 cup slices	35	*	*	*	*	3	12	2	5	2	*	2	3	383	3	2	3	2	*	3
1 medium	21	*	*	*	*	2	8	*	3	*	2	*	*	226	2	*	2	*	*	2
boiled w/ salt																				
1/2 cup slices	35	*	*	*	*	3	—	10	5	2	*	2	3	383	3	2	3	2	*	3
CARROT, CANNED																				
cut																				
(Del Monte) 1/2 cup	35	*	*	*	*	3	12	13	—	2	2	—	—	300	6	—	—	—	—	—
low salt																				
drained																				
(generic) 1/2 cup slices	17	*	*	*	*	*	—	*	4	2	3	*	*	201	3	*	*	2	*	2
solid & liquid																				
(generic) 1/2 cup slices	28	*	*	*	*	2	16	2	6	3	4	2	3	324	6	2	2	3	*	3
sliced																				
(Bush Bros) 1/2 cup	30	2	*	*	*	2	8	10	—	2	6	—	—	200	*	—	—	—	—	—
(Del Monte) 1/2 cup	35	*	*	*	*	3	12	13	—	2	2	—	—	300	6	—	—	—	—	—
drained																				
(generic) 1/2 cup slices	17	*	*	*	*	*	4	7	4	2	3	*	*	201	3	*	*	2	*	2
solid & liquid																				
(generic) 1/2 cup slices	28	*	*	*	*	2	4	12	6	3	4	2	3	324	6	2	2	3	*	3
CARROT, FROZEN																				
baby, whole																				
(Bird's Eye Deluxe) 1/2 cup	40	2	*	*	*	3	—	2	—	2	4	2	2	300	10	2	2	4	*	2
(Green Giant Harvest Fresh) 1/2 cup	18	2	*	*	*	2	8	3	3	2	*	—	—	190	2	*	*	*	—	—
(Green Giant Select) 1/2 cup	20	2	*	*	*	2	8	*	4	2	*	—	—	250	2	*	*	2	—	—
boiled																				
(generic) 1/2 cup slices	26	*	*	*	*	2	12	2	3	2	2	*	2	258	3	*	2	2	*	2
boiled w/ salt																				
(generic) 1/2 cup slices	26	*	*	*	*	2	—	9	3	2	2	*	2	258	3	*	2	2	*	2
CARROT JUICE																				
canned																				
6 fl oz	74	3	*	*	*	6	4	2	15	4	5	2	6	948	26	11	6	4	*	2
CASABA MELON																				
1 cup cubed	44	3	*	*	*	3	4	*	10	*	4	—	3	*	45	7	2	3	*	—
1/10 fruit	43	2	*	*	*	3	4	*	10	*	4	—	3	*	44	7	2	3	*	—
CASHEW																				
(Frito-Lay) 1 1/2 oz	270	15	34	20	*	3	4	11	—	—	—	—	—	—	—	—	—	—	—	—
dry roasted																				
(generic) 1 oz	163	7	20	—	*	3	4	*	5	*	9	11	18	*	*	4	3	—	—	—

	Calories	Protein	Fat	Sat. Fat	Cholesterol	Carbohydrates	Fiber	Sodium	Potassium	Calcium	Iron	Zinc	Magnesium	Vitamin A	Vitamin C	Thiamin	Riboflavin	Niacin	Vitamin B₁₂	Folic acid
CASHEW (continued)																				
(Planter's) 1 oz	170	8	22	14	*	3	5	5	4	*	10	10	15	*	*	—	—	—	—	—
w/ salt (generic) 1 oz	163	7	20	13	*	3	4	8	5	*	9	11	18	*	*	4	3	2	*	5
halves (Fisher) 1 oz	170	8	23	13	*	3	2	7	—	*	10	—	—	*	*	—	—	—	—	—
jumbo (Fisher) 1 oz	170	8	23	13	*	3	2	4	—	*	10	—	—	*	*	—	—	—	—	—
oil roasted w/ salt (generic) 1 oz	164	8	21	14	*	3	4	7	4	*	6	9	18	*	*	8	3	3	*	5
CASHEW BUTTER																				
salted 1 oz	167	8	22	14	*	3	4	7	4	*	8	10	18	*	*	6	3	2	*	5
CASSAVA																				
raw 3 oz	102	4	*	*	*	8	4	*	18	8	17	*	14	*	68	13	5	6	*	5
CATFISH, CHANNEL																				
breaded & fried 1 fillet	199	26	18	15	23	2	—	10	8	4	7	5	6	*	*	4	7	10	27	*
CATFISH, FARMED																				
raw 1 fillet	215	41	19	14	25	*	*	3	14	*	4	8	9	2	2	38	7	18	65	*
broiled/baked 1 fillet	217	45	18	13	30	*	*	5	13	*	7	10	9	*	2	40	6	18	66	*
CATFISH, WILD																				
raw 1 fillet	151	43	7	6	31	*	*	3	16	2	3	5	9	2	2	22	7	15	59	*
broiled/baked 1 fillet	150	44	6	6	34	*	*	3	17	2	3	6	10	*	2	22	6	17	69	*
CATFISH, FROZEN																				
(Gorton's Select) 1 fillet	190	35	17	10	20	*	—	37	—	*	2	—	—	*	*	15	6	10	—	—
CATSUP see **KETCHUP**																				
CAULIFLOWER																				
raw 1/2 cup	13	2	*	*	*	*	4	*	4	*	*	*	2	*	39	2	2	*	*	7
3 florets	14	2	*	*	*	*	4	*	5	*	*	*	2	*	43	2	2	*	*	8
boiled 1/2 cup	14	2	*	*	*	*	8	*	3	*	*	*	*	*	46	2	2	*	*	7
3 florets	12	2	*	*	*	*	4	*	2	*	*	*	*	*	40	2	2	*	*	6
boiled w/ salt 1/2 cup	14	2	*	*	*	*	8	6	3	*	*	*	*	*	46	2	2	*	*	7
CAULIFLOWER, BOTTLED																				
hot & spicy (Vlasic) 1 oz	35	*	*	*	*	3	*	19	—	*	*	2	—	*	*	*	*	*	*	*
sweet (Vlasic) 1 oz	35	*	*	*	*	3	*	11	—	*	*	*	—	*	*	*	*	*	*	*
CAULIFLOWER, FROZEN																				
boiled (generic) 1/2 cup	17	2	*	*	*	*	8	*	4	2	2	*	2	*	47	2	3	*	*	9
(Green Giant) 1/2 cup	12	2	*	*	*	*	8	*	3	—	—	*	—	*	40	*	2	2	*	—
boiled w/ salt (generic) 1/2 cup	17	2	*	*	*	—	10	4	2	2	*	2	*	47	2	3	*	*	9	
in cheese flavored sauce (Bird's Eye Deluxe) 1/2 cup	60	7	5	5	2	2	—	16	—	*	8	—		6	30	50	2	6	*	—
(Green Giant) 1/2 cup	60	3	3	3	*	3	8	21	6	6	2	—	—	6	50	2	8	2	*	—
(Green Giant One Serving) 5 1/2 oz	80	5	3	3	2	5	8	27	8	8	2	—	—	30	50	2	6	4	*	—

	Calories	Protein	Fat	Sat. Fat	Cholesterol	Carbohydrates	Fiber	Sodium	Potassium	Calcium	Iron	Zinc	Magnesium	Vitamin A	Vitamin C	Thiamin	Riboflavin	Niacin	Vitamin B12	Folic acid
CAULIFLOWER, GREEN																				
raw 1/2 cup	16	2	*	*	*	*	8	*	4	2	2	2	3	2	73	3	3	2	*	7
cooked 1/2 cup	20	3	*	*	*	*	8	*	5	2	2	3	3	2	75	3	4	2	*	6
cooked, w/ salt 1/2 cup	20	3	*	*	*	*	8	7	5	2	2	3	3	2	75	3	4	2	*	6
CAVIAR																				
black raw 1 oz	71	11	8	6	55	*	*	17	*	8	18	2	21	10	*	4	10	*	93	*
red raw 1 oz	71	11	8	6	55	*	*	17	*	8	18	2	21	10	*	4	10	*	93	*
CELERIAC																				
raw 1/2 cup	30	2	*	*	*	2	4	3	7	3	3	2	4	*	10	3	3	3	*	2
boiled 3 oz	21	*	*	*	*	2	—	2	4	2	2	*	3	*	5	2	2	2	*	*
boiled w/ salt 3 oz	21	*	*	*	*	2	—	10	4	2	2	*	3	*	5	2	2	2	*	*
CELERY																				
raw 1/2 cup diced	10	*	*	*	*	*	4	2	5	2	*	*	2	2	7	2	2	*	*	4
1 stalk	6	*	*	*	*	*	4	*	3	2	*	*	*	*	5	*	*	*	*	3
boiled 1/2 cup diced	14	*	*	*	*	*	4	3	6	3	2	*	2	2	8	2	2	*	*	4
boiled w/ salt 1/2 cup diced	14	*	*	*	*	*	—	10	6	3	2	*	2	2	8	2	2	*	*	4
CELERY SEED 1 tbsp	25	2	2	—	*	*	4	*	3	11	16	3	7	*	2	*	*	*	*	*
CELTUCE																				
raw 3 oz	19	*	*	*	*	*	—	*	8	3	3	2	6	60	28	3	3	2	*	10
CEREAL BAR *see* **GRANOLA BAR**																				
CEREAL, COLD																				
100% bran (generic) 1 cup	178	14	5	3	*	16	80	19	23	5	45	38	78	*	104	105	105	105	104	12
100% natural plain (Quaker) 1 cup	489	20	34	75	*	22	36	2	15	18	17	16	31	*	*	21	33	12	2	8
w/ raisins & dates (Quaker) 1 cup	496	19	31	69	*	24	28	2	15	16	14	14	31	*	*	21	38	10	2	11
40% bran (generic) 1 cup	127	8	*	*	*	10	20	13	7	2	137	34	18	34	*	34	34	34	34	35
(Post) 1 cup	152	9	*	*	*	12	36	18	7	2	41	17	25	41	*	41	41	41	41	42
(Ralston) 1 cup	159	9	*	*	*	13	28	19	8	2	43	14	29	43	43	42	43	43	43	43
All-bran (Kellogg's) 1 1/4 oz	88	8	*	*	*	9	52	17	12	3	31	31	33	31	31	31	31	31	*	31
Almond Flavor O's (Health Valley) 1/2 cup	100	4	*	*	*	7	12	*	2	2	6	—	—	10	*	10	2	6	—	—
Alpha-bits marshmallow 1 oz	110	2	2	*	*	8	4	6	*	*	15	10	4	25	*	25	25	25	25	25
original 1 oz	110	4	2	*	*	8	4	7	2	*	15	10	6	25	*	25	25	25	25	25
Apple Cinnamon O's (Health Valley) 1/2 cup	100	4	*	*	*	7	12	*	2	2	6	—	—	10	*	10	2	6	—	—
Bran Buds 1 cup	217	19	3	—	*	21	124	21	40	6	74	74	67	74	74	73	74	74	*	74

	Calories	Protein	Fat	Sat. Fat	Cholesterol	Carbohydrates	Fiber	Sodium	Potassium	Calcium	Iron	Zinc	Magnesium	Vitamin A	Vitamin C	Thiamin	Riboflavin	Niacin	Vitamin B12	Folic acid
CEREAL, COLD (continued)																				
Bran Flakes																				
(Post) 1 oz	90	4	*	*	*	8	20	9	5	*	45	10	15	25	*	25	25	25	25	25
C.W. Post																				
plain																				
1 cup	432	15	23	57	*	23	28	7	6	5	86	11	17	86	*	84	86	85	85	86
w/ raisins																				
1 cup	446	15	23	55	*	25	56	7	7	5	91	11	19	91	*	89	91	91	91	91
Cap'n Crunch																				
regular																				
1 cup	156	3	5	11	*	10	4	12	*	*	55	27	4	*	*	44	42	43	39	60
w/ crunchberries																				
1 cup	146	3	4	10	*	9	4	10	*	*	50	24	3	*	*	40	40	41	42	32
w/ peanut butter																				
1 cup	154	4	7	10	*	9	*	11	2	*	51	25	5	*	*	40	41	45	38	61
Cheerios																				
honey nut																				
1 cup	125	6	*	*	*	9	4	12	3	2	29	6	10	29	29	29	29	29	29	5
plain																				
1 oz	111	7	3	*	*	7	8	13	3	5	25	5	10	25	25	25	25	25	25	2
Chex																				
corn																				
1 oz (1 cup)	110	2	*	*	*	8	2	12	*	*	45	—	—	*	25	25	2	25	25	25
double																				
1 oz (2/3 cup)	110	2	*	*	*	8	*	11	*	*	45	—	—	*	25	25	*	25	25	25
graham																				
1 oz (2/3 cup)	110	2	2	—	*	8	4	9	*	*	30	20	4	*	25	25	*	25	25	25
juniors																				
1 oz (3/4 cup)	110	2	*	*	*	8	—	8	*	*	25	—	—	*	25	25	*	25	25	25
multi-bran																				
1 oz (2/3 cup)	100	4	2	—	*	8	16	8	4	*	45	25	10	*	25	25	4	25	25	25
rice																				
1 oz (1 1/8 cup)	110	2	*	*	*	8	2	10	*	*	45	2	—	*	25	25	*	25	25	25
whole grain wheat																				
1 oz (2/3 cup)	100	4	2	—	*	8	12	10	3	*	45	4	8	*	25	25	4	25	25	25
Cocoa Krispies																				
1 cup	139	3	*	*	*	11	*	11	2	*	13	13	3	32	32	31	32	32	*	32
Cookie Crisp																				
chocolate chip																				
1 oz (1 cup)	110	2	2	—	*	8	—	6	*	*	25	15	—	*	*	25	15	25	25	25
corn bran																				
1 cup	125	4	2	—	*	10	28	13	2	4	68	27	5	2	*	25	41	54	23	58
corn flakes																				
(Kellogg's) 1 oz	110	4	*	*	*	8	4	12	*	*	10	*	*	25	25	25	25	25	*	25
(Ralston) 1 cup	98	3	*	*	*	7	*	10	*	*	3	*	*	2	*	8	*	5	*	*
honey nut																				
(Kellogg's) 1 oz	113	3	2	—	*	8	*	9	*	*	10	*	*	25	25	25	25	25	*	25
low sodium																				
(generic) 1 cup	100	2	*	*	*	7	*	*	*	*	3	*	*	2	*	*	*	3	*	*
Cracklin' Bran																				
1 cup	229	9	14	—	*	14	40	20	10	4	21	21	29	53	53	52	53	53	*	53
Crispy Mini-Grahams																				
1 oz (2/3 cup)	110	2	2	—	*	8	4	9	*	*	30	20	4	*	25	25	*	25	25	25
Crispy Rice																				
(generic) 1 cup	111	3	*	*	*	8	*	9	*	*	4	3	3	*	2	7	2	10	*	*
low sodium																				
(generic) 1 cup	105	2	*	*	*	8	—	*	*	2	4	3	3	*	*	*	3	2	*	*
Crispy Wheats 'n Raisins																				
1 cup	150	5	*	*	*	12	12	8	5	7	38	3	9	38	*	37	38	38	38	4

	Calories	Protein	Fat	Sat. Fat	Cholesterol	Carbohydrates	Fiber	Sodium	Potassium	Calcium	Iron	Zinc	Magnesium	Vitamin A	Vitamin C	Thiamin	Riboflavin	Niacin	Vitamin B₁₂	Folic acid
CEREAL, COLD (continued)																				
Fiber Flakes																				
plain (Health Valley) 1/2 cup	90	6	*	*	*	7	20	*	*	*	6	—	—	10	*	2	2	8	—	—
w/ raisins (Health Valley) 1/2 cup	90	6	*	*	*	7	20	*	*	*	6	—	—	10	*	2	2	8	—	—
Froot Loops 1 oz	111	3	*	*	*	8	4	6	*	*	25	25	2	25	25	25	25	25	*	25
Frosted Mini-Wheats 1 oz	102	5	*	*	*	8	8	*	3	*	10	10	6	25	25	25	25	25	*	25
Frosted Rice Krinkles 1 oz	109	2	*	*	*	9	*	7	*	*	10	10	2	25	*	25	25	25	25	25
Fruit & Fibre																				
dates, raisins & walnuts 1 1/4 oz	120	4	3	—	*	9	20	7	6	*	35	10	10	30	*	30	30	30	30	30
peaches, raisins & almonds 1 1/4 oz	120	4	3	—	*	9	20	7	6	*	30	10	15	30	*	30	30	30	30	30
pineapple, bananas & coconut 1 1/4 oz	120	4	5	—	*	9	20	7	6	*	30	10	15	30	*	30	30	30	30	30
Fruit Lites																				
brown rice (Health Valley) 1/2 cup	50	2	*	*	*	4	2	*	*	*	*	—	—	*	*	2	*	2	—	—
golden corn (Health Valley) 1/2 cup	50	2	*	*	*	4	3	*	*	*	2	—	—	*	*	4	*	*	—	—
wheat (Health Valley) 1/2 cup	50	4	*	*	*	4	4	*	*	*	4	—	—	*	*	4	*	2	—	—
Golden Crisp (Post) 1 oz	100	2	*	*	*	9	2	2	*	*	10	10	4	25	*	25	25	25	25	25
Golden Grahams 1 cup	150	4	2	5	*	11	4	16	2	2	34	2	4	34	34	34	34	34	34	2
Graham Crackos 1 cup	108	4	*	*	*	9	8	8	3	*	10	11	6	26	26	26	26	26	*	27
granola (homemade) 1 cup	594	25	51	29	*	22	52	*	17	8	27	30	35	*	—	49	18	11	*	25
(Nature Valley) 1 cup	503	19	30	65	*	25	24	10	11	7	21	15	29	*	—	26	11	4	*	21
cinnamon raisin (Health Valley) 1 oz dry	90	4	*	*	*	7	12	*	2	*	2	—	—	*	*	4	*	2	—	—
date & almond (Health Valley) 1 oz dry	90	4	*	*	*	7	12	*	2	*	2	—	—	*	*	4	*	2	—	—
tropical fruit (Health Valley) 1 oz dry	90	4	*	*	*	7	12	*	3	*	2	—	—	*	*	4	*	2	—	—
Grape-Nuts																				
original 1 oz	110	4	*	*	*	8	12	7	3	*	45	8	6	25	*	25	25	25	25	25
raisin 1 oz	100	4	*	*	*	8	8	6	3	*	10	8	6	25	*	25	25	25	25	25
Grape-Nuts Flakes 1 oz	100	5	2	*	*	8	12	5	2	*	45	8	8	25	*	25	25	25	25	25
Great Grains																				
double pecan 1 oz	120	5	5	—	*	7	12	2	3	*	15	8	10	25	*	25	25	25	25	25
raisins, dates & pecans 1 1/4 oz	140	5	5	—	*	9	12	3	4	*	20	8	10	30	*	30	30	30	30	30
Heartland Natural																				
plain 1 cup	499	19	27	—	*	26	28	12	11	7	24	20	37	*	—	24	9	8	*	16
w/ coconut 1 cup	463	18	26	—	*	24	28	9	11	7	30	18	34	*	—	23	9	9	*	14
w/ raisin 1 cup	468	18	24	—	*	25	24	9	12	7	22	19	35	*	—	21	8	8	*	11

	Calories	Protein	Fat	Sat. Fat	Cholesterol	Carbohydrates	Fiber	Sodium	Potassium	Calcium	Iron	Zinc	Magnesium	Vitamin A	Vitamin C	Thiamin	Riboflavin	Niacin	Vitamin B₁₂	Folic acid
CEREAL, COLD (continued)																				
High Fiber O's (Health Valley) 1 oz dry	90	4	*	*	*	6	20	*	3	2	6	6	—	10	*	10	2	6	—	—
Honey Almond Delight 1 oz (3/4 cup)	110	2	3	—	*	8	4	8	—	*	10	10	—	*	25	25	*	25	25	25
Honey Bran 1 cup	119	5	*	*	*	10	16	8	4	2	31	6	11	31	31	30	31	31	31	6
Honey Bunches of Oats honey roasted 1 oz	110	3	3	—	*	8	8	7	2	*	15	2	4	25	*	25	25	25	25	25
w/ almonds 1 oz	110	3	3	—	*	8	8	6	*	*	15	2	4	25	*	25	25	25	25	25
Honeycomb 1 oz	110	2	*	*	*	8	2	7	*	*	15	10	2	25	*	25	25	25	25	25
King Vitaman 1 cup	85	2	2	4	*	6	*	7	*	*	71	*	2	48	55	62	62	65	68	72
Kix 1 oz	110	4	*	*	*	8	4	12	*	*	45	2	3	25	25	25	25	25	25	25
Life cinnamon 1 cup	162	13	*	*	*	10	12	10	6	15	65	10	4	*	—	—	59	58	*	9
plain 1 cup	162	13	*	*	*	10	12	10	6	15	65	10	4	*	—	—	59	58	*	9
Lucky Charms 1 cup	125	5	2	*	*	9	4	9	2	4	28	4	7	28	28	28	28	28	28	2
Most 1 cup	175	12	*	*	*	13	28	11	10	8	183	18	26	183	184	184	183	183	183	184
muesli banana-walnut (Ralston) 1 1/2 oz (1/2 cup)	150	6	5	—	*	10	12	6	4	*	20	10	10	25	*	25	25	25	25	25
cranberry-walnut (Ralston) 1 1/2 oz (1/2 cup)	150	6	5	—	*	10	12	6	4	*	20	10	8	25	*	25	25	25	25	25
date-almond (Ralston) 1 1/2 oz (1/2 cup)	140	6	3	—	*	11	12	4	6	*	20	10	8	25	*	25	25	25	25	25
peach-pecan (Ralston) 1 1/2 oz (1/2 cup)	150	6	5	—	*	10	12	6	5	*	20	10	8	25	*	25	25	25	25	25
raspberry-almond (Ralston) 1 1/2 oz (1/2 cup)	150	6	5	—	*	10	12	6	5	*	20	10	8	25	*	25	25	25	25	25
Nutri-Grain barley 1 cup	153	7	*	*	*	11	8	12	3	*	8	36	8	36	36	35	36	36	36	36
corn 1 cup	160	6	2	—	*	12	12	11	3	*	5	37	7	37	37	36	37	37	37	37
rye 1 cup	144	6	*	*	*	11	12	11	2	*	6	35	8	35	35	35	35	35	35	35
wheat 1 cup	158	6	*	*	*	12	12	12	3	*	7	39	9	39	39	38	39	39	39	39
Oat Flakes (Post) 1 oz	110	6	2	*	*	7	8	5	4	*	45	10	10	25	*	25	25	25	25	25
fortified (generic) 1 cup	177	15	*	*	*	12	4	18	10	7	76	10	14	42	*	42	42	42	42	42
Pebbles cocoa 1 oz	110	*	2	*	*	8	2	6	*	*	10	10	2	25	*	25	25	25	25	25
dino 1 oz	110	*	2	*	*	8	2	6	*	*	10	10	*	25	*	25	25	25	25	25
fruity 1 oz	110	*	2	*	*	8	2	6	*	*	10	10	*	25	*	25	25	25	25	25
Post Toasties 1 oz	110	2	*	*	*	8	2	12	*	*	2	*	*	25	*	25	25	25	25	25

CEREAL, COLD (continued)

	Calories	Protein	Fat	Sat. Fat	Cholesterol	Carbohydrates	Fiber	Sodium	Potassium	Calcium	Iron	Zinc	Magnesium	Vitamin A	Vitamin C	Thiamin	Riboflavin	Niacin	Vitamin B$_{12}$	Folic acid
Product 19 1 cup	126	5	*	*	*	9	4	16	*	*	116	3	3	116	117	116	116	116	116	117
Quisp 1 cup	124	2	3	8	*	8	4	10	*	*	35	*	3	*	*	36	45	29	43	2
raisin bran (Kellogg's) 1 1/3 oz	115	7	*	*	*	9	16	8	5	*	93	25	12	25	*	25	26	25	25	25
(Post) 1 3/8 oz	120	4	2	*	*	10	24	8	7	*	35	15	15	35	*	35	35	35	35	35
(Ralston) 1 cup	178	7	*	*	*	15	32	20	8	3	152	11	21	37	3	37	36	37	37	37
Raisins, Rice & Rye 1 cup	155	4	*	*	*	13	12	15	4	*	31	31	5	31	*	31	32	31	31	31
Rice Krispies 1 oz	112	3	*	*	*	8	*	14	*	*	10	3	3	25	25	25	25	25	*	25
frosted 1 oz	109	2	*	*	*	9	*	10	*	*	10	2	*	25	25	25	25	25	*	25
rice, puffed fortified (generic) 1 cup	56	*	*	*	*	4	—	*	*	*	25	*	*	*	*	24	15	25	*	*
unfortified (generic) 1 cup	56	*	*	*	*	4	*	*	*	*	*	*	*	*	*	*	*	2	*	*
Special K 1 oz	111	9	*	*	*	7	4	11	*	*	25	25	4	25	25	25	25	25	*	25
Sprouts 7 w/ bananas & hawaiian fruit (Health Valley) 1 oz dry	90	4	*	*	*	5	17	*	5	*	6	—		*		6	8	10	10	—
w/ raisins (Health Valley) 1 oz dry	90	4	*	*	*	5	19	*	4	*	8	—		2	*	4	4	8	—	—
Sugar Corn Pops 1 oz	108	2	*	*	*	9	*	4	*	*	10	10	*	25	25	25	25	25	*	25
sugar frosted flakes (generic) 1 oz	109	2	*	*	*	9	*	7	2	*	2	*	*	25	*	25	25	25	25	25
(Kellogg's) 1 cup	133	3	*	*	*	11	4	12	*	*	12	*	*	31	31	30	31	31	*	31
(Ralston) 1 cup	149	3	*	*	*	11	4	10	*	*	5	5	*	34	34	33	34	33	33	*
Sugar Smacks 1 oz	106	3	*	*	*	8	*	3	*	*	10	2	3	25	25	25	25	25	*	25
Sunflakes 1 oz (1 cup)	100	2	2	—	*	8	*	10	—	*	10	—	—	25	25	25	*	25	25	25
Super Sugar Krisp 1 cup	123	4	*	*	*	10	*	*	4	*	12	12	5	29	*	29	29	29	29	29
Tasteeos 1 cup	94	5	*	*	*	6	12	8	2	*	21	5	7	21	21	21	21	21	21	2
Team 1 cup	164	4	*	*	*	12	4	11	2	*	14	4	5	37	37	36	37	37	37	2
Teenage Mutant Ninja Turtles 1 oz (1 cup)	110	2	*	*	*	9	—	8	—	*	10	—	—	*	25	25	4	25	25	25
Total 1 cup	116	5	*	*	*	9	16	14	4	28	116	5	9	116	117	116	116	116	116	117
Trix 1 cup	108	3	*	*	*	8	*	7	*	*	25	*	2	25	25	24	25	25	25	*
Waffleos 1 cup	122	3	2	—	*	9	—	5	*	*	26	2	2	26	26	26	26	26	26	*
wheat, puffed fortified (generic) 1 cup	44	3	*	*	*	3	—	*	*	*	21	2	4	*	*	21	13	21	*	*
unfortified (generic) 1 cup	44	3	*	*	*	3	4	*	*	*	3	2	4	*	*	2	2	6	*	*
wheat, shredded (generic) 1 oz	102	5	*	*	*	8	12	*	3	*	7	7	9	*	*	5	5	7	*	4
(generic) 1 large biscuit	83	4	*	*	*	6	8	*	2	*	4	4	10	*	*	4	4	5	*	3
Wheaties 1 cup	101	5	*	*	*	8	12	11	3	4	26	4	8	26	26	25	26	26	26	26

	Calories	Protein	Fat	Sat. Fat	Cholesterol	Carbohydrates	Fiber	Sodium	Potassium	Calcium	Iron	Zinc	Magnesium	Vitamin A	Vitamin C	Thiamin	Riboflavin	Niacin	Vitamin B$_{12}$	Folic acid
CEREAL, HOT																				
cream of rice																				
(generic) 1 cup	127	4	*	*	*	9	*	*	*	*	3	3	2	*	*	*	*	5	*	2
salted																				
(generic) 1 cup	127	4	*	*	*	9	—	18	*	*	3	3	2	*	*	*	*	5	*	2
cream of wheat																				
(generic) 1 cup	133	6	*	*	*	9	8	*	*	5	57	2	3	*	*	17	*	8	*	3
salted																				
1 cup	133	6	*	*	*	9	—	14	*	5	57	2	3	*	*	17	*	8	*	3
cream of wheat, instant																				
salted																				
1 cup	154	7	*	*	*	11	—	15	*	6	67	3	4	*	*	16	*	8	*	2
cream of wheat, quick																				
1 cup	129	6	*	*	*	9	4	6	*	5	57	2	3	*	*	16	*	7	*	2
salted																				
1 cup	129	6	*	*	*	9	—	19	*	5	57	2	3	*	*	16	*	7	*	2
farina																				
(H-O) 3 tbsp uncooked	120	4	*	*	*	9	12	*	3	*	4	—	—	*	*	10	4	6	—	—
(Pillsbury) 1 cup	80	7	*	*	*	6	—	11	*	*	2	—	—	*	*	6	2	2	—	—
enriched																				
(generic) 1 cup	117	5	*	*	*	8	12	*	*	*	6	*	*	*	—	12	7	6	*	*
enriched, salted																				
(generic) 1 cup	117	5	*	*	*	8	12	32	*	*	6	*	*	*	*	12	7	6	*	*
unenriched																				
(generic) 1 cup	117	5	*	*	*	8	12	*	*	*	*	*	*	*	*	2	*	*	*	*
unenriched, salted																				
(generic) 1 cup	117	5	*	*	*	8	12	32	*	*	*	*	*	*	*	2	*	*	*	*
granola																				
(H-O) 1/2 cup, uncooked	200	10	5	*	*	14	20	2	—	2	—	—	—	*	*	—	—	3	—	—
grits																				
all types																				
(generic) 1 cup	145	6	*	*	*	10	*	*	2	*	9	*	2	*	—	16	9	10	*	*
white, enriched salted																				
(generic) 1 cup	145	6	*	*	*	10	*	22	2	*	9	*	2	*	—	16	9	10	*	*
white, unenriched																				
(generic) 1 cup	145	6	*	*	*	10	*	22	2	*	3	*	2	*	*	3	*	2	*	*
salted																				
(generic) 1 cup	145	6	*	*	*	10	*	*	2	*	3	*	2	*	—	3	*	2	*	*
yellow, enriched																				
(generic) 1 cup	145	6	*	*	*	10	*	*	2	*	9	*	2	3	*	16	9	10	*	*
salted																				
(generic) 1 cup	145	6	*	*	*	10	*	22	2	*	9	*	2	3	*	16	9	10	*	*
yellow, unenriched																				
(generic) 1 cup	145	6	*	*	*	10	*	*	2	*	3	*	2	3	*	3	*	2	*	*
salted																				
(generic) 1 cup	145	6	*	*	*	10	*	22	2	*	3	*	2	3	*	3	*	2	*	*
grits, instant																				
plain																				
(generic) 1 packet	82	3	*	*	*	6	*	14	*	*	6	*	*	*	*	12	5	7	*	*
w/ bacon																				
(generic) 1 packet	104	5	*	*	*	7	*	22	2	*	7	*	2	*	*	13	7	8	*	2
w/ cheese																				
(generic) 1 packet	107	4	2	—	*	7	*	20	*	*	6	*	2	*	*	11	8	7	*	*
w/ ham																				
(generic) 1 packet	103	5	*	*	*	7	*	27	*	*	8	*	2	*	*	17	9	9	*	2
grits, quick																				
(Alber's) 3 tbsp	140	5	*	*	*	10	4	*	—	*	6	*	*	*	*	—	—	—	—	—
high fiber																				
(Ralston) 1 oz (1/3 cup uncooked)	90	4	2	—	*	7	16	*	3	*	4	4	10	*	*	8	2	10	—	—

CEREAL, HOT (continued)

	Calories	Protein	Fat	Sat. Fat	Cholesterol	Carbohydrates	Fiber	Sodium	Potassium	Calcium	Iron	Zinc	Magnesium	Vitamin A	Vitamin C	Thiamin	Riboflavin	Niacin	Vitamin B₁₂	Folic acid
														PERCENTAGE DAILY VALUE →						
Malt cereal																				
(Malt-o-Meal) 1 cup	122	6	*	*	*	9	4	*	*	*	53	*	*	*	*	32	14	29	*	*
(Maltex) 1 cup	179	10	2	—	*	13	—	8	8	2	10	12	14	*	*	17	6	12	*	6
maple (maypo) 1 cup	170	10	4	—	*	11	24	*	6	12	47	10	13	47	48	48	42	47	48	2
salted (maypo) 1 cup	170	10	4	—	*	11	—	11	6	12	47	10	13	47	48	48	42	47	48	2
maple brown sugar (H-O) 1 packet, uncooked	160	6	3	*	*	11	12	12	3	2	6	—	—	*	*	10	4	*	—	—
multigrain (Mothers) 1/2 cup	130	8	2	*	*	9	20	*	5	*	6	—	—	*	*	6	2	6	—	—
oat bran (Mothers) 1/2 cup	150	13	5	5	*	6	24	*	7	2	15	—	—	*	*	25	6	*	—	—
(Quaker) 1/2 cup	150	13	5	5	*	6	24	*	7	2	15	—	—	*	*	25	6	*	—	—
oatmeal (generic) 1 cup	145	10	4	2	*	8	16	16	4	*	10	8	14	*	*	17	3	2	*	2
old fashioned (Quaker) 1/2 cup	150	8	5	3	*	8	16	*	4	*	10	—	—	*	*	10	2	*	—	—
quick (H-O) 1/3 cup, uncooked	100	6	3	*	*	6	12	*	3	*	6	—	—	*	*	10	*	*	—	—
(Quaker) 1/2 cup	150	8	5	3	*	8	16	*	4	*	10	—	—	*	*	10	2	*	—	—
rolled oats (generic) 1 cup	145	10	4	2	*	8	16	*	4	2	9	8	14	*	—	17	3	2	*	2
oatmeal, instant (H-O) 1/3 cup, uncooked	100	6	3	*	*	6	12	*	3	*	6	—	—	*	*	10	*	*	—	—
(Mothers) 1/2 cup	150	8	5	3	*	7	16	*	4	*	10	—	—	*	*	10	2	*	—	—
apple & cinnamon (Quaker) 1 packet prep	35	7	2	3	*	4	12	4	3		30	—	—	15	*	20	10	15	—	—
apple, raisin & walnut (Quaker) 1 packet prep	37	5	4	3	*	4	12	7	4	15	30	—	—	20	*	20	10	15	—	—
blueberry & cream (Quaker) 1 packet prep	35	5	4	3	*	5	8	6	3	10	30	—	—	20	*	20	10	15	—	—
cinnamon graham cookie (Quaker) 1 packet prep	40	7	4	3	*	5	12	7	3	15	30	—	—	25	*	20	10	15	—	—
cinnamon spice (Quaker) 1 packet prep	46	7	3	*	*	6	12	12	3	15	50	—	—	20	*	25	15	20	—	—
cinnamon toast (Quaker) 1 packet prep	35	5	3	*	*	5	8	7	3	15	35	—	—	20	*	20	10	15	—	—
date & walnut (Quaker) 1 packet prep	37	5	4	3	*	4	12	10	4	15	30	—	—	20	*	20	10	15	—	—
fortified (generic) 1 packet prep	104	7	3	—	*	6	12	12	3	16	35	6	11	30	*	35	17	27	*	38
honey nut (Quaker) 1 packet prep	35	5	5	3	*	5	8	9	3	10	25	—	—	20	*	15	10	15	—	—
low sodium (Quaker) 1 packet prep	34	8	4	3	*	6	12	4	4	25	80	—	—	30	*	30	15	20	—	—
maple & brown sugar (Quaker) 1 packet prep	43	7	3	3	*	6	12	10	3	15	50	—	—	20	*	25	10	20	—	—
peaches & cream (Quaker) 1 packet prep	35	5	3	3	*	4	8	6	4	10	30	—	—	20	*	20	10	15	—	—
raisin-spice (Quaker) 1 packet prep	160	8	3	3	*	5	12	10	5	15	30	—	—	20	*	20	10	15	—	—
raspberry (Quaker) 1 packet prep	40	7	5	3	*	5	12	7	3	15	30	—	—	25	*	20	10	15	—	—
strawberries & cream (Quaker) 1 packet prep	130	5	3	3	*	4	8	7	4	15	30	—	—	15	*	20	10	15	—	—

	Calories	Protein	Fat	Sat. Fat	Cholesterol	Carbohydrates	Fiber	Sodium	Potassium	Calcium	Iron	Zinc	Magnesium	Vitamin A	Vitamin C	Thiamin	Riboflavin	Niacin	Vitamin B₁₂	Folic acid

PERCENTAGE DAILY VALUE

	Calories	Protein	Fat	Sat. Fat	Cholesterol	Carbohydrates	Fiber	Sodium	Potassium	Calcium	Iron	Zinc	Magnesium	Vitamin A	Vitamin C	Thiamin	Riboflavin	Niacin	Vitamin B12	Folic acid
CEREAL, HOT (continued)																				
strawberries & stuff (Quaker) 1 packet prep	150	5	3	3	*	5	12	7	3	15	30	—	—	25	*	20	10	15	—	—
oats 'n fiber																				
apple & bran (H-O) 1 packet	130	6	3	*	*	9	12	6	3	2	6	—	—	*	*	8	2	*	—	—
plain (H-O) 1 packet	110	8	3	*	*	6	12	6	3	2	6	—	—	*	*	10	4	*	—	—
raisin & bran (H-O) 1 packet	150	6	3	*	*	11	12	6	3	2	8	—	—	*	*	8	4	*	—	—
old fashioned (H-O) 1/3 cup	100	6	3	*	*	6	12	*	3	*	6	—	—	*	*	10	*	*	—	—
raisin & spice (H-O) 1 packet	150	—	3	*	*	11	12	10	4	2	8	—	—	*	*	8	4	*	—	—
(Ralston) 1 cup	134	9	*	*	*	9	24	*	4	*	9	9	15	*	*	13	10	10	2	4
salted (Ralston) 1 cup	134	9	*	*	*	9	—	20	4	*	9	9	15	*	*	13	10	10	2	4
Roman meal 1 cup	147	11	2	—	*	11	—	*	9	3	12	12	27	*	*	16	7	15	*	6
salted 1 cup	147	11	2	—	*	11	—	8	9	3	12	12	27	*	*	16	7	15	*	6
w/ oats 1 cup	170	12	3	—	*	11	—	*	7	3	8	13	19	*	—	21	13	16	*	6
salted 1 cup	170	12	3	—	*	11	—	22	7	3	8	13	19	*	—	21	13	16	*	6
Super Bran (H-O) 1/3 cup	110	10	3	*	*	6	32	*	3	*	6	—	—	*	*	8	2	*	—	—
Sweet 'n Mellow (H-O) 1 packet	150	6	3	*	*	10	12	11	3	2	6	—	—	*	*	10	4	*	—	—
Wheatena 1 cup	136	8	2	—	*	10	28	*	5	*	8	11	12	*	*	2	3	7	*	4
salted 1 cup	136	8	2	—	*	10	—	24	5	*	8	11	12	*	*	2	3	7	*	4
whole wheat (generic) 1 cup	150	8	2	—	*	11	16	*	5	2	8	8	13	*	*	11	7	11	*	7
(Mothers) 1/2 cup	130	8	2	x	x	9	16	*	5	*	6	—	—	*	*	8	2	8	—	—
whole wheat natural salted (generic) 1 cup	150	8	2	—	*	11	—	23	5	2	8	8	13	*	*	11	7	11	*	7
CHARD, SWISS																				
raw																				
1/2 cup chopped	3	*	*	*	*	*	*	2	2	*	2	*	4	12	9	*	*	*	*	*
1 leaf	10	2	*	*	*	*	4	5	6	3	5	*	11	36	27	*	3	*	*	2
boiled																				
1/2 cup chopped	18	3	*	*	*	*	8	7	14	5	11	2	19	55	26	2	4	2	*	2
boiled w/ salt																				
1/2 cup chopped	18	3	*	*	*	*	—	15	14	5	11	2	19	55	26	2	4	2	*	2
CHARDONNAY SAUCE																				
from mix (Knorr) 1 1/2 oz	190	60	11	—	23	2	—	31	—	2	6	—	—	*	*	4	6	50	*	*
CHASSEUR SAUCE																				
from mix (Knorr) 3 3/4 oz	270	60	9	—	23	4	—	36	—	2	6	—	—	*	*	4	6	50	*	*
CHAYOTE																				
raw																				
1/2 cup	16	*	*	*	*	*	8	*	3	*	*	2	2	*	12	*	2	2	*	5
1 medium fruit	49	3	*	*	*	4	24	*	9	4	5	5	7	2	37	4	5	5	*	14
boiled																				
1/2 cup	19	*	*	*	*	*	—	*	4	*	*	2	2	*	11	*	2	2	*	4

	Calories	Protein	Fat	Sat. Fat	Cholesterol	Carbohydrates	Fiber	Sodium	Potassium	Calcium	Iron	Zinc	Magnesium	Vitamin A	Vitamin C	Thiamin	Riboflavin	Niacin	Vitamin B₁₂	Folic acid
CHAYOTE, FROZEN																				
boiled w/ salt 1/2 cup	19	*	*	*	*	*	—	8	4	*		2	2	*	11	*	2	2	*	4
CHEESE																				
American (generic) 1 oz	94	9	10	22	6	*	*	11	3	14	*	6	2	4	*	*	*	*	6	*
blue (Kraft) 1 oz	100	15	14	40	10	*	*	14	*	15	*	—	—	6	*	*	8	*	—	—
brick (generic) 1 oz	105	11	13	27	9	*	*	7	*	19	*	5	2	6	*	*	*	*	6	2
(Kraft) 1 oz	110	15	14	40	10	*	*	7	*	20	*	—	—	6	*	*	6	*	—	—
brie (generic) 1 oz	95	10	12	25	9	*	*	7	*	5	*	4	*	4	*	*	3	*	8	5
camembert (generic) 1 oz	85	9	10	22	7	*	*	10	2	11	*	4	*	5	*	*	*	*	6	4
caraway (generic) 1 oz	107	12	13	27	9	*	*	8	*	19	*	6	2	6	*	*	*	*	*	*
cheddar (generic) 1 oz	114	12	14	30	10	*	*	7	*	20	*	6	2	6	*	*	*	*	4	*
(Kraft) 1 oz	110	15	14	40	10	*	*	7	*	20	*	—	—	6	*	*	6	*	—	—
low salt 1 oz	113	12	14	30	9	*	*	*	*	20	*	6	2	6	*	*	6	*	4	*
lowfat 1 oz	49	12	3	6	2	*	*	7	*	12	*	3	*	*	*	*	4	*	2	*
mild (Weight Watchers) 1 oz	80	13	8	13	5	*	*	7	*	25	*	—	—	4	*	—	—	—	—	—
low sodium (Weight Watchers) 1 oz	80	13	8	13	5	*	*	3	*	25	*	—	—	4	*	—	—	—	—	—
reduced fat (Kraft Light Naturals) 1 oz	80	20	8	15	7	*	*	9	*	25	*	—	—	6	*	*	8	*	—	—
sharp (Weight Watchers) 1 oz	80	13	8	15	5	*	*	3	*	25	*	—	—	4	*	—	—	—	—	—
reduced fat (Kraft Light Naturals) 1 oz	80	20	8	15	7	*	*	9	*	25	*	—	—	6	*	*	8	*	—	—
sharp white reduced fat (Cracker Barrel Light) 1 oz	80	20	8	15	7	*	*	9	*	25	*	—	—	6	*	*	8	*	—	—
shredded reduced fat (Sargento) 1/4 cup	70	13	7	11	5	*	0	7	—	20	*	—	—	8	*	—	—	—	—	—
white, sharp (Weight Watchers) 1 oz	80	13	8	13	5	*	*	7	*	25	*	—	—	4	*	—	—	—	—	—
cheddar ball w/ almonds (Cracker Barrel) 1 oz	100	10	11	15	7	*	*	10	3	15	*	—	—	4	*	*	10	*	—	—
w/ almonds, smokey (Cracker Barrel) 1 oz	90	10	9	30	5	*	*	10	4	15	*	—	—	2	*	*	10	*	—	—
smokey (Cracker Barrel) 1 oz	90	10	9	30	5	*	*	10	5	15	*	—	—	2	*	*	10	*	—	—
cheddar log port wine, w/ almonds (Cracker Barrel) 1 oz	90	10	9	15	5	*	*	11	4	15	*	—	—	2	*	*	10	*	—	—
cheshire (generic) 1 oz	110	11	13	28	10	*	*	8	*	18	*	5	*	6	*	*	*	*	4	*
colby (generic) 1 oz	112	11	14	29	9	*	*	7	*	19	*	6	2	6	*	*	*	*	4	*
(Kraft) 1 oz	110	15	14	40	10	*	*	7	*	20	*	—	—	6	*	*	6	*	—	—
(Weight Watchers) 1 oz	80	13	8	13	5	*	*	7	*	25	*	—	—	4	*	—	—	—	—	—
low salt 1 oz	113	12	14	30	9	*	*	*	*	20	*	6	2	6	*	*	6	*	4	*
low fat 1 oz	49	12	3	6	2	*	*	7	*	12	*	3	*	*	*	*	4	*	2	*

CHEESE (continued)

	Calories	Protein	Fat	Sat. Fat	Cholesterol	Carbohydrates	Fiber	Sodium	Potassium	Calcium	Iron	Zinc	Magnesium	Vitamin A	Vitamin C	Thiamin	Riboflavin	Niacin	Vitamin B$_{12}$	Folic acid
reduced fat (Kraft Light Naturals) 1 oz	80	20	8	15	7	*	*	9	*	25	*	—	—	6	*	*	8	*	—	—
colby / monterey jack blend **reduced fat** (Kraft Light Naturals) 1 oz	80	20	8	15	7	*	*	9	*	25	*	—	—	6	*	*	8	*	—	—
cottage **1% fat** (generic) 4 oz	82	23	2	4	2	*	*	19	3	7	*	3	2	*	*	2	*	*	12	3
(Light 'n Lively) 1/2 cup	80	27	2	5	5	*	*	16	—	10	*	—	—	*	*	—	—	—	—	—
(Weight Watchers) 1/2 cup	90	23	2	3	2	*	*	19	2	6	*	—	—	*	*	—	—	—	—	—
w/salad (Light 'n Lively) 1/2 cup	90	26	2	5	5	2	*	17	—	10	*	—	—	4	*	—	—	—	—	—
2% fat (Friendship) 1/2 cup	90	77	2	3	3	*	*	*	—	10	*	—	—	2	*	—	—	—	—	—
(generic) 4 oz	101	26	3	7	3	*	*	19	3	8	*	3	2	2	*	2	*	*	13	4
(Sealtest) 1/2 cup	100	26	4	8	5	*	*	16	—	8	*	—	—	*	*	—	—	—	—	—
(Weight Watchers) 1/2 cup	90	20	3	8	5	*	*	2	2	8	*	—	—	2	*	—	—	—	—	—
large curd (Breakstone) 1/2 cup	90	27	4	8	5	*	*	16	—	8	*	—	—	*	*	—	—	—	—	—
4% fat large curd (Breakstone) 1/2 cup	120	28	8	18	8	*	*	17	—	10	*	—	—	4	*	—	—	—	—	—
creamed (generic) 4 oz	117	24	8	16	6	*	*	19	3	7	*	3	*	4	*	2	*	*	12	3
dry curd (generic) 4 oz	96	33	*	*	3	*	*	*	*	4	*	4	*	*	*	2	*	*	15	4
w/ fruit (generic) 4 oz	140	19	6	12	4	5	*	19	2	5	*	2	*	3	*	*	*	*	9	3
cream (generic) 1 oz	99	4	15	31	10	*	*	3	*	2	2	*	*	8	*	*	*	*	2	*
(Weight Watchers) 1 oz	35	5	3	5	3	*	*	2	*	2	*	—	—	*	*	—	—	—	—	—
regular (Philadelphia) 1 oz	100	4	15	30	10	*	*	4	*	2	*	—	—	6	*	*	2	*	—	—
w/ chives (Philadelphia) 1 oz	90	4	14	25	10	*	*	6	*	2	*	—	—	8	*	*	2	*	—	—
w/ pimento (Philadelphia) 1 oz	90	4	14	25	10	*	*	5	*	2	*	—	—	8	*	*	2	*	—	—
soft **regular** (Philadelphia) 1 oz	100	2	15	25	10	*	*	4	2	4	*	—	—	6	*	*	4	*	—	—
w/ chives & onions (Philadelphia) 1 oz	100	6	14	25	10	*	*	4	*	2	*	—	—	8	*	*	2	*	—	—
w/ herb & garlic (Philadelphia) 1 oz	100	2	14	25	8	*	*	7	2	4	*	—	—	6	*	*	4	*	—	—
w/ olives & pimento (Philadelphia) 1 oz	90	2	12	25	8	*	*	7	*	2	*	—	—	8	*	*	2	*	—	—
w/ pineapple (Philadelphia) 1 oz	90	2	12	25	8	*	*	4	*	2	*	—	—	6	*	*	2	*	—	—
w/ smoked salmon (Philadelphia) 1 oz	90	4	14	25	8	*	*	7	*	2	*	—	—	6	*	*	2	*	—	—
w/ strawberries (Philadelphia) 1 oz	90	2	12	25	7	*	*	3	2	2	*	—	—	4	*	*	2	*	—	—
whipped **plain** (Philadelphia) 1 oz	100	4	15	30	10	*	*	4	*	2	*	—	—	8	*	*	2	*	—	—
w/ chives (Philadelphia) 1 oz	90	4	12	25	10	*	*	6	*	2	*	—	—	8	*	*	2	*	—	—
w/ onions (Philadelphia) 1 oz	90	4	12	25	8	*	*	7	*	2	*	—	—	6	*	*	2	*	—	—

	Calories	Protein	Fat	Sat. Fat	Cholesterol	Carbohydrates	Fiber	Sodium	Potassium	Calcium	Iron	Zinc	Magnesium	Vitamin A	Vitamin C	Thiamin	Riboflavin	Niacin	Vitamin B₁₂	Folic acid
CHEESE (continued)																				
w/ smoked salmon (Philadelphia) 1 oz	90	4	12	25	10	*	*	7	*	2	*	—	—	8	*	*	2	*	—	—
edam (generic) 1 oz	101	12	12	25	8	*	*	11	2	21	*	7	2	5	*	*	*	*	7	*
(Kraft) 1 oz	90	15	11	20	7	*	*	13	*	25	*	—	—	4	*	*	6	*	—	—
feta (generic) 1 oz	75	7	9	21	8	*	*	13	*	14	*	5	*	3	*	3	*	*	8	2
fontina (generic) 1 oz	110	12	13	27	11	*	*	9	*	16	*	7	*	7	*	*	17	*	8	*
gjetost (generic) 1 oz	132	5	13	27	9	4	*	7	11	11	*	2	5	6	*	6	*	*	11	*
goat																				
high moisture (generic) 1 oz	76	9	9	21	4	*	*	4	*	4	3	2	*	3	*	*	57	*	*	*
low moisture (generic) 1 oz	128	14	15	35	10	*	*	4	*	25	3	3	4	3	*	3	17	3	*	*
medium moisture (generic) 1 oz	103	10	13	30	7	*	*	6	*	8	3	*	2	3	*	*	2	*	*	*
gouda (generic) 1 oz	101	12	12	25	11	*	*	10	*	20	*	7	2	4	*	*	*	*	7	2
(Kraft) 1 oz	110	15	14	40	10	*	*	8	*	20	*	—	—	6	*	*	4	*	—	—
gruyere (generic) 1 oz	117	14	14	27	10	*	*	4	*	29	*	7	3	7	*	*	*	*	8	*
havarti (Casino) 1 oz	120	15	17	35	12	*	*	6	*	20	*	—	—	6	*	*	6	*	—	—
jarlsberg (Sargento) 1 slice	120	15	14	25	7	*	*	2	—	30	*	—	—	8	*	—	—	—	—	—
limburger (generic) 1 oz	93	9	12	24	8	*	*	9	*	14	*	4	*	7	*	2	2	*	5	4
(Mohawk Valley) 1 oz	90	15	12	40	8	*	*	10	*	15	*	—	—	6	*	*	6	*	—	—
monterey jack (generic) 1 oz	106	12	13	27	8	*	*	6	*	21	*	6	2	5	*	*	33	*	4	*
(Kraft) 1 oz	110	15	14	40	10	*	*	8	*	20	*	—	—	6	*	*	6	*	—	—
(Weight Watchers) 1 oz	80	13	8	13	5	*	*	7	*	25	*	—	—	4	*	—	—	—	—	—
reduced fat (Kraft Light Naturals) 1 oz	80	20	8	15	7	*	*	9	*	25	*	—	—	6	*	*	6	*	—	—
w/ caraway seeds (Kraft) 1 oz	100	15	12	40	10	*	*	7	*	15	*	—	—	6	*	*	6	*	—	—
w/ jalapeños (Kraft) 1 oz	110	15	14	40	10	*	*	8	*	20	*	—	—	8	*	*	6	*	—	—
w/ peppers reduced fat (Kraft Light Naturals) 1 oz	80	20	8	15	7	*	*	9	*	25	*	—	—	8	*	*	6	*	—	—
mozzarella (Kraft) 1 oz	90	15	11	20	7	*	*	8	*	15	*	—	—	4	*	*	4	*	—	—
part skim (Kraft) 1 oz	80	15	8	15	5	*	*	8	*	20	*	—	—	2	*	*	4	*	—	—
part skim, low moisture (generic) 1 oz	79	13	7	16	5	*	*	6	*	21	*	6	2	4	*	*	*	*	4	*
reduced fat (Kraft Light Naturals) 1 oz	80	20	6	15	5	*	*	8	*	25	*	—	—	2	*	*	6	*	—	—
skim milk (generic) 1 oz	72	11	7	15	5	*	*	5	*	18	*	5	2	3	*	*	*	*	4	*
whole milk (generic) 1 oz	80	9	9	19	7	*	*	4	*	15	*	4	*	4	*	*	*	*	3	*
whole milk, low moisture (generic) 1 oz	90	10	11	22	8	*	*	5	*	16	*	5	*	5	*	*	*	*	3	*
reduced fat (Sargento) 1 slice	90	—	8	15	5	*	*	10	—	35	*	—	—	10	*	—	—	—	—	—

CHEESE (continued)

	Calories	Protein	Fat	Sat. Fat	Cholesterol	Carbohydrates	Fiber	Sodium	Potassium	Calcium	Iron	Zinc	Magnesium	Vitamin A	Vitamin C	Thiamin	Riboflavin	Niacin	Vitamin B₁₂	Folic acid
shredded reduced fat (Sargento) 1/4 cup	60	—	5	11	3	*	*	6	—	25	*	—	—	6	*	—	—	—	—	—
muenster (Dorman's) 1 slice	160	17	20	39	14	*	*	12	—	30	*	—	—	10	*	—	—	—	—	—
(generic) 1 oz	104	11	13	27	9	*	*	7	*	20	*	5	2	6	*	*	*	*	7	*
low sodium (Dorman's) 1 slice	160	17	20	41	13	*	*	8	—	25	*	—	—	6	*	—	—	—	—	—
for nachos (Snyder) 2 tbsp	48	2	5	5	*	2	*	11	—	3	*	—	—	*	*	—	—	—	—	—
neufchatel (generic) 1 oz	74	5	10	21	7	*	*	5	*	2	*	*	*	6	*	*	*	*	*	*
parmesan (Kraft) 1 oz	100	20	11	20	7	*	*	12	*	30	*	—	—	4	*	*	*	6	*	—
grated (generic) 1 tbsp	23	3	2	5	*	*	*	4	*	7	*	*	*	*	*	*	*	*	*	*
(Kraft) 1 oz	130	25	14	25	10	*	*	18	*	40	*	—	—	4	*	*	*	6	*	—
(Progresso) 1 tbsp	23	3	3	5	*	*	*	4	*	6	*	—	—	*	*	*	*	*	—	—
hard (generic) 1 oz	111	17	11	24	6	*	*	19	*	34	*	5	3	3	*	*	*	*	6	*
shredded (generic) 1 tbsp	21	3	2	5	*	*	*	4	*	6	*	*	*	*	*	*	*	*	*	*
pizza cheese shredded reduced fat (Sargento) 1/4 cup	60	—	5	11	3	*	*	6	—	20	*	—	—	6	*	—	—	—	—	—
port du salut (generic) 1 oz	100	11	12	24	12	*	*	6	*	18	*	5	2	8	*	*	33	*	7	*
provolone (Dorman's) 1 slice	100	12	12	22	7	*	*	10	—	20	*	—	—	4	*	—	—	—	—	—
(generic) 1 oz	100	12	12	24	6	*	*	10	*	21	*	6	2	5	*	*	*	*	7	*
(Kraft) 1 oz	100	15	11	20	8	*	*	11	*	20	*	—	—	6	*	*	4	*	—	—
queso anejo (generic) 1 oz	106	10	13	27	10	*	*	13	*	19	*	6	2	*	*	*	3	*	6	*
queso asajerdo (generic) 1 oz	101	11	12	26	10	*	*	8	*	19	*	6	2	*	*	*	4	*	5	*
queso chihuahua (generic) 1 oz	106	10	13	27	10	*	*	7	*	18	*	7	2	*	*	*	4	*	5	*
ricotta part skim (generic) 1/2 cup	171	24	15	31	13	2	*	6	4	34	3	11	5	11	*	2	*	*	6	4
whole milk (generic) 1/2 cup	216	23	25	52	21	*	*	4	4	26	3	10	4	12	*	*	*	*	7	4
romano (generic) 1 oz	110	15	12	25	10	*	*	14	*	30	*	5	3	3	*	*	*	*	5	*
(Kraft) 1 oz	100	20	11	20	7	*	*	10	*	30	*	—	—	4	*	*	6	*	—	—
grated (Kraft) 1 oz	130	25	14	30	10	*	*	15	*	35	*	—	—	4	*	*	6	*	—	—
(Progresso) 1 tbsp	23	3	3	5	2	*	*	3	*	6	*	—	—	*	*	*	*	*	—	—
string (Sorrento) 1 oz	80	13	8	15	5	*	*	6	—	25	*	—	—	4	*	—	—	—	—	—
(Sorrento) 1 oz	80	13	8	15	5	*	*	6	—	25	*	—	—	4	*	—	—	—	—	—
w/ jalapeños (Kraft) 1 oz	80	15	8	15	7	*	*	10	*	20	*	—	—	4	*	*	4	*	—	—
Swiss (Casino) 1 oz	110	15	12	25	10	*	*	*	*	25	*	—	—	6	*	*	4	*	—	—
(generic) 1 oz	107	13	12	25	9	*	*	3	*	27	*	7	3	5	*	*	*	*	8	*
aged (Kraft) 1 oz	110	20	12	25	8	*	*	2	*	30	*	—	—	6	*	*	4	*	—	—

	Calories	Protein	Fat	Sat. Fat	Cholesterol	Carbohydrates	Fiber	Sodium	Potassium	Calcium	Iron	Zinc	Magnesium	Vitamin A	Vitamin C	Thiamin	Riboflavin	Niacin	Vitamin B₁₂	Folic acid
CHEESE (continued)																				
baby (Cracker Barrel) 1 oz	110	15	14	25	8	*	*	3	*	20	*	—	—	6	*	*	6	*	—	—
low sodium (Dorman's) 1 slice	130	17	14	28	11	*	*	3	—	35	*	—	—	6	*		—	—	—	—
(Kraft) 1 oz	110	20	12	25	8	*	*	*	*	25	*	—	—	6	*	*	6	*	—	—
reduced fat (Kraft Light Naturals) 1 oz	90	20	8	15	7	*	*	3	*	35	*	—	—	6	*	*	6	*	—	—
reduced fat (Sargento) 1 slice	80	—	7	11	5	*	*	3	—	35	*	—	—	6	*	*	—	—	—	—
regular (Kraft) 1 oz	110	20	12	25	8	*	*	2	*	30	*	—	—	6	*	*	4	*	—	—
taco cheese																				
shredded (Kraft) 1 oz	110	15	14	25	10	*	*	8	*	20	*	—	—	8	*	*	6	*	—	—
reduced fat (Sargento) 1/4 cup	80	—	7	11	5	*	*	3	*	20	*	—	—	10	*					
tilsit																				
whole milk (generic) 1 oz	96	12	11	24	10	*	*	9	*	20	*	7	*	6	*	*	*	*	10	*
CHEESE FOOD																				
American																				
(generic) 1 oz	93	9	11	22	6	*	*	19	2	16	*	6	2	5	*	*	*	*	5	*
(Nippy) 1 oz	90	10	11	20	7	*	*	16	2	20	*	—	—	4	*	*	6	*	—	—
grated (Kraft) 1 oz	130	20	11	20	8	3	*	31	7	25	*	—	—	6	*	*	20	*	—	—
imitation (Golden Image) 1 oz	90	15	9	10	2	*	*	15	2	20	*	—	—	10	*	*	6	*	—	—
pasteurized process (generic) 1 oz	92	10	43	22	8	*	*	18	2	21	*	7	2	5	*	*	*	*	11	*
no salt (generic) 1 oz	106	10	14	28	9	*	*	8	*	17	*	6	2	7	*	*	*	*	3	*
shredded (Velveeta) 1 oz	100	15	11	20	7	*	*	17	2	15	*	—	—	10	*	*	8	*	—	—
singles (Kraft) 1 oz	90	10	11	20	8	*	*	16	2	15	*	—	—	6	*	*	6	*	—	—
white (Kraft) 1 oz	90	10	11	20	7	*	*	17	2	15	*	—	—	4	*	*	8	*	—	—
cheddar																				
extra sharp (Cracker Barrel) 1 oz	90	10	11	20	7	*	*	10	3	15	*	—	—	6	*	*	8	*	—	—
port wine (Cracker Barrel) 1 oz	100	10	11	20	7	*	*	10	3	15	*	—	—	4	*	*	8	*	—	—
sharp (Cracker Barrel) 1 oz	100	10	11	20	7	*	*	10	3	15	*	—	—	4	*	*	8	*	—	—
Cheez & Bacon																				
singles (Kraft) 1 oz	90	10	11	20	8	*	*	17	2	15	*	—	—	6	*	*	8	*	—	—
jalapeño																				
singles (Kraft) 1 oz	90	10	11	20	8	*	*	19	2	15	*	—	—	10	*	*	8	*	—	—
Mexican																				
hot (Velveeta) 1 oz	100	15	11	20	8	*	*	18	2	20	*	—	—	10	*	*	8	*	—	—
mild (Velveeta) 1 oz	100	15	11	20	8	*	*	17	2	15	*	—	—	10	*	*	8	*	—	—
monterey jack																				
singles (Kraft) 1 oz	90	10	11	20	8	*	*	16	2	15	*	—	—	4	*	*	8	*	—	—
mozzarella																				
(generic) 1 oz	70	5	43	6	*	2	*	8	4	17	*	4	3	8	*	*	*	*	4	*

	Calories	Protein	Fat	Sat. Fat	Cholesterol	Carbohydrates	Fiber	Sodium	Potassium	Calcium	Iron	Zinc	Magnesium	Vitamin A	Vitamin C	Thiamin	Riboflavin	Niacin	Vitamin B12	Folic acid
CHEESE FOOD (continued)																				
pimento																				
singles																				
(Kraft) 1 oz	90	10	11	20	8	*	*	16	2	15	*	—	—	8	*	*	6	*	—	—
sharp																				
singles																				
(Kraft) 1 oz	100	15	12	25	8	*	*	17	*	15	*	—	—	10	*	*	6	*	—	—
Swiss																				
pasteurized process																				
(generic) 1 oz	82	8	9	19	5	*	*	16	2	16	*	5	2	4	*	*	*	*	2	*
no salt																				
(generic) 1 oz	95	12	11	23	8	*	*	8	2	22	*	7	2	5	*	*	*	*	6	*
singles																				
(Kraft) 1 oz	90	10	11	20	8	*	*	18	2	20	*	—	—	4	*	*	6	*	—	—
w/ bacon																				
(Cracker Barrel) 1 oz	90	10	11	20	7	*	*	12	2	15	*	—	—	4	*	*	8	*	—	—
w/ garlic																				
(Kraft) 1 oz	90	10	11	20	7	*	*	15	2	15	*	—	—	4	*	*	6	*	—	—
w/ jalapeños																				
(Kraft) 1 oz	90	10	11	20	7	*	*	16	2	15	*	—	—	4	*	*	6	*	—	—
CHEESE PRODUCT																				
American																				
(generic) 1 oz	106	10	14	28	9	*	*	17	*	17	*	6	2	7	*	*	*	*	3	*
(Harvest Moon) 1 oz	70	15	6	10	5	*	*	17	2	20	*	—	—	4	*	*	6	*	—	—
(Kraft Light) 1 oz	70	15	6	15	5	*	*	17	2	20	*	—	—	6	*	*	8	*	—	—
(Light 'N' Lively) 1 oz	70	15	6	15	5	*	*	17	2	20	*	—	—	6	*	*	8	*	—	—
(Light 'N' Lively) 1 oz	70	15	6	10	5	*	*	17	2	20	*	—	—	6	*	*	6	*	—	—
(Velveeta) 1 oz	70	10	6	10	5	*	*	20	3	15	*	—	—	4	*	*	6	*	—	—
fat free																				
(Smartbeat) 1 oz	30	10	*	*	*	*	*	7	—	15	*	—	—	4	*	*	4	*	—	—
loaf																				
(Kraft) 1 oz	110	15	14	25	8	*	*	18	*	15	*	—	—	6	*	*	6	*	—	—
low sodium																				
(Smartbeat) 1 oz	35	10	3	3	*	*	*	4	—	15	*	—	—	4	*	*	4	*	—	—
(Weight Watchers)																				
2 slices (3/4 oz)	50	8	3	5	2	*	*	5	8	15	*	—	—	4	*	—	—	—	—	—
sharp																				
loaf																				
(Old English) 1 oz	110	15	14	25	10	*	*	17	*	20	*	—	—	8	*	*	6	*	—	—
slices																				
(Old English) 1 oz	110	15	14	25	10	*	*	18	*	15	*	—	—	6	*	*	6	*	—	—
slices																				
(Kraft) 1 oz	110	15	14	25	8	*	*	19	*	15	*	—	—	6	*	*	6	*	—	—
white																				
(Kraft Light) 1 oz	70	15	6	10	5	*	*	17	2	20	*	—	—	6	*	*	6	*	—	—
low sodium																				
(Weight Watchers)																				
2 slices (3/4 oz)	50	8	3	5	2	*	*	5	8	15	*	—	—	4	*	—	—	—	—	—
cheddar																				
(Kraft Light) 1 oz	70	15	6	10	5	*	*	16	2	20	*	—	—	6	*	*	6	*	—	—
(Light 'N' Lively) 1 oz	70	15	6	10	5	*	*	16	2	20	*	—	—	6	*	*	6	*	—	—
fat free																				
(Weight Watchers)																				
2 slices (3/4 oz)	30	8	*	*	*	*	*	13	2	10	*	—	—	4	*	—	—	—	—	—
medium																				
(Spreadery) 1 oz	70	10	6	10	5	*	*	10	4	15	*	—	—	2	*	*	8	*	—	—
mellow																				
fat free																				
(Smartbeat) 1 oz	30	10	*	*	*	*	*	7	—	15	*	—	—	4	*	*	4	*	—	—

	Calories	Protein	Fat	Sat. Fat	Cholesterol	Carbohydrates	Fiber	Sodium	Potassium	Calcium	Iron	Zinc	Magnesium	Vitamin A	Vitamin C	Thiamin	Riboflavin	Niacin	Vitamin B12	Folic acid
CHEESE PRODUCT (continued)																				
mild																				
(Golden Image) 1 oz	110	15	14	10	2	*	*	8	*	20	*	—	—	4	*	*	6	*	—	—
sharp																				
(Spreadery) 1 oz	70	10	6	10	5	*	*	10	5	15	*	—	—	2	*	*	10	*	—	—
Vermont white																				
(Spreadery) 1 oz	70	10	6	10	5	*	*	10	4	15	*	—	—	2	*	*	10	*	—	—
colby																				
imitation																				
(Golden image) 1 oz	110	15	14	10	2	*	*	8	*	20	*	—	—	6	*	*	4	*	—	—
cream																				
light																				
(Philadelphia) 1 oz	60	6	8	15	3	*	*	7	2	4	*	—	—	6	*	*	4	*	—	—
mexican																				
w/ jalapeños																				
(Spreadery) 1 oz	70	10	6	15	5	*	*	11	4	15	*	—	—	2	*	*	8	*	—	—
nacho																				
(Spreadery) 1 oz	70	10	6	10	5	*	*	10	5	15	*	—	—	2	*	*	10	*	—	—
nonfat																				
(Kraft Free) 1 oz	56	15	*	*	2	*	*	17	2	20	*	—	—	10	*	*	8	*	—	—
parmesan																				
fat free grated																				
(Weight Watchers) 1 tbsp	15	3	*	*	2	*	*	2	*	4	*	—	—	*	*					
pimento																				
(generic) 1 oz	106	10	13	28	9	*	*	17	*	17	*	6	2	7	*	*	*	*	3	*
(Kraft) 1 oz	100	15	12	25	8	*	*	18	*	15	*	—	—	6	*	*	6	*	—	—
port wine																				
(Spreadery) 1 oz	70	10	6	10	5	*	*	10	4	15	*	—	—	2	*	*	8	*	—	—
sandwich slices																				
made w/ vegetable oil																				
(Lunch Wagon) 1 oz	90	10	11	10	2	*	*	15	2	20	*	—	—	10	*	*	8	*	—	—
sharp																				
fat free																				
(Smartbeat) 1 oz	30	10	*	*	*	*	*	10	—	15	*	—	—	4	*	*	4	*	—	—
Swiss																				
(generic) 1 oz	95	12	11	23	8	*	*	16	2	22	*	7	2	5	*	*	*	*	6	*
(Kraft Light) 1 oz	70	15	5	10	5	*	*	15	2	20	*	—	—	2	*	*	6	*	—	—
(Light 'N' Lively) 1 oz	70	15	5	10	5	*	*	15	2	20	*	—	—	2	*	*	6	*	—	—
fat free																				
(Smartbeat) 1 oz	30	10	*	*	*	*	*	7	—	15	*	—	—	4	*	*	4	*	—	—
(Weight Watchers) 2 slices (3/4 oz)	30	8	*	*	*	*	*	12	2	10	*	—	—	4	*	—	—	—	—	—
slices																				
(Kraft) 1 oz	90	15	11	20	8	*	*	17	*	20	*	—	—	6	*	*	4	*	—	—
white																				
fat free																				
(Weight Watchers) 2 slices (3/4 oz)	30	8	*	*	*	*	*	13	2	10	*	—	—	4	*	—	—	—	—	—
yellow																				
fat free																				
(Weight Watchers) 2 slices (3/4 oz)	30	8	*	*	*	*	*	13	2	10	*	—	—	4	*	—	—	—	—	—
CHEESE DIP																				
blue																				
premium																				
(Kraft) 2 tbsp	50	2	6	10	3	*	*	9	*	4	*	—	—	2	*	*	2	*	—	—
cheddar																				
jalapeño																				
(Frito-Lay) 2 tbsp	50	3	5	5	2	*	*	12	—	—	—	—	—	—	—	—	—	—	—	—
mild																				
(Frito-Lay) 2 tbsp	50	3	5	5	2	*	*	10	—	—	—	—	—	—	—	—	—	—	—	—

	Calories	Protein	Fat	Sat. Fat	Cholesterol	Carbohydrates	Fiber	Sodium	Potassium	Calcium	Iron	Zinc	Magnesium	Vitamin A	Vitamin C	Thiamin	Riboflavin	Niacin	Vitamin B₁₂	Folic acid
CHEESE DIP																				
conqueso (Tostitos) 2 tbsp.	40	2	31	3	*	2	2	27			—			—					—	—
fiesta (Chi-Chi's) 1 oz	41	2	5	5	3	*	—	12	2	4	*	2	*	2	4	*	4	*	—	—
jalapeño premium (Kraft) 2 tbsp	50	2	6	15	5	*	*	7	2	4	*	—	—	2	*	*	4	*	—	—
nacho (Kraft) 2 tbsp	55	2	6	10	3	*	*	8	2	4	*	—	—	2	2	*	4	*	—	—
CHEESE ENTREE																				
fondue (homemade) 1/2 cup	247	26	22	47	16	*	*	6	3	51	2	14	6	9	*	2	12	*	15	*
CHEESE ENTREE, FROM MIX																				
nacho (Hamburger Helper) 1 cup	360	35	23	—		12	—	44	10	8	15			2	*	20	20	25		
CHEESE ENTREE, FROZEN																				
broccoli & cheese puff pastry (Pepperidge Farm) 3 2/3 oz	230	8	25	—		6		16	—	6	8			8	20	10	10	8	—	—
grilled cheese sandwiches (Swanson Kids') 6 1/2 oz	300	25	18	—		16	—	16		25	8			*	10	4	8	8		
mozzarella cheese nuggets (Banquet Entree) 2.5 oz	230	23	18	—		5	—	21	2	35	*			*	*	4	6	*		
Welsh rarebit (Stouffer's Side Dishes) 10 oz	120	22	14	20	7	2	—	12	2	15	*			*	*	2	20	*		
CHEESE PUFFS & SNACKS																				
cheese & pretzels (Moo Town Snackers) 1 snack	90	—	5	10	3	12	0	13	—	6	4			4	*	—	—	—	—	—
cheese & sticks (Moo Town Snackers) 1 snack	100	—	6	13	3	4	0	11	—	6	4			4	*	—	—	—	—	—
Cheez ums (Pringle's) 1 oz	150	3	15	13	*	5	4	8	—	*	—			*	6	—	—	—	—	—
crunchy (Chee-tos) 1 oz	150	3	14	10	*	5	2	12	—	—	—			—	—	—	—	—	—	—
curls (Chee-tos) 1 oz	150	3	14	13	*	5	4	12	—	—	—			—	—	—	—	—	—	—
(Slim-Fast) 1 oz	110	10	5	—	*	7	12	3	*	10	2	4	*	10	10	10	10	10	10	10
(Weight Watchers) 1 bag (1/2 oz)	70	2	4	5	*	3	*	4	3	*	*			*	*	—	—	—	—	—
Flamin' hot (Chee-tos) 1 oz	160	3	14	10	*	5	2	10	—	—	—			—	—	—	—	—	—	—
green onion (Health Valley) 1 oz	100	6	*	*	*	7	—	9	3	*	2	—	—	2	*	2	*	*	—	—
original (Health Valley) 1 oz	100	6	*	*	*	7	9	9	3	*	2	—	—	2	*	2	*	*	—	—
Paws (Chee-tos) 1 oz	160	3	15	13	*	5	2	12	—	—	—			—	—	—	—	—	—	—
puffed balls (Chee-tos) 1 oz	160	3	15	13	*	4	2	15	—	—	—			—	—	—	—	—	—	—
puffs (Chee-tos) 1 oz	160	3	15	13	*	5	2	2	—	—	—			—	—	—	—	—	—	—
puffs, jumbo (Chee-tos) 1 oz	160	3	15	13	*	5	4	14	—	—	—			—	—	—	—	—	—	—
Wild Fangs (Chee-tos) 1 oz	160	3	15	8	*	5	2	10	—	—	—			—	—	—	—	—	—	—
zesty chili (Health Valley) 1 oz	100	6	*	*	*	7	—	3	*	*	2	—	—	2	*	2	*	*	—	—

	Calories	Protein	Fat	Sat. Fat	Cholesterol	Carbohydrates	Fiber	Sodium	Potassium	Calcium	Iron	Zinc	Magnesium	Vitamin A	Vitamin C	Thiamin	Riboflavin	Niacin	Vitamin B12	Folic acid
CHEESE SAUCE																				
from mix																				
prep. w/ milk																				
(generic) 1 cup	307	27	26	—	—	8	4	65	16	57	2	6	12	8	4	10	33	2	19	3
homemade																				
2 tbsp	59	5	7	12	4	*	*	6	*	9	*	3	*	4	*	*	4	*	2	*
CHEESE SPREAD																				
American																				
(Cheez Whiz) 1 oz	80	10	9	15	7	*	*	20	2	10	*	—	—	6	*	*	6	*	—	—
(generic) 1 oz	82	8	9	19	5	*	*	19	2	16	*	5	2	4	*	*	*	*	2	*
(Kraft) 1 oz	80	10	9	15	5	*	*	20	2	15	*	—	—	4	*	*	6	*	—	—
(Nabisco Easy Cheese) 1 oz	80	7	9	20	7	*	—	14	2	10	*	—	—	*	*	*	6	*	—	—
(Squeez-A-Snak) 1 oz	80	10	11	20	7	*	*	18	*	15	*	—	—	2	*	*	2	*	—	—
(Velveeta) 1 oz	80	10	9	20	7	*	*	18	3	15	*	—	—	6	*	*	8	*	—	—
w/ bacon																				
(Squeez-A-Snak) 1 oz	80	10	11	20	7	*	*	21	*	15	*	—	—	2	*	*	2	*	—	—
blue																				
(Roka) 2 tbsp	70	4	9	20	7	*	*	11	2	6	*	—	—	4	*	*	4	*	—	—
cheddar																				
medium																				
(Kraft) 2 tbsp	60	8	8	15	5	*	*	12	—	15	*	—	—	2	*	—	—	—	—	—
(Kraft) 2 tbsp	80	8	8	15	5	*	*	12	—	15	*	—	—	2	*	—	—	—	—	—
mild																				
(Nabisco Easy Cheese) 1 oz	80	7	9	20	7	*	—	15	2	10	*	—	—	*	*	*	6	*	—	—
port wine																				
(WisPride) 2 tbsp	100	7	11	15	7	*	*	9	—	*	*	—	—	5	*	15	*	*	—	—
sharp																				
(Nabisco Easy Cheese) 1 oz	80	7	9	20	7	*	—	15	2	10	*	—	—	*	*	*	6	*	—	—
(WisPride) 2 tbsp	100	13	11	20	7	*	*	10	—	15	*	—	—	6	*	—	—	—	—	—
cheese & bacon																				
(Nabisco Easy Cheese) 1 oz	80	7	9	20	7	*	—	14	2	10	*	—	—	*	*	*	6	*	—	—
garlic flavor																				
(Squeez-A-Snak) 1 oz	80	10	11	20	7	*	*	18	*	15	*	—	—	2	*	*	2	*	—	—
hickory smoke flavor																				
(Squeez-A-Snak) 1 oz	80	10	11	20	7	*	*	18	*	15	*	—	—	2	*	*	2	*	—	—
jalapeño																				
(Kraft) 2 tbsp	70	2	8	15	5	*	*	4	*	4	*	—	—	4	*	*	4	*	—	—
(Squeez-A-Snak) 1 oz	80	10	9	20	7	*	*	17	*	15	*	—	—	2	*	*	2	*	—	—
loaf																				
(Kraft) 1 oz	80	10	9	20	7	*	*	20	3	15	*	—	—	10	*	*	8	*	—	—
slices																				
(Cheez Whiz) 1 oz	80	10	9	20	7	*	*	18	*	10	*	—	—	6	*	*	4	*	—	—
limburger																				
(Mohawk Valley) 1 oz	70	10	9	15	7	*	*	17	*	10	*	—	—	4	*	*	2	*	—	—
(Mohawk Valley) 2 tbsp	80	7	11	20	7	*	*	21	—	15	*	—	—	6	*	—	—	—	—	—
Mexican																				
(Cheez Whiz) 1 oz	80	10	9	20	7	*	*	18	*	10	*	—	—	4	*	*	4	*	—	—
hot																				
(Velveeta) 1 oz	80	10	9	15	7	*	*	22	3	15	*	—	—	10	*	*	8	*	—	—
mild																				
(Velveeta) 1 oz	80	10	9	15	7	*	*	18	3	15	*	—	—	8	*	*	8	*	—	—
nacho																				
(Nabisco Easy Cheese) 1 oz	80	7	9	20	7	*	—	14	2	10	*	—	—	*	*	*	6	*	—	—
neufchatel																				
(WisPride) 2 tbsp	60	5	8	15	5	*	*	7	—	*	*	—	—	8	4	15	*	*	—	—

	Calories	Protein	Fat	Sat. Fat	Cholesterol	Carbohydrates	Fiber	Sodium	Potassium	Calcium	Iron	Zinc	Magnesium	Vitamin A	Vitamin C	Thiamin	Riboflavin	Niacin	Vitamin B₁₂	Folic acid
CHEESE SPREAD (continued)																				
light (Philadelphia) 1 oz	80	6	11	20	8	*	*	5	*	2	*	—	—	6	*	*	2	*	—	—
w/ french onion (Spreadery) 1 oz	70	4	9	15	7	*	*	9	*	2	*	—	—	8	*	*	2	*	—	—
w/ garden vegetables (Spreadery) 1 oz	70	4	9	20	7	*	*	6	*	2	*	—	—	4	*	*	2	*	—	—
w/ garlic & herb (Spreadery) 1 oz	70	4	9	20	7	*	*	6	*	2	*	—	—	4	*	*	2	*	—	—
w/ ranch flavor (Spreadery) 1 oz	70	6	11	20	7	*	*	8	*	2	*	—	—	4	*	*	2	*	—	—
w/ strawberries (Spreadery) 1 oz	70	4	8	15	5	—	*	11	*	2	*	—	—	4	*	*	2	*	—	—
olive & pimento (Kraft) 2 tbsp	60	2	8	15	5	*	*	7	*	4	*	—	—	4	*	*	4	*	—	—
pimento (Kraft) 2 tbsp	70	2	8	15	5	*	*	5	2	4	*	—	—	4	*	*	4	*	—	—
(Velveeta) 1 oz	80	10	9	15	7	*	*	17	3	15	*	—	—	15	*	*	8	*	—	—
w/ pineapple (Kraft) 2 tbsp	70	2	8	15	5	*	*	3	2	4	*	—	—	4	*	*	4	*	—	—
sharp (Old English) 1 oz	80	10	11	20	7	*	*	20	*	15	*	—	—	10	*	*	2	*	—	—
slices (Velveeta) 1 oz	90	10	9	20	7	*	*	17	3	15	*	—	—	4	*	*	8	*	—	—
w/ bacon (Squeez-A-Snak) 1 oz	80	10	11	20	7	*	*	21	*	15	*	—	—	2	*	*	2	*	—	—
CHERIMOYA 1 fruit	514	12	3	—	*	44	52	—	—	13	15	—	—	*	82	36	35	36	*	—
CHERRY DRINK (Kool-Aid) 8 1/2 fl oz	140	*	*	*	*	13	*	*	*	*	*	*	*	*	10	*	*	*	*	*
from mix (Kool-Aid) 8 fl oz	70	*	*	*	*	6	*	*	*	*	*	*	*	*	10	*	*	*	*	*
(Tang) 8 1/2 fl oz	130	*	*	*	*	11	*	*	*	*	*	—	—	*	100	*	10	10	*	20
sugar-free (Kool-Aid) 8 fl oz	4	*	*	*	*	*	*	*	*	*	*	*	*	*	10	*	*	*	*	*
unsweetened (Kool-Aid) 8 fl oz prep. w/ out sugar	2	*	*	*	*	*	*	*	*	*	*	*	*	*	10	*	*	*	*	*
unsweetened (Kool-Aid) 8 fl oz prep. w/ sugar	100	*	*	*	*	8	*	*	*	*	*	*	*	*	10	*	*	*	*	*
organic (Santa Cruz Natural) 8 fl oz	110	*	*	*	*	9	*	*	3	4	4	—	—	6	4	—	—	—	—	—
CHERRY-CRANBERRY DRINK (Ocean Spray Cran-Cherry) 8 fl oz	160	—	*	*	*	13	*	*	*	*	*	—	—	*	100	—	—	—	—	—
CHERRY JUICE (Farmer's Market) 8 fl oz	120	*	*	*	*	10	*	*	*	*	—	—	—	*	2	—	—	—	—	—
CHERVIL, DRIED 1 tbsp	4	*	*	*	*	*	*	*	3	3	3	*	*	—	—	—	—	—	*	—
CHESTNUT, EUROPEAN roasted (generic) 1 oz	70	*	*	*	*	5	16	*	5	*	*	*	2	*	12	5	3	2	*	5
CHESTNUT, JAPANESE raw (generic) 1 oz	44	*	*	*	*	3	—	*	3	*	2	2	3	*	12	7	3	2	*	3
boiled (generic) 1 oz	16	*	*	*	*	*	—	*	*	*	*	*	*	*	4	2	*	*	*	*
dried (generic) 1 oz	102	2	*	*	*	8	*	*	6	2	5	5	8	*	29	15	6	5	*	8
roasted (generic) 1 oz	57	*	*	*	*	4	*	*	3	*	3	3	5	*	13	9	—	*	*	4

Food	Calories	Protein	Fat	Sat. Fat	Cholesterol	Carbohydrates	Fiber	Sodium	Potassium	Calcium	Iron	Zinc	Magnesium	Vitamin A	Vitamin C	Thiamin	Riboflavin	Niacin	Vitamin B₁₂	Folic acid
CHEWING GUM see **CANDY**																				
CHIA SEED																				
dried																				
(generic) 1 oz	134	8	12	15	*	5	—	*	8	15	16	10	5	*	7	16	3	8	*	8
CHICK PEA																				
dry, cooked																				
(generic) 1/2 cup	134	12	3	*	*	7	—	8	7	4	13	8	10	*	2	6	3	2	*	35
salted																				
(generic) 1/2 cup	134	12	3	*	*	7	—	*	7	4	13	8	10	*	2	6	3	2	*	35
canned																				
(generic) 1/2 cup	143	10	2	*	*	9	20	15	6	4	9	8	9	*	8	2	2	*	*	20
(Hain) 1/2 cup	80	7	3	3	*	6	24	10	8	4	10	—	—	*	*	6	*	2	*	—
(Old El Paso) 1/2 cup	190	8	*	*	*	5	—	10	7	—	—	—	—	*	*	*	*	*	*	—
(Progresso) 1/2 cup	110	15	2	—	*	7	24	8	4	4	4	—	—	*	*	4	2	*	*	—
dry, canned in brine (Green Giant/Joan of Arc) 1/2 cup	45	10	2	*	*	3	10	7	3	2	3	—	—	*	*	*	*	*	*	—
50% less salt (Green Giant/Joan of Arc) 1/2 cup	45	10	2	*	*	3	10	4	3	2	3	—	—	*	*	*	*	*	*	—
CHICKEN, BROILER/ FRYER																				
back w/ out skin																				
fried																				
1/2 back	167	29	14	12	18	*	*	2	4	2	5	11	4	*	*	4	9	22	3	*
roasted																				
1/2 back	96	19	8	7	12	*	*	2	3	*	3	7	2	*	*	2	5	14	2	*
stewed																				
1/2 back	88	18	7	7	12	*	*	*	2	*	3	7	2	*	*	*	4	10	*	*
back w/ skin																				
batter-fried																				
1/2 back	397	44	40	35	35	4	—	16	6	3	10	16	6	—	*	10	15	35	5	3
flour-fried																				
1/2 back	238	33	23	20	21	2	—	3	5	2	6	12	4	—	*	5	10	26	3	2
roasted																				
3 oz	255	37	27	25	25	*	*	3	5	2	7	13	4	6	*	3	10	29	4	*
stewed																				
3 oz	219	31	24	22	22	*	*	2	4	2	6	11	3	5	*	2	8	18	3	*
breast w/ out skin																				
fried																				
1/2 breast	161	48	6	6	26	*	*	3	7	*	5	6	7	*	*	5	6	64	5	*
roasted																				
1/2 breast	142	44	5	5	24	*	*	3	6	*	5	6	6	*	*	4	6	59	5	*
stewed																				
1/2 breast	143	46	4	4	24	*	*	2	5	*	5	6	6	*	*	3	7	40	4	*
breast w/ skin																				
batter-fried																				
1/2 breast	364	58	28	25	40	4	*	16	8	3	10	9	8	2	*	11	12	74	7	2
flour-fried																				
1/2 breast	218	52	13	12	29	*	—	3	7	2	6	7	7	—	*	5	8	67	6	*
roasted																				
1/2 breast	193	49	12	11	27	*	*	3	7	*	6	7	7	2	*	4	7	62	5	*
stewed																				
1/2 breast	202	50	13	12	27	*	*	3	6	*	6	7	6	2	*	3	7	43	4	*
dark meat w/ out skin																				
fried																				
3 oz	203	41	15	14	27	*	*	3	6	2	7	16	5	*	*	5	12	30	5	2
roasted																				
3 oz	174	39	13	12	26	*	*	3	6	*	6	16	5	*	*	4	11	28	5	2
stewed																				
3 oz	163	37	12	11	25	*	*	3	4	*	6	15	4	*	*	3	10	20	3	2

	Calories	Protein	Fat	Sat. Fat	Cholesterol	Carbohydrates	Fiber	Sodium	Potassium	Calcium	Iron	Zinc	Magnesium	Vitamin A	Vitamin C	Thiamin	Riboflavin	Niacin	Vitamin B$_{12}$	Folic acid
CHICKEN, BROILER/FRYER (continued)																				
dark meat w/ skin																				
batter-fried 3 oz	253	31	24	21	25	3	—	10	4	2	7	12	4	—	*	7	11	24	4	2
flour-fried 3 oz	242	39	22	20	26	*	—	3	6	*	7	15	5	—	*	5	12	29	4	2
roasted 3 oz	215	37	21	19	26	*	*	3	5	*	6	14	5	3	*	4	10	27	4	2
stewed 3 oz	198	33	19	18	23	*	*	2	4	*	6	13	4	3	*	3	9	19	3	*
drumstick w/ out skin																				
fried 1 drumstick	82	20	5	5	13	*	*	2	3	*	3	9	3	*	*	2	6	13	2	*
roasted 1 drumstick	76	21	4	4	14	*	*	2	3	*	3	9	3	*	*	2	6	13	2	*
stewed 1 drumstick	78	21	4	4	13	*	*	2	3	*	3	9	2	*	*	2	6	10	2	*
drumstick w/ skin																				
batter-fried 1 drumstick	193	26	17	15	21	2	—	8	4	*	5	11	4	—	*	5	9	18	3	2
flour-fried 1 drumstick	120	22	10	9	15	*	—	2	3	*	4	9	3	*	*	3	6	15	3	*
roasted 1 drumstick	112	23	9	8	16	*	*	2	3	*	4	10	3	*	*	2	7	16	3	*
stewed 1 drumstick	116	24	9	9	16	*	*	2	3	*	4	10	3	*	*	2	6	12	2	*
fat																				
1 tbsp	115	*	22	19	4	*	*	*	*	*	*	*	*	*	*	*	*	*	*	*
giblets																				
fried 1 cup	402	79	30	28	215	2	*	7	14	3	83	61	9	346	21	9	130	80	320	138
simmered 3 oz	133	37	6	7	111	*	*	2	4	*	30	26	4	126	11	5	48	17	143	80
gizzard																				
simmered 3 oz	130	38	5	5	55	*	*	2	4	*	20	25	4	3	2	2	12	17	27	11
heart																				
simmered 1 cup	268	64	18	17	117	*	*	3	5	3	73	70	7	*	4	7	63	20	175	29
leg w/ out skin																				
fried 1 leg	196	44	14	12	31	*	*	4	7	*	7	19	6	*	*	5	14	31	5	2
roasted 1 leg	181	43	12	11	30	*	*	4	7	*	7	18	6	*	*	5	13	30	5	2
stewed 1 leg	187	44	12	11	30	*	*	3	5	*	8	19	5	*	*	4	13	24	4	2
leg w/ skin																				
batter-fried 1 leg	431	57	39	34	47	5	—	18	9	3	12	23	8	—	*	12	21	43	7	4
flour-fried 1 leg	284	50	25	22	35	*	—	4	7	*	9	20	7	—	*	7	15	37	6	2
roasted 1 leg	264	49	24	21	35	*	*	4	7	*	8	20	7	3	*	5	14	35	6	2
light meat w/ out skin																				
fried 3 oz	163	46	7	7	25	*	*	3	6	*	5	7	6	*	*	4	6	57	5	*
roasted 3 oz	147	44	6	6	24	*	*	3	6	*	5	7	6	*	*	4	6	53	5	*
stewed 3 oz	135	41	5	5	22	*	*	2	4	*	4	7	5	*	*	2	6	33	3	*

CHICKEN, BROILER/FRYER (continued)

	Calories	Protein	Fat	Sat. Fat	Cholesterol	Carbohydrates	Fiber	Sodium	Potassium	Calcium	Iron	Zinc	Magnesium	Vitamin A	Vitamin C	Thiamin	Riboflavin	Niacin	Vitamin B12	Folic acid
light meat w/ skin																				
batter-fried 3 oz	235	33	20	18	24	3	—	10	4	2	6	6	5	—	*	6	7	39	4	*
flour-fried 3 oz	209	43	16	14	25	*	*	3	6	*	6	7	6	*	*	4	7	51	5	*
roasted 3 oz	189	41	14	13	24	*	*	3	6	*	5	7	5	2	*	3	6	47	5	*
stewed 3 oz	171	37	13	12	21	*	*	2	4	*	5	6	4	2	*	2	6	29	3	*
liver																				
simmered 1 cup	220	57	12	13	294	*	*	3	6	2	66	40	7	459	37	14	144	31	451	270
neck w/ out skin																				
fried 1 neck	50	10	4	4	8	*	*	*	*	*	4	6	*	*	*	*	4	6	*	*
stewed 1 neck	32	7	2	2	5	*	*	*	*	*	3	5	*	*	*	*	3	4	*	*
neck w/ skin																				
batter-fried 1 neck	172	17	19	16	16	*	—	6	2	2	6	9	2	—	*	3	7	12	2	*
flour-fried 1 neck	120	14	13	12	11	*	—	*	2	*	5	7	2	*	*	2	5	10	2	*
stewed 1 neck	94	12	11	10	9	*	*	*	*	*	5	7	*	*	*	*	6	6	*	*
skin																				
roasted 3 oz	386	29	53	49	24	*	*	2	3	*	7	7	3	4	*	2	6	24	3	*
stewed 3 oz	309	22	43	40	18	*	*	2	3	*	5	5	3	3	*	2	5	16	2	*
thigh w/ out skin																				
fried 1 thigh	113	24	8	7	18	*	*	2	4	*	4	10	3	*	*	3	8	19	3	*
roasted 1 thigh	109	22	9	8	16	*	*	2	4	*	4	9	3	*	*	3	7	17	3	*
stewed 1 thigh	107	23	8	8	16	*	*	2	3	*	4	9	3	*	*	2	7	14	2	*
thigh w/ skin																				
batter-fried 1 thigh	238	31	22	19	27	3	—	10	5	2	7	12	5	—	*	7	11	25	4	2
flour-fried 3 oz	223	38	20	18	27	*	—	3	6	*	7	14	5	—	*	5	12	30	4	2
roasted 1 thigh	153	26	15	14	19	*	*	2	4	*	5	10	3	2	*	3	8	20	3	*
stewed 1 thigh	158	26	15	14	19	*	*	2	3	*	5	10	3	2	*	3	8	17	2	*
whole w/ out skin																				
fried 3 oz	186	43	12	11	27	*	*	3	6	*	6	13	6	*	*	5	10	41	5	2
roasted 3 oz	162	41	10	9	25	*	*	3	6	*	6	12	5	*	*	4	9	39	5	*
stewed 3 oz	150	39	9	8	24	*	*	2	4	*	6	11	4	*	*	3	8	26	3	*
whole, w/ skin																				
batter-fried 3 oz	247	32	23	20	29	3	—	10	5	2	8	11	4	—	*	6	12	30	12	5
flour-fried 3 oz	427	27	56	50	21	3	—	2	3	*	7	7	4	—	*	5	8	25	3	*

	Calories	Protein	Fat	Sat. Fat	Cholesterol	Carbohydrates	Fiber	Sodium	Potassium	Calcium	Iron	Zinc	Magnesium	Vitamin A	Vitamin C	Thiamin	Riboflavin	Niacin	Vitamin B₁₂	Folic acid
CHICKEN, BROILER/FRYER (continued)																				
roasted 3 oz	203	39	18	16	25	*	*	3	5	*	6	11	5	3	*	4	8	36	4	*
stewed 3 oz	186	35	16	15	22	*	*	2	4	*	5	10	4	2	*	3	7	24	3	*
wing flour-fried 1 wing	54	10	5	4	7	*	—	*	*	*	2	3	*	—	*	*	3	9	4	2
wing w/out skin fried 1 wing	44	11	3	3	6	*	*	*	*	*	*	3	*	*	*	*	2	8	*	*
roasted 1 wing	49	12	3	3	7	*	*	*	*	*	2	3	*	*	*	*	2	9	*	*
stewed 1 wing	52	13	3	3	7	*	*	*	*	*	2	4	*	*	*	*	2	8	*	*
wing w/ skin batter-fried 1 wing	159	16	16	15	13	2	—	7	2	*	4	5	2	—	*	3	4	13	2	*
flour-fried 1 wing	103	14	11	10	9	*	—	*	2	*	2	4	2	—	*	*	3	11	*	*
roasted 1 wing	116	18	12	11	11	*	*	*	2	*	3	5	2	*	*	*	3	13	2	*
stewed 3 oz	212	32	22	20	20	*	*	2	3	*	5	9	3	2	*	2	5	20	3	*
CHICKEN, CAPON																				
w/out skin whole raw 3 oz	197	26	22	21	25	*	*	2	5	*	7	7	4	15	4	4	9	30	14	6
w/skin whole roasted 3 oz	195	41	15	14	24	*	*	2	6	*	7	10	5	*	*	4	8	38	5	*
CHICKEN, ROASTER																				
dark meat w/skin roasted 1 cup	249	54	19	17	35	*	*	6	9	2	10	20	7	2	*	6	16	40	6	2
giblets stewed 1 cup	239	65	12	12	172	*	*	4	7	2	49	45	7	236	16	7	69	29	203	110
light meat w/skin roasted 1 cup	214	63	9	8	35	*	*	3	9	2	8	7	8	*	*	6	8	73	7	*
meat w/skin roasted 1 cup	234	58	14	13	35	*	*	4	9	2	9	14	7	*	*	6	12	55	7	2
CHICKEN, STEWING																				
dark meat w/skin stewed 1 cup	361	66	33	29	44	*	*	6	8	2	13	29	8	4	*	12	29	32	6	3
giblets stewed 3 oz	143	25	12	11	68	*	*	3	5	*	28	17	4	178	16	5	55	36	153	75
light meat w/skin stewed 1 cup	298	77	17	14	33	*	*	3	8	2	9	8	8	2	*	9	16	60	6	*
meat w/out skin stewed 1 cup	332	71	26	22	39	*	*	5	8	2	11	19	8	3	*	10	23	45	6	2
whole stewed 3 oz	242	38	25	22	22	*	*	3	4	*	6	10	4	2	*	5	12	25	3	*

	Calories	Protein	Fat	Sat. Fat	Cholesterol	Carbohydrates	Fiber	Sodium	Potassium	Calcium	Iron	Zinc	Magnesium	Vitamin A	Vitamin C	Thiamin	Riboflavin	Niacin	Vitamin B$_{12}$	Folic acid
CHICKEN, CANNED																				
chunk																				
(Hormel) 2 1/2 oz	100	25	6	5	13	*	—	10	4	1	3	6	—	*	*	*	6	15	—	*
breast																				
(Hormel) 2 1/2 oz	90	25	5	5	10	*	—	13	4	1	2	3	—	*	*	*	4	20	—	*
no salt																				
(Hormel) 2 1/2 oz	90	27	5	5	12	*	—	*	3	*	1	3	2	*	*	*	4	18	—	*
white meat																				
(Swanson) 2 1/2 oz	100	30	6	—	—	—	—	10	—	*	2	—	—	*	*	*	4	20	—	*
w/ broth																				
(generic) 1/2 can	117	26	9	8	15	*	*	15	3	*	6	7	2	2	2	*	5	22	3	*
CHICKEN, COLD CUTS																				
breast																				
(Oscar Mayer) 1 slice	25	8	*	*	4	*	*	12	4	*	*	*	*	*	*	*	—	—	—	*
(Oscar Mayer Healthy Favorites)																				
1 slice	12	4	*	*	2	*	*	5	2	*	*	*	*	*	*	*	—	—	—	*
deluxe																				
(Oscar Mayer) 1 slice	29	8	*	*	5	*	*	14	2	*	2	*	2	*	*	*	—	—	—	*
roasted																				
(Oscar Mayer) 1 slice	13	4	*	*	2	*	*	7	*	*	*	*	*	*	*	*	—	—	—	*
roasted																				
(Bryan Thin Sliced) 1 oz	30	10	2	—	5	—	*	4	—	—	—	—	—	—	—	—	—	—	—	*
smoked																				
(Bryan Thin Sliced) 1 oz	30	10	2	—	5	—	*	4	—	—	—	—	—	—	—	—	—	—	—	*
(Oscar Mayer) 1 slice	30	8	*	*	*	*	*	15	2	*	*	*	*	*	*	*	—	—	—	*
roll																				
light																				
(generic) 3 oz	135	28	10	9	14	*	*	21	6	4	5	4	4	*	*	4	6	22	2	*
light meat																				
(generic) 1 1 oz slice	45	9	3	3	5	*	*	7	2	*	2	*	*	*	*	*	2	7	*	*
white meat slices																				
(Oscar Mayer) 1 slice	38	7	3	3	5	*	*	15	2	*	3	*	2	*	*	*	—	—	—	*
CHICKEN DINNER, FROZEN																				
à la king																				
(Armour Classics Lite)																				
11 1/4 oz	290	32	11	—	18	13	—	26	11	6	10			45	100	10	10	15		
(Swanson) 5 1/4 oz	190	20	18	—	—	3	—	29	—	4	2	—		*	*	2	8	10	—	—
(Top Shelf) 10 oz	360	30	15	20	12	16	—	37	14	6	2	8	8	25	2	8	10	45	—	—
w/ almonds																				
(Swanson) 10 oz	310	35	14	—	—	13	—	26	—	8	8			20	30	6	20	30	—	—
baked																				
(Swanson Hungry-Man)																				
15 oz	740	80	58	—	—	19	—	56	—	8	20			*	8	10	25	20	—	—
barbecue flavored																				
(Swanson) 10 oz	550	50	35	—	—	20	—	49	—	8	20			15	6	15	15	25	—	—
w/ barbecue sauce																				
(Healthy Choice) 12 3/4 oz	380	40	9	10	13	19	—	23	19	6	15	—		10	20	8	8	45	—	—
boneless																				
(Swanson Hungry-Man)																				
17 1/4 oz	670	70	42	—	—	24	—	52	—	8	20			35	15	25	40	50	—	—
breast																				
glazed																				
(Top Shelf) 10 oz	170	32	3	5	12	6	—	32	23	4	4	7	10	40	6	4	10	40	—	—
teriyaki																				
(Budget Gourmet																				
Light & Healthy)																				
11 oz	300	30	12	5	10	14	—	20	14	4	4	—		25	45	15	15	45	—	—

CHICKEN DINNER, FROZEN (continued)

	Calories	Protein	Fat	Sat. Fat	Cholesterol	Carbohydrates	Fiber	Sodium	Potassium	Calcium	Iron	Zinc	Magnesium	Vitamin A	Vitamin C	Thiamin	Riboflavin	Niacin	Vitamin B$_{12}$	Folic acid
w/ fettucini (Budget Gourmet Light & Healthy) 11 oz	240	35	9	10	15	10	—	18	11	15	10	—	—	80	50	25	25	35	—	—
w/ Spanish rice (Top Shelf) 10 oz	400	45	23	35	25	13	—	34	17	10	4	11	10	10	6	6	15	40	—	—
burgundy (Armour Classics Lite) 10 oz	210	38	3	—	15	8	—	32	15	4	10	—	—	40	40	10	10	30	—	—
cacciatore (Top Shelf) 10 oz	210	35	5	—	17	8	—	34	—	10	4	—	—	10	4	10	15	35	—	—
chunks (Country Skillet) 6 oz	260	33	25	—	8	6	—	20	3	2	6	—	—	*	*	6	4	6	—	—
southern fried (Country Skillet) 6 oz	170	37	28	—	10	5	—	24	3	2	6	—	—	*	*	6	4	6	—	—
cordon bleu (Le Menu) 11 1/2 oz	390	45	25	—	—	11	—	40	—	20	10	—	—	150	15	10	10	40	—	—
dijon (Healthy Choice) 11 oz	250	35	5	5	13	13	—	20	10	2	10	—	—	10	15	15	8	50	—	—
w/ fettucini (Armour Classics) 11 oz	260	28	14	—	17	9	—	27	11	15	10	—	—	30	100	10	10	15	—	—
fried (Banquet Extra Helping) 14 1/4 oz	790	55	66	—	50	23	—	62	21	10	20	—	—	*	20	15	15	30	—	—
southern style (Banquet Extra Helping) 13 1/4 oz	790	58	60	—	45	25	—	99	20	15	25	—	—	*	10	25	20	35	—	—
fried, dark meat (Swanson Hungry-Man) 14 1/4 oz	860	60	69	—	—	26	—	69	—	6	20	—	—	*	8	20	25	50	—	—
large (Swanson) 9 3/4 oz	560	45	43	—	—	19	—	47	—	6	15	—	—	2	6	15	15	25	—	—
regular (Swanson) 7 1/4 oz	420	40	34	—	—	12	—	43	—	4	20	—	—	2	35	15	20	35	—	—
fried, mostly white meat (Swanson Hungry-Man) 14 1/4 oz	870	60	71	—	—	27	—	89	—	8	20	—	—	*	8	25	20	60	—	—
fried, white meat (Banquet Extra Helping) 14 1/4 oz	760	60	58	—	40	23	—	74	23	15	15	—	—	*	20	20	15	45	—	—
(Swanson) 10 1/4 oz	550	50	38	—	—	20	—	59	—	6	15	—	—	*	6	20	15	35	—	—
w/ garlic (Swanson Hungry-Man) 16 1/2 oz	500	60	29	—	—	18	—	60	—	8	15	—	—	180	30	15	15	50	—	—
glazed (Armour Classics) 10 3/4 oz	300	25	25	—	20	8	—	40	11	4	10	—	—	6	15	10	15	20	—	—
(Le Menu Healthy) 10 1/2 oz	330	38	5	5	10	17	—	17	—	10	4	—	—	60	4	8	20	35	—	—
grilled (Swanson Hungry-Man) 17 oz	660	70	37	—	—	26	—	73	—	10	20	—	—	15	20	20	35	20	—	—
herb roasted (Healthy Choice) 11 1/2 oz	380	43	11	15	20	19	—	20	19	6	8	—	—	40	2	15	15	35	—	—
(Le Menu Healthy) 11 oz	300	37	6	10	17	14	—	20	—	10	4	—	—	10	10	10	25	45	—	—
w/ homestyle gravy (Budget Gourmet Light & Healthy) 11 oz	280	30	12	10	12	12	—	23	18	10	10	—	—	70	20	30	20	50	—	—
honey mustard (Le Menu) 11 1/2 oz	390	33	18	—	—	17	—	28	—	4	8	—	—	220	10	6	10	25	—	—
imperial (Chun King) 13 oz	300	28	2	—	10	18	—	64	7	5	10	—	—	25	15	10	25	10	—	—

Encyclopedia of Daily Values

CHICKEN DINNER, FROZEN (continued)

	Calories	Protein	Fat	Sat. Fat	Cholesterol	Carbohydrates	Fiber	Sodium	Potassium	Calcium	Iron	Zinc	Magnesium	Vitamin A	Vitamin C	Thiamin	Riboflavin	Niacin	Vitamin B12	Folic acid
marsala																				
(Armour Classics Lite) 10 1/2 oz	250	33	11	—	27	9	—	39	13	6	15	—	—	6	30	20	15	25	—	—
mesquite																				
(Armour Classics) 9 1/2 oz	370	37	25	—	18	14	—	27	23	2	10	—	—	8	25	15	10	20	—	—
(Budget Gourmet Light & Healthy) 11 oz	250	35	9	5	13	11	—	23	20	6	6	—	—	90	25	20	15	50	—	—
(Healthy Choice) 10 1/2 oz	300	35	5	5	13	18	—	20	12	4	6	—	—	8	80	15	8	6	—	—
(Le Menu Healthy) 10 1/4 oz	300	40	5	5	10	16	—	12	—	15	6	—	—	35	60	8	20	45	—	—
w/ noodles																				
(Armour Classics) 11 oz	230	32	11	—	17	8	—	27	15	8	10	—	—	90	90	10	10	20	—	—
nuggets																				
(Banquet Extra Helping) 10 oz	540	53	29	—	27	23	—	97	20	6	15	—	—	*	10	20	10	45	—	—
(Country Skillet) 6 oz	250	43	23	—	13	5	—	24	4	2	6	—	—	*	2	6	4	8	—	—
(Kid Cuisine) 6 3/4 oz	360	18	26	—	18	13	—	27	8	2	10	—	—	8	*	8	8	8	—	—
(Swanson) 8 3/4 oz	470	45	35	—	—	16	—	28	—	2	10	—	—	2	4	10	10	15	—	—
w/ sweet & sour sauce																				
(Banquet Extra Helping) 10 oz	540	53	29	—	27	23	—	97	20	6	15	—	—	*	10	20	10	45	—	—
oriental style																				
(Armour Classics Lite) 10 oz	180	30	2	—	12	9	—	27	15	4	10	—	—	10	70	10	10	25	—	—
(Healthy Choice) 11 1/4 oz	200	32	2	3	12	11	—	18	11	4	8	—	—	25	60	10	8	40	—	—
(Stouffer's Lunch Express) 9 3/4 oz	80	—	14	8	13	15	8	39	11	2	6	—	—	15	15	—	—	—	—	—
parmigiana																				
(Armour Classics) 11 1/2 oz	370	37	29	—	25	9	—	44	15	15	15	—	—	15	15	30	15	20	—	—
(Budget Gourmet Light & Healthy) 11 oz	270	35	14	15	17	10	—	22	15	10	8	—	—	20	8	30	15	45	—	—
(Healthy Choice) 11 1/2 oz	290	38	9	15	18	14	—	14	15	10	10	—	—	70	10	15	15	30	—	—
(Le Menu) 10 1/4 oz	340	37	25	—	—	9	—	36	—	15	15	—	—	100	50	15	20	35	—	—
homestyle																				
(Stouffer's) 10 7/8 oz	320	47	15	10	25	10	16	37	22	10	10	—	—	10	10	20	25	45	—	—
large																				
(Swanson) 11 1/2 oz	400	35	29	—	—	14	—	44	—	15	15	—	—	20	45	8	15	15	—	—
regular																				
(Swanson) 10 oz	300	15	23	—	—	12	—	32	—	6	10	—	—	50	20	8	10	20	—	—
pasta divan																				
(Healthy Choice) 12 oz	300	42	6	10	17	14	—	22	14	15	10	—	—	80	120	25	15	25	—	—
pasta primavera																				
(Le Menu) 11 1/2 oz	330	35	15	—	—	13	—	35	—	15	10	—	—	110	40	10	25	35	—	—
patties																				
(Country Skillet) 6 oz	230	40	23	—	13	5	—	23	3	2	6	—	—	*	2	6	4	8	—	—
southern fried																				
(Country Skillet) 6 oz	240	37	23	—	12	5	—	22	3	2	6	—	—	*	6	6	4	4	—	—
w/ salsa																				
(Healthy Choice) 11 1/4 oz	240	33	3	5	17	12	—	19	15	8	6	—	—	20	110	15	10	25	—	—
(Le Menu Healthy) 10 1/4 oz	300	45	6	5	8	15	—	14	—	10	6	—	—	8	100	10	20	45	—	—
santa fe grilled																				
(Le Menu) 10 1/4 oz	320	33	15	—	—	12	—	36	—	8	10	—	—	100	35	8	10	25	—	—
southwestern style																				
(Healthy Choice) 12 1/2 oz	340	42	8	10	20	17	—	23	16	4	10	—	—	8	50	6	6	40	—	—
stir fry w/ pasta																				
(Healthy Choice Homestyle) 12 oz	300	38	8	5	10	14	—	23	8	2	4	—	—	10	15	*	6	4	—	—
sweet & sour																				
(Armour Classics Lite) 11 oz	240	30	3	—	12	13	—	34	14	4	8	—	—	20	40	10	10	20	—	—
(Healthy Choice) 11 1/2 oz	280	33	3	3	12	17	—	13	14	4	10	—	—	25	50	10	10	45	—	—
(Le Menu) 11 oz	360	37	14	—	—	16	—	30	—	6	8	—	—	140	15	6	10	25	—	—

	Calories	Protein	Fat	Sat. Fat	Cholesterol	Carbohydrates	Fiber	Sodium	Potassium	Calcium	Iron	Zinc	Magnesium	Vitamin A	Vitamin C	Thiamin	Riboflavin	Niacin	Vitamin B$_{12}$	Folic acid
CHICKEN DINNER, FROZEN (continued)																				
teriyaki																				
(Healthy Choice) 12 1/4 oz	290	40	6	5	18	13	—	23	15	4	8	—	—	2	10	6	6	40	—	—
tomato garden																				
(Le Menu) 10 1/4 oz	240	37	9	—		8	—	32	—	10	8	—	—	25	25	6	10	30	—	—
vegetable w/ pot pie																				
(Banquet) 7 oz	550	25	55	—	12	13	—	36	5	2	10	—	—	6	*	20	15	30	—	—
w/ wine & mushroom sauce																				
(Armour Classics) 10 3/4 oz	280	37	17	—	17	8	—	37	16	8	8	—	—	35	35	10	10	30	—	—
CHICKEN ENTREE, CANNED																				
stew																				
(Dinty Moore) 7 1/2 oz	260	18	28	20	27	5	—	35	15	4	6	7	6	40	3	3	14	16		
(Swanson) 7 2/3 oz	160	20	11	—	—	5	—	41	—	2	4	—	—	110	10	2	4	15		
microwave																				
(Dinty Moore) 7 1/2 oz	260	18	28	20	27	5	—	35	15	4	6	7	6	40	3	3	14	16		
sweet & sour																				
(La Choy) 3/4 cup	240	13	3	3	6	16	4	59	7	2	10	—	—	*	4	2	4	10		
bi-pack																				
(La Choy) 3/4 cup	120	12	3	2	4	6	8	18	11	2	10	—	—	*	15	2	2	8		
teriyaki																				
bi-pack																				
(La Choy) 3/4 cup	85	13	3	3	7	3	4	35	7	2	6	—	—	*	12	2	4	10		
w/ dumplings																				
(Swanson) 7 1/2 oz	220	20	17	—	—	6	—	41	—	2	4	—	—	8	*	2	6	10		
CHICKEN ENTREE, FROM MIX																				
cheesy broccoli																				
(Chicken Helper) 7 oz	310	40	14	15	22	11	—	33	9	8	10	—	—	2	*	10	10	25		
creamy																				
(Chicken Helper) 8 1/4 oz	330	43	20	20	33	10	—	34	10	8	10	—	—	20	*	20	20	30		
creamy mushroom																				
(Chicken Helper) 8 oz	320	42	17	15	30	10	—	34	10	8	10	—	—	4	*	20	20	30		
stir-fried																				
(Chicken Helper) 7 oz	370	42	22	15	48	12	—	40	8	6	10	—	—	8	*	10	15	30		
CHICKEN ENTREE, FROZEN																				
à l'orange																				
(Healthy Choice) 9 oz	260	38	3	3	13	13	—	14	12	2	8	—	—	15	45	10	6	30		
(Stouffer's Lean Cuisine) 8 oz	280	45	6	5	18	11	—	12	14	4	4	—	—	8	20	15	10	50		
(Weight Watchers) 8 oz	200	20	2	*	5	12	8	13	9	4	4	—	—	10	8	—	—	—		
à la king																				
(Light & Elegant) 9 oz	240	23	11	—	13	10	—	32	6	6	8	—	—	*	8	10	10	10		
(Stouffer's) 9 1/2 oz	320	30	15	15	18	14	12	31	8	10	4	—	—	2	6	10	15	20		
alfredo																				
(Stouffer's Lunch Express) 9 5/8 oz	150	—	26	30	20	11	12	26	10	15	6	—	—	20	10	—	—	—		
au gratin																				
(Budget Gourmet Light & Healthy) 9 oz	230	30	12	25	13	8	—	34	11	15	6	—	—	70	15	10	20	35		
baked																				
(Stouffer's) 8 7/8 oz	270	—	18	15	25	6	8	31	16	2	4	—	—	*	2	—	—	—		
barbecue glazed																				
(Weight Watchers) 7 1/2 oz	190	30	4	5	7	7	4	14	17	4	10	—	—	8	10	—	—	—		
barbecue sauce w/ rice pilaf																				
(Stouffer's Lean Cuisine) 8 3/4 oz	260	33	9	5	17	11	—	21	19	6	8	—	—	25	30	10	10	30		
biscuit sandwich																				
(Hormel Quickmeal) 1 sandwich	310	22	20	—	17	12	—	37	—	8	8	—	—	*	*	15	15	25		
breast, glazed																				
(Healthy Choice) 8 1/2 oz	220	35	5	5	15	9	—	21	11	*	6	—	—	*	2	10	8	35	—	—

PERCENTAGE DAILY VALUE

	Calories	Protein	Fat	Sat. Fat	Cholesterol	Carbohydrates	Fiber	Sodium	Potassium	Calcium	Iron	Zinc	Magnesium	Vitamin A	Vitamin C	Thiamin	Riboflavin	Niacin	Vitamin B12	Folic acid
CHICKEN ENTREE, FROZEN (continued)																				
breast, oven baked & breaded (Stouffer's Lean Cuisine) 8 oz	200	28	8	10	12	7	—	20	16	2	8	—	—	35	10	10	10	40	—	—
breast tenders (Banquet) 2.25 oz	150	18	9	—	—	4	—	12	5	*	2	—	—	*	2	6	2	15	—	—
southern fried (Banquet) 2.25 oz	160	17	11	—	—	4	—	14	5	*	2	—	—	*	*	6	2	15	—	—
breast tenders & o'brien potatoes homestyle (Stouffer's) 6 5/8 oz	380	33	28	15	17	11	16	44	17	2	6	—	—	2	6	15	8	30	—	—
cacciatore (Stouffer's Lean Cuisine) 10 7/8 oz	280	37	11	10	15	10	—	24	16	4	8	—	—	10	15	15	10	30	—	—
cajun (Chicken by George) 5 oz	180	42	12	5	27	*	—	37	20	2	6	5	9	3	4	7	12	68	—	—
chicken biscuits (Jimmy Dean) 1 sandwich	150	7	9	—	—	5	—	17	—	4	6	—	—	*	*	10	6	10	—	—
chicken, sweet & sour (Stouffer's Lean Cuisine) 9 oz	280	28	9	5	17	13	—	20	11	2	4	—	—	25	20	10	10	25	—	—
cordon bleu (Weight Watchers) 9 oz	220	28	9	10	7	12	—	21	10	15	8	—	—	20	10	—	—	—	—	—
creamed (Stouffer's) 6 1/2 oz	280	32	31	35	27	3	4	30	6	8	2	—	—	*	*	4	15	15	—	—
crunchy walnut (Chun King) 13 oz	310	27	8	—	15	16	—	71	6	4	10	—	—	*	8	100	10	10	—	—
divan (Stouffer's) 8 oz	210	40	15	20	22	3	4	24	14	15	2	—	—	2	40	10	20	25	—	—
drum-snackers (Banquet) 2.5 oz	210	15	22	—	—	4	—	21	4	*	2	—	—	*	2	4	4	8	—	—
drumlets (Swanson Kids') 9 1/4 oz	530	40	40	—	—	18	—	30	—	8	10	—	—	*	8	10	15	20	—	—
w/ egg noodles (Budget Gourmet) 10 oz	440	35	40	—	30	9	—	37	9	20	15	—	—	20	15	15	20	20	—	—
(Light & Elegant) 9 oz	240	28	11	—	17	9	—	24	9	10	10	—	—	25	*	15	15	15	—	—
(Swanson) 9 oz	310	25	23	—	—	10	—	41	—	6	8	—	—	10	*	8	10	15	—	—
escalloped (Stouffer's) 10 oz	440	35	45	30	27	9	8	37	9	10	10	—	—	*	*	10	20	20	—	—
homestyle (Stouffer's) 10 oz	310	37	22	25	27	8	8	43	13	15	6	—	—	35	2	10	25	15	—	—
fajitas (Healthy Choice) 7 oz	200	30	5	5	12	8	—	13	10	8	15	—	—	15	15	15	10	20	—	—
w/ fettucini (Budget Gourmet) 10 oz	400	35	32	—	28	10	—	29	10	20	2	—	—	20	6	15	25	40	—	—
(Healthy Choice) 8 1/2 oz	240	37	6	10	15	10	—	16	5	8	10	—	—	*	*	15	10	15	—	—
(Stouffer's Lean Cuisine) 9 oz	280	38	9	15	12	11	—	21	12	15	8	—	—	*	*	20	25	30	—	—
(Stouffer's Lean Cuisine) 10 1/4 oz	60	—	9	13	12	11	16	22	12	15	4	—	—	10	40	—	—	—	—	—
homestyle (Stouffer's) 10 1/2 oz	380	37	23	20	22	11	12	52	17	30	10	—	—	4	2	10	20	30	—	—
fiesta (Stouffer's Lean Cuisine) 8 1/2 oz	240	32	8	10	13	10	—	23	17	2	2	—	—	15	15	15	8	30	—	—
(Weight Watchers) 8 oz	200	22	2	3	5	11	12	19	15	4	4	—	—	10	20	—	—	—	—	—
Francais (Weight Watchers) 8 1/2 oz	150	23	2	*	3	7	16	16	13	15	8	—	—	10	15	—	—	—	—	—
French recipe (Budget Gourmet Light & Healthy) 10 oz	220	25	14	20	13	7	—	36	19	6	4	—	—	50	15	15	15	60	—	—
fried (Kid Cuisine) 7 1/2 oz	430	27	34	—	28	14	—	37	12	4	8	—	—	*	8	10	10	15	—	—

CHICKEN ENTREE, FROZEN (continued)

	Calories	Protein	Fat	Sat. Fat	Cholesterol	Carbohydrates	Fiber	Sodium	Potassium	Calcium	Iron	Zinc	Magnesium	Vitamin A	Vitamin C	Thiamin	Riboflavin	Niacin	Vitamin B$_{12}$	Folic acid
breast & whipped potatoes homestyle (Stouffer's) 7 1/8 oz	330	28	25	20	18	10	12	32	11	2	4	—	—	2	2	10	8	35		
dark meat (Swanson Kids') 9 3/4 oz	690	60	52	—	—	—	—	49	—	6	25	—	—	*	4	10	20	40		
w/ whipped potatoes (Swanson) 7 oz	400	40	32	—	—	11	—	45	—	4	10	—	—	*	6	10	10	25		
glazed w/ vegetable rice (Stouffer's Lean Cuisine) 8 1/2 oz	250	35	11	10	17	8	—	25	17	2	2	—	—	2	6	10	10	40		
grilled & glazed (Weight Watchers) 8 oz	130	20	2	*	3	7	132	19	9	4	6	—	—	2	2					
half breast (Swanson) 4 1/2 oz	360	50	31	—	—	7	—	33	—	4	8	—	—	*	*	10	10	30		
honey mustard (Healthy Choice) 9 1/2 oz	250	40	5	5	13	12	—	20	3	2	8	—	—	10	6	10	2	8		
(Stouffer's Lean Cuisine) 7 1/2 oz	230	30	6	5	13	10	—	22	10	2	4	—	—	20	4	10	10	20		
(Weight Watchers) 7 1/2 oz	140	18	2	3	5	7	28	14	10	4	15	—	—	2	6					
imperial (Weight Watchers) 8 1/2 oz	200	30	5	5	8	8	16	17	12	4	6	—	—	8	6					
Italiano (Stouffer's Lean Cuisine) 9 oz	270	37	9	5	13	11	—	25	17	10	8	—	—	10	40	20	15	30		
lemon herb (Chicken by George) 5 oz	170	40	9	5	23	2	—	36	23	1	3	5	8	*	2	7	10	64		
mandarin (Budget Gourmet Light & Healthy) 10 oz	240	25	8	5	13	13	—	30	7	2	2	—	—	25	25	10	15	35		
(Healthy Choice) 10 oz	240	35	3	3	15	12	—	15	10	2	10	—	—	25	15	10	8	20		
(Stouffer's Lean Cuisine) 9 3/4 oz	50	—	9	5	10	14	8	22	10	25	6	—	—	8	60	—	—	—		
marsala (Budget Gourmet) 9 oz	260	25	12	—	30	10	—	30	6	4	10	—	—	35	6	15	15	35		
(Weight Watchers) 8 oz	110	17	2	*	3	5	4	*	10	2	8	—	—	6	10	—	—	—		
w/ vegetables (Stouffer's Lean Cuisine) 8 1/8 oz	180	37	6	5	18	4	—	18	11	4	8	—	—	40	10	15	10	45		
mesquite (Chicken by George) 5 oz	170	42	9	5	23	2	—	33	21	2	7	6	10	3	1	9	12	71		
mirabella (Weight Watchers) 9 1/4 oz	160	20	2	*	3	8	20	20	10	4	8	—	—	15	25	—	—	—		
monterey homestyle (Stouffer's) 9 3/8 oz	410	—	31	45	25	12	16	29	10	35	6	—	—	10	15	—	—	—		
nibbles w/ french fries (Swanson) 4 1/4 oz	330	20	29	—	—	10	—	30	—	2	8	—	—	*	4	8	6	15		
nuggets (Banquet) 2.5 oz	200	17	20	—	—	3	—	22	4	*	4	—	—	*	2	4	6	8		
(Swanson) 3 oz	230	30	22	—	—	5	—	15	—	*	4	—	—	*	*	4	4	20		
hot 'n' spicy (Banquet) 2.5 oz	240	17	26	—	—	3	—	15	4	*	4	—	—	*	2	4	6	8		
southern fried (Banquet) 2.5 oz	210	17	22	—	—	4	—	21	4	*	2	—	—	*	2	4	4	8		
w/ cheddar (Banquet) 2.5 oz	240	17	26	—	—	3	—	22	3	8	2	—	—	*	2	2	6	6		
w/ french fries (Swanson) 4 3/4 oz	290	25	22	—	—	10	—	23	—	2	8	—	—	*	*	8	6	20		

CHICKEN ENTREE, FROZEN (continued)

	Calories	Protein	Fat	Sat. Fat	Cholesterol	Carbohydrates	Fiber	Sodium	Potassium	Calcium	Iron	Zinc	Magnesium	Vitamin A	Vitamin C	Thiamin	Riboflavin	Niacin	Vitamin B₁₂	Folic acid
orange glazed (Budget Gourmet Light & Healthy) 9 oz	270	25	5	5	8	15	—	36	10	2	4	—	—	10	15	10	8	35	—	—
oriental style (Healthy Choice) 9 1/2 oz	280	48	8	5	15	10	—	17	10	4	4	—	—	8	10	15	15	35	—	—
(Stouffer's Lean Cuisine) 9 oz	280	37	11	10	12	10	—	20	13	4	10	—	—	4	10	15	10	35	—	—
w/ vegetables (Budget Gourmet Light & Healthy) 9 oz	280	30	9	5	7	15	—	29	7	4	15	—	—	10	6	30	15	35	—	—
(Budget Gourmet Light & Healthy) 10 oz	280	15	11	5	3	16	—	25	9	6	4	—	—	25	25	15	15	20	—	—
parmigiana (Stouffer's Lean Cuisine) 10 7/8 oz	260	40	11	10	20	8	—	24	27	10	10	—	—	25	10	15	15	40	—	—
(Weight Watchers) 9 oz	230	32	9	15	17	8	8	20	18	15	10	—	—	8	8	—	—	—	—	—
patties (Banquet) 2.5 oz	190	18	18			4	—	18	5	*	2	—	—	*	*	4	*	15	—	—
southern fried (Banquet) 2.5 oz	200	17	18	—		4	—	25	4	*	2	—	—	*	*	6	2	15	—	—
piccata lemon herb (Weight Watchers) 7 1/2 oz	170	18	2	*	5	9	12	22	8	4	6	—	—	20	8	—	—	—	—	—
plump & juicy assortment (Swanson) 3 1/4 oz	270	35	25	—		5	—	27		*	*	—	—	*	*	6	8	20	—	—
pot pie (Mrs. Paterson's) 1 pie (5 1/2 oz)	440	22	37	40	27	14	—	32	9	3	9	9	6	30	1	24	16	25	—	—
(Stouffer's) 10 oz	520	37	51	40	23	12	12	42	11	8	10	—	—	50	4	20	25	25	—	—
(Swanson) 7 oz	390	20	35	—	—	8	—	32	—	2	10	—	—	25	*	15	10	15	—	—
(Swanson Hungry-Man) 16 oz	700	50	62	—	—	13	—	65	—	8	10	—	—	170	6	30	25	40	—	—
deluxe (Swanson) 9 oz	290	40	25	—	—	6	—	47	—	15	10	—	—	*	2	6	20	10	—	—
pot pie, w/ vegetables (Morton) 7 oz	420	23	43	—	12	9	—	31	5	2	10	—	—	6	*	20	15	30	—	—
w/ rice stir-fry (Stouffer's Lean Cuisine) 9 oz	80	—	14	5	5	13	12	25	9	4	4	—	—	35	25	—	—	—	—	—
roast glazed (Weight Watchers) 9 oz	200	28	8	13	5	8	16	21	17	8	8	—	—	4	2	—	—	—	—	—
sandwich (Hormel Quickmeal) 4 3/4 oz	300	35	14	—	20	12	—	26	—	6	10	—	—	2	*	50	15	40	—	—
(Kid Cuisine) 8 1/4 oz	470	27	26	—	13	20	—	35	10	10	15	—	—	6	4	20	20	30	—	—
(Weight Watchers) 4 oz	270	38	9	13	8	10	12	22	6	8	8	—	—	*	*	—	—	—	—	—
w/ broccoli & cheddar (Weight Watchers) 5 oz	250	22	9	13	8	13	4	13	6	6	4	—	—	10	4	—	—	—	—	—
southern fried (Weight Watchers) 8 oz	280	32	17	23	22	8	4	25	16	8	6	—	—	15	*	—	—	—	—	—
spicy fried (Swanson) 3 1/4 oz	290	30	28	—	—	6	—	25	—	*	8	—	—	*	*	6	6	15	—	—
sticks (Banquet) 2.5 oz	210	17	22	—	—	3	—	14	4	*	2	—	—	*	*	4	4	8	—	—
suiza (Weight Watchers) 8 1/2 oz	240	37	9	10	12	8	12	25	17	15	10	—	—	15	8	—	—	—	—	—
sweet & sour (Budget Gourmet) 10 oz	340	25	8	—	10	18	—	26	7	6	6	—	—	45	20	10	15	25	—	—

	Calories	Protein	Fat	Sat. Fat	Cholesterol	Carbohydrates	Fiber	Sodium	Potassium	Calcium	Iron	Zinc	Magnesium	Vitamin A	Vitamin C	Thiamin	Riboflavin	Niacin	Vitamin B₁₂	Folic acid
CHICKEN ENTREE, FROZEN (continued)																				
tenderloins																				
in herb cream sauce																				
(Stouffer's Lean Cuisine)																				
9 1/2 oz	240	48	8	10	20	6	—	20	21	15	4	—		20	8	15	20	40	—	—
in peanut sauce																				
(Stouffer's Lean Cuisine) 9 oz	290	38	11	10	15	11	—	22	14	8	10	—		8	8	20	20	30	—	—
teriyaki																				
(Chicken by George) 5 oz	180	42	8	5	23	3	—	31	21	1	4	6	9	*	4	7	10	66	—	—
tex-mex																				
(Weight Watchers) 8 1/3 oz	260	35	6	8	12	12	4	18	19	4	15	—		30	20				—	—
thighs & drumsticks																				
(Swanson) 3 1/4 oz	280	30	25	—		6	—	29	—	2	6	—		*	*	6	6	15	—	—
w/ vegetables																				
(Healthy Choice) 11 1/2 oz	280	40	5	5	8	13	—	16	11	4	15	—		15	15	20	10	20	—	—
(Stouffer's Lean Cuisine) 11 3/4 oz	240	30	8	5	10	10	—	21	14	8	10	—		15	10	20	15	30	—	—
Italian style																				
(Budget Gourmet Light & Healthy) 10 1/4 oz	310	20	12	10	10	17	—	29	7	8	4	—		40	15	15	90	15	—	—
w/ vegetables & teriyaki																				
(Weight Watchers) 9 oz	150	23	3	5	7	6	16	18	18	8	6	—		8	10	—	—	—	—	—
wing nibbles																				
(Swanson) 3 1/4 oz	300	25	29	—		6	—	29	—	2	8	—		*	*	8	6	15	—	—
CHICKEN GRAVY																				
canned																				
(Franco-American) 1/4 cup	45	*	6	—	—	*	*	10	—	*	*	—		*	*	*	*	*	—	—
(generic) 1/4 cup	47	2	5	—	*	*	*	29	2	*	*	3	*	5	*	*	*	*	*	*
golden																				
(Pepperidge Farm) 1/4 cup	25	4	2	—	—	*	*	15	—	*	*	—		*	*	*	6	*	—	—
w/ giblets																				
(Franco-American) 1/4 cup	30	*	3	—	—	*	*	13	—	*	*	—		*	*	*	*	*	—	—
from mix																				
(Pillsbury) 1/4 cup	25	*	*	*	*	*	*	7	*	2	*	—		*	*	*	*	*	*	*
(Weight Watchers) 1/4 cup	10	2	*	*	—	*	—	17	—	*	*	—		*	*	—	—	—	—	—
CHICKEN HOT DOG see **HOT DOG**																				
CHICKEN LIVER PATE																				
(generic) 1 oz	57	6	6	6	37	*	*	5	*	*	14	4	*	4	5	*	23	11	38	23
CHICKEN SALAD																				
canned																				
(Libby's) 2 oz	90	10	9	5	5	2	*	10	2	*	*	2	2	*	*	*	2	6	*	*
CHICKEN SPREAD																				
canned																				
(generic) 2 oz	108	14	10	10	10	*	*	8	*	8	8	4	*	*	*	*	4	8	*	*
light, chunky																				
(Underwood) 2 1/8 oz	100	18	8	5	10	*	*	14	3	*	5	—	—	*	*	*	2	10	—	—
regular																				
(Underwood) 2 1/8 oz	150	17	14	15	13	*	*	18	3	*	4	—	—	*	*	*	2	10	—	—
CHICORY GREENS																				
raw																				
1/2 cup chopped	21	3	*	*	*	*	16	2	11	9	4	3	7	72	36	4	5	2	*	25
CHICORY ROOT																				
raw																				
1/2 cup	7	*	—	—	*	—	—	*	*	*	*	*	*	*	*	*	*	*	*	*
1 root	44	*	*	*	*	3	—	*	5	2	3	*	3	*	5	2	*	*	*	3
CHICORY, WITLOOF																				
raw																				
1/2 cup	8	*	*	*	*	*	4	*	3	*	*	*	*	*	2	2	*	*	*	4

	Calories	Protein	Fat	Sat. Fat	Cholesterol	Carbohydrates	Fiber	Sodium	Potassium	Calcium	Iron	Zinc	Magnesium	Vitamin A	Vitamin C	Thiamin	Riboflavin	Niacin	Vitamin B12	Folic acid
CHILI, CANNED																				
(Gebhardt) 1 cup	530	35	66	80	50	7	4	41	19	6	28	—	—	*	11	14	34	19	—	—
w/ beans																				
(Chef Boyardee) 7 1/2 oz	330	25	26	—	—	10	—	42	—	6	20	—	—	20	4	8	10	6	—	—
(generic) 1/2 cup	143	12	11	15	7	5	24	28	13	6	24	17	14	9	4	4	8	2	*	7
(Just Rite) 1 cup	200	33	17	20	11	5	4	21	12	4	12	—	—	*	4	9	8	10	—	—
(Libby's) 1 cup	420	27	42	65	17	10	16	50	—	6	20	—	—	15	*	—	—	—	—	—
(Libby's) 7 3/4 oz	360	25	38	55	12	8	36	43	—	6	15	—	—	15	2	—	—	—	—	—
(Old El Paso) 1 cup	217	25	15	—	11	6	24	20	16	4	20	—	—	55	—	10	10	10	—	—
hot																				
(Gebhardt) 1 cup	470	27	42	49	22	16	24	42	41	10	36	—	—	*	40	29	18	22	—	—
(Just Rite) 1 cup	195	37	15	18	11	5	4	21	13	4	13	—	—	*	4	9	8	8	—	—
mild																				
(Gebhardt) 1 cup	495	33	43	50	31	16	24	42	42	10	41	—	—	*	40	30	30	25	—	—
(Hormel) 7 1/2 oz	300	25	23	25	18	9	—	43	22	6	16	14	14	21	*	6	10	9	—	—
w/ out beans																				
(Just Rite) 1 cup	180	43	17	19	14	3	*	21	11	3	12	—	—	*	5	5	9	17	—	—
hot																				
(Hormel) 7 1/2 oz	360	27	42	55	20	5	—	36	14	5	14	18	10	33	*	3	13	13	—	—
(Hormel) 7 1/2 oz	360	27	42	55	20	5	—	36	14	5	14	18	10	33	*	3	13	13	—	—
(Libby's) 1 cup	280	35	57	85	25	5	4	66	—	8	20	—	—	25	*	—	—	—	—	—
chili-mac																				
(Chef Boyardee) 7 1/2 oz	230	13	17	—	7	9	—	59	—	*	—	—	—	15	2	10	15	10	—	—
vegetarian																				
mild																				
(Health Valley) 7 1/2 oz	105	23	*	*	*	5	48	11	16	12	30	—	—	150	6	15	23	12	—	—
w/ black beans																				
(Health Valley) 7 1/2 oz	105	15	*	*	*	4	48	11	16	9	23	—	—	150	6	12	23	12	—	—
spicy																				
(Health Valley) 7 1/2 oz	105	15	*	*	*	4	48	11	16	9	23	—	—	150	6	12	23	12	—	—
CHILI, FROM MIX																				
(Manwich Chili Fixin's) 1 cup prepared	290	33	22	27	22	7	20	41	2	6	25	—	—	*	24	13	10	25	—	—
CHILI, FROZEN																				
w/ beans																				
con carne																				
(Stouffer's) 1 cup	270	33	15	20	12	10	32	47	19	10	15	—	—	15	6	10	15	15	—	—
microwave																				
(Hormel Micro Cup) 7 1/3 oz	250	25	17	20	16	8	—	41	19	6	19	18	13	19	*	9	9	9	—	—
(Hormel Micro Cup) 7 1/3 oz	250	25	17	20	16	8	—	41	19	6	19	18	13	19	*	9	9	9	—	—
w/ out beans																				
microwave																				
(Hormel Micro Cup) 7 1/3 oz	290	30	26	40	20	5	—	35	14	6	16	26	10	40	*	5	14	13	—	—
chili mac																				
microwave																				
(Hormel Micro Cup) 7 1/2 oz	192	17	14	20	7	6	—	41	13	—	15	14	10	21	*	5	10	11	—	—
turkey w/ beans																				
(Healthy Choice) 7 1/2 oz	200	30	8	—	15	7	—	23	22	6	15	—	—	30	20	15	15	15	—	—
microwave																				
(Healthy Choice) 7 1/2 oz	200	30	8	—	15	7	—	23	22	6	15	—	—	30	20	15	15	15	—	—
CHILI POWDER																				
(Gebhardt) 1 tbsp	40	*	*	*	*	*	*	*	6	*	6	*	*	*	*	*	*	*	—	—
(generic) 1 tbsp	24	2	2	31	*	*	12	3	4	2	6	*	3	52	8	2	4	3	*	—
CHILI SAUCE																				
(Del Monte) 1 tbsp	20	*	*	*	*	2	*	20	—	*	*	—	—	10	2	—	—	—	—	—
CHILI SEASONING MIX																				
(Gebhardt Chili Quik) 1 tbsp	30	*	*	*	*	*	*	21	*	*	6	—	—	*	*	*	*	*	—	—
(Hain) 1/4 pkg	30	2	2	—	*	2	*	12	3	4	2	*	*	*	10	*	*	4	*	*
(Old El Paso) 1/5 pkg	21	2	2	—	*	*	4	30	2	2	4	—	—	6	2	*	—	—	—	—

	Calories	Protein	Fat	Sat. Fat	Cholesterol	Carbohydrates	Fiber	Sodium	Potassium	Calcium	Iron	Zinc	Magnesium	Vitamin A	Vitamin C	Thiamin	Riboflavin	Niacin	Vitamin B₁₂	Folic acid
CHIVES																				
raw																				
1 tbsp chopped	1	*	*	*	*	*	*	*	*	*	*	*	*	3	3	*	*	*	*	*
freeze-dried																				
1 tbsp	1	*	*	*	*	*	—	*	*	*	*	*	*	3	2	*	*	*	*	*
CHOCOLATE, BAKING																				
liquid																				
(Nestlé Choco-Bake) 1 oz	160	4	24	50	*	4	24	*	—	*	8	—	*	*	*	*	—	—	—	—
semi-sweet																				
(Baker's) 1 oz	140	2	14	—	*	6	*	*	3	*	6	4	10	*	*	*	*	*	—	—
(Nestlé) 1 oz	140	*	12	26	*	6	16	*	—	*	4	—	—	*	*	—	—	—	—	—
made w/ butter																				
(generic) 1 oz	101	*	10	19	*	5	—	*	2	*	4	2	6	*	*	*	*	*	*	*
sweet																				
(German's) 1 oz	140	*	15	—	*	6	*	*	2	*	4	2	6	*	*	*	*	*	—	—
unsweetened																				
(Baker's) 1 oz	140	4	23	—	*	3	*	*	7	2	10	*	20	*	*	*	*	4	2	—	—
(Hershey's) 1 oz	185	2	25	49	*	2	—	*	7	*	11	8	21	*	*	*	7	*	*	*
(Nestlé) 1 oz	160	6	22	20	*	4	24	*	—	*	8	—	*	*	*	—	—	—	—	—
liquid																				
(generic) 1 packet	134	6	21	36	*	3	—	*	9	2	7	7	19	*	*	*	2	3	*	*
square																				
(generic) 1 square	148	5	24	46	*	3	16	*	7	2	10	8	22	*	*	2	3	2	*	*
white																				
(generic) 1 bar	453	9	40	76	6	17	*	3	7	18	*	5	*	4	*	3	14	*	11	3
(Nestlé) 1 oz	160	4	16	30	*	6	*	*	—	8	*	—	—	*	*	—	—	—	—	—
chips																				
(generic) 1 cup	906	17	80	151	12	35	*	6	15	35	2	10	2	7	*	6	28	*	21	6
CHOCOLATE BAR *see* **CANDY BAR**																				
CHOCOLATE CANDY *see* **CANDY**																				
CHOCOLATE CHIPS																				
w/ butter																				
(generic) 1 oz	136	2	13	25	2	6	—	*	3	*	5	3	8	—	*	*	2	*	*	*
milk																				
(Baker's) 1 oz	140	2	12	—	*	6	*	*	3	4	*	*	4	*	*	*	4	*	—	—
(Nestlé) 1 oz	140	2	12	20	*	6	*	*	—	*	4	—	—	*	*	—	—	—	—	—
mint																				
(Nestlé) 1 oz	140	2	12	20	*	6	16	*	—	*	4	—	—	*	*	—	—	—	—	—
rainbow																				
(Nestlé) 1 oz	140	2	10	20	*	6	8	*	—	*	4	—	—	*	*	—	—	—	—	—
semi-sweet																				
(Baker's) 1/4 cup	200	2	17	—	*	9	*	*	4	*	6	4	10	*	*	*	2	*	—	—
(generic) 1 oz	136	2	13	25	*	6	—	*	3	*	5	3	8	—	*	*	2	*	*	*
(Nestlé) 1 oz	140	*	12	20	*	6	16	*	—	*	4	—	—	*	*	—	—	—	—	—
chocolate flavored																				
(Baker's) 1 oz	140	*	10	—	*	4	*	*	4	4	3	*	6	*	*	*	4	*	—	—
w/ butter																				
(generic) 1 oz	136	2	13	25	2	6	—	*	3	*	5	3	8	—	*	*	2	*	*	*
minis																				
(Nestlé) 1 oz	140	*	12	20	*	6	16	*	—	*	4	—	—	*	*	—	—	—	—	—
CHOCOLATE MILK																				
from mix																				
(generic) 1 cup milk + 2-3 heaping tsp	226	15	14	*	11	10	*	7	14	30	4	9	13	6	4	7	25	2	15	3
(Quik) 2 tbsp & 1 cup low fat milk	210	16	8	16	6	10	4	6	—	30	*	7	9	10	—	7	*	*	16	22
chocolate malt unfortified																				
(generic) 1 cup milk + 3 heaping tsp	228	15	14	*	11	10	*	7	14	30	3	7	12	7	4	9	26	3	15	4

	Calories	Protein	Fat	Sat. Fat	Cholesterol	Carbohydrates	Fiber	Sodium	Potassium	Calcium	Iron	Zinc	Magnesium	Vitamin A	Vitamin C	Thiamin	Riboflavin	Niacin	Vitamin B₁₂	Folic acid
CHOCOLATE MILK continued																				
malt fortified (generic) 1 cup milk + 4–5 heaping tsp	225	15	13	*	11	10	*	10	18	38	21	8	13	61	57	49	74	55	15	8
ready-to-drink lowfat, 1% (generic) 1 cup	158	13	4	8	2	9	*	6	12	29	3	7	8	10	4	6	*	2	14	3
lowfat, 2% (generic) 1 cup	179	13	8	16	6	9	16	6	12	28	3	7	8	10	4	6	*	2	14	3
whole (generic) 1 cup	208	13	13	27	10	9	16	6	12	28	3	7	8	6	4	6	*	2	14	3
from syrup fortified (generic) 1 cup milk + 2 tbsp syrup	197	14	13	*	11	8	*	6	13	29	15	6	8	23	4	6	32	33	14	3
unfortified (generic) 1 cup milk + 1 tbsp syrup	231	15	13	*	11	11	*	6	13	30	5	8	14	6	4	6	24	2	15	3
CHOCOLATE SYRUP																				
(Bosco) 2 tbsp	75	*	*	*	*	9	*	*	—	*	*	—	*	*	*	*	—	—	—	*
(generic) 2 tbsp	73	2	4	6	*	4	*	*	*	2	*	*	3	*	*	*	3	*	*	*
CHOCOLATE TOPPING																				
(Kraft) 2 tbsp	100	*	*	*	*	8	*	*	*	*	*	—	—	*	*	*	4	*	—	—
chocolate flavored (Smucker's) 2 tbsp	130	2	*	*	*	9	*	*	—	*	2	*	*	*	*	*	*	*	—	*
dark (Smucker's Special Recipe) 2 tbsp	130	2	2	—	*	10	*	2	—	2	*	*	*	*	*	*	2	*	*	*
fudge (Hershey's) 2 tbsp	95	2	6	*	*	5	*	3	3	2	2	4	*	*	*	*	4	*	—	*
(Smucker's) 2 tbsp	130	2	2	—	*	10	*	2	—	2	*	*	*	*	*	*	2	*	—	*
magic shell (Smucker's) 2 tbsp	190	2	23	—	*	5	*	—	—	*	*	*	*	*	*	*	*	*	—	*
fudge (Smucker's) 2 tbsp	190	2	23	—	*	5	*	2	—	*	*	*	*	*	*	*	*	*	—	*
nut (Smucker's) 2 tbsp	200	3	25	—	*	8	*	2	—	*	*	*	*	*	*	*	*	2	—	*
Swiss milk (Smucker's) 2 tbsp	140	5	2	—	*	10	*	3	—	4	*	*	*	*	*	*	6	*	—	*
CHORIZO																				
pork & beef (generic) 1 oz	129	11	17	21	8	*	*	15	3	*	3	6	*	*	*	*	12	5	7	9	*
CHOW MEIN, CANNED																				
beef (La Choy) 3/4 cup	40	8	3	4	5	2	8	40	4	8	8	—	—	*	2	4	6	6	—	—
bi-pack (La Choy) 3/4 cup	70	12	2	*	7	3	4	35	7	2	8	—	—	*	18	2	4	6	—	—
chicken (La Choy) 3/4 cup	70	10	6	5	5	2	8	35	5	8	6	—	—	*	3	4	6	6	—	—
pork bi-pack (La Choy) 3/4 cup	80	8	6	7	5	2	8	40	8	2	4	—	—	*	12	4	4	6	—	—
CHOW MEIN, CANNED																				
shrimp (La Choy) 3/4 cup	35	7	2	*	17	*	8	39	8	8	4	—	—	*	6	2	2	2	—	—
bi-pack (La Choy) 3/4 cup	70	12	2	*	6	2	4	36	6	4	6	—	—	*	15	4	4	4	—	—
vegetarian (La Choy) 3/4 cup	25	2	*	*	*	2	8	36	5	6	4	—	—	*	5	2	2	2	—	—

	Calories	Protein	Fat	Sat. Fat	Cholesterol	Carbohydrates	Fiber	Sodium	Potassium	Calcium	Iron	Zinc	Magnesium	Vitamin A	Vitamin C	Thiamin	Riboflavin	Niacin	Vitamin B$_{12}$	Folic acid
CHOW MEIN, FROZEN																				
chicken																				
(Chun King) 13 oz	370	42	9	—	28	18	—	65	7	2	10	—		10	6	100	10	15	—	—
(Healthy Choice) 9 oz	240	33	8	10	15	10	—	22	8	2	8	—		8	6	10	8	20	—	—
(Light & Elegant) 9 oz	180	17	3	—	10	10	—	27	5	2	6	—		*	8	8	10	8	—	—
(Stouffer's) 10 5/8 oz	260	22	6	5	10	14	12	39	8	2	6	—		6	10	2	10	10	—	—
(Stouffer's Lean Cuisine) 9 oz	240	23	8	5	10	11	—	22	10	4	6	—		6	10	10	10	25	—	—
(Stouffer's Lunch Express) 10 5/8 oz	35	—	6	5	10	14	12	39	8	2	6	—		6	10	—	—	—	—	—
(Weight Watchers) 9 oz	200	22	2	*	7	11	24	20	10	4	8	—		10	35	—	—	—	—	—
CHRYSANTHEMUM																				
raw																				
1/2 cup	2	*	*	*	*	*	*	*	2	*	2	*	*	38	8	*	2	*	*	3
boiled																				
1/2 cup	10	*	*	*	*	*	4	*	8	3	10	*	2	51	20	*	5	2	*	6
boiled w/ salt																				
1/2 cup	10	*	*	*	*	*	—	6	8	3	10	*	2	51	20	*	5	2	*	6
CILANTRO see **CORIANDER, FRESH**																				
CINNAMON, GROUND																				
1 tbsp	18	*	*	*	*	2	16	*	*	8	14	*	*	*	3	*	*	*	*	—
CINNAMON ROLL																				
97% fat free																				
(Hostess) 1 roll	120	3	2	3	*	9	5	5	*	10	6	—	—	*	*	8	6	4	—	—
frozen																				
(Pepperidge Farm) 1 roll	280	—	22	*	*	11	—	8	—	2	6	—	—	*	*	10	6	10	—	—
(Rich's) 1 roll	310	5	29	20	3	11	8	4	*	9	17	*	2	*	2	7	65	*	—	—
(Weight Watchers) 1 roll	180	7	8	5	2	10	12	7	2	4	4	—	—	*	*	—	—	—	—	—
w/ icing																				
from refrigerated dough																				
(Pillsbury) 1 roll	110	2	8	5	*	6	—	11	*	*	2	—	—	*	*	4	2	2	—	—
minis																				
original																				
(Hostess Cinnaminis) 4 rolls	300	5	26	20	7	12	4	10	*	2	8	—	—	*	*	10	15	8	—	—
pecan																				
(Hostess Cinnaminis) 4 rolls	300	5	26	20	7	12	4	8	*	2	8	—	—	*	*	10	15	8	—	—
sweet																				
(Hostess) 1 roll	140	5	6	10	7	8	4	7	*	10	6	—	—	*	*	8	6	6	—	—
CISCO																				
raw																				
1 fillet	77	25	2	*	13	*	*	2	8	*	2	2	3	2	*	5	5	10	13	*
smoked																				
3 oz	150	23	16	8	9	*	*	17	7	2	2	2	4	16	*	3	8	10	60	*
CITRUS DRINK see also **FRUIT PUNCH & FRUIT DRINK**																				
Citrus Cruz, organic																				
(Santa Cruz Natural) 8 fl oz	120	2	*	*	*	9	*	*	5	4	*			20	8	—	—	—	—	—
CITRUS-CRANBERRY DRINK																				
(Ocean Spray Refreshers) 8 fl oz	140	—	*	*	*	12	*	*	*	*	*			*	100	—	—	—	—	—
CITRUS-PEACH DRINK																				
(Ocean Spray Refreshers) 8 fl oz	120	—	*	*	*	10	*	*	2	*	*	—	—	6	100	—	—	—	—	—
CLAM																				
raw																				
9 lg or 20 sm clams	133	38	3	*	20	2	*	4	16	8	140	16	4	11	39	10	23	16	1477	*
breaded & fried																				
20 small clams	380	45	32	25	38	6	—	28	17	12	145	18	7	11	31	13	27	19	1257	*
steamed/poached																				
20 small clams	133	38	3	*	20	2	*	4	16	8	140	16	4	10	33	9	23	15	1477	*

PERCENTAGE DAILY VALUE

	Calories	Protein	Fat	Sat. Fat	Cholesterol	Carbohydrates	Fiber	Sodium	Potassium	Calcium	Iron	Zinc	Magnesium	Vitamin A	Vitamin C	Thiamin	Riboflavin	Niacin	Vitamin B12	Folic acid
CLAM, CANNED																				
minced																				
(generic) 1/2 cup	118	17	*	*	9	*	*	2	4	4	62	7	2	5	15	4	10	7	1313	*
(Gorton's) 1/2 can	40	12	*	*	7	*	—	25	*	*	8	—	—	*	*	2	2	2	—	—
(Progresso) 1/2 cup	90	30	2	*	15	*	*	17	*	*	15	*	*	*	*	*	*	*	—	—
CLAM, FROZEN																				
fried																				
(Mrs. Paul's) 2 1/2 oz	200	28	14	5	5	7	*	19	—	*	6			*	*	15	6	6		
strips, microwave																				
(Gorton's) 1/2 package (3 oz)	270	15	26	25	8	7	*	15	—	*	6			*	*	2	2	2		
CLAM DIP																				
(Kraft) 2 tbsp	60	*	6	5	3	*	*	10	*	*	*			*	*	*	*	*		
premium																				
(Kraft) 2 tbsp	45	2	6	10	7	*	*	9	*	2				2	*	*	2	*		
CLAM SAUCE *see* **PASTA SAUCE**																				
CLOVES, GROUND																				
1 tbsp	21	*	2	*	*	*	8	*	2	4	3	*	4	*	9	*	*	*	*	—
COCKTAIL SAUCE																				
(Del Monte) 1 tbsp	13	*	*	*	*	*	*	5	—	*	*			3	*	—	—	—		
(Sauceworks) 1 tbsp	14	*	*	*	*	*	*	7	2	*	*			2	2	—	—	—		
COCOA DRINK																				
(homemade) 8 fl oz	193	16	9	18	7	10	12	5	14	32	6	10	18	10	4	7	26	2	15	25
COCOA DRINK, FROM MIX																				
(Kayo) 6 fl oz	100	2	—	—	—	8	*	9	3	*	2	*	*	*	*	*	—	*	*	*
(Weight Watchers) 1 packet	70	10	*	*	*	3	4	7	11	*	*	—	—	6	*	—	—	—	—	—
Bavarian chocolate																				
(Swiss Miss) 6 fl oz	110	2	5	7	*	7	*	7	4	4	4			*	*	*	4	*		
diet																				
(Swiss Miss) 6 fl oz	20	3	*	*	*	*	*	7	5	8	2	—	—	*	*	2	8	*	—	—
double rich																				
(Swiss Miss) 6 fl oz	110	3	2	3	*	7	*	6	4	6	4			*	*	*	6	*		
fortified																				
(generic) 6 fl oz & 1/2 oz pkt	119	3	4	*	*	8	*	9	12	10	10	2	6	10	10	10	10	10	7	*
lite																				
(Kayo) 6 fl oz	50	8	2	—	—	3	*	8	9	*	2	*	*	*	*	*	—	*	*	*
(Swiss Miss) 6 fl oz	70	2	*	*	*	6	*	7	6	4	*	—	—	*	*	*	4	*	—	—
low-calorie																				
(generic) 6 fl oz	48	6	*	*	*	3	*	7	12	9	4	4	8	*	*	3	12	*	5	*
prep. w/ milk																				
(generic) 6 fl oz	48	6	*	*	*	3	*	4	12	22	4	4	8	5	*	3	12	*	5	*
w/ mini marshmallows																				
(Swiss Miss) 6 fl oz	110	2	2	2	2	8	*	7	6	2	2	—	—	*	*	*	6	*	—	—
w/ marshmallows																				
(Weight Watchers) 1 packet	70	10	*	*	*	3	4	6	11	*	*	—	—	6	*	—	—	—	—	—
milk chocolate flavor																				
(Swiss Miss) 6 fl oz	110	3	2	2	2	8	*	5	4	4	2	—	—	*	*	*	5	*	—	—
sugar free																				
(Swiss Miss) 6 fl oz	60	5	*	*	*	3	*	5	5	8	2	—	—	*	*	*	10	*	—	—
sugar free w/ sugar free marshmallows																				
(Swiss Miss) 6 fl oz	50	5	*	*	*	3	*	5	6	8	2	—	—	*	*	*	10	*	—	—
Swiss style																				
(Kayo) 6 fl oz	100	—	—	—	—	8	*	5	3	6	2	*	*	*	*	*	—	*	*	*
unfortified																				
(generic) 6 fl oz & 3–4 heaping tsp	95	5	*	*	*	7	*	6	6	9	2	3	6	*	*	2	9	*	6	*
COCOA POWDER																				
(generic) 1 tbsp	11	2	*	2	*	*	8	*	2	*	4	2	6	*	*	*	*	*	*	—
(Nestlé) 1 oz (1/3 cup)	80	10	8	—	*	2	40	*	15	4	25	—	—	*	*	4	2	2	—	—

	Calories	Protein	Fat	Sat. Fat	Cholesterol	Carbohydrates	Fiber	Sodium	Potassium	Calcium	Iron	Zinc	Magnesium	Vitamin A	Vitamin C	Thiamin	Riboflavin	Niacin	Vitamin B12	Folic acid
COCOA POWDER (continued)																				
alkali process (generic) 1 tbsp	11	2	*	2	*	*	4	*	4	*	4	2	6	*	*	*	*	*	*	*
baking (Nestlé) 1 tbsp	15	2	2	*	*	*	8	*	—	*	—	*	*	*	*	—	—	—	—	—
European style (generic) 1 tbsp	10	2	*	*	*	*	—	*	7	*	10	2	7	*	*	*	*	*	*	*
COCONUT																				
creamed (generic) 1 oz	194	3	30	87	*	2	—	*	4	*	5	4	7	*	*	*	2	*	*	*
flaked sweetened (generic) 1 cup	351	4	37	106	*	12	12	8	7	*	7	9	9	*	*	*	*	*	*	2
shredded bag (Baker's) 1/3 cup	120	*	12	—	*	3	*	3	2	*	2	*	2	*	*	*	*	*	—	—
can (Baker's) 1/3 cup	110	*	14	—	*	3	*	2	2	*	2	*	2	*	*	*	*	*	—	—
premium (Baker's) 1/3 cup	140	*	14	—	*	4	*	4	2	*	2	*	2	*	*	*	*	*	*	*
sweetened (generic) 1 cup	466	4	51	147	*	15	16	10	9	*	10	11	12	*	*	2	*	2	*	2
toasted (generic) 1 oz	168	3	20	59	*	4	—	*	4	*	5	4	7	*	*	*	2	*	*	*
COCONUT CREAM																				
raw 1 cup	792	15	128	369	*	5	—	*	22	3	30	15	17	*	11	5	*	11	*	14
canned 1 cup	568	13	81	233	*	8	28	6	9	*	8	12	13	*	9	4	7	*	*	11
COCONUT MILK																				
raw 1 cup	552	9	88	254	*	4	20	*	18	4	22	11	22	*	11	4	*	9	*	10
canned 1 cup	445	8	74	214	*	2	—	*	14	4	41	8	26	*	4	3	*	7	*	8
frozen 1 cup	485	6	77	222	*	4	—	*	16	*	11	9	19	*	4	4	*	8	*	9
COCONUT NECTAR (Knudsen Tropical Blend) 8 fl oz	140	2	*	*	*	9	*	2	2	*	—	*	*	*	*	*	—	—	—	—
COCONUT OIL 1 tbsp	117	*	5	59	*	*	*	*	*	*	*	*	*	*	*	*	*	*	*	*
COCONUT WATER 1 cup	46	3	*	2	*	3	12	10	17	6	4	2	15	*	10	5	8	*	*	2
COD, ATLANTIC																				
raw 1 fillet	189	69	2	*	33	*	*	5	27	4	5	7	18	2	4	12	9	24	35	*
baked/broiled 1 fillet	189	68	2	*	33	*	*	6	13	3	5	7	19	2	3	11	8	23	31	*
dried & salted 3 oz	247	89	3	2	43	*	*	248	35	14	12	9	28	2	5	15	12	32	141	*
COD, PACIFIC																				
raw 1 fillet	95	35	*	*	14	*	*	3	13	*	2	3	7	*	6	2	3	12	17	*
broiled/baked 1 fillet	95	34	*	*	14	*	*	3	13	*	2	3	7	*	4	*	3	11	16	*
COD, CANNED																				
Atlantic (generic) 1/2 can	164	30	*	*	14	*	*	7	12	2	2	8	*	*	*	5	4	10	27	*
cakes (Gorton's) 2 cakes	100	13	*	*	5	5	—	27	9	2	4	—	—	*	*	*	2	4	—	—

	Calories	Protein	Fat	Sat. Fat	Cholesterol	Carbohydrates	Fiber	Sodium	Potassium	Calcium	Iron	Zinc	Magnesium	Vitamin A	Vitamin C	Thiamin	Riboflavin	Niacin	Vitamin B$_{12}$	Folic acid
COD, FROZEN																				
fillet (Mrs. Paul's Light) 4 1/4 oz	240	30	17	10	17	7	*	18	—	2	6	—	—	*	*	10	8	10	—	—
light (Van de Kamp's) 1 fillet	250	28	17	10	12	7	—	21	7	2	8	—	—	*	*	15	15	15	—	—
lemon thyme seasoned (Gorton's Select) 1 fillet	90	20	3	—	13	2	—	11	—	2	*	—	—	*	*	2	2	6	—	—
COD LIVER OIL																				
1 tbsp	123	*	20	16	26	*	*	*	*	*	*	*	*	*	*	—	*	*	*	*
COFFEE																				
(generic) 6 fl oz	4	*	*	*	*	*	*	*	3	*	*	*	2	*	*	*	*	2	*	*
from mix cappuccino (Superior) 6 fl oz	120	*	6	—	*	8	*	6	—	*	*	*	*	*	*	*	—	*	*	*
instant (generic) 6 fl oz & 1 tsp	4	*	*	*	*	*	*	*	2	*	*	*	2	*	*	*	*	3	*	*
decaffinated (generic) 6 fl oz & 1 tsp	4	*	*	*	*	*	*	*	2	*	*	*	2	*	*	*	*	3	*	*
COFFEE, FLAVORED																				
amaretto (General Foods) 6 fl oz	50	*	5	—	*	2	*	4	4	*	*	*	*	*	*	*	*	4	*	*
cappuccino prep. w/ water (generic) 6 fl oz & 2 tsp	61	*	3	—	*	4	*	4	3	*	*	*	2	*	*	*	*	2	*	*
cappuccino, hot cinnamon (Maxwell House) 6 fl oz	60	2	2	—	—	4	*	4	4	4	*	—	—	*	*	*	2	*	—	—
coffee (Maxwell House) 6 fl oz	60	*	2	—	—	4	*	5	4	2	*	—	—	*	*	*	2	2	—	—
mocha (Maxwell House) 6 fl oz	70	2	3	—	—	4	*	3	4	4	*	—	—	*	*	*	2	*	—	—
cappuccino, iced cinnamon (Maxwell House Cappio) 8 fl oz	130	4	5	—	—	8	*	3	8	8	*	—	—	*	*	*	8	*	—	—
coffee (Maxwell House Cappio) 8 fl oz	120	4	5	—	—	8	*	3	9	8	*	—	—	*	*	*	8	*	—	—
mocha (Maxwell House Cappio) 8 fl oz	130	4	3	—	—	8	*	3	8	8	*	—	—	*	*	*	8	*	—	—
w/ chicory (generic) 6 fl oz & 1 tsp	7	*	*	*	*	*	*	*	2	*	*	*	*	*	*	*	*	2	*	*
Double Dutch Chocolate (General Foods) 6 fl oz	50	*	3	—	*	3	*	*	4	*	*	*	*	*	*	*	*	—	*	*
Francais (General Foods) 6 fl oz	60	*	5	—	*	2	*	*	7	*	*	*	*	*	*	*	*	4	*	*
French prep. w/ water (generic) 6 fl oz & 2 tsp	57	*	5	*	*	2	*	*	4	*	*	*	*	*	*	*	*	3	*	*
French vanilla (General Foods) 6 fl oz	60	*	5	—	*	3	*	2	3	*	*	*	*	*	*	*	*	—	*	*
Hazelnut Belgian (General Foods) 6 fl oz	60	*	3	—	*	3	*	2	3	*	*	*	*	*	*	*	*	2	*	*
mocha prep. w/ water (generic) 6 fl oz & 2 tsp	56	*	3	—	*	3	*	2	4	*	*	*	3	*	*	*	*	*	*	*
orange cappuccino (General Foods) 6 fl oz	60	*	3	—	*	3	*	4	4	*	*	*	*	*	*	*	*	*	*	*
sugar-free (General Foods) 6 fl oz	30	*	3	—	*	*	*	2	4	*	*	*	*	*	*	*	*	2	*	*

PERCENTAGE DAILY VALUE

	Calories	Protein	Fat	Sat. Fat	Cholesterol	Carbohydrates	Fiber	Sodium	Potassium	Calcium	Iron	Zinc	Magnesium	Vitamin A	Vitamin C	Thiamin	Riboflavin	Niacin	Vitamin B$_{12}$	Folic acid
COFFEE, FLAVORED (continued)																				
Suisse mocha (General Foods) 6 fl oz	50	*	5	—	*	2	*	2	4	*	*	*	*	*	*	*	*	*	*	*
decaffeinated (General Foods) 6 fl oz	50	*	5	—	*	2	*	2	4	*	*	*	*	*	*	*	*	*	*	*
decaffeinated and sugar-free (General Foods) 6 fl oz	30	*	3	—	*	*	*	*	4	*	*	*	*	*	*	*	*	*	*	*
sugar-free (General Foods) 6 fl oz	30	*	3	—	*	*	*	2	3	*	*	*	*	*	*	*	*	*	*	*
Viennese chocolate (General Foods) 6 fl oz	50	*	3	—	*	3	*	*	2	*	*	*	*	*	*	*	*	—	*	*
Vienna (General Foods) 6 fl oz	60	*	3	—	*	3	*	4	4	*	*	*	*	*	*	*	*	4	*	*
sugar-free (General Foods) 6 fl oz	30	*	3	—	*	*	*	3	3	*	*	*	*	*	*	*	*	2	*	*
COFFEE CAKE *see* **CAKE, SNACK**																				
COFFEE CREAMER																				
liquid (generic) 1/2 oz	20	*	2	7	*	*	*	*	*	*	*	*	*	*	*	*	*	*	*	*
(N-Rich) 1/2 oz	20	*	*	*	*	*	*	*	*	*	*	*	*	*	*	*	*	*	*	*
non-dairy (Farm Rich) 1/2 oz	20	*	3	*	*	*	*	*	*	*	*	*	*	*	*	*	*	*	*	*
light (Farm Rich Light) 1/2 oz	10	*	*	*	*	*	*	*	*	*	*	*	*	*	*	*	*	*	*	*
soybean based (generic) 1/2 oz	20	*	2	*	*	*	*	*	*	*	*	*	*	*	*	*	*	*	*	*
powder (generic) 1/2 oz	22	*	*	8	*	*	*	*	*	*	*	*	*	*	*	*	*	*	*	*
kosher (Coffee Rich) 1/2 oz	25	*	3	*	*	*	*	*	*	*	*	*	*	*	*	*	*	*	*	*
light (Coffee Rich) 1/2 oz	12	*	*	*	*	*	*	*	*	*	*	*	*	*	*	*	*	*	*	*
COFFEE SUBSTITUTE *see* **GRAIN BEVERAGE**																				
COLD CUTS *see* **SPECIFIC MEATS**																				
COLESLAW																				
1/2 cup	41	*	2	*	2	2	—	*	3	3	2	*	*	8	33	3	2	*	*	4
COLLARD GREENS																				
raw 1/2 cup chopped	6	*	*	*	*	*	*	4	*	*	*	*	*	12	7	*	*	*	*	*
boiled 1/2 cup chopped	17	*	*	*	*	*	*	4	*	2	*	*	*	35	13	*	2	*	*	*
boiled w/ salt 1/2 cup chopped	17	*	*	*	*	*	—	7	2	*	*	*	*	35	13	*	2	*	*	*
canned (Bush Bros) 1/2 cup	30	3	*	*	*	*	8	17	—	15	4	—		70	15	—	—	—	*	—
frozen *boiled* (generic) 1/2 cup chopped	31	4	*	*	*	2	—	2	6	18	5	2	6	102	37	3	6	3	*	16
boiled w/ salt (generic) 1/2 cup chopped	31	4	*	*	*	2	—	10	6	18	5	2	6	102	37	3	6	3	*	16
COOKIE																				
Almond Toast (Stella d'Oro) 2 cookies	110	3	4	—	10	7	—	4	—	—	—	—	—	—	—	—	—	—	—	—
Angel Bar (Stella d'Oro) 2 cookies	150	3	15	—	*	5	—	*	—	—	—	—	—	—	—	—	—	—	—	—
Angel Wing (Stella d'Oro) 2 cookies	140	3	14	—	*	4	—	3	—	—	—	—	—	—	—	—	—	—	—	—
Angelica Goodie (Stella d'Oro) 1 cookie	100	3	6	—	5	5	—	2	—	—	—	—	—	—	—	—	—	—	—	—

COOKIE (continued)

	Calories	Protein	Fat	Sat. Fat	Cholesterol	Carbohydrates	Fiber	Sodium	Potassium	Calcium	Iron	Zinc	Magnesium	Vitamin A	Vitamin C	Thiamin	Riboflavin	Niacin	Vitamin B$_{12}$	Folic acid
Anginetti (Stella d'Oro) 4 cookies	140	3	6	—	13	8	—	*	—	—	—	—	—	—	—	—	—	—	—	—
Animal Cracker (Barnum's) 5 (1/2 oz)	60	2	3	3	*	4	—	3	*	*	2	—	—	*	*	4	4	4	—	—
anisette sponge (Stella d'Oro) 2 cookies	90	3	2	—	13	6	—	3	—	—	—	—	—	—	—	—	—	—	—	—
anisette toast (Stella d'Oro) 3 cookies	130	3	2	—	12	9	—	6	—	—	—	—	—	—	—	—	—	—	—	—
apple (Health Valley) 1 bar	140	4	*	*	*	10	12	*	4	2	20	6	10	2	*	2	4	2	—	—
fruit centers (Health Valley) 1 cookie	80	4	*	*	*	6	8	3	2	2	4	—	—	10	4	6	2	2	—	—
apple bar (Newtons) 1 bar (1/2 oz)	70	2	3	3	*	5	—	3	*	*	2	—	—	*	*	2	2	2	—	—
(Stella d'Oro) 1 cookie	100	2	4	—	2	7	—	*	—	—	—	—	—	—	—	—	—	—	—	—
fat free (Newtons) 1 bar (1/2 oz)	70	2	*	*	*	5	—	2	*	*	2	—	—	*	*	2	2	*	—	—
apple cinnamon fruit centers, mini (Health Valley) 2 cookies	90	4	*	*	*	7	8	2	2	2	4	—	—	10	6	6	2	2	—	—
apple filled (Weight Watchers) 3/4 oz	70	2	*	*	*	5	*	2	*	*	*	—	—	*	*	—	—	—	—	—
apple raisin fruit centers (Health Valley) 1 cookie	70	4	*	*	*	5	14	*	5	2	4	—	—	10	4	6	2	2	—	—
fruit chunks (Health Valley) 3 cookies	85	4	*	*	*	6	12	3	3	2	4	—	—	10	6	6	2	2	—	—
apple raisin bar (Weight Watchers) 1 oz	100	2	5	5	*	6	8	5	2	*	2	—	—	*	*	—	—	—	—	—
apple raisin jumbo (Health Valley) 1 cookie	80	4	*	*	*	6	8	3	3	2	4	—	—	10	4	6	2	2	—	—
apple spice (Health Valley) 3 cookies	80	4	*	*	*	6	12	3	3	2	4	—	—	10	4	6	2	2	—	—
apricot (Health Valley) 1 bar	140	4	*	*	*	10	12	*	4	2	20	6	10	2	*	2	4	2	—	—
fruit centers (Health Valley) 1 cookie	80	4	*	*	*	6	8	3	2	2	4	—	—	10	4	6	2	2	—	—
apricot apple fruit chunks (Health Valley) 3 cookies	85	4	*	*	*	6	12	3	3	2	4	—	—	10	6	6	2	2	—	—
apricot delight (Health Valley) 3 cookies	80	4	*	*	*	6	12	3	3	2	4	—	—	10	4	6	2	2	—	—
arrowroot biscuit (National) 1 (1/2 oz)	20	*	*	*	*	*	—	*	*	*	*	—	—	*	*	5	5	5	—	—
banana spice fruit chunks (Health Valley) 3 cookies	85	4	*	*	*	6	12	3	3	2	4	—	—	10	6	6	2	2	—	—
Beacon Hill Chocolate Walnut (Pepperidge Farm) 1 cookie	120	2	11	10	2	5	4	3	—	*	4	—	—	*	*	*	*	*	—	—
Biscottini Cashews (Stella d'Oro) 1 cookie	110	2	9	—	2	4	—	2	—	—	—	—	—	—	—	—	—	—	—	—
biscuit (Nabisco Social Tea) 3 (1/2 oz)	70	2	3	3	2	4	—	2	*	*	2	—	—	*	*	4	2	2	—	—
blueberry (Health Valley) 1 bar	100	4	*	*	*	8	12	2	4	2	4	6	6	10	4	6	2	2	—	—
blueberry-apple bars (Health Valley) 1 bar	90	4	*	*	*	7	12	2	4	2	4	6	6	10	4	6	2	2	—	—
Bordeaux (Pepperidge Farm) 2 cookies	70	*	5	5	*	4	*	2	—	*	*	—	—	*	*	*	*	*	*	—

COOKIE (continued)

	Calories	Protein	Fat	Sat. Fat	Cholesterol	Carbohydrates	Fiber	Sodium	Potassium	Calcium	Iron	Zinc	Magnesium	Vitamin A	Vitamin C	Thiamin	Riboflavin	Niacin	Vitamin B₁₂	Folic acid
Breakfast Treat (Stella d'Oro) 1 cookie	100	2	5	—		3		5	—	3	—	—	—	—	—	—	—	—	—	—
Brown Edge Wafer (Nabisco) 2 (3/8 oz)	70	*	5	3	*	3	—	2	*	*	2	—	*	*	2	2	2	—	—	—
brownie chocolate nut (Pepperidge Farm Old Fashioned) 2 cookies	110	2	11	10	3	4	*	2	—	*	4	—	*	*	*	*	*	*	—	—
Brussels (Pepperidge Farm) 2 cookies	110	*	8	10	*	4	*	3	—	*	*	—	*	*	*	*	*	*	*	—
Brussels Mint (Pepperidge Farm) 2 cookies	130	*	11	10	*	6	*	2	—	*	*	—	*	*	*	*	*	*	*	—
candied animals (Grandma's) 5 cookies	140	2	2	20	*	6	2	3			—	—	—	—	—	—	—	—	—	—
caramel bar (Heyday) 1 bar (1/2 oz)	110	3	9	10	13	4	—	2	2	2	2	—	*	*	*	*	2	6	—	—
Castelet (Stella d'Oro) 2 cookies	130	3	9	—	*	6		3	—	—	—	—	—	—	—	—	—	—	—	—
Chantilly (Pepperidge Farm) 1 cookie	80	*	3	5	*	5		*	—	*	*	—	*	*	*	*	*	*	*	—
Chesapeake Chocolate Chunk Pecan (Pepperidge Farm) 1 cookie	120	2	11	10	2	5	4	2	—	*	—	*	*	*	*	*	*	*	—	—
Chessmen (Pepperidge Farm) 2 cookies	90	*	6	10	3	4	*	2	—	*	*	—	*	*	*	*	*	*	*	—
Cheyenne Peanut Butter Chocolate (Pepperidge Farm) 3/4 oz	110	4	9	10	2	4	4	3	—	*	2	—	*	*	*	*	*	*	2	—
Chinese dessert (Stella d'Oro) 1 cookie	170	3	14	—	2	7	—	4	—	—	—	—	—	—	—	—	—	—	—	—
chocolate (Weight Watchers) 3/4 oz	80	2	5	5	*	4	8	3	*	*	4	—	*	—	*	*	*	*	—	—
bits (Grandma's) 9 cookies	170	3	12	10	*	8	4	10			—	—	—	—	—	—	—	—	—	—
Chocolate Chantilly (Pepperidge Farm) 1 cookie	90	*	5	5	*	5		*	—	*	*	—	*	*	*	*	*	*	*	—
chocolate chip (Grandma's) 1 cookie	190	3	14	13	*	8	4	5			—	—	—	—	—	—	—	—	—	—
(Keebler Rainbow Chip) 2 cookies	160	3	12	20	2	7	—	2	*	—	4	—	—	—	—	4	4	4	—	—
(Pepperidge Farm Family Request) 2 cookies	90	*	8	5	*	5	4	2	4	*	*	—	*	*	*	*	*	*	—	—
(Pepperidge Farm Old Fashioned) 2 cookies	100	*	8	10	2	4	*	2	—	*	*	—	*	*	*	*	*	*	—	—
(Snackwell's) 1 cookie (1/2 oz)	60	*	2	3	*	4	—	4	*	*	4	—	*	*	*	2	2	2	—	—
(Sunshine) 2 cookies	120	2	9	10	*	5	—	4	—	*	4	—	*	*	*	*	*	*	—	—
(Weight Watchers) 1 oz	140	3	8	10	*	7	4	4	*	2	4	—	*	*	*	—	—	—	—	—
bite size (Chips Ahoy) 1 (1/2 oz)	70	2	5	5	*	3	—	2	*	*	2	—	*	*	*	2	2	2	—	—
chewy (Chips Ahoy) 1 (1/2 oz)	60	2	5	5	*	3	—	2	*	*	*	—	*	*	*	*	*	*	—	—
chocolate chunk pecan (Chips Ahoy) 1 (1/2 oz)	100	2	9	10	3	3	—	3	*	*	2	—	*	*	*	2	2	2	—	—
Heath toffee chunk (Chips Ahoy) 1 (1/2 oz)	90	2	8	10	2	4	—	4	*	2	2	—	*	*	*	2	2	2	—	—
real chocolate (Chips Ahoy) 1 (1/2 oz)	50	2	3	3	*	2	—	2	*	*	2	—	*	*	*	2	*	*	—	—
rockers (Chips Ahoy) 1 (1/2 oz)	60	2	5	3	*	3	—	2	*	*	2	—	*	*	*	*	*	*	—	—

	Calories	Protein	Fat	Sat. Fat	Cholesterol	Carbohydrates	Fiber	Sodium	Potassium	Calcium	Iron	Zinc	Magnesium	Vitamin A	Vitamin C	Thiamin	Riboflavin	Niacin	Vitamin B₁₂	Folic acid

COOKIE (continued)

	Calories	Protein	Fat	Sat. Fat	Cholesterol	Carbohydrates	Fiber	Sodium	Potassium	Calcium	Iron	Zinc	Magnesium	Vitamin A	Vitamin C	Thiamin	Riboflavin	Niacin	Vit. B₁₂	Folic acid
snaps (Nabisco) 3 (1/2 oz)	70	2	3	3	*	4	—	2	*	*	2	—	—	*	*	2	2	2	—	—
sprinkled (Chips Ahoy) 1 (1/2 oz)	60	2	5	3	*	3	—	2	*	*	2	—	—	*	*	2	*	*	—	—
striped (Chips Ahoy) 1 (1/2 oz)	90	2	8	10	*	3	—	2	*	*	2	—	—	*	*	2	2	2	—	—
white fudge chunk (Chips Ahoy) 1 (1/2 oz)	90	2	8	10	*	3	—	3	*	*	2	—	—	*	*	2	2	*	—	—
chocolate chip snap (Nabisco) 3 cookies (1/2 oz)	70	2	3	—	*	4	—	2	*	*	2	—	—	*	*	2	2	2	—	—
chocolate chunk (Pepperidge Farm Soft Baked) 1 oz	130	2	9	10	3	6	*	2	—	*	4	—	—	*	*	2	*	*	—	—
chocolate laced pirouettes (Pepperidge Farm) 2 cookies	70	*	6	5	—	3	*	*	*	*	*	—	—	*	*	*	*	*	—	—
chocolate marshmallow (Mallowmar) 1 cookie (1/2 oz)	60	2	5	5	*	3	*	*	*	*	2	—	—	*	*	*	*	*	—	—
(Pinwheels) 1 (1 oz)	130	2	8	15	*	7	—	*	*	*	2	—	—	*	*	2	2	*	—	—
chocolate middles (Nabisco) 1 (1/2 oz)	80	2	8	10	*	3	*	*	*	*	2	—	—	*	*	*	2	2	—	—
chocolate sandwich (Grandma's Value Line) 3 cookies	180	3	8	8	*	10	2	8				—	—	—	—	—	—	—	—	—
(Hydrox) 3 cookies	150	3	11	10	*	7	4	5	—	*	6	—	—	*	*	2	4	2	—	—
(Oreo) 1 (1/2 oz)	50	2	3	3	*	3	—	3	*	*	2	—	—	*	*	*	*	*	—	—
(Weight Watchers) 1 oz	140	3	5	5	*	8	4	7	2	*	6	—	—	*	*	—	—	—	—	—
double stuffed (Oreo) 1 (1/2 oz)	70	2	6	5	*	3	—	3	*	*	2	—	—	*	*	*	*	*	—	—
fudge covered (Oreo) 1 (3/4 oz)	110	2	9	5	*	4	—	3	*	*	2	—	—	*	*	2	2	*	—	—
low fat (Keebler Elfin Delights) 3 cookies	150	3	6	5	*	9	3	7	—	*	6	—	—	*	*	—	—	—	—	—
reduced fat (Hydrox) 3 cookies	130	2	6	5	*	8	4	6	—	*	6	—	—	*	*	2	4	2	—	—
white fudge covered (Oreo) 1 (3/4 oz)	110	2	9	5	*	5	—	3	2	2	*	—	—	*	*	2	2	*	—	—
chocolate snap (Nabisco) 4 cookies (1/2 oz)	60	2	3	5	*	3	—	3	*	*	2	—	—	*	*	2	2	2	—	—
chocolate toffee chip (Pepperidge Farm Old Fashioned) 2 cookies	100	*	8	10	2	4	*	3	—	*	2	—	—	*	*	2	*	*	—	—
chocolate wafer (Nabisco) 2 cookies (1/2 oz)	60	2	3	3	*	4	—	4	*	*	4	—	—	*	*	2	2	2	—	—
chocolate walnut (Pepperidge Farm Soft Baked) 1 oz	130	2	9	10	2	6	*	2	—	*	2	—	—	*	*	2	*	*	—	—
cinnamon graham snacks (Snackwell's) 9 (1/2 oz)	50	2	*	*	*	4	—	2	*	*	2	—	—	*	*	2	2	2	—	—
cinnamon sugar (Pepperidge Farm Family Request) 2 cookies	80	*	6	5	5	4	*	2	—	*	*	—	—	*	*	*	*	*	—	—
combination sandwich (Grandma's Value Line) 3 cookies	150	3	6	5	*	8	4	7				—	—	—	—	—	—	—	—	—
Como Delight (Stella d'Oro) 1 cookie	140	3	11	—	13	6	—	2				—	—	—	—	—	—	—	—	—

COOKIE (continued)

	Calories	Protein	Fat	Sat. Fat	Cholesterol	Carbohydrates	Fiber	Sodium	Potassium	Calcium	Iron	Zinc	Magnesium	Vitamin A	Vitamin C	Thiamin	Riboflavin	Niacin	Vitamin B$_{12}$	Folic acid
creme sandwich																				
(Nabisco Cameo) 1 cracker (1/2 oz)	70	2	5	5	*	3	—	2	*	*	2	—	—	*	*	4	2	2	—	—
crisped rice bar																				
almond (generic) 1 oz bar	130	3	9	6	*	6	4	3	2	2	10	10	5	15	5	25	25	25	*	*
chocolate chip (generic) 1 oz bar	115	2	6	8	*	7	4	3	*	*	10	2	3	10	*	10	10	10	*	10
Dakota Milk Chocolate Oatmeal (Pepperidge Farm) 3/4 oz	110	22	9	10	2	5	4	3	—	*	*	—	—	*	*	*	*	*	—	—
Danish (Nabisco) 2 cookies (1/2 oz)	70	2	6	—	5	3	—	*	—	*	2	—	—	*	*	2	2	2	—	—
date (Health Valley) 1 bar	140	4	*	*	*	10	12	*	4	2	20	6	10	2	*	2	4	2	—	—
fruit centers (Health Valley) 1 cookie	70	4	*	*	*	5	14	*	5	2	4	—	—	10	4	6	2	2	—	—
fruit centers, mini (Health Valley) 3 cookies	85	4	*	*	*	6	8	3	2	2	4	—	—	10	6	6	2	2	—	—
date delight (Health Valley) 3 cookies	80	4	*	*	*	6	12	3	3	2	4	—	—	10	4	6	2	2	—	—
devil's food (Nabisco) 1 cookie (1/2 oz)	70	2	2	3	*	5	—	2	*	*	2	—	—	*	*	2	2	*	—	—
(Snackwell's) 1 (1/2 oz)	50	2	*	*	*	4	—	*	*	*	2	—	—	*	*	2	2	2	—	—
egg biscuit																				
roman (Stella d'Oro) 1 cookie	120	2	5	—	5	7	—	2												
sugared (Stella d'Oro) 1 cookie	80	3	2	—	5	6	—	2												
egg jumbo (Stella d'Oro) 2 cookies	90	3	2	—	10	6	—	2												
fig bar (Newtons) 1 bar (1/2 oz)	60	2	2	3	*	4	—	2	*	*	2	—	—	*	*	2	2	*	—	—
(Sunshine) 2 cookies	110	2	4	3	*	7	4	3	—	*	2	—	—	*	*	—	—	—	—	—
fat free (Newtons) 1 bar (1/2 oz)	70	2	*	*	*	5	—	3	2	*	2	—	—	*	*	2	2	2	—	—
fig filled (Weight Watchers) 3/4 oz	70	2	*	*	*	5	*	2	*	2	2	—	—	*	*	—	—	—	—	—
fortune cookies (La Choy) 2	15	*	*	*	*	*	*	*	*	*	*	—	—	*	*	*	*	*	—	—
fruit slice (Stella d'Oro) 2 cookies	130	3	8	—	*	7	—	4	—	—	—	—	—	*	*	—	—	—	—	—
fudge (Heyday) 1 bar (1/2 oz)	110	3	9	10	13	4	—	2	2	2	2	—	—	*	*	*	2	6	—	—
deep (Stella d'Oro) 2 cookies	130	3	9	—	3	6	—	3	—											
nutty (Grandma's) 1 cookie	190	5	12	8	*	8	4	6	—											
Swiss (Stella d'Oro) 2 cookies	130	2	9	—	5	6	—	3	—											
fudge brownie (Grandma's) 1 brownie	360	7	20	15	7	19	4	7	—											
fudge chocolate chip (Grandma's) 1 cookie	170	3	9	10	*	9	4	7	—											
fudge coated wafers (Keebler) 3 cookies	150	2	12	23	*	7	3	2	—	*	2	—	—	*	*	—	—	—	—	—
fudge stripes (Keebler) 3 cookies	160	2	12	23	*	7	3	6	—	*	4	—	—	*	*	—	—	—	—	—
Geneva (Pepperidge Farm) 2 cookies	130	*	9	10	*	5	*	2	—	*	22	—	—	*	*	*	*	*	—	—

COOKIE (continued)

	Calories	Protein	Fat	Sat. Fat	Cholesterol	Carbohydrates	Fiber	Sodium	Potassium	Calcium	Iron	Zinc	Magnesium	Vitamin A	Vitamin C	Thiamin	Riboflavin	Niacin	Vitamin B12	Folic acid
ginger snap (Nabisco) 2 (1/2 oz)	60	*	2	3	*	4	—	3	2	*	4	—	—	*	*	2	2	2	—	—
(Sunshine) 7 cookies	130	3	7	5	*	7	2	6	—	*	6	—	—	*	*	—	—	—	—	—
gingerman (Pepperidge Farm Old Fashioned) 2 cookies	70	*	5	*	2	3	*	2	—	*	*	*	—	*	*	*	*	*	—	—
Golden Bar (Stella d'Oro) 1 cookie	110	3	5	—	7	6	—	3	—	—	—	—	—	—	—	—	—	—	—	—
graham cracker (Nabisco) 2 cookies (1/2 oz)	60	2	2	3	*	4	—	4	*	*	2	—	—	*	*	2	2	2	—	—
(Nabisco Bugs Bunny) 5 crackers (1/2 oz)	60	2	3	3	*	4	—	3	*	*	2	—	—	*	*	2	2	2	—	—
chocolate covered (Cookies'n' Fudge) 2 (1/2 oz)	45	2	3	3	*	2	—	*	*	*	*	—	—	*	*	2	*	*	—	—
(Nabisco) 1 cookie (1/2 oz)	50	2	5	—	*	2	—	*	*	*	2	—	—	*	*	*	*	*	—	—
cinnamon (Honey Maid) 2 crackers (1/2 oz)	60	2	2	3	*	4	—	4	*	*	2	—	—	*	*	2	2	2	—	—
(Sunshine) 2 cookies	120	3	8	6	*	7	3	6	—	2	4	—	—	*	*	2	4	6	—	—
honey (Honey Maid) 2 (1/2 oz)	60	2	2	3	*	4	—	4	*	*	2	—	—	*	*	2	2	2	—	—
(Sunshine) 2 cookies	120	3	6	5	*	7	4	5	—	2	6	—	—	*	*	2	4	6	—	—
graham peanut butter (Frito-Lay) 1 pkg	200	3	14	13	*	9	4	7	—	—	—	—	—	—	—	—	—	—	—	—
graham sandwich chocolate/ peanut butter (T.G. Bearwich) 2 cookies (1/2 oz)	70	2	5	3	*	3	—	3	2	2	4	—	—	*	*	2	2	2	—	—
chocolate/ vanilla (T.G. Bearwich) 2 cookies (1/2 oz)	70	2	5	3	*	3	—	2	*	2	2	—	—	*	*	2	2	2	—	—
cinnamon/ vanilla (T.G. Bearwich) 2 cookies (1/2 oz)	70	2	5	3	*	3	—	2	*	2	2	*	—	*	*	2	2	2	—	—
vanilla/ chocolate (T.G. Bearwich) 2 cookies (1/2 oz)	70	2	5	3	*	3	—	3	*	2	2	—	—	*	*	2	2	2	—	—
graham vanilla (Frito-Lay) 1 pkg	210	8	17	13	*	7	8	8	—	—	—	—	—	—	—	—	—	—	—	—
Hawaiian fruit (Health Valley) 3 cookies	80	4	*	*	*	6	12	3	3	2	4	—	—	10	4	6	2	2	—	—
hazelnut (Pepperidge Farm Old Fashioned) 2 cookies	110	*	9	10	*	5	*	3	—	*	*	—	—	*	*	*	*	*	—	—
Healthy Chips (Health Valley) 3 cookies	80	4	*	*	*	6	12	3	2	2	4	—	—	10	6	6	2	2	—	—
Holiday Rings (Stella d'Oro) 3 cookies	140	2	5	—	*	9	—	*	—	—	—	—	—	—	—	—	—	—	—	—
Irish oatmeal (Pepperidge Farm Old Fashioned) 2 cookies	90	*	8	5	2	4	*	3	—	*	*	*	—	*	*	*	*	*	—	—
lemon bits (Grandma's) 9 cookies	150	3	9	13	*	7	2	4	—	—	—	—	—	—	—	—	—	—	—	—
lemon nut crunch (Pepperidge Farm Old Fashioned) 2 cookies	110	*	11	10	*	4	*	2	—	*	2	—	—	*	*	*	*	*	—	—
Lido (Pepperidge Farm) 1 cookie	90	*	8	5	*	3	*	*	—	*	*	—	—	*	*	*	*	*	—	—

COOKIE (continued)

	Calories	Protein	Fat	Sat. Fat	Cholesterol	Carbohydrates	Fiber	Sodium	Potassium	Calcium	Iron	Zinc	Magnesium	Vitamin A	Vitamin C	Thiamin	Riboflavin	Niacin	Vitamin B12	Folic acid
linzer (Pepperidge Farm) 1 cookie	120	2	6	5	*	7	*	2	—	*	2	—	—	*	*	*	2	*	—	—
Margherite chocolate (Stella d'Oro) 2 cookies	150	3	11	—	*	6	—	3												
vanilla (Stella d'Oro) 2 cookies	140	3	8	—	5	7	—	4												
marshmallow fudge cakes (Nabisco) 1 cookie (1/2 oz)	90	2	6	5	*	5	—	2	*	*	4	—	—	*	*	2	2	*	—	—
marshmallow puff (Nabisco) 1 cookie (1/2 oz)	90	2	6	5	*	5	—	2	*	*	4	—	—	*	*	2	2	*	—	—
marshmallow twirl (Nabisco) 1 cookie (1/2 oz)	130	2	8	5	*	7	—	2	*	*	4	—	—	*	*	2	2	2	—	—
Milano (Pepperidge Farm) 2 cookies	120	*	9	10	2	5	*	2	—	*	*	—	—	*	*	*	*	*	—	—
milk chocolate macadamia (Pepperidge Farm Soft Baked) 1 oz	130	2	11	10	3	5	*	2	—	*	*	—	—	*	*	2	*	*	—	—
Mint Milano (Pepperidge Farm) 2 cookies	150	2	11	10	2	6	*	2	—	*	2	—	—	*	*	*	*	*	—	—
mint sandwich (Mystic) 1 (1/2 oz)	90	2	6	5	*	4	—	3	*	*	4	—	—	*	*	2	2	*	—	—
molasses (Grandma's) 1 cookie	160	3	6	5	*	10	4	11	—	—	—	—	—	—	—	—	—	—	—	—
molasses crisps (Pepperidge Farm Old Fashioned) 2 cookies	70	*	5	*	*	3	*	2	—	*	*	—	—	*	*	*	*	*	—	—
Nantucket Chocolate Chunk (Pepperidge Farm) 1 cookie	120	2	9	10	2	5	4	2	—	2	*	—	—	*	*	*	*	*	—	—
oatmeal (Baker's Bonus) 1 (1/2 oz)	80	2	5	3	*	4	—	3	*	*	2	—	—	*	*	4	2	2	—	—
(Pepperidge Farm Family Request) 1 cookie	90	*	6	5	3	4	4	3	—	*	*	—	—	*	*	*	*	*	—	—
fat-free (generic) 1 oz (2 cookies)	92	3	*	*	*	7	8	3	2	*	3	*	2	*	*	3	4	2	*	*
w/ raisins (Snackwell's) 1 (1/2 oz)	60	2	2	3	*	3	—	3	*	*	4	—	—	*	*	2	2	*	—	—
oatmeal apple spice (Grandma's) 1 cookie	170	3	9	8	*	9	8	9	—	—	—	—	—	—	—	—	—	—	—	—
oatmeal chocolate chip (Sunshine) 2 cookies	170	5	12	15	*	8	8	5	—	*	4	—	—	*	*	*	*	*	—	—
oatmeal raisin (Health Valley) 3 cookies	80	4	*	*	*	6	12	3	3	2	4	—	—	10	4	6	2	2	—	—
(Keebler) 2 cookies	140	3	9	10	*	7	—	4	*	—	2	—	—	*	*	*	*	*	—	—
(Pepperidge Farm Old Fashioned) 2 cookies	110	*	8	10	3	5	*	5	—	*	2	—	—	*	*	*	*	*	—	—
(Sunshine) 2 cookies	170	3	11	8	*	8	4	7	—	*	4	—	—	*	*	*	*	*	—	—
(Weight Watchers) 1 oz	120	3	3	*	*	7	4	4	2	*	2	—	—	*	*					
oatmeal raisin cinnamon fruit chunks (Health Valley) 3 cookies	85	4	*	*	*	6	12	3	3	2	4	—	—	10	6	6	2	2	—	—
oatmeal spice (Weight Watchers) 3/4 oz	80	3	3	5	*	4	4	3	*	*	2	—	—	*	*					
Orange Milano (Pepperidge Farm) 2 cookies	150	2	11	10	2	6	*	2	—	*	2	—	—	*	*	*	*	*	—	—
orange pineapple fruit centers, mini (Health Valley) 2 cookies	90	4	*	*	*	7	8	2	2	2	4	—	—	10	6	6	2	2	—	—

COOKIE (continued)	Calories	Protein	Fat	Sat. Fat	Cholesterol	Carbohydrates	Fiber	Sodium	Potassium	Calcium	Iron	Zinc	Magnesium	Vitamin A	Vitamin C	Thiamin	Riboflavin	Niacin	Vitamin B$_{12}$	Folic acid
Orleans (Pepperidge Farm) 2 cookies	90	*	9	10	*	4	*	*	—	*	2	—	—	*	*	*	*	*	—	—
Orleans Sandwich (Pepperidge Farm) 2 cookies	120	*	12	10	*	5	*	2	—	*	*	—	—	*	*	*	*	*	—	—
peach apricot fruit centers, mini (Health Valley) 2 cookies	90	4	*	*	*	7	8	2	2	2	4	—	—	10	6	6	2	2	—	—
peanut bar (Heyday) 1 bar (1/2 oz)	110	3	9	10	13	4	—	2	2	2	2	—	—	*	*	*	2	6	—	—
peanut butter (Grandma's) 1 cookie	190	7	14	10	*	7	4	7	—	*	—	—	—	—	—	—	—	—	—	—
(Pepperidge Farm Family Request) 2 cookies	80	6	8	10	*	3	4	3	—	6	6	—	—	10	15	2	8	10	—	—
bits (Grandma's) 9 cookies	150	5	9	8	*	7	4	6	—	*	—	—	—	—	—	—	—	—	—	—
peanut butter bar (Grandma's) 1 bar	180	5	14	13	*	7	4	2	—	*	—	—	—	—	—	—	—	—	—	—
peanut butter sandwich (Grandma's) 5 cookies	210	7	14	10	*	10	4	8	—	*	—	—	—	—	—	—	—	—	—	—
(Nutter Butter) 1 (1/2 oz)	70	2	5	3	*	3	—	2	*	*	2	—	—	*	*	4	2	2	—	—
(Nutter Butter Bites) 5 cookies (1/2 oz)	70	2	5	3	*	3	—	2	*	*	2	—	—	*	*	2	2	2	—	—
peanut creme patty (Nutter Butter) 2 (1/2 oz)	80	3	6	3	*	3	—	2	*	*	2	—	—	*	*	4	2	2	—	—
pecan (Nabisco) 1 (1/2 oz)	80	2	8	5	*	3	*	2	*	*	2	—	—	*	*	2	2	2	—	—
pecan shortbread (Pepperidge Farm Old Fashioned) 1 cookie	70	*	8	10	*	2	*	*	—	*	*	—	—	*	*	*	*	*	—	—
raisin (Health Valley) 1 bar	140	6	*	*	*	11	15	*	8	2	20	6	10	*	*	2	4	2	—	—
raisin bran (Pepperidge Farm Old Fashioned) 2 cookies	110	*	8	10	*	4	*	2	—	*	*	—	—	*	*	*	*	*	—	—
raisin jumbo (Health Valley) 1 cookie	80	4	*	*	*	6	8	3	3	2	4	—	—	10	4	6	2	2	—	—
raspberry fruit centers (Health Valley) 1 cookie	80	4	*	*	*	6	8	3	2	2	4	—	—	10	4	6	2	2	—	—
raspberry apple fruit centers, mini (Health Valley) 2 cookies	90	4	*	*	*	7	8	2	2	2	4	—	—	10	6	6	2	2	—	—
fruit chunks (Health Valley) 3 cookies	85	4	*	*	*	6	12	3	3	2	4	—	—	10	6	6	2	2	—	—
raspberry bar (Health Valley) 1 bar	90	4	*	*	*	7	12	2	4	4	6	6	6	10	4	6	2	2	—	—
(Newtons) 1 bar (1/2 oz)	70	2	3	3	*	5	—	3	*	*	2	—	—	*	*	2	2	*	—	—
raspberry filled (Weight Watchers) 3/4 oz	70	2	*	*	*	5	*	2	*	*	*	—	—	*	*	*	*	*	—	—
raspberry jumbo (Health Valley) 1 cookie	80	4	*	*	*	6	8	3	3	2	4	—	—	10	4	6	2	2	—	—
rich & chewy (Grandma's) 1 bar	270	5	17	20	3	13	4	6	—	*	—	—	—	—	—	—	—	—	—	—
Santa Fe Oatmeal Raisin (Pepperidge Farm) 1 cookie	100	2	6	5	*	5	4	3	—	*	*	—	—	*	*	*	*	*	—	—
Sausalito Milk Chocolate Macadamia (Pepperidge Farm) 1 cookie	120	*	11	10	2	5	*	3	—	*	*	—	—	*	*	*	*	*	—	—

COOKIE (continued)

	Calories	Protein	Fat	Sat. Fat	Cholesterol	Carbohydrates	Fiber	Sodium	Potassium	Calcium	Iron	Zinc	Magnesium	Vitamin A	Vitamin C	Thiamin	Riboflavin	Niacin	Vitamin B12	Folic acid
sesame (Stella d'Oro) 3 cookies	140	3	8	—	7	7	—	5	—	—	—	—	—	—	—	—	—	—	—	—
shortbread (Lorna Doone) 2 (1/2 oz)	70	2	6	3	*	3	—	3	*	*	4	—	—	*	*	2	2	4	—	—
(Pepperidge Farm Old Fashioned) 2 cookies	150	*	12	10	*	6	*	4	—	*	*	—	—	*	*	*	*	*	—	—
(Weight Watchers) 3/4 oz	80	2	3	5	*	4	4	4	*	*	2	—	—	*	*	—	—	—	—	—
fudge striped (Cookies & Fudge) 1 cookie (1/2 oz)	60	2	5	5	*	2	—	2	*	*	2	—	—	*	*	2	2	*	—	—
strawberry fruit centers, mini (Health Valley) 2 cookies	90	4	*	*	*	7	8	2	3	2	4	—	—	10	6	6	2	2	—	—
strawberry bar (Health Valley) 1 bar	90	4	*	*	*	7	12	2	4	4	4	6	6	10	4	6	2	2	—	—
(Newtons) 1 bar (1/2 oz)	70	2	3	3	*	5	—	3	*	*	2	—	—	*	*	2	2	2	—	—
strawberry wafer (Grandma's Value Line) 1 pkg	230	3	12	10	*	13	2	3	—	—	—	—	—	—	—	—	—	—	—	—
striped wafer (Nabisco Cookies'n 'Fudge) 1 (1/2 oz)	70	2	6	3	*	3	—	*	*	*	2	—	—	*	*	*	2	*	—	—
sugar (Pepperidge Farm Old Fashioned) 2 cookies	100	*	8	10	3	4	*	2	—	*	*	—	—	*	*	*	*	*	—	—
sugar wafer (Biscos) 4 cookies (1/2 oz)	70	*	5	3	*	3	—	*	*	*	*	—	—	*	*	*	*	*	—	—
(Nabisco Nilla) 4 (1 1/8 oz)	60	2	3	3	*	4	—	2	*	*	2	—	—	*	*	2	2	2	—	—
(Sunshine) 4 wafers	180	3	6	5	*	4	—	2	—	*	*	*	*	*	*	*	*	*	*	*
peanut butter (Sunshine) 4 wafers	170	5	14	10	*	6	4	3	—	*	2	—	—	*	*	*	4	8	—	—
toffee chip (Keebler) 2 cookies	140	3	12	10	*	5	—	4	*	—	—	—	—	—	—	—	—	4	—	—
tropical fruit centers (Health Valley) 1 cookie	80	4	*	*	*	6	8	3	2	2	4	—	—	10	4	6	2	2	—	—
vanilla (Keebler) 8 cookies	160	2	9	10	*	7	—	5	*	—	4	—	—	—	—	—	—	4	—	—
(Nilla) 4 cookies (1/2 oz)	60	2	3	3	*	4	—	2	*	*	2	—	—	*	*	2	2	2	—	—
(Sunshine) 7 cookies	150	3	11	9	1	7	2	5	—	*	4	—	—	*	*	2	2	4	—	—
bits (Grandma's) 9 cookies	150	3	11	8	*	7	2	7	—	—	—	—	—	—	—	—	—	—	—	—
vanilla sandwich (Grandma's) 5 cookies	210	5	14	13	*	10	4	5	—	—	—	—	—	—	—	—	—	—	—	—
(Grandma's Value Line) 3 cookies	180	3	8	8	*	11	2	7	—	—	—	—	—	—	—	—	—	—	—	—
(Sunshine Vienna Fingers) 2 cookies	140	3	9	8	*	7	3	4	—	*	4	—	—	*	*	*	4	4	—	—
(Weight Watchers) 1 oz	140	2	5	5	*	8	4	3	*	*	4	—	—	*	*	—	—	—	—	—
reduced fat (Sunshine Vienna Fingers) 2 cookies	130	3	5	3	*	8	4	4	—	*	4	—	—	*	*	*	4	4	—	—
vanilla wafer (Grandma's Value Line) 1 pkg	230	3	12	10	*	13	4	3	—	—	—	—	—	—	—	—	—	—	—	—
waffle creme (Bisco) 1 cracker (1/2 oz)	40	*	3	3	*	2	—	*	*	*	*	—	—	*	*	*	*	*	—	—
Zürich (Pepperidge Farm) 1 cookie	60	*	3	5	*	3	*	*	—	*	*	—	—	*	*	*	*	*	—	—

	Calories	Protein	Fat	Sat. Fat	Cholesterol	Carbohydrates	Fiber	Sodium	Potassium	Calcium	Iron	Zinc	Magnesium	Vitamin A	Vitamin C	Thiamin	Riboflavin	Niacin	Vitamin B$_{12}$	Folic acid
COOKIE, FROM MIX																				
chocolate chip																				
basic recipe (Duncan Hines) 2 cookies	150	3	11	5	3	6	4	4	—	*	4	—	—	*	*	—	—	—	—	—
no cholesterol recipe (Duncan Hines) 2 cookies	140	3	11	5	*	6	4	4	—	*	4	—	—	*	*	—	—	—	—	—
peanut butter																				
basic recipe (Duncan Hines) 2 cookies	140	5	12	8	3	5	4	5	—	*	4	—	—	*	*	—	—	—	—	—
no cholesterol recipe (Duncan Hines) 2 cookies	140	5	12	8	*	5	4	5	—	*	4	—	—	*	*	—	—	—	—	—
sugar																				
(Pillsbury) 2 cookies	130	2	8	6	1	6	*	5	—	*	4	—	—	*	*	—	—	—	—	—
basic recipe (Duncan Hines) 2 cookies	120	2	9	8	3	6	4	3	—	*	4	—	—	*	*	—	—	—	—	—
from refrigerated dough (Pillsbury) 2 cookies (1 oz)	70	3	5	3	*	3	—	3	*	*	*	—	—	*	*	*	2	*	—	—
no cholesterol recipe (Duncan Hines) 2 cookies	120	2	8	8	*	6	4	3	—	*	4	—	—	*	*	—	—	—	—	—
COOKIE, FROM REFRIGERATED DOUGH																				
candy																				
(Pillsbury Oven Lovin') 2 cookies (1 oz)	70	2	5	5	*	3	—	2	*	*	*	—	—	*	*	*	2	*	—	—
chocolate chip																				
(Pillsbury) 2 cookies	140	2	10	9	1	6	2	4	—	*	2	—	—	*	*	—	—	—	—	—
(Pillsbury Oven Lovin') 2 cookies (1 oz)	70	2	5	5	2	3	—	2	*	*	*	—	—	*	*	*	2	*	—	—
chocolate chocolate chip																				
(Pillsbury) 2 cookies (1 oz)	70	3	5	3	*	3	—	*	*	*	2	—	—	*	*	2	*	*	—	—
oatmeal raisin																				
(Pillsbury) 2 cookies (1 oz)	60	3	3	3	*	3	—	2	*	*	2	—	—	*	*	*	2	*	—	—
peanut butter																				
(Pillsbury) 2 cookies (1 oz)	70	3	5	3	2	3	—	3	*	*	*	—	—	*	*	*	2	2	—	—
COOKING SPRAY																				
butter flavor																				
aerosol (Pam) 1/2 second spray	0	*	*	*	*	*	*	*	*	*	*	*	*	*	*	*	*	*	*	*
canola oil																				
aerosol (Pam) 1/2 second spray	0	*	*	*	*	*	*	*	*	*	*	*	*	*	*	*	*	*	*	*
(Wesson Lite) 1 tbsp	4	*	*	*	*	*	*	*	*	*	*	*	*	*	*	*	*	*	*	*
pump bottle (Pam) 2 pumps	0	*	*	*	*	*	*	*	*	*	*	*	*	*	*	*	*	*	*	*
olive oil																				
aerosol (Pam) 2 pumps	0	*	*	*	*	*	*	*	*	*	*	*	*	*	*	*	*	*	*	*
CORIANDER, FRESH																				
1/2 cup	2	*	*	*	*	*	*	*	*	*	*	*	*	4	*	*	*	*	*	*
CORIANDER LEAF, DRIED																				
1 tbsp	5	*	*	*	*	*	*	*	2	2	4	—	3	—	17	2	2	*	*	—
CORIANDER SEED																				
1 tbsp	15	*	*	*	*	*	—	*	2	4	5	2	4	*	—	*	*	*	*	*
CORN																				
white																				
raw 1/2 cup cut	66	4	*	*	*	5	8	*	6	*	2	2	7	*	9	10	3	7	*	9
boiled w/ salt 1/2 cup	89	5	2	*	*	7	—	9	6	*	3	3	7	*	8	12	3	7	*	10
sweet																				
boiled 1/2 cup cut	89	5	2	*	*	7	20	*	6	*	3	3	7	*	8	12	3	7	*	10

	Calories	Protein	Fat	Sat. Fat	Cholesterol	Carbohydrates	Fiber	Sodium	Potassium	Calcium	Iron	Zinc	Magnesium	Vitamin A	Vitamin C	Thiamin	Riboflavin	Niacin	Vitamin B$_{12}$	Folic acid
CORN (continued)																				
yellow																				
raw																				
1/2 cup cut	66	4	*	*	*	5	8	*	6	*	2	2	7	4	9	10	3	7	*	9
1 ear	77	5	2	*	*	6	8	*	7	*	3	3	8	5	10	12	3	8	*	10
boiled																				
1/2 cup cut	89	5	2	*	*	7	8	*	6	*	3	3	7	4	8	12	3	7	*	10
1 ear	83	4	2	*	*	6	8	*	5	*	3	2	6	3	8	11	3	6	*	9
boiled w/ salt																				
1/2 cup cut	89	5	2	*	*	7	—	9	6	*	3	3	7	4	8	12	3	7	*	10
1 ear	76	4	*	*	*	6	—	8	6	*	3	3	6	3	7	10	3	6	*	6
CORN, CANNED																				
cream style																				
(Bush Bros) 1/2 cup	110	5	2	*	*	7	8	17	—	*	*	—	—	2	*	—	—	—	—	—
no salt added																				
(Del Monte) 1/2 cup	90	3	*	*	*	7	8	*	—	*	2	—	—	*	10	—	—	—	—	—
reduced salt																				
(Del Monte) 1/2 cup	90	3	*	*	*	7	8	8	—	*	2	—	—	*	10	—	—	—	—	—
supersweet																				
(Del Monte) 1/2 cup	60	2	*	*	*	5	7	15	—	*	2	—	—	*	10	—	—	—	—	—
white																				
(Del Monte) 1/2 cup	100	3	*	*	*	7	8	15	—	*	2	—	—	*	6	—	—	—	—	—
(generic) 1/2 cup	92	4	*	*	*	8	8	15	5	*	3	5	5	*	10	2	4	6	*	14
low salt																				
(generic) 1/2 cup	92	4	*	*	*	8	—	*	5	*	3	5	5	*	10	2	4	6	*	14
yellow																				
(Del Monte) 1/2 cup	90	3	*	*	*	7	8	15	—	*	2	—	—	*	10	—	—	—	—	—
(generic) 1/2 cup	92	4	*	*	*	8	8	15	5	*	3	5	5	2	10	2	4	6	*	14
(generic) 1/2 cup	92	4	*	*	*	8	28	*	5	*	3	5	5	2	10	2	4	6	*	14
(Green Giant) 1/2 cup	100	3	*	*	*	8	8	20	5	*	*	—	—	2	4	2	4	4	—	—
supersweet																				
no salt added																				
(Del Monte) 1/2 cup	60	3	2	*	*	4	10	*	—	*	2	—	—	*	10	—	—	—	—	—
no sugar																				
(Del Monte) 1/2 cup	60	3	2	*	*	4	10	15	—	*	2	—	—	*	10	—	—	—	—	—
reduced salt																				
(Del Monte) 1/2 cup	60	3	2	*	*	4	10	5	—	*	2	—	—	*	10	—	—	—	—	—
vacuum pack																				
(Del Monte) 1/2 cup	70	3	2	*	*	4	12	11	—	*	4	—	—	*	10	—	—	—	—	—
white																				
drained																				
(generic) 1/2 cup	66	4	*	*	*	5	4	11	5	*	4	2	4	*	12	2	4	5	*	10
no salt added																				
(Del Monte) 1/2 cup	70	3	2	*	*	4	12	*	—	*	4	—	—	*	10	—	—	—	—	—
solid & liquid																				
(generic) 1/2 cup	78	4	*	*	*	6	—	13	6	*	2	3	5	*	14	2	5	6	*	12
sweet																				
(Del Monte) 1/2 cup	80	3	*	*	*	6	8	15	—	*	2	—	—	*	15	—	—	—	—	—
vacuum pack																				
(generic) 1/2 cup	83	4	*	*	*	7	—	12	6	*	2	3	6	*	14	3	5	6	*	13
low salt																				
(generic) 1/2 cup	83	4	*	*	*	7	—	*	6	*	2	3	6	*	14	3	5	6	*	13
whole kernel																				
(Bush Bros) 1/2 cup	80	3	*	*	*	5	8	14	—	*	4	—	—	4	*	—	—	—	—	—
(Del Monte) 1/2 cup	90	3	2	*	*	6	10	15	—	*	2	—	—	*	10	—	—	—	—	—
yellow																				
Delicorn																				
(Green Giant) 1/2 cup	80	3	*	*	*	6	8	15	6	*	2	—	—	6	*	*	2	6	—	—

	Calories	Protein	Fat	Sat. Fat	Cholesterol	Carbohydrates	Fiber	Sodium	Potassium	Calcium	Iron	Zinc	Magnesium	Vitamin A	Vitamin C	Thiamin	Riboflavin	Niacin	Vitamin B12	Folic acid
CORN, CANNED (continued)																				
golden sweet, whole kernel (Green Giant) 1/2 cup	70	3	*	*	*	6	8	15	5	*	2	—	—	2	6	2	2	4	—	—
50% less salt (Green Giant) 1/2 cup	70	3	*	*	*	5	8	7	5	*	*	—	—	*	4	*	2	4	—	—
Mexicorn (Green Giant) 1/2 cup	70	3	*	*	*	6	12	24	5	*	2	—	—	*	*	*	2	6	—	—
niblets (Green Giant) 1/2 cup	80	3	*	*	*	7	8	13	6	*	2	—	—	4	10	2	4	6	—	—
niblets, no salt or sugar added (Green Giant) 1/2 cup	80	3	*	*	*	6	8	*	5	*	2	—	—	2	4	2	6	8	—	—
solid & liquid (generic) 1/2 cup	78	4	*	*	*	6	4	*	6	*	2	3	5	3	14	2	5	6	*	12
sweet select (Green Giant) 1/2 cup	60	3	*	*	*	5	12	12	6	*	2	—	—	2	*	*	6	6	—	—
vacuum pack (generic) 1/2 cup	83	4	*	*	*	7	—	*	6	*	2	3	6	5	14	3	5	6	*	13
CORN, FROZEN																				
cob																				
boiled (generic) 1/2 cup kernels	76	4	*	*	*	6	20	*	6	*	3	3	6	*	7	10	3	6	*	6
cream style (Green Giant) 1/2 cup	110	5	2	*	*	8	10	15	5	*	*	—	—	2	8	6	2	2	—	—
in butter sauce (Bird's Eye Deluxe) 1/2 cup	90	3	3	—	2	6	—	7	5	*	2	—	—	4	6	2	2	4	—	—
microwave																				
golden whole kernel (Green Giant) 1/2 cup	80	3	*	*	*	6	4	9	5	*	*	—	—	6	2	*	2	10	—	—
niblets in butter sauce (Green Giant) 1/2 cup	100	5	3	5	2	6	8	13	4	*	2	—	—	*	4	4	2	2	—	—
shoepeg white in butter sauce (Green Giant) 1/2 cup	100	3	3	3	2	7	8	12	7	*	10	—	—	*	8	2	2	8	—	—
sweet (Bird's Eye Deluxe) 3 1/3 oz	80	5	2	*	*	7	—	*	—	*	2	2	2	4	8	4	4	8	4	8
(generic) 1/2 cup	72	4	*	*	*	6	8	*	5	*	2	2	4	*	9	5	3	7	*	7
tendersweet (Bird's Eye Deluxe) 3 1/3 oz	70	5	2	*	*	6	—	*	—	*	2	2	6	4	8	6	4	8	*	10
white (Green Giant) 1/2 cup	80	3	*	*	*	7	8	13	6	*	2	—	—	*	15	*	4	6	—	—
boiled (generic) 1/2 cup	66	4	*	*	*	6	—	*	3	*	*	2	4	4	4	4	4	5	*	5
boiled w/ salt (generic) 1/2 cup	66	4	*	*	*	6	—	8	3	*	*	2	4	4	4	4	4	5	*	5
cob boiled w/ salt (generic) 1 ear	59	3	*	*	*	5	—	6	5	*	2	3	5	*	5	7	3	5	*	5
shoepeg (Green Giant Harvest Fresh) 1/2 cup	90	5	2	*	*	6	8	2	5	*	*	—	—	*	10	2	2	6	—	—
(Green Giant Select) 1/2 cup	90	3	*	*	*	6	8	*	5	*	*	—	—	*	10	2	2	6	—	—
yellow																				
boiled (generic) 1/2 cup	66	4	*	*	*	6	8	*	3	*	*	2	4	4	4	4	4	5	*	5
w/ salt (generic) 1/2 cup	66	4	*	*	*	6	—	8	3	*	*	2	4	4	4	4	4	5	*	5
cob (generic) 1 ear	80	4	*	*	*	6	8	*	7	*	3	4	7	4	10	6	4	7	*	8

	Calories	Protein	Fat	Sat. Fat	Cholesterol	Carbohydrates	Fiber	Sodium	Potassium	Calcium	Iron	Zinc	Magnesium	Vitamin A	Vitamin C	Thiamin	Riboflavin	Niacin	Vitamin B12	Folic acid
CORN, FROZEN (continued)																				
boiled *(generic)* 1 ear	76	4	*	*	*	6	—	*	6	*	3	3	6	3	7	10	3	6	*	6
in butter sauce niblets *(Green Giant One Serving)* 4 1/2 oz	120	5	3	5	2	8	12	11	6	*	2	—	—	2	4	4	2	8	—	—
nibblers *(Green Giant)* 1 ear	120	3	2	*	*	9	8	*	7	*	4	—	—	2	8	4	6	10	—	—
nibblers *(Green Giant One Serving)* 2 half ears	120	7	2	3	*	9	8	*	7	*	4	—	—	2	*	*	4	10	—	—
niblets *(Green Giant)* 1/2 cup	90	3	*	*	*	6	8	*	5	*	*	—	—	*	6	2	2	6	—	—
(Green Giant Harvest Fresh) 1/2 cup	80	3	2	*	*	6	8	2	4	*	*	—	—	*	6	2	*	6	—	—
sweet select *(Green Giant)* 1/2 cup	60	3	2	*	*	4	8	*	4	*	4	—	—	2	*	*	4	8	—	—
niblet ears *(Green Giant)* 1 ear	120	7	2	*	*	9	8	*	7	*	4	—	—	2	8	4	6	10	—	—
sweet select *(Green Giant)* 1 ear	90	5	3	*	*	6	8	*	7	*	2	—	—	4	4	4	6	8	—	—
CORN COMBINATION, CANNED																				
corn w/ red & green peppers *(generic)* 1/2 cup	86	4	*	*	*	7	—	16	5	*	5	3	7	5	17	2	5	5	*	10
CORN DISH, FROZEN																				
corn soufflé *(Stouffer's Side Dishes)* 12 oz	170	12	11	8	22	7	4	20	7	4	2	—	—	2	4	10	15	6	—	—
CORN BREAD see BREAD																				
CORN CHIPS (see also TORTILLA CHIPS)																				
barbecue *(Fritos)* 1 oz	150	3	15	8	*	5	4	12			—	—	—	—	—	—	—	—	—	—
(generic) 2 oz	296	6.6	29	12	*	10	12	18	4	7	5	4	11	7	*	3	7	5	*	5
chili cheese *(Fritos)* 1 oz	160	3	15	8	*	5	4	11			—	—	—	—	—	—	—	—	—	—
corn cones plain *(generic)* 2 oz	289	5.3	23	64	*	12	—	24	*	*	8	*	*	4	*	12	8	4	*	*
corn snacks onion flavor *(generic)* 2 oz	284	7	20	13	*	12	8	23	2	2	12	*	4	*	2	8	10	9	*	2
crisp 'n' thin *(Fritos)* 1 oz	160	3	15	10	*	5	4	8			—	—	—	—	—	—	—	—	—	—
dip size *(Fritos)* 1 oz	160	3	15	8	*	5	4	6			—	—	—	—	—	—	—	—	—	—
Flamin' Hot *(Doritos)* 1 oz	140	3	11	5	*	6	4	7			—	—	—	—	—	—	—	—	—	—
nacho *(Doritos)* 1 oz	130	3	6	5	*	7	4	10			—	—	—	—	—	—	—	—	—	—
plain *(Fritos)* 1 oz	160	3	15	8	*	5	4	7			—	—	—	—	—	—	—	—	—	—
(generic) 1 oz	152	3	15	7	*	5	5	8	*		2	3	6	*	*	*	3	*	*	*
ranch *(Doritos)* 1 oz	140	3	11	5	*	6	4	7			—	—	—	—	—	—	—	—	—	—
ranch, choice *(Doritos)* 1 oz	130	3	6	5	*	7	4	8			—	—	—	—	—	—	—	—	—	—
salsa 'n' cheese *(Doritos)* 1 oz	140	3	11	8	*	6	4	9			—	—	—	—	—	—	—	—	—	—
salsa, zesty *(Doritos)* 1 oz	140	3	11	8	*	6	4	7			—	—	—	—	—	—	—	—	—	—

	Calories	Protein	Fat	Sat. Fat	Cholesterol	Carbohydrates	Fiber	Sodium	Potassium	Calcium	Iron	Zinc	Magnesium	Vitamin A	Vitamin C	Thiamin	Riboflavin	Niacin	Vitamin B12	Folic acid
CORN CHIPS (continued)																				
scoops (Fritos) 1 oz	150	3	14	8	*	5	4	6	—	—	—	—	—	—	—	—	—	—	—	—
taco (Doritos) 1 oz	140	3	11	8	*	6	4	8	—	—	—	—	—	—	—	—	—	—	—	—
thin																				
original (Doritos) 1 oz	140	3	11	5	*	6	4	6	—	—	—	—	—	—	—	—	—	—	—	—
salsa 'n cheese (Doritos) 1 oz	150	3	11	8	*	6	4	7	—	—	—	—	—	—	—	—	—	—	—	—
sour cream & onion (Doritos) 1 oz	150	3	12	5	*	6	2	7	—	—	—	—	—	—	—	—	—	—	—	—
toasted (Doritos) 1 oz	140	3	9	5	*	6	4	3	—	—	—	—	—	—	—	—	—	—	—	—
Wild 'n' Mild (Fritos) 1 oz	160	3	15	8	*	5	4	7	—	—	—	—	—	—	—	—	—	—	—	—
CORN FLAKE CRUMBS (Kellogg's) 1/4 cup	100	3	*	*	*	8	4	12	*	—	10	—	—	—	—	25	25	25	—	25
CORN FRITTER																				
frozen (Mrs. Paul's) 4 oz	240	10	14	5	3	12	—	23		2				4	*	10	8	2		
CORN GRITS see CEREAL, HOT																				
CORN MEAL																				
white (Alber's) 3 tbsp	110	3	*	*	*	11	—	*	—	*	6	*	*	4	*	—	—	—	—	—
yellow (Alber's) 3 tbsp	110	3	*	*	*	11	—	*	—	*	6	*	*	4	*	—	—	—	—	—
CORN NUTS																				
(Frito-Lay) 1/3 cup	150	5	8	5	*	8	8	10	—	—	—	—	—	—	—	—	—	—	—	—
(generic) 2 oz	249	8	12	7	*	14	16	13	5	*	5	7	16	*	*	2	4	5	*	*
barbecue flavor (generic) 2 oz	247	9	12	8	*	14	20	23	5	*	5	7	15	4	*	13	5	4	*	*
nacho flavor (generic) 2 oz	248	9	12	8	*	14	20	15	5	2	5	7	15	*	15	14	3	3	*	2
CORN OIL (Wesson) 1 tbsp	120	*	22	10	*	*	*	*	*	*	*	*	*	*	*	*	*	*	*	—
CORN & CANOLA OIL BLEND (Mazola Rightblend) 1 tbsp	120	*	22	5	*	*	*	*	—	*	*	*	*	*	*	*	*	*	*	*
CORN PUDDING 1/2 cup	136	9	10	16	42	5	—	3	6	5	4	4	5	6	6	34	9	6	2	8
CORN STARCH (Argo) 1 tbsp	30	*	*	*	*	2	*	*	*	*	*	*	*	*	*	*	*	*	*	*
CORN SYRUP																				
dark (generic) 1 tbsp	56	*	*	*	*	5	*	*	*	*	*	*	*	*	*	*	*	*	*	*
(Karo) 1 tbsp	60	*	*	*	*	5	*	2	—	*	*	—	—	*	*	*	*	*	*	*
high-fructose (generic) 1 tbsp	53	*	*	*	*	5	*	*	*	*	*	*	*	*	*	*	*	*	*	*
light (generic) 1 tbsp	56	*	*	*	*	5	—	*	*	*	*	*	*	*	*	*	*	*	*	*
(Karo) 1 tbsp	60	*	*	*	*	5	*	2	—	*	*	—	—	*	*	*	*	*	*	*
CORNED BEEF																				
canned																				
(generic) 1 slice	53	9	5	7	*	*	*	9	*	*	2	5	*	*	*	*	2	3	6	*
(Libby's) 3 oz	180	37	16	21	23	*	*	30	—	*	12	—	—	*	*	—	—	—	—	—
cooked (generic) 3 oz	213	26	25	27	—	*	*	40	4	*	9	26	3	*	23	*	8	13	23	*
sliced (Hormel) 1 slice	62	13	5	5	7	*	—	10	2	*	4	13	1	1	*	*	3	3	—	—

	Calories	Protein	Fat	Sat. Fat	Cholesterol	Carbohydrates	Fiber	Sodium	Potassium	Calcium	Iron	Zinc	Magnesium	Vitamin A	Vitamin C	Thiamin	Riboflavin	Niacin	Vitamin B₁₂	Folic acid
CORNED BEEF HASH																				
microwave																				
(Dinty Moore) 7 1/2 oz	350	32	34	45	22	6	—	35	15	4	13	22	7	1	2	—	9	17	—	—
CORNED BEEF LOAF, JELLIED																				
sliced																				
(generic) 1 slice	43	11	3	4	4	*	*	11	*	*	3	8	*	*	4	*	2	2	6	*
CORNISH GAME HEN																				
flesh only																				
roasted																				
1/2 bird	72	21	3	3	19	*	*	*	4	*	2	6	3	*	*	3	7	17	3	*
flesh & skin																				
roasted																				
1/2 bird	296	42	32	29	50	*	*	3	8	*	6	11	5	2	*	5	13	34	5	*
CORNSALAD																				
raw																				
1/2 cup	6	*	*	*	*	*	—	*	4	*	3	*	*	40	18	*	*	*	*	*
COTTONSEED FLOUR																				
lowfat																				
(generic) 1 oz	94	24	*	*	*	3	—	*	14	13	20	22	51	2	*	40	7	6	*	16
partially defatted																				
(generic) 1 tbsp	18	3	*	*	*	*	*	*	3	2	4	4	9	*	*	7	*	*	*	3
COTTONSEED KERNEL																				
roasted																				
(generic) 1 tbsp	51	5	6	5	*	*	4	*	4	*	3	4	11	*	*	5	*	*	*	6
COTTONSEED MEAL																				
partially defatted																				
(generic) 1 oz	104	23	2	*	*	4	—	*	15	14	21	23	54	3	*	42	7	6	*	17
COUSCOUS see RICE DISH																				
COWBOY PEA																				
(Bush Bros) 1/2 cup	120	12	2	*	*	6	20	21	—	2	10	—	—	—	*	*	—	—	—	*
COWPEA																				
catjang																				
cooked																				
salted																				
(generic) 1/2 cup	101	12	*	*	*	6	—	9	9	2	15	11	21	*	*	9	2	3	*	31
unsalted																				
(generic) 1/2 cup	101	12	*	*	*	6	—	*	9	2	15	11	21	*	*	9	2	3	*	31
common																				
raw																				
1/2 cup	65	4	*	*	*	5	16	*	9	9	4	5	9	12	3	5	6	5	*	30
boiled																				
1/2 cup	80	4	*	*	*	6	16	*	10	10	5	6	11	13	3	6	7	6	*	26
boiled w/ salt																				
1/2 cup	80	4	*	*	*	6	—	8	10	10	5	6	11	13	3	6	7	6	*	26
cooked																				
(generic) 1/2 cup	100	11	*	*	*	6	—	9	7	2	12	7	11	*	*	12	3	2	*	45
cooked w/ salt																				
(generic) 1/2 cup	100	11	*	*	*	6	24	*	7	2	12	7	11	*	*	12	3	2	*	45
COWPEA, CANNED																				
blackeye																				
dry, canned in brine																				
(Green Giant/Joan of Arc)																				
1/2 cup	45	12	*	*	*	3	8	6	4	3	4	—	—	*	*	2	*	*	*	—
common																				
(generic) 1/2 cup	92	9	*	*	*	5	16	15	6	2	6	6	8	*	5	6	5	2	*	15
w/ pork																				
(generic) 1/2 cup	100	5	3	4	3	7	16	17	6	2	9	8	13	*	*	5	4	3	*	15
COWPEA, FROZEN																				
common, frozen																				
boiled																				
1/2 cup	112	12	*	*	*	7	—	*	9	2	10	8	11	*	4	15	3	3	*	30

	Calories	Protein	Fat	Sat. Fat	Cholesterol	Carbohydrates	Fiber	Sodium	Potassium	Calcium	Iron	Zinc	Magnesium	Vitamin A	Vitamin C	Thiamin	Riboflavin	Niacin	Vitamin B12	Folic acid
COWPEA, FROZEN (continued)																				
boiled w/ salt																				
1/2 cup	112	12	*	*	*	7	—	9	9	2	10	8	11	*	4	15	3	3	*	30
COWPEA LEAF																				
raw																				
1/2 cup chopped	5	*	*	*	*	*	—	*	2	*	2	*	2	3	11	4	2	*	*	5
boiled																				
1/2 cup chopped	6	2	*	*	*	*	—	*	3	2	2	*	4	3	8	4	2	*	*	4
boiled w/ salt																				
1/2 cup chopped	6	2	*	*	*	*	—	3	3	2	2	*	4	3	8	4	2	*	*	4
COWPEA POD																				
raw																				
1/2 cup	21	3	*	*	*	*	—	*	3	3	3	*	7	15	26	5	4	3	*	6
boiled																				
1/2 cup	16	*	*	*	*	*	—	*	3	3	2	*	5	13	13	3	2	2	*	3
boiled w/ salt																				
1/2 cup	16	2	*	*	*	*	—	5	3	3	2	*	5	13	13	3	2	2	*	3
CRAB, ALASKA KING																				
raw																				
1 leg	144	52	2	*	24	*	*	60	10	8	6	68	21	*	20	5	4	9	257	*
CRAB, BLUE																				
raw																				
1 crab	18	6	*	*	5	*	*	3	2	2	*	5	2	*	*	*	*	*	3	31	*
canned																				
1/2 cup	66	12	*	*	10	*	*	5	4	3	2	9	3	*	2	2	2	2	5	*
steamed/poached																				
1/2 cup	68	11	*	*	11	*	*	4	3	4	2	9	3	*	2	2	*	6	87	*
CRAB, DUNGENESS																				
raw																				
1 crab	140	47	2	*	32	*	*	20	16	7	3	46	18	3	10	5	16	26	244	*
steamed/poached																				
1 crab	140	47	2	*	32	*	*	20	15	7	3	46	18	3	8	5	15	23	219	*
CRAB, KING																				
steamed/poached																				
1 leg	130	43	3	*	24	*	*	60	10	8	6	68	21	*	17	5	4	9	256	*
CRAB, QUEEN																				
raw																				
3 oz	77	26	2	*	16	*	*	19	4	2	12	16	10	3	10	5	10	11	127	*
steamed/poached																				
3 oz	98	34	2	*	20	*	*	24	5	3	14	20	13	3	10	5	12	12	146	*
CRAB, FROZEN																				
deviled																				
(Mrs. Paul's) 3 oz	180	20	14	5	7	6	*	20	—	6	6	—	—	*	*	8	10	6	—	—
miniatures																				
(Mrs. Paul's) 3 1/2 oz	240	20	18	10	7	8	*	22	—	6	6	—	—	*	*	10	10	8	—	—
CRAB, IMITATION see SURIMI																				
CRAB CAKE																				
all types																				
1 cake	160	19	16	11	27	2	*	20	5	20	6	14	6	6	*	4	4	6	73	2
blue																				
1 cake	93	20	7	5	30	*	*	8	6	6	4	16	5	3	3	4	3	9	59	*
CRABAPPLE																				
with skin																				
1 cup slices	84	*	*	*	*	7	—	*	6	2	2	—	2	*	15	2	*	—	—	—
CRACKER																				
bacon																				
(Nabisco) 7 crackers (1/2 oz)	70	2	6	3	*	3	—	9	*	2	2	—	—	*	*	4	2	2	—	—
bacon cheddar																				
(Frito-Lay) 1 pkg	200	5	15	15	*	8	4	16	—	—	—	—	—	—	—	—	—	—	—	—

CRACKER (continued)

	Calories	Protein	Fat	Sat. Fat	Cholesterol	Carbohydrates	Fiber	Sodium	Potassium	Calcium	Iron	Zinc	Magnesium	Vitamin A	Vitamin C	Thiamin	Riboflavin	Niacin	Vitamin B12	Folic acid
biscuit																				
unsalted tops (Uneeda) 2 crackers (1/2 oz)	60	2	3	3	*	3	—	4	*	*	4	—	—	*	*	4	*	4	—	—
cheddar																				
(Keebler Munch 'Ems) 28 small crackers	150	5	9	5	*	6	3	15	—	*	2	—	—	*	*	—	—	—	—	—
(Snorkels) 27 crackers (1/2 oz)	60	3	3	3	*	3	—	5	*	2	6	—	—	*	*	4	6	6	—	—
(Sunshine) 30 crackers	160	5	14	10	1	6	2	12	—	*	6	—	—	*	*	8	6	6	—	—
cheese																				
(Hain) 6	70	3	5	—	—	3	—	4	*	*	*	—	—	*	*	6	2	4	—	—
(Nabisco Better Cheddars) 10 crackers (1/2 oz)	70	3	6	3	*	3	—	5	*	2	2	—	—	*	*	4	4	2	—	—
(Nabisco Cheddar Wedges) 31 wedges (1/2 oz)	70	2	5	3	*	3	—	6	*	*	4	—	—	*	*	4	4	4	—	—
(Nabisco Nips) 13 crackers (1/2 oz)	70	2	5	3	*	3	—	6	*	*	4	—	—	*	*	4	4	4	—	—
(Snackwell's) 18 crackers (1/2 oz)	60	3	2	3	*	4	—	7	*	*	6	—	—	*	*	4	6	6	—	—
(Sunshine) 30 crackers	160	7	13	9	*	3	4	10	—	4	6	—	—	*	*	10	8	6	—	—
hot & spicy																				
(Sunshine) 24 crackers	140	3	12	10	*	5	—	13	—	*	2	—	—	*	*	2	2	2	—	—
low salt																				
(Nabisco Better Cheddars) 10 crackers (1/2 oz)	70	3	6	3	*	3	—	3	*	*	2	—	—	*	*	4	4	2	—	—
(Sunshine) 27 crackers	160	7	12	10	0	5	3	3	—	4	6	—	—	*	*	10	8	6	—	—
reduced fat																				
(Sunshine) 30 crackers	140	7	8	5	x	6	3	12	—	4	6	—	—	*	*	10	8	6	—	—
cheese peanut butter																				
(Frito-Lay) 1 pkg	200	10	15	10	*	7	4	17												
Chicken in a Biskit																				
(Nabisco) 7 crackers (1/2 oz)	80	2	8	3	*	3	—	5	*	*	2	—	—	*	*	2	2	2	—	—
chips																				
cheddar (Nabisco Zings) 15 chips (1/2 oz)	70	2	5	3	*	3	—	5	*	*	2	—	—	*	*	2	2	2	—	—
original (Nabisco Zings) 15 chips (1/2 oz)	70	2	5	3	*	3	—	5	*	*	2	—	—	*	*	2	2	2	—	—
ranch (Nabisco Zings) 15 chips (1/2 oz)	70	2	5	3	*	3	—	6	*	*	2	—	—	*	*	2	2	2	—	—
cracked wheat (American Classic) 4 crackers (1/2 oz)	70	2	6	3	*	3	—	6	*	*	2	—	—	*	*	4	2	2	—	—
crispbread																				
dark (Finncrisp) 2 slices	40	2	*	*	*	3	—	5	—	*	2	2	2	*	*	*	*	*	—	—
dark, seeded (Finncrisp) 2 slices	40	2	*	*	*	3	—	5	—	*	2	2	2	*	*	*	*	*	—	—
fiber plus (Wasa) 1 slice	35	2	2	*	*	2	12	2	—	*	4	—	—	*	*	—	—	—	—	—
fruit & nut (Wasa) 1 slice	50	3	2	*	*	3	8	2	—	*	3	—	—	*	*	—	—	—	—	—
multigrain (Wasa) 1 slice	40	13	1	1	*	4	2	4	—	*	4	—	—	*	*	—	—	—	—	—
rye light (Wasa) 1 slice	25	2	*	*	*	2	4	2	—	2	2	—	—	*	*	—	—	—	—	—

	Calories	Protein	Fat	Sat. Fat	Cholesterol	Carbohydrates	Fiber	Sodium	Potassium	Calcium	Iron	Zinc	Magnesium	Vitamin A	Vitamin C	Thiamin	Riboflavin	Niacin	Vitamin B12	Folic acid
CRACKER (continued)																				
sesame (Wasa) 1 slice	30	3	1	*	*	2	12	2	—	2	4	—	—	*	*	—	—	—	—	—
toasted wheat (Wasa) 1 slice	50	7	2	*	*	3	2	2	—	*	2	—	—	*	*	—	—	—	—	—
Crown Pilot (Nabisco) 3 crackers (1/2 oz)	70	2	6	3	*	3	—	5	*	*	2	—	—	*	*	4	2	2	—	—
dairy butter (Nabisco American Classic) 4 crackers (1/2 oz)	70	2	5	3	*	3	—	6	*	*	2	—	—	*	*	4	2	2	—	—
Escort (Nabisco) 3 crackers (1/2 oz)	70	2	6	3	*	3	—	5	*	*	2	—	—	*	*	4	2	2	—	—
five grain (Nabisco Harvest Crisps) 6 crackers (1/2 oz)	60	2	3	3	*	3	—	6	*	2	6	—	—	*	*	4	4	4	—	—
garlic flavor (Keebler Club) 4 crackers	60	2	3	3	*	3	*	6	—	*	*	—	—	*	*	—	—	—	—	—
golden sesame (Nabisco American Classic) 4 crackers (1/2 oz)	70	2	5	3	*	3	—	5	*	2	4	—	—	*	*	4	2	2	—	—
herb fat free (Hain) 5 crackers	60	3	*	*	*	4	—	5	2	*	2	—	—	*	*	*	4	4	—	—
jalapeño & cheddar (Frito-Lay) 1 pkg	200	7	15	13	*	8	4	20												
milk (Nabisco Royal Lunch) 1 cracker (1/2 oz)	60	2	3	3	*	3	—	3	*	2	2	—	—	*	*	4	2	2	—	—
multigrain (Nabisco Wheat Thins) 8 crackers (1/2 oz)	60	2	3	3	*	3	—	6	*	2	4	—	—	*	*	2	2	4	—	—
oat (Nabisco Harvest Crisps) 6 crackers (1/2 oz)	60	2	3	3	*	3	—	6	*	2	2	—	—	*	*	4	2	2	—	—
(Nabisco Oat Thins) 8 crackers (1/2 oz)	70	2	5	3	*	3	—	4	*	*	2	—	—	*	*	4	2	2	—	—
(Ralston) 2 crackers	50	2	3	*	*	2	12	6	—	*	2	—	—	*	*	2	2	*	—	—
onion fat free (Hain) 5 crackers	60	3	*	*	*	4	—	4	2	*	2	—	—	*	*	*	4	4	—	—
oyster (Nabisco Oysterettes) 18 crackers (1/2 oz)	60	2	2	3	*	3	—	6	*	*	4	—	—	*	*	4	4	4	—	—
(Premium) 20 crackers (1/2 oz)	60	2	2	3	*	3	—	9	*	*	4	—	—	*	*	4	4	4	—	—
pizza (Snorkels) 27 crackers (1/2 oz)	60	2	3	3	*	3	—	5	*	2	6	—	—	*	*	4	6	4	—	—
poppy (American Classic) 4 crackers (1/2 oz)	70	2	5	3	*	3	—	6	*	4	6	—	—	*	*	4	2	2	—	—
ranch (Snorkels) 27 crackers (1/2 oz)	60	2	3	3	*	3	—	5	*	2	6	—	—	*	*	4	6	4	—	—
rich (Hain) 4 crackers	70	3	5	—	*	3	—	2	3	*	2	—	—	*	*	2	2	4	—	—
Ritz (Nabisco) 4 crackers (1/2 oz)	70	2	6	3	*	3	—	5	*	*	2	—	—	*	*	4	2	2	—	—
bits (Nabisco) 22 bits (1/2 oz)	70	2	6	3	*	3	—	5	*	2	2	—	—	*	*	4	2	2	—	—
bits w/ cheese (Nabisco) 22 bits (1/2 oz)	70	2	6	3	*	3	—	5	*	2	2	—	—	*	*	4	2	2	—	—
cheese pizza sandwich bits (Nabisco) 5 crackers (1/2 oz)	80	2	8	5	*	3	—	6	2	2	2	—	—	*	*	2	2	2	—	—

CRACKER (continued)

	Calories	Protein	Fat	Sat Fat	Cholesterol	Carbohydrates	Fiber	Sodium	Potassium	Calcium	Iron	Zinc	Magnesium	Vitamin A	Vitamin C	Thiamin	Riboflavin	Niacin	Vitamin B12	Folic acid
cheese sandwich bits (Nabisco) 6 crackers (1/2 oz)	80	2	8	5	*	2	—	6	*	2	2	—	—	*	*	4	2	2	—	—
low salt (Nabisco) 4 crackers (1/2 oz)	70	2	6	3	*	3	—	2	*	2	2	—	—	*	*	4	2	2	—	—
low salt bits (Nabisco) 22 bits (1/2 oz)	70	2	6	3	*	3	—	2	*	2	2	—	—	*	*	4	2	2	—	—
nacho cheese sandwich bits (Nabisco) 6 crackers (1/2 oz)	80	2	8	5	*	3	—	6	*	2	2	—	—	*	*	2	2	2	—	—
peanut butter sandwich bits (Nabisco) 6 crackers (1/2 oz)	70	2	6	3	*	3	—	5	*	2	4	—	—	*	*	2	2	6	—	—
w/ whole wheat (Nabisco) 5 crackers (1/2 oz)	60	2	3	3	*	3	—	6	*	2	2	—	—	*	*	2	2	2	—	—
rye																				
plain (Ralston Rykrisp) 2 crackers	40	2	*	*	*	4	12	3	2	*	2	—	—	*	*	*	*	2	*	—
seasoned (Ralston Rykrisp) 2 crackers	45	2	2	*	*	4	12	4	2	*	2	—	—	*	*	*	*	2	*	—
sesame (Ralston Rykrisp) 2 crackers	50	2	3	*	*	3	12	4	2	*	*	—	—	*	*	*	*	2	*	—
Saltine																				
bits (Premium) 5 crackers (1/2 oz)	70	2	5	3	*	3	—	7	*	2	4	—	—	*	*	6	4	4	—	—
fat free (Premium) 5 crackers (1/2 oz)	50	2	*	*	*	4	—	5	*	*	4	—	—	*	*	6	4	4	—	—
fat free low sodium (generic) 6 saltines	118	5	*	*	*	8	4	8	*	*	13	2	2	*	*	10	10	9	*	*
low salt (Premium) 5 crackers (1/2 oz)	60	2	3	3	*	3	—	5	3	2	4	—	—	*	*	6	4	4	—	—
multigrain (Premium) 5 crackers (1/2 oz)	60	2	3	3	*	3	—	7	*	*	6	—	—	*	*	4	4	4	—	—
unsalted tops (Premium) 5 crackers (1/2 oz)	60	2	3	3	*	3	—	6	*	2	4	—	—	*	*	6	4	4	—	—
sesame (Hain) 6 crackers	70	2	5	—	*	3	—	3	*	*	2	—	—	*	*	6	2	4	—	—
sesame/cheese (Twigs) 7 crackers (1/2 oz)	70	2	6	3	*	3	—	6	*	4	2	—	—	*	*	4	*	2	—	—
toast & cheddar (Frito-Lay) 1 pkg	230	5	20	20	2	8	4	21			—	—	—	—	—	—	—	—	—	—
toast peanut butter (Frito-Lay) 1 pkg	190	8	14	8	*	8	4	16			—	—	—	—	—	—	—	—	—	—
vegetable (Hain) 6 crackers	60	2	5	—	*	3	—	4	*	*	2	—	—	*	*	6	2	4	—	—
(Nabisco) 6 crackers (1/2 oz)	70	2	6	3	*	3	—	6	*	2	2	—	—	*	*	4	2	2	—	—
(Nabisco Garden Crisps) 7 crackers (1/2 oz)	60	2	3	3	*	4	—	6	*	2	2	—	—	*	*	2	2	2	—	—
fat free (Hain) 5 crackers	60	3	*	*	*	4	—	6	2	*	2	—	—	*	*	*	4	4	—	—
no salt added (Hain) 6 crackers	70	2	5	—	*	3	—	*	*	*	2	—	—	*	*	6	2	4	—	—
Waverly (Nabisco) 4 crackers (1/2 oz)	70	2	5	3	*	3	—	7	*	*	2	—	—	*	*	4	4	2	—	—
low salt (Nabisco) 4 crackers (1/2 oz)	70	2	5	3	*	3	—	3	*	*	2	—	—	*	*	4	4	2	—	—
wheat (Keebler Town House) 9 crackers	150	3	12	8	*	6	4	13	—	*	6	—	—	*	*	*	—	—	—	—
(Nabisco Wheat Thins) 8 crackers (1/2 oz)	70	2	5	3	*	3	—	5	*	*	2	—	—	*	*	4	2	4	—	—

	Calories	Protein	Fat	Sat. Fat	Cholesterol	Carbohydrates	Fiber	Sodium	Potassium	Calcium	Iron	Zinc	Magnesium	Vitamin A	Vitamin C	Thiamin	Riboflavin	Niacin	Vitamin B12	Folic acid
CRACKER (continued)																				
(Ralston) 2 crackers	50	2	2	*	*	4	6	9	3	*	2	—	—	*	*	*	*	*	—	—
(Snackwell's) 5 crackers (1/2 oz)	50	2	*	3	*	4	—	7	*	2	4	—	—	*	*	4	4	4	—	—
(Wheatables) 26 small crackers	150	5	11	10	*	6	4	13	—	*	6	—	—	*	*	—	—	—	—	—
cheddar *(Frito-Lay)* 1 pkg	210	5	18	15	*	8	4	13												
cheese *(Frito-Lay)* 1 pkg	200	7	14	10	*	8	4	18												
low salt *(Nabisco Wheat Thins)* 8 crackers (1/2 oz)	70	2	5	3	*	3	—	7	*	*	2	—	—	*	*	4	2	4	—	—
(Triscuit) 3 crackers (1/2 oz)	60	2	3	3	*	3	—	*	2	*	2	—	—	*	*	2	*	2	—	—
low sodium *(Keebler Town House)* 8 crackers	140	3	12	5	*	5	—	5	*	*	4	—	—	*	*	4	4	4	—	—
(Wheatables) 24 small crackers	140	3	9	10	*	5	—	6	3	*	4	—	—	*	*	4	4	8	—	—
nutty *(Nabisco Wheat Thins)* 7 crackers (1/2 oz)	70	2	6	3	*	3	—	3	*	*	2	—	—	*	*	4	2	4	—	—
plain *(Triscuit)* 3 crackers (1/2 oz)	60	2	3	3	*	3	—	3	2	*	2	—	—	*	*	2	*	2	—	—
stone ground *(Wheatsworth)* 4 crackers (1/2 oz)	70	2	5	3	*	6	*	6	*	*	4	—	—	*	*	4	2	4	—	—
w/ bran *(Triscuit)* 3 crackers (1/2 oz)	60	2	3	3	*	3	—	3	2	*	2	—	—	*	*	2	*	2	—	—
w/ rye *(Triscuit)* 3 crackers (1/2 oz)	60	2	3	3	*	3	—	3	2	*	2	—	—	*	*	4	*	4	—	—
whole wheat w/ cheese *(Health Valley)* 5 crackers	45	2	*	*	*	3	8	3	2	*	2	—	—	6	*	4	*	2	—	—
fat free *(Hain)* 5 crackers	50	3	*	*	*	4	—	4	2	*	2	—	—	*	*	*	4	4	—	—
w/ herbs *(Health Valley)* 5 crackers	45	2	*	*	*	3	8	3	2	*	2	—	—	6	*	4	*	2	—	—
w/ onion *(Health Valley)* 5 crackers	45	2	*	*	*	3	8	3	2	*	2	—	—	6	*	4	*	2	—	—
organic *(Health Valley)* 5 crackers	45	2	*	*	*	3	8	3	2	*	2	—	—	6	*	4	*	2	—	—
w/ vegetables *(Health Valley)* 5 crackers	45	2	*	*	*	3	8	*	2	*	2	—	—	6	*	4	*	2	—	—
zweiback *(Nabisco)* 2 crackers (1/2 oz)	60	3	2	3	*	3	—	*	*	*	2	—	—	*	*	2	2	2	—	—
CRACKER CRUMBS *fat free* *(Premium)* 1/4 cup (1/2 oz)	100	3	*	*	*	7	—	*	2	8	4	—	—	*	*	4	8	8	—	—
Saltine *(Nabisco)* 1/4 cup	100	5	*	*	*	8	—	*	*	*	10	—	—	*	*	8	8	10	—	—
(Premium) 1/4 cup	100	4	*	*	*	8	—	*	*	*	12	—	—	*	*	4	8	8	—	—
CRACKER MEAL *(Nabisco)* 1/4 cup (1/2 oz)	100	5	*	3	*	8	—	*	*	*	10	—	—	*	*	8	8	10	—	—
CRANBERRY 1 cup	54	*	*	*	*	5	20	*	2	*	*	*	*	*	25	2	*	*	*	*
CRANBERRY BEAN *canned* 1/2 cup	108	12	*	*	*	7	—	18	10	4	11	7	10	*	2	3	3	3	*	25

	Calories	Protein	Fat	Sat. Fat	Cholesterol	Carbohydrates	Fiber	Sodium	Potassium	Calcium	Iron	Zinc	Magnesium	Vitamin A	Vitamin C	Thiamin	Riboflavin	Niacin	Vitamin B12	Folic acid
CRANBERRY BEAN (continued)																				
cooked 1/2 cup	120	14	*	*	*	7	—	*	10	4	10	7	11	*	*	12	4	2	*	46
salted 1/2 cup	120	14	*	*	*	7	—	9	10	4	10	7	11	*	*	12	4	2	*	46
CRANBERRY DRINK																				
organic (Santa Cruz Natural) 8 fl oz	110	*	*	*	*	9	*	*	2	2	4	—	—	—	2	—	—	—	—	—
Yankee (Knudsen Exotic Blends) 8 fl oz	120	*	*	*	*	10	*	*	3	*	2	—	*		10	—	—	—	—	—
CRANBERRY JUICE																				
(generic) 8 fl oz	116	*	*	*	*	10	—	*	*	*	2	*	*	*	120	*	*	*	*	*
100% (Farmer's Market) 8 fl oz	120	*	*	*	*	10	*	*	*	*	*	—	—	*	4	—	—	—	—	—
(Heinke's) 8 fl oz	60	*	*	*	*	5	*	*	2	2	15	—	—	*	*	—	—	—	—	—
(Knudsen Just Cranberry) 8 fl oz	60	*	*	*	*	5	*	*	2	2	15	—	—	*	*	—	—	—	—	—
from concentrate (Knudsen Exotic Blends) 8 fl oz	70	*	*	*	*	6	*	*	4	*	15	—	—	*	*	—	—	—	—	—
CRANBERRY JUICE COCKTAIL																				
(generic) 6 fl oz	105	*	*	*	*	9	*	*	*	*	2	*	*	*	109	*	*	*	*	*
(Ocean Spray) 8 fl oz	140	—	*	*	*	11	*	*	—	*	*	—	*	*	100	—	—	—	—	—
from concentrate (Welch's) 6 fl oz	100	*	*	*	*	9	*	*	*	*	*	*	*	*	45	*	*	*	*	*
light (Welch's) 6 fl oz	40	*	*	*	*	3	*	*	*	*	2	*	*	*	*	*	*	*	*	*
low calorie (generic) 6 fl oz	36	*	*	*	*	3	*	*	*	*	2	*	*	*	102	*	*	*	*	*
(Lightstyle) 8 fl oz	40	—	*	*	*	3	*	*	*	*	*	*	*	*	100	—	—	—	—	—
(Ocean Spray) 8 fl oz	50	*	*	*	*	4	*	*	*	*	*	*	*	*	100	—	—	—	—	—
CRANBERRY NECTAR																				
(Heinke's) 8 fl oz	120	*	*	*	*	10	*	*	6	2	4	—	—	*	2	—	—	—	—	—
(Knudsen Exotic Blends) 8 fl oz	150	2	*	*	*	13	*	2	3	2	4	—	—	*	2	—	—	—	—	—
from concentrate (Knudsen) 8 fl oz	150	2	*	*	*	13	*	2	3	2	4	—	—	*	2	—	—	—	—	—
CRANBERRY SAUCE																				
canned sweetened 1/2 cup	208	*	*	*	*	18	4	2	*	*	2	*	*	*	5	*	2	*	*	—
CRANBERRY-APPLE DRINK																				
(generic) 6 fl oz	119	*	*	*	*	10	*	*	*	*	*	*	*	*	94	*	2	*	*	*
CRANBERRY-APPLE JUICE																				
from concentrate (Welch's) 6 fl oz	120	*	*	*	*	10	*	*	*	*	*	*	*	*	45	*	*	*	*	*
CRANBERRY-APRICOT DRINK																				
(generic) 6 fl oz	118	*	*	*	*	10	*	*	3	2	2	*	*	17	*	*	*	*	*	*
(Ocean Spray Cranicot) 8 fl oz	160	—	*	*	*	13	*	*	4	*	*	—	—	30	*	—	—	—	—	—
CRANBERRY-CHERRY JUICE																				
from concentrate (Welch's) 6 fl oz	110	*	*	*	*	9	*	*	—	*	*	*	*	*	45	*	*	*	*	*
CRANBERRY-GRAPE DRINK																				
(generic) 6 fl oz	103	*	*	*	*	9	*	*	*	*	*	*	*	*	98	*	2	*	*	*
CRANBERRY-LEMON JUICE																				
organic (Santa Cruz Natural) 8 fl oz	120	*	*	*	*	10	*	*	2	*	—	—	—	*	8	—	—	—	—	—
CRANBERRY-ORANGE JUICE																				
from concentrate (Welch's) 6 fl oz	110	*	*	*	*	9	*	*	2	*	*	*	*	*	45	*	*	*	*	*
CRANBERRY-RASPBERRY JUICE																				
(Knudsen Exotic Blends) 8 fl oz	140	*	*	*	*	12	*	*	2	2	2	—	—	*	4	—	—	—	—	—
(Tropicana Twister) 6 fl oz	110	*	*	*	*	9	—	*	*	*	*	—	*	*	*	*	*	*	—	—

	Calories	Protein	Fat	Sat. Fat	Cholesterol	Carbohydrates	Fiber	Sodium	Potassium	Calcium	Iron	Zinc	Magnesium	Vitamin A	Vitamin C	Thiamin	Riboflavin	Niacin	Vitamin B₁₂	Folic acid
CRANBERRY-RASPBERRY JUICE (continued)																				
from concentrate																				
(Welch's) 6 fl oz	110	*	*	*	*	9	*	*	2	*	*	*	*	*	45	*	*	*	*	*
light																				
(Welch's) 6 fl oz	40	*	*	*	*	3	*	*	—	*	*	*	*	*	*	*	*	*	*	*
CRANBERRY-STRAWBERRY DRINK																				
(Ocean Spray) 8 fl oz	140	—	*	*	*	12	2	*	—	*	*	—	—	*	100	—	—	—	—	—
CRAYFISH, FARMED																				
raw																				
8 crayfish	19	7	*	*	10	*	*	*	2	*	*	2	2	*	*	*	*	3	9	*
steamed/poached																				
3 oz	74	25	2	*	39	*	*	3	6	4	5	8	7	*	*	3	4	7	44	*
CRAYFISH, WILD																				
raw																				
8 crayfish	21	7	*	*	10	*	*	*	2	*	*	2	2	*	*	*	*	3	9	*
steamed/poached																				
3 oz	75	24	2	*	38	*	*	3	7	5	4	10	7	*	*	3	4	10	30	*
CREAM																				
half & half																				
1 tbsp	20	*	3	6	2	*	*	*	*	2	*	*	*	*	*	*	*	*	*	*
heavy, whipping																				
1 tbsp	52	*	9	18	7	*	*	*	*	*	*	*	*	4	*	*	*	9	*	*
light																				
1 tbsp	29	*	4	9	3	*	*	*	*	*	*	*	*	2	*	*	*	*	*	*
light, whipping																				
1 tbsp	44	*	7	15	6	*	*	*	*	*	*	*	*	3	*	*	*	*	*	*
medium																				
25 % fat																				
1 tbsp	37	*	6	12	4	*	*	*	*	*	*	*	*	3	*	*	*	*	*	*
whipped																				
pressurized																				
1 tbsp	8	*	*	2	*	*	*	*	*	*	*	*	*	*	*	*	*	*	*	*
CREAM GRAVY																				
canned																				
(Franco-American) 1/4 cup	70	*	6	—	—	*	*	18	—	*	*	—	—	*	*	*	*	*	—	—
CREAM PUFF																				
Bavarian																				
(Rich's) 1 puff	140	3	11	25	8	6	*	2	*	*	2	*	*	*	*	3	12	*	—	—
CREAM, SOUR																				
(generic) 1 tbsp	26	*	4	8	2	*	*	*	*	*	*	*	*	2	*	*	*	*	*	*
half & half																				
(generic) 1 tbsp	20	*	22	6	2	*	*	*	2	*	*	*	*	*	*	*	*	*	*	*
imitation																				
(generic) 1 tbsp	30	*	4	13	*	*	*	*	*	*	*	*	*	*	*	*	*	*	*	*
light																				
(Weight Watchers) 1 oz	35	3	3	*	2	*	*	6	2	6	*	—	—	15	*	—	—	—	—	—
CREAM TOPPING																				
frozen																				
(generic) 1 tbsp	13	*	2	5	*	*	*	*	*	*	*	*	*	*	*	*	*	*	*	*
whipped																				
(Rich Prewhip) 2 tbsp	12	*	2	5	*	*	*	*	*	*	*	*	*	*	*	*	*	*	—	—
(Richwhip) 1/4 oz	20	*	3	10	*	*	*	*	*	*	*	*	*	*	*	*	*	*	—	—
from mix																				
prep w/ whole milk																				
(Dream-Whip) 1 tbsp	10	*	*	*	*	*	*	*	*	*	*	*	*	*	*	*	*	*	*	*
reduced calorie																				
(D-Zerta) 1 tbsp	8	*	2	—	*	*	*	*	*	*	*	—	—	*	*	*	*	*	—	—
pressurized																				
(generic) 1 tbsp	11	*	*	4	*	*	*	*	*	*	*	*	*	*	*	*	*	*	*	*
(Rich's) 1/4 oz	20	*	3	—	*	*	*	*	*	*	*	*	*	*	*	*	*	*	—	—

PERCENTAGE DAILY VALUE

	Calories	Protein	Fat	Sat. Fat	Cholesterol	Carbohydrates	Fiber	Sodium	Potassium	Calcium	Iron	Zinc	Magnesium	Vitamin A	Vitamin C	Thiamin	Riboflavin	Niacin	Vitamin B₁₂	Folic acid
CREAM TOPPING (continued)																				
ready-to-eat (generic) 1 tbsp	8	*	*	2	*	*	*	*	*	*	*	*	*	*	*	*	*	*	*	*
(La Creme) 1 tbsp	16	*	2	—	*	*	*	*	*	*	*	*	*	*	*	*	*	*	*	*
(Pet Whip) 1 tbsp	14	*	2	—	*	*	*	*	*	*	*	*	*	*	*	*	*	*	—	—
real cream (Kraft) 1 tbsp	15	*	*	5	*	*	*	*	*	*	*	*	*	*	*	*	*	*	—	—
whipped (Kraft) 1 tbsp	18	*	3	8	*	*	*	*	—	*	*	*	*	*	*	*	*	*	—	—
dairy (Cool-Whip) 1 tbsp	14	*	2	—	*	*	*	*	*	*	*	*	*	*	*	*	*	*	—	—
lite (Cool-Whip) 1 tbsp	8	*	2	—	*	*	*	*	*	*	*	*	*	*	*	*	*	*	—	—
non-dairy (Cool-Whip) 1 tbsp	12	*	2	—	*	*	*	*	*	*	*	*	*	*	*	*	*	*	—	—
CREME DE MENTHE																				
1 1/2 fl oz	186	*	*	*	*	7	*	*	*	*	*	*	*	*	*	*	*	*	*	*
CRESS, GARDEN																				
raw 1/2 cup	8	*	*	*	*	*	*	*	4	2	2	*	2	47	29	*	4	*	*	5
1 sprig	0	*	*	*	*	*	*	*	*	*	*	*	*	2	*	*	*	*	*	*
boiled 1/2 cup	16	2	*	*	*	*	*	*	7	4	3	*	4	105	26	3	6	3	*	6
boiled w/ salt 1/2 cup	16	2	*	*	*	*	—	7	7	4	3	*	4	105	26	3	6	3	*	6
CROAKER, ATLANTIC																				
raw 1 fillet	82	23	4	5	16	*	*	2	8	*	2	2	8	*	*	4	4	17	33	*
breaded & fried 1 fillet	192	26	17	15	24	2	—	13	8	3	4	3	9	*	*	5	7	19	30	*
CROISSANT																				
petite (Pepperidge Farm) 1 croissant	120	4	9	10	5	4	*	7	—	2	4	—	—	*	*	10	4	4	—	—
(Sara Lee) 2 croissants	230	—	*	20	2	9	4	11	—	*	8	—	—	4	4	—	—	—	—	—
regular (Sara Lee) 1 croissant	170	—	12	15	*	7	4	8	—	*	6	—	—	4	2	—	—	—	—	—
CROOKNECK SQUASH see SQUASH																				
CROUTON																				
caesar (Brownberry) 1/2 oz	60	2	5	—	*	3	—	7	—	*	2	—	—	*	*	4	2	2	—	—
homestyle (Pepperidge Farm) 1/2 oz	70	2	5	5	*	3	—	7	—	*	4	—	—	*	*	4	2	4	—	—
cheddar cheese (Brownberry) 1/2 oz	60	2	5	5	*	3	4	7	—	*	2	—	—	*	*	2	2	2	—	—
cheddar & romano cheese (Pepperidge Farm) 1/2 oz	60	2	3	*	*	3	—	8	—	2	4	—	—	*	*	4	4	4	—	—
cheese & garlic (Brownberry) 1/2 oz	60	2	5	5	*	3	4	7	—	*	2	—	—	*	*	4	2	2	—	—
(Pepperidge Farm) 1/2 oz	70	2	5	5	*	3	—	7	—	2	2	—	—	*	*	4	4	4	—	—
crispy (Arnold) 1/2 oz	60	2	3	5	*	3	4	5	—	*	2	—	—	*	*	2	2	2	—	—
fine herb crispy (Arnold) 1/2 oz	50	2	2	*	*	3	4	6	—	*	4	—	—	*	*	4	4	4	—	—
Italian (Progresso) 1/2 oz	30	3	2	—	*	*	—	5	*	2	4	—	—	*	*	4	2	15	—	—
crispy (Arnold) 1/2 oz	60	2	5	5	*	3	4	6	—	*	2	—	—	*	*	4	2	2	—	—

	Calories	Protein	Fat	Sat. Fat	Cholesterol	Carbohydrates	Fiber	Sodium	Potassium	Calcium	Iron	Zinc	Magnesium	Vitamin A	Vitamin C	Thiamin	Riboflavin	Niacin	Vitamin B12	Folic acid
CROUTON (continued)																				
homestyle (Pepperidge Farm) 1/2 oz	70	2	5	5	*	3	—	7	—	*	4	—	—	*	*	4	2	4	—	—
restaurant style (Pepperidge Farm) 1/2 oz	70	2	5	5	*	3	—	7	—	*	4	—	—	*	*	4	2	4	—	—
olive oil & garlic (Pepperidge Farm) 1/2 oz	60	2	3	*	*	3	4	7	—	*	2	—	—	*	*	4	2	4	—	—
onion & garlic (Brownberry) 1/2 oz	60	2	3	5	*	3	4	8	—	*	2	—	—	*	*	2	2	2	—	—
(Pepperidge Farm) 1/2 oz	70	2	5	5	*	3	—	7	—	*	2	—	—	*	*	6	4	4	—	—
crispy (Arnold) 1/2 oz	60	2	3	5	*	3	—	8	—	*	2	—	—	*	*	2	2	2	—	—
plain (Arnold) 1/2 oz	50	2	2	*	*	3	4	5	—	*	4	—	—	*	*	4	2	2	—	—
(Brownberry) 1/2 oz	60	2	—	*	*	3	4	5	—	*	4	—	—	*	*	4	2	2	—	—
(Croutettes) 1 cup	100	7	*	*	*	7	*	15	*	2	8	—	—	*	*	8	2	8	—	—
ranch (Brownberry) 1/2 oz	60	2	3	—	*	3	—	7	—	*	4	—	—	*	*	4	4	4	—	—
seasoned (Brownberry) 1/2 oz	60	2	3	5	*	3	4	7	—	*	2	—	—	*	*	4	2	2	—	—
(Pepperidge Farm) 1/2 oz	70	2	5	5	*	3	—	7	—	2	2	—	—	*	*	4	4	4	—	—
crispy (Arnold) 1/2 oz	60	2	5	5	*	3	4	7	—	*	2	—	—	*	*	4	2	4	—	—
wheat (Brownberry) 1/2 oz	60	2	5	—	*	3	4	7	—	*	4	—	—	*	*	2	2	*	—	—
sourdough cheese (Pepperidge Farm) 1/2 oz	70	2	5	5	*	3	—	7	—	2	4	—	—	*	*	6	4	4	—	—
toasted (Brownberry) 1/2 oz	60	2	2	*	*	3	4	6	—	*	4	—	—	*	*	4	4	4	—	—
CROWDER PEA (Bush Bros) 1/2 cup	110	12	2	*	*	6	20	21	—	2	8	—	—	*	*	—	—	—	—	—
CUCUMBER																				
raw w/ peel 1/2 cup slices	7	*	*	*	*	*	*	2	*	*	*	*	*	2	5	*	*	*	*	2
1 medium	39	3	*	*	*	3	8	*	12	4	4	4	8	13	27	5	4	3	*	10
CUCUMBER DIP																				
creamy premium (Kraft) 2 tbsp	50	2	6	15	3	*	*	5	*	2	*	—	—	*	*	2	*	*	—	—
CUMIN SEED 1 tbsp	22	2	2	21	*	*	4	*	3	6	22	2	5	2	*	3	*	*	*	—
CUPCAKE																				
chocolate (Hostess) 1 cake	180	3	9	15	2	10	4	12	2	10	6	*	*	*	*	4	4	2	*	*
lowfat (generic) 1 cake	131	3	2	3	*	10	8	7	3	2	4	2	3	*	*	*	3	2	*	*
chocolate, light w/ creme filling (Hostess) 1 cake	130	3	3	3	*	9	4	8	3	2	4	*	*	*	*	*	3	2	*	*
chocolate w/ chocolate fudge frosting from mix (Pillsbury) 1 cake	160	2	11	10	3	8	—	8	4	2	6	—	—	*	*	2	2	*	—	—
devil's food w/ chocolate frosting from mix (Duncan Hines) 1 cake	180	2	11	8	*	10	4	8	—	*	6	—	—	*	*	—	—	—	—	—
orange (Hostess) 1 cake	160	2	8	5	3	9	2	6	*	8	4	*	*	*	*	4	4	*	*	*
yellow w/ vanilla frosting from mix (Pillsbury) 1 cake	180	2	11	10	3	9	—	7	*	4	2	—	—	*	*	2	2	2	—	—

	Calories	Protein	Fat	Sat. Fat	Cholesterol	Carbohydrates	Fiber	Sodium	Potassium	Calcium	Iron	Zinc	Magnesium	Vitamin A	Vitamin C	Thiamin	Riboflavin	Niacin	Vitamin B₁₂	Folic acid
CUPCAKE, FROM MIX																				
yellow w/ chocolate frosting from mix (Duncan Hines) 1 cake	200	2	12	10	*	10	2	6	—	*	4	—	—	*	*	—	—	—	—	—
CUPU ASSU OIL																				
1 tbsp	120	*	22	36	*	*	*	*	*	*	—	*	*	*	*	*	*	*	*	—
CURRANT																				
black 1/2 cup	35	*	*	*	*	3	—	*	5	3	5	*	3	3	169	2	2	*	*	—
red/white 1/2 cup	31	*	*	*	*	3	8	*	4	2	3	*	2	*	38	*	2	*	*	—
zante dried 1/2 cup	204	5	*	*	*	18	20	*	18	6	13	3	7	*	6	8	6	6	*	2
CURRY POWDER																				
1 tbsp	20	*	*	*	*	*	8	*	3	3	10	2	4	*	*	*	*	*	*	—
CURRY SAUCE																				
from mix (Knorr) 1/4 oz	70	4	6	—		3	2	—	10	—	8					2	6	*		
CUSK																				
raw 1 fillet	106	39	*	*	17	*	*	2	14	*	6	3	9	*	*	3	10	16	21	*
broiled/baked 1 fillet	106	39	*	*	17	*	*	2	14	*	6	3	10	*	*	3	9	16	19	
CUSTARD see PUDDING																				
CUSTARD-APPLE																				
3 1/2 oz	101	3	*	*	*	8	—	*	11	3	4	—	5	*	32	5	6	3	*	—
CUTTLEFISH																				
raw 3 oz	67	23	*	*	32	*	*	13	9	8	28	10	6	6	8	*	45	5	42	*
steamed/poached 3 oz	134	46	2	*	63	*	*	26	15	15	51	20	13	11	12	*	86	9	76	*
DAIKON see RADISH, DAIKON																				
DAIQUIRI																				
homemade 1 cocktail (2 fl oz)	112	*	*	*	*	*	*	*	*	*	*	*	*	*	*	*	*	*	*	*
canned 6 3/4 fl oz can	259	*	*	*	*	11	*	3	*	*	*	*	*	*	*	*	*	*	*	*
DANDELION GREENS																				
raw 1/2 cup chopped	13	*	*	*	*	*	4	*	3	5	5	*	3	78	16	4	4	*	*	2
boiled 1/2 cup chopped	17	2	*	*	*	*	8	*	3	7	5	*	3	122	16	5	5	*	*	2
boiled w/ salt 1/2 cup chopped	17	2	*	*	*	*	—	6	3	7	5	*	3	122	16	5	5	*	*	2
DANISH PASTRY																				
apple (Hostess) 1 danish	400	7	34	50	7	15	7	14	3	8	8	—	—	*	*	10	8	8	—	—
97% fat free (Hostess) 1 danish	120	3	2	3	*	8	4	5	*	6	6	—	—	*	*	8	6	4	—	—
frozen (Pepperidge Farm) 1 danish	220	—	12	—	—	12	—	5	—	4	4	—	—	*	*	15	8	10	—	—
cheese frozen (Pepperidge Farm) 1 danish	260	—	22	—	—	8	—	10	—	4	6	—	—	*	*	15	8	10	—	—
cherry 97% fat free (Hostess) 1 danish	120	3	2	3	*	8	4	5	*	6	6	—	—	*	*	8	6	4	—	—

	Calories	Protein	Fat	Sat. Fat	Cholesterol	Carbohydrates	Fiber	Sodium	Potassium	Calcium	Iron	Zinc	Magnesium	Vitamin A	Vitamin C	Thiamin	Riboflavin	Niacin	Vitamin B₁₂	Folic acid
DANISH PASTRY (continued)																				
cinnamon raisin																				
from refrigerated dough																				
(Pillsbury) 1 danish	150	3	11	10	*	7	—	10	*	*	2	—	—	*	*	4	2	2	—	—
frozen																				
(Pepperidge Farm) 1 danish	250	—	17	—	—	12	—	7	—	4	4	—	—	*	*	15	6	10	—	—
orange w/ icing																				
from refrigerated dough																				
(Pillsbury) 1 danish	150	3	11	10	*	6	—	10	*	*	4	—	—	*	*	6	2	4	—	—
raspberry																				
(Hostess) 1 danish	390	7	31	50	7	16	7	12	3	10	8	—	—	*	*	10	8	8	—	—
frozen																				
(Pepperidge Farm) 1 danish	220	—	14	—	—	10	—	6	—	4	8	—	—	*	*	6	10	4	—	—
DATE																				
domestic																				
dried																				
1/2 cup	245	3	*	*	*	22	28	*	17	3	6	2	8	*	*	5	5	10	—	3
DEER see VENISON																				
DEMI-GLACE SAUCE																				
mix																				
(Knorr) 1/4 oz	25	*	2	—	*	*	—	15	—	*	*	*	*	*	*	2	*	*	*	*
DESSERT TOPPING see CREAM TOPPING																				
DIET BAR																				
chocolate																				
(Figurines) 1 bar	100	3	8	5	*	4	4	2	3	6	15	10	10	10	15	10	6	10	10	15
(Slim-Fast) 1 bar	130	10	6	—	2	6	24	4	4	10	35	35	10	35	35	35	35	35	35	20
chocolate caramel																				
(Figurines) 1 bar	100	3	9	5	*	4	4	3	3	6	10	10	8	10	10	10	6	10	10	15
chocolate chip																				
(Ultra Slim-Fast Crunch) 1 bar	120	4	6	—	*	6	12	*	3	15	15	4	6	15	15	15	15	15	15	15
chocolate peanut butter																				
(Figurines) 1 bar	100	5	9	5	*	3	4	2	3	6	10	10	10	10	10	10	6	15	10	20
cocoa almond																				
(Ultra Slim-Fast Crunch) 1 bar	110	4	6	—	*	6	12	*	3	15	15	4	6	15	15	15	15	15	15	15
mint chocolate																				
(Ultra Slim-Fast Crunch) 1 bar	120	4	6	—	*	6	12	*	3	15	15	4	6	15	15	15	15	15	15	15
peanut butter																				
(Slim-Fast) 1 bar	140	10	6	—	2	5	28	4	5	10	35	35	10	35	35	35	35	35	35	20
(Ultra Slim-Fast Crunch) 1 bar	120	4	6	—	*	7	12	2	3	15	15	4	6	15	15	15	15	15	15	15
s'mores																				
(Figurines) 1 bar	100	3	8	5	*	4	4	2	3	6	10	10	8	10	10	10	6	10	10	15
vanilla																				
(Figurines) 1 bar	100	3	8	5	*	4	4	2	3	6	10	10	8	10	15	10	6	10	10	15
vanilla almond																				
(Ultra Slim-Fast Crunch) 1 bar	110	4	6	—	*	6	12	*	3	15	15	4	10	15	15	15	15	15	15	15
DIET DRINK																				
canned																				
chocolate fudge																				
(Nestlé) 10 fl oz	200	25	5	5	*	11	*	9	15	50	35	35	35	35	35	35	35	35	35	35
(Ultra Slim-Fast) 8 fl oz skim milk & powder	200	30	3	—	5	12	20	10	21	45	35	35	30	60	35	35	35	35	35	30
chocolate royale																				
(Ultra Slim-Fast) 11 fl oz.	230	25	5	—	2	14	20	9	34	50	35	35	35	35	35	35	35	35	35	30
coffee																				
(Ultra Slim-Fast) 11 fl oz	200	25	5	—	3	13	20	10	35	50	35	35	35	35	35	35	35	35	35	30
French vanilla																				
(Ultra Slim-Fast) 11 fl oz	230	25	8	—	2	13	20	8	33	50	35	35	35	35	35	35	35	35	35	30

	Calories	Protein	Fat	Sat. Fat	Cholesterol	Carbohydrates	Fiber	Sodium	Potassium	Calcium	Iron	Zinc	Magnesium	Vitamin A	Vitamin C	Thiamin	Riboflavin	Niacin	Vitamin B₁₂	Folic acid

DIET DRINK (continued)

	Calories	Protein	Fat	Sat. Fat	Cholesterol	Carbohydrates	Fiber	Sodium	Potassium	Calcium	Iron	Zinc	Magnesium	Vitamin A	Vitamin C	Thiamin	Riboflavin	Niacin	Vitamin B12	Folic acid
strawberry (Sego Lite) 10 fl oz	150	18	6	—	—	6	*	16	17	50	25	—	—	25	25	25	25	25	—	—
strawberry (Sego Very) 10 fl oz	225	18	8	—	—	11	*	15	17	50	25	—	—	25	25	25	25	25	—	—
vanilla (Sego Lite) 10 fl oz	150	18	6	—	—	6	*	16	17	50	25	—	—	25	25	25	25	25	—	—
vanilla (Sego Very) 10 fl oz	225	18	8	—	—	11	*	15	17	50	25	—	—	25	25	25	25	25	—	—
milk chocolate (Nestlé) 10 fl oz	200	25	5	5	*	11	*	10	15	50	35	35	35	35	35	35	35	35	35	35
(Ultra Slim-Fast) 11 fl oz	200	25	5	—	2	12	20	7	17	40	35	35	35	35	35	35	35	35	35	30
strawberry supreme (Ultra Slim-Fast) 11 fl oz	210	25	5	—	2	13	20	9	31	50	35	35	35	35	35	35	35	35	35	30
from mix																				
cafe mocha (Ultra Slim-Fast) 1 scoop w/ 8 fl oz nonfat milk	200	30	2	—	3	13	24	12	23	45	35	35	35	35	35	35	35	35	35	30
chocolate royale (Ultra Slim-Fast) 1 scoop w/ 8 fl oz nonfat milk	200	30	2	—	3	12	20	10	23	45	35	35	35	35	35	35	35	35	35	30
chocolate malt (Slim-Fast) 1 scoop w/ 8 fl oz nonfat milk	190	30	2	—	3	11	8	10	20	45	35	35	35	35	35	35	35	35	35	30
chocolate (Slim-Fast) 1 scoop w/ 8 fl oz nonfat milk	190	30	2	—	3	11	8	9	21	45	35	35	35	35	35	35	35	35	35	30
chocolate almond (Nestlé) 1 scoop w/ 8 fl oz nonfat milk	180	35	3	5	2	8	*	12	21	50	35	35	35	35	35	35	35	35	35	35
chocolate chip (Nestlé) 1 scoop w/ 8 fl oz nonfat milk	180	35	3	5	2	8	*	12	17	50	35	35	35	35	35	35	35	35	35	35
chocolate fantasy (Ultra Slim-Fast) 12 fl oz skim milk & juice + powder	250	35	3	—	3	17	32	14	24	50	50	50	50	80	100	50	50	50	50	50
chocolate fudge (Nestlé) 1 scoop w/ 8 fl oz nonfat milk	180	35	3	5	2	8	*	12	21	50	35	35	35	35	35	35	35	35	35	35
chocolate malt (Ultra Slim-Fast) 1 scoop w/ 8 fl oz nonfat milk	200	30	2	—	5	12	20	10	19	45	35	35	30	60	35	35	35	35	35	30
chocolate raspberry truffle (Nestlé) 1 scoop w/ 8 fl oz nonfat milk	180	35	3	5	2	8	*	12	22	50	35	35	35	35	35	35	35	35	35	35
chocolate royale (Ultra Slim-Fast) 11 fl oz	230	25	5	—	2	14	20	9	34	50	35	35	35	35	35	35	35	35	35	30
coffee (Ultra Slim-Fast) 11 fl oz	200	25	5	—	3	13	20	10	35	50	35	35	35	35	35	35	35	35	35	30
French vanilla (Ultra Slim-Fast) 8 fl oz skim milk & powder	190	30	2	—	3	12	16	10	21	45	35	35	35	35	35	35	35	35	35	30
(Ultra Slim-Fast) 11 fl oz	230	25	8	—	2	13	20	8	33	50	35	35	35	35	35	35	35	35	35	30

	Calories	Protein	Fat	Sat. Fat	Cholesterol	Carbohydrates	Fiber	Sodium	Potassium	Calcium	Iron	Zinc	Magnesium	Vitamin A	Vitamin C	Thiamin	Riboflavin	Niacin	Vitamin B₁₂	Folic acid
DIET DRINK (continued)																				
milk chocolate (Nestlé) 1 scoop w/ 8 fl oz nonfat milk	180	35	3	5	2	8	*	12	21	50	35	35	35	35	35	35	35	35	35	35
(Ultra Slim-Fast) 11 fl oz	200	25	5	—	2	12	20	7	17	40	35	35	35	35	35	35	35	35	35	30
strawberry (Slim-Fast) 8 fl oz skim milk & powder	190	30	2	—	3	11	8	9	21	45	35	35	35	35	35	35	35	35	35	30
strawberry supreme (Ultra Slim-Fast) 8 fl oz skim milk & powder	190	30	2	—	3	12	16	10	20	45	35	35	35	35	35	35	35	35	35	30
(Ultra Slim-Fast) 11 fl oz	210	25	5	—	2	13	20	9	31	50	35	35	35	35	35	35	35	35	35	30
vanilla (Slim-Fast) 8 fl oz skim milk & powder	190	30	2	—	2	11	8	9	21	45	35	35	35	35	35	35	35	35	35	30
liquid protein chocolate (Sego Lite) 10 fl oz	150	18	5	—	—	7	*	20	20	50	25	—	—	25	25	25	25	25	—	—
chocolate (Sego Very) 10 fl oz	225	18	2	—	—	14	*	19	20	50	25	—	—	25	25	25	25	25	—	—
chocolate malt (Sego Very) 10 fl oz	225	18	2	—	—	14	*	15	17	50	25	—	—	25	25	25	25	25	—	—
Dutch chocolate (Sego Lite) 10 fl oz	150	18	5	—	—	7	*	20	20	50	25	—	—	25	25	25	25	25	—	—
French vanilla (Sego Lite) 10 fl oz	150	18	6	—	—	6	*	16	17	50	25	—	—	25	25	25	25	25	—	—
DILL DIP																				
from mix (Knorr) 1 tbsp	50	*	2	—	3	*	—	4	*	*	*	*	*	*	*	*	*	*	*	*
DILL SEED																				
1 tbsp	20	2	2	*	*	*	4	*	2	10	6	2	4	*	—	2	*	*	*	—
DILL WEED																				
fresh 1 tbsp	4	*	*	*	*	*	—	*	2	2	3	*	*	14	13	*	2	*	*	3
dried 1 tbsp	8	*	*	*	*	*	—	*	3	6	8	*	3	—	—	*	*	*	*	—
DOCK																				
raw 1/2 cup chopped	15	2	*	*	*	*	8	*	7	3	9	*	17	54	54	2	4	2	*	2
boiled 3 oz	17	3	*	*	*	*	—	*	8	3	10	*	19	59	37	2	4	2	*	2
boiled w/ salt 3 oz	17	3	*	*	*	*	—	*	8	3	10	*	19	59	37	2	4	2	*	2
DOLPHINFISH																				
raw 1 fillet	173	63	2	2	50	*	*	7	24	3	13	6	15	7	*	3	8	62	20	*
broiled/baked 1 fillet	173	63	2	2	50	*	*	7	24	3	13	6	15	7	*	2	8	59	18	*
DOUGHNUT																				
cinnamon 8-pack (Hostess) 1 doughnut	140	3	9	15	2	5	2	6	*	*	4	—	—	*	*	4	4	2	—	—
Apple Filled Donette (Hostess) 2 doughnuts	70	3	5	5	2	3	*	3	*	*	2	—	—	*	*	2	2	2	—	—
Donette (Hostess) 2 doughnuts	60	3	5	10	2	2	*	3	*	*	2	—	—	*	*	2	2	2	—	—
family pack (Hostess) 1 doughnut	140	3	9	15	2	5	2	6	*	*	4	—	—	*	*	4	4	2	—	—
pantry (Hostess) 1 doughnut	190	5	15	25	3	8	4	10	2	2	6	—	—	*	*	6	6	4	—	—

	Calories	Protein	Fat	Sat. Fat	Cholesterol	Carbohydrates	Fiber	Sodium	Potassium	Calcium	Iron	Zinc	Magnesium	Vitamin A	Vitamin C	Thiamin	Riboflavin	Niacin	Vitamin B₁₂	Folic acid
DOUGHNUT (continued)																				
crumb																				
(Hostess) 1 doughnut	160	2	15	25	3	5	4	6	*	4	4	—	—	*	*	6	4	4	—	—
Donette																				
(Hostess) 2 doughnuts	80	3	8	10	2	3	2	3	*	2	2	—	—	*	*	2	2	2	—	—
frosted																				
(Hostess) 1 doughnut	160	3	15	30	2	6	4	6	3	*	6	—	—	*	*	6	4	4	—	—
(Hostess O's) 1 doughnut	260	5	22	45	2	11	7	10	5	2	8	—	—	*	*	6	6	4	—	—
Donette																				
(Hostess) 2 doughnuts	80	3	8	15	*	3	2	3	2	*	2	—	—	*	*	2	2	2	—	—
Strawberry Filled Donette																				
(Hostess) 2 doughnuts	80	3	6	15	*	3	2	3	*	*	2	—	—	*	*	2	2	*	—	—
glazed																				
(Rich's) 1 doughnut	140	3	12	10	*	5	2	*	*	*	2	*	—	*	*	3	29	*	—	—
glazed whirl																				
(Hostess O's) 1 doughnut	190	5	11	15	2	9	4	10	3	4	6	—	—	*	*	8	4	4	—	—
honey wheat																				
(Hostess O's) 1 doughnut	250	5	18	30	8	11	5	12	2	15	6	—	—	*	*	8	6	6	—	—
old fashioned																				
(Hostess) 1 doughnut	170	5	14	20	3	7	4	10	2	2	6	—	—	*	*	8	6	4	—	—
old fashioned glazed																				
(Hostess O's) 1 doughnut	250	5	18	25	5	11	6	10	2	10	8	—	—	*	*	15	10	8	—	—
plain																				
(Hostess O's) 1 doughnut	230	5	15	20	2	11	4	10	2	2	6	—	—	*	*	10	8	4	—	—
8-pack																				
(Hostess) 1 doughnut	130	3	11	15	3	5	2	7	*	*	4	—	—	*	*	6	4	4	—	—
Donette																				
(Hostess) 2 doughnuts	60	3	5	10	2	2	*	3	*	*	2	—	—	*	*	2	2	2	—	—
family pack																				
(Hostess) 1 doughnut	120	3	9	15	2	4	2	7	*	*	4	—	—	*	*	6	4	4	—	—
pantry																				
(Hostess) 1 doughnut	190	5	17	25	3	7	4	11	2	2	6	—	—	*	*	10	6	6	—	—
powdered sugar																				
8-pack																				
(Hostess) 1 doughnut	140	3	11	20	3	6	2	7	*	*	2	—	—	*	*	6	2	2	—	—
Donette																				
(Hostess) 2 doughnuts	60	3	5	10	2	2	*	3	*	*	2	—	—	*	*	2	2	2	—	—
family pack																				
(Hostess) 1 doughnut	120	2	9	15	2	5	2	6	*	*	4	—	—	*	*	4	2	2	—	—
pantry																				
(Hostess) 1 doughnut	190	3	15	25	3	8	3	10	2	2	6	—	—	*	*	8	4	4	—	—
Strawberry Filled Donette																				
(Hostess) 2 doughnuts	70	3	5	5	2	3	*	3	*	*	4	—	—	*	*	4	2	2	—	—
sugar & spice minis																				
(Rich's) 3 donuts	200	3	17	10	3	8	2	12	*	2	2	*	*	*	*	2	18	*	—	—
DRUM, FRESHWATER																				
raw																				
1 fillet	236	58	15	11	42	*	*	6	16	12	10	9	15	7	3	9	20	23	66	*
broiled/baked																				
1 fillet	236	58	15	11	42	*	*	6	16	12	10	9	15	6	3	8	19	22	59	*
DUCK																				
meat w/ skin																				
raw																				
3 oz	343	16	51	56	22	*	*	2	5	*	11	8	3	3	4	11	10	17	4	3
fat																				
1 tbsp	115	*	20	21	4	*	*	*	*	*	*	*	*	*	*	*	*	*	*	*
meat w/ skin																				
roasted																				
(generic) 3 oz	286	27	37	41	24	*	*	2	5	*	13	11	3	4	*	10	13	21	4	*

	Calories	Protein	Fat	Sat. Fat	Cholesterol	Carbohydrates	Fiber	Sodium	Potassium	Calcium	Iron	Zinc	Magnesium	Vitamin A	Vitamin C	Thiamin	Riboflavin	Niacin	Vitamin B12	Folic acid
DUCK SAUCE																				
(La Choy) 1 tbsp	25	*	*	*	*	2	*	2	*	*	—	*	*	*	*	*	*	*	—	—
DUTCH LOAF																				
pork & beef																				
(generic) 1 1 oz slice	68	6	8	9	4	*	*	15	3	2	2	3	*	*	9	6	4	3	6	*
ECLAIR, FROZEN																				
chocolate																				
(Weight Watchers) 2 oz	150	5	8	8	*	8	8	6	2	4	*	—	—	*	*	—	—	—	—	—
EEL																				
raw																				
1 fillet	375	63	37	24	86	*	*	4	16	4	6	22	10	142	6	20	5	36	102	*
baked/broiled																				
1 fillet	375	63	37	24	85	*	*	4	16	4	6	22	10	120	5	19	5	36	76	*
EGG																				
chicken																				
raw																				
1 large	75	10	8	8	71	*	*	3	2	2	4	4	*	6	*	2	*	*	8	6
dried																				
1 tbsp	30	4	3	3	32	*	*	*	*	*	2	2	*	2	*	*	*	*	8	2
poached																				
1 large	75	10	8	8	70	*	*	6	2	2	4	4	*	6	*	2	*	*	7	4
scrambled																				
1 large	100	11	11	11	70	*	*	7	2	4	4	4	2	8	*	2	*	*	8	5
whole fried																				
1 large	92	10	11	10	70	*	*	7	2	3	4	4	*	8	*	2	*	*	7	4
hard-boiled																				
1 large	78	10	8	8	71	*	*	3	2	3	3	3	*	6	*	2	*	*	9	6
white																				
dried powder																				
1 cup	402	147	*	*	*	2	*	55	34	10	*	*	19	*	*	3	*	4	9	26
yolk																				
raw																				
1 large	59	5	8	8	71	*	*	*	*	2	3	3	*	6	*	2	*	*	9	6
dried																				
1 tbsp	27	2	4	4	39	*	*	*	*	*	2	2	*	3	*	*	*	*	5	2
duck																				
1 egg	130	15	15	13	206	*	*	4	4	4	15	7	3	19	*	7	*	*	63	14
goose																				
1 egg	267	33	29	26	408	*	*	8	9	9	29	13	6	37	*	14	*	*	122	27
turkey																				
1 egg	135	18	14	15	245	*	*	5	3	8	18	8	3	9	*	6	46	*	22	14
EGG SUBSTITUTE																				
frozen																				
(generic) 1/4 cup	96	11	10	6	*	*	*	5	4	4	7	4	2	16	*	5	71	*	3	2
liquid																				
(Egg Beaters) 1/4 cup	30	17	*	*	*	*	*	4	—	2	6	4	—	6	*	4	60	4	10	8
(Healthy Choice) 1/4 cup	30	8	*	*	*	—		4	2	2	4	—	—	10	*	4	15	*	—	—
EGG ROLL																				
almond chicken																				
(La Choy) 3 oz	120	8	5	—	2	6	—	12	—	*	6	—	—	8	10	12	8	8	—	—
chicken																				
(La Choy Snack Size) 1 1/2 oz	90	5	5	—	*	4	—	6	—	*	4	—	—	*	4	8	4	6	—	—
lobster																				
(La Choy Snack Size) 1 1/2 oz	75	3	3	—	*	4	—	6	—	*	4	—	—	*	4	8	4	4	—	—
meat & shrimp																				
(La Choy Snack Size) 1 1/2 oz	80	5	5	—	*	4	—	5	—	*	4	—	—	*	4	8	4	4	—	—
pork																				
(La Choy Restaurant Style) 3 oz	150	12	8	—	2	7	—	20	—	10	10	—	—	6	30	15	10	35	—	—

	Calories	Protein	Fat	Sat. Fat	Cholesterol	Carbohydrates	Fiber	Sodium	Potassium	Calcium	Iron	Zinc	Magnesium	Vitamin A	Vitamin C	Thiamin	Riboflavin	Niacin	Vitamin B12	Folic acid
EGG ROLL (continued)																				
shrimp																				
(La Choy Restaurant Style) 3 oz	130	8	6	—	2	6	—	11	—	2	8	—	—	6	10	10	8	8	—	—
(La Choy Snack Size) 1 1/2 oz	75	3	3	—	*	4	—	5	—	*	4	—	—	*	6	8	4	4	—	—
sweet & sour chicken																				
(La Choy) 3 oz	150	7	6	—	2	8	—	12	—	*	6	—	—	*	15	10	8	8	—	—
EGGNOG																				
(generic) 1 cup	342	16	29	57	50	11	*	6	12	33	3	8	12	18	6	6	*	*	19	*
from mix																				
(generic) 1 cup milk + 2 heaping tsp	261	14	13	*	11	13	*	7	11	29	2	6	8	6	4	6	23	*	14	3
EGGPLANT																				
raw																				
1/2 cup	11	*	*	*	*	*	4	*	3	*	*	*	*	*	*	*	*	*	*	2
1 medium	119	8	*	*	*	9	44	*	28	3	7	4	16	8	13	16	9	14	*	22
boiled																				
1/2 cup	13	*	*	*	*	*	4	*	3	*	*	*	2	*	*	2	*	*	*	2
boiled w/ salt																				
1/2 cup	13	*	*	*	*	*	—	5	3	*	*	*	2	*	*	2	*	*	*	2
bottled																				
caponata (Progresso) 1/4 cup	70	3	6	5	*	*	2	11	4	*	6	—	—	8	*	*	*	2	—	—
ELDERBERRY																				
1/2 cup	106	2	*	*	*	9	40		12	6	13			17	87	7	5	—	—	—
ELK																				
roasted																				
4 oz	165	57	3	4	27	*	*	3	11	*	23	24	7	*	*	—	—	—		
ENCHANADA, FROZEN																				
beef & bean																				
(Stouffer's Lean Cuisine) 9 1/4 oz	240	25	9	15	15	11	—	20	13	10	10	—	—	8	10	15	15	10	—	—
chicken																				
(Stouffer's Lean Cuisine) 9 7/8 oz	290	28	14	15	18	11	—	21	13	15	15	—	—	25	10	15	20	15	—	—
ENCHILADA, FROZEN																				
beef																				
(Healthy Choice) 13 1/3 oz	370	25	8	10	10	22	—	19	17	15	10	—	—	25	40	20	15	10	—	—
(Patio) 13 1/4 oz	520	27	37	—	13	20	—	75	20	15	20	—	—	15	*	20	10	8	—	—
(Weight Watchers) 9 oz	190	30	8	10	7	6	20	21	16	20	10	—	—	15	15	—	—	—	—	—
cheese																				
(Patio) 12 oz	370	23	15	—	7	19	—	82	17	15	15	—	—	8	*	15	10	4	—	—
(Stouffer's) 9 3/4 oz	370	38	22	25	8	16	20	37	9	20	8	—	—	20	20	6	20	8	—	—
chicken																				
(Healthy Choice) 13 1/3 oz	320	22	9	15	10	19	—	23	12	10	20	—	—	15	90	45	20	35	—	—
(Healthy Choice) 9 1/2 oz	310	23	14	15	12	15	—	20	11	10	8	—	—	8	35	10	10	25	—	—
(Stouffer's) 10 oz	370	35	22	18	10	15	12	40	15	10	25	6	—	—	10	10	6	20	15	—	—
nacho grande																				
(Weight Watchers) 9 oz	190	25	12	13	7	14	16	23	17	30	6	—	—	30	20	—	—	—	—	—
suiza																				
(Weight Watchers) 9 oz	230	27	11	8	13	8	32	22	13	20	8	—	—	4	4	—	—	—	—	—
nacho cheese																				
(Weight Watchers) 9 oz	150	17	9	13	8	13	20	22	17	25	8	—	—	25	30	—	—	—	—	—
regular																				
(Gebhardt) 2 enchiladas	310	8	37	45	19	7	8	19	6	2	10	—	—	*	3	13	7	9	—	—
ENCHILADA SAUCE																				
green																				
(Old El Paso) 1/4 cup	22	*	*	*	*	*	*	16	*	*	*	*	*	*	*	*	*	*	*	*
hot																				
(Old El Paso) 1/4 cup	30	*	2	—	*	*	*	10	—	*	20	—	—	*	*	*	4	*	—	—

	Calories	Protein	Fat	Sat. Fat	Cholesterol	Carbohydrates	Fiber	Sodium	Potassium	Calcium	Iron	Zinc	Magnesium	Vitamin A	Vitamin C	Thiamin	Riboflavin	Niacin	Vitamin B₁₂	Folic acid
ENCHILADA SAUCE (continued)																				
mild																				
(Gebhardt) 1/4 cup	33	*	3	5	*	*	*	10	*	12	4	—	—	*	*	3	5	5	—	—
(Old El Paso) 1/4 cup	25	*	2	—	*	*	*	10	—	*	6	*	*	*	*	*	2	2	*	*
(Rosarita) 1/4 cup	40	*	4	*	*	*	*	16	4	*	6	—	—	*	9	*	3	3	—	—
ENCHILADA SEASONING MIX																				
(Old El Paso) 1/18 pkg	6	*	*	*	*	*	*	3	*	*	*	*	*	*	*	*	*	*	—	—
ENDIVE																				
raw																				
1/2 cup chopped	4	*	*	*	*	*	4	*	2	*	*	*	*	10	3	*	*	*	*	9
1 head	87	11	2	*	*	6	64	5	46	27	24	27	19	210	56	27	23	10	*	183
EPPAW																				
raw																				
1/2 cup	75	4	*	*	*	5	—	*	5	6	3	4	4	*	11	4	4	*	*	3
FALAFEL																				
(generic) 3 patties	170	11	14	6	*	5	—	6	8	3	10	5	10	*	*	5	5	3	*	10
from mix																				
(Near East) 3 patties	310	22	27	15	*	7	28	31	—	6	20	—	—	*	*	—	—	—	—	—
FARINA see CEREAL, HOT																				
FAST FOOD, BURGER KING																				
bacon double cheeseburger																				
1 sandwich	470	45	43	65	33	9	—	33	—	20	20	—	—	8	*	—	—	—	—	—
bacon double cheeseburger deluxe																				
1 sandwich	570	50	58	75	37	9	—	41	—	20	20	—	—	10	4	—	—	—	—	—
big fish sandwich																				
1 sandwich	710	35	66	40	20	19	—	46	—	8	20	—	—	2	2	—	—	—	—	—
Breakfast Buddy																				
1 sandwich	255	17	25	30	42	5	—	20	—	8	10	—	—	5	*	—	—	—	—	—
broiler chicken sandwich																				
1 sandwich	280	30	15	10	17	6	—	32	—	4	10	—	—	2	6	—	—	—	—	—
butterfly shrimp																				
1 serving	300	25	26	25	45	7	—	25	—	15	6	—	—	*	4	—	—	—	—	—
cheeseburger																				
1 sandwich	300	25	22	30	15	9	—	27	—	10	15	—	—	6	4	—	—	—	—	—
chef salad																				
1 serving	178	26	14	20	34	2	—	24	—	16	9	—	—	95	25	—	—	—	—	—
chicken salad																				
1 serving	142	31	6	5	16	3	—	18	—	4	7	—	—	92	34	—	—	—	—	—
chicken sandwich																				
1 sandwich	700	40	65	40	20	18	—	60	—	8	20	—	—	*	*	—	—	—	—	—
Chicken Tenders																				
6 pieces	236	25	20	15	13	5	—	23	—	*	4	—	—	2	*	—	—	—	—	—
Croissan'wich																				
bacon, egg & cheese																				
1 sandwich	353	24	35	40	77	6	—	32	—	14	10	—	—	10	4	—	—	—	—	—
ham, egg & cheese																				
1 sandwich	351	29	34	35	79	7	—	57	—	14	12	—	—	10	*	—	—	—	—	—
sausage, egg & cheese																				
1 sandwich	534	32	62	70	86	7	—	41	—	15	16	—	—	10	*	—	—	—	—	—
dinner roll																				
1 roll	80	4	3	*	*	4	—	6	—	1	5	—	—	*	*	—	—	—	—	—
dinner salad																				
1 serving	20	*	*	*	*	*	—	*	—	*	2	—	—	90	15	—	—	—	—	—
double cheeseburger																				
1 sandwich	450	40	38	60	30	10	—	35	—	20	20	—	—	10	4	—	—	—	—	—
double Whopper																				
1 sandwich	860	70	85	95	57	15	—	40	—	8	40	—	—	10	20	—	—	—	—	—
double Whopper w/ cheese																				
1 sandwich	950	80	97	115	65	15	—	52	—	25	40	—	—	20	20	—	—	—	—	—

	Calories	Protein	Fat	Sat. Fat	Cholesterol	Carbohydrates	Fiber	Sodium	Potassium	Calcium	Iron	Zinc	Magnesium	Vitamin A	Vitamin C	Thiamin	Riboflavin	Niacin	Vitamin B12	Folic acid
FAST FOOD, BURGER KING (continued)																				
Dutch apple pie 1 pie	308	4	23	15	*	13	—	9	—	*	6	—	—	*	8	—	—	—	—	—
french fries medium	372	8	31	25	*	14	—	10	—	*	7	—	—	*	5	—	—	—	—	—
French toast sticks 1 serving	440	6	42	35	*	20	—	20	—	6	15	—	—	*	*	—	—	—	—	—
garden salad 1 serving	95	9	8	15	5	3	—	5	—	15	6	—	—	100	58	—	—	—	—	—
hamburger 1 sandwich	260	20	15	20	10	9	—	21	—	2	15	—	—	2	4	—	—	—	—	—
hash browns 1 serving	213	3	18	15	*	8	—	13	—	*	2	—	—	12	9	—	—	—	—	—
mini muffin blueberry 1 muffin	292	7	22	15	24	12	—	10	—	4	7	—	—	*	*	—	—	—	—	—
onion rings 1 medium	339	7	29	25	*	13	—	26	—	11	3	—	—	15	*	—	—	—	—	—
orange juice 1 medium	82	*	*	*	*	7	—	*	—	*	*	—	—	3	119	—	—	—	—	—
popcorn 1 serving	130	4	9	15	5	6	—	22	—	*	2	—	—	*	*	—	—	—	—	—
potato, baked 1 potato	210	8	*	*	*	16	—	*	—	2	15	—	—	*	50	—	—	—	—	—
sauce honey 1 oz	91	*	*	*	*	8	—	*	—	*	*	—	—	*	*	—	—	—	—	—
AM express 1 oz	84	*	*	*	*	7	—	*	—	*	*	—	—	*	*	—	—	—	—	—
barbecue 1 oz	36	*	*	*	*	3	—	17	—	*	*	—	—	3	4	—	—	—	—	—
ranch 1 oz	171	*	28	15	*	*	—	9	—	*	*	—	—	*	*	—	—	—	—	—
sweet & sour 1 oz	45	*	*	*	*	4	—	2	—	*	*	—	—	*	*	—	—	—	—	—
shake chocolate 1 medium	320	10	11	25	7	11	—	10	—	20	10	—	—	4	*	—	—	—	—	—
chocolate w/ syrup 1 medium	400	15	14	25	7	23	—	15	—	30	2	—	—	6	6	—	—	—	—	—
strawberry 1 medium	370	15	9	20	7	22	—	10	—	30	*	—	—	6	6	—	—	—	—	—
vanilla 1 medium	310	15	9	20	7	12	—	10	—	30	*	—	—	6	6	—	—	—	—	—
side salad 1 serving	20	*	*	*	*	*	—	*	—	*	2	—	—	90	15	—	—	—	—	—
Whopper 1 sandwich	630	40	58	55	30	15	—	37	—	8	30	—	—	10	20	—	—	—	—	—
Whopper w/ cheese 1 sandwich	720	50	71	80	38	15	—	50	—	20	30	—	—	20	20	—	—	—	—	—
Whopper jr. 1 sandwich	330	20	29	25	13	9	—	21	—	4	15	—	—	4	8	—	—	—	—	—
Whopper jr. w/ cheese 1 sandwich	380	25	34	35	17	10	—	27	—	10	15	—	—	8	8	—	—	—	—	—
FAST FOOD, KENTUCKY FRIED CHICKEN																				
baked beans 1 serving	132	8	3	5	*	8	16	22	—	4	4	—	—	5	*	—	—	—	—	—
biscuit, buttermilk 1 biscuit	220	8	18	15	*	9	—	22	—	4	10	—	—	*	*	—	—	—	—	—
breadstick 1 piece	110	5	5	*	*	6	*	*	—	3	3	—	—	*	*	—	—	—	—	—

PERCENTAGE DAILY VALUE

FAST FOOD, KENTUCKY FRIED CHICKEN (continued)

	Calories	Protein	Fat	Sat. Fat	Cholesterol	Carbohydrates	Fiber	Sodium	Potassium	Calcium	Iron	Zinc	Magnesium	Vitamin A	Vitamin C	Thiamin	Riboflavin	Niacin	Vitamin B₁₂	Folic acid
chicken, fried, extra crispy																				
breast, center 1 piece	330	43	29	20	25	5	*	31	—	2	4	—	—	*	*	—	—	—	—	—
breast, side 1 piece	400	35	42	30	25	6	*	30	—	2	4	—	—	*	*	—	—	—	—	—
drumstick 1 piece	190	23	18	15	22	2	*	13	—	2	4	—	—	*	*	—	—	—	—	—
thigh 1 piece	380	38	45	35	30	2	*	22	—	2	6	—	—	2	*	—	—	—	—	—
wing 1 piece	240	22	26	20	22	3	*	13	—	2	2	—	—	2	*	—	—	—	—	—
chicken, fried, hot & spicy																				
breast, center 1 piece	360	47	34	25	27	4	*	31	—	2	4	—	—	*	*	—	—	—	—	—
breast, side 1 piece	400	37	43	30	27	5	*	35	—	4	6	—	—	*	*	—	—	—	—	—
drumstick 1 piece	180	23	18	10	18	2	*	13	—	2	4	—	—	*	*	—	—	—	—	—
thigh 1 piece	370	40	42	30	33	3	*	28	—	2	6	—	—	*	*	—	—	—	—	—
wing 1 piece	220	23	25	20	22	2	*	18	—	2	4	—	—	2	*	—	—	—	—	—
chicken, fried, original recipe																				
breast, center 1 piece	260	42	22	20	31	3	*	25	—	3	4	—	*	*	*	—	—	—	—	—
breast, side 1 piece	245	30	23	20	26	3	*	25	—	4	4	—	*	*	*	—	—	—	—	—
drumstick 1 piece	152	23	14	10	25	*	*	11	—	*	4	—	*	*	*	—	—	—	—	—
thigh 1 piece	287	30	32	25	37	3	*	25	—	4	6	—	*	*	*	—	—	—	—	—
wing 1 piece	172	20	17	15	20	2	*	16	—	3	3	—	*	*	*	—	—	—	—	—
Chicken Littles sandwich 1 sandwich	169	10	15	10	6	5	—	14	—	2	10	—	—	*	*	—	—	—	—	—
chicken nugget sauce																				
barbeque 1 oz	35	*	2	*	*	2	*	19	—	*	*	—	—	7	*	—	—	—	—	—
honey 1/2 oz	49	*	*	*	*	4	*	*	—	*	*	—	—	*	*	—	—	—	—	—
chicken nuggets 6 pieces	284	27	28	20	22	5	—	36	—	2	4	—	—	*	*	—	—	—	—	—
chicken, rotisserie gold																				
dark quarter as served 1 serving	333	50	36	33	54	*	*	41	—	*	*	—	—	*	*	—	—	—	—	—
skin removed 1 serving	217	45	19	18	43	*	*	32	—	*	*	—	—	*	*	—	—	—	—	—
white quarter as served 1 serving	335	67	29	27	52	*	*	46	—	*	*	—	—	*	*	—	—	—	—	—
skin & wing removed 1 serving	199	62	9	9	32	*	*	28	—	*	*	—	—	*	*	—	—	—	—	—
chicken sandwich 1 sandwich	482	35	42	30	16	13	—	44	—	5	7	—	—	*	*	—	—	—	—	—
coleslaw 1 serving	114	2	9	5	*	4	—	7	—	3	2	—	—	*	45	—	—	—	—	—
corn on the cob 1 ear	176	8	5	3	*	11	—	*	—	7	*	—	—	5	2	—	—	—	—	—
cornbread 1 piece	228	5	20	10	14	8	4	8	—	6	6	—	—	*	*	—	—	—	—	—

THE HEALTH NUTRIENT BIBLE

	Calories	Protein	Fat	Sat. Fat	Cholesterol	Carbohydrates	Fiber	Sodium	Potassium	Calcium	Iron	Zinc	Magnesium	Vitamin A	Vitamin C	Thiamin	Riboflavin	Niacin	Vitamin B12	Folic acid
FAST FOOD, KENTUCKY FRIED CHICKEN (continued)																				
french fries 1 regular serving	294	7	26	20	*	11	—	32	—	3	5	—	—	*	4	—	—	—	—	—
garden salad 1 serving	16	2	*	*	*	*	4	*	—	*	2	—	—	23	20	—	—	—	—	—
green beans 1 serving	36	2	2	*	*	2	8	23	—	4	4	—	—	3	3	—	—	—	—	—
Hot Wings pieces 6 pieces	471	45	51	40	50	6	—	51	—	4	8	—	—	*	*	—	—	—	—	—
Italian dressing 1 serving	15	*	2	*	*	*	*	17	—	*	*	—	—	*	*	—	—	—	—	—
macaroni & cheese 1 serving	162	12	12	15	5	5	*	22	—	12	12	—	—	19	*	—	—	—	—	—
macaroni salad 1 serving	248	7	26	15	4	7	4	*	—	*	6	—	—	*	2	—	—	—	—	—
Mean Greens 1 serving	52	5	3	5	2	3	12	20	—	14	14	—	—	43	8	—	—	—	—	—
pasta salad 1 serving	135	3	12	5	*	5	4	28	—	2	6	—	—	11	12	—	—	—	—	—
potato, mashed w/ gravy 1 serving	70	5	2	5	*	5	—	15	—	2	2	—	—	*	*	—	—	—	—	—
potato salad 1 serving	180	5	17	10	4	6	8	18	—	*	12	—	—	8	*	—	—	—	—	—
potato wedges 1 serving	192	5	14	15	*	8	12	18	—	1	6	—	—	*	*	—	—	—	—	—
red beans & rice 1 serving	114	7	5	5	*	6	12	13	—	*	*	—	—	*	*	—	—	—	—	—
rice 1 serving	75	3	2	*	*	5	4	24	—	*	*	—	—	7	9	—	—	—	—	—
sourdough roll 1 piece	128	7	3	*	*	8	4	10	—	4	4	—	—	*	*	—	—	—	—	—
vegetable medley salad 1 serving	126	2	6	5	*	7	12	10	—	2	2	—	—	75	9	—	—	—	—	—
FAST FOOD, MCDONALD'S																				
apple bran muffin fat free 1 muffin	180	8	*	*	*	13	—	8	—	4	6	—	—	*	*	10	10	10	—	—
apple pie 1 serving	280	5	23	—	*	12	—	4	—	2	6	—	—	*	*	6	4	10	—	—
barbecue sauce 1 order	50	*	*	*	*	4	—	14	—	*	2	—	—	4	4	*	*	*	—	—
Big Mac 1 burger	500	42	40	45	33	14	—	37	—	25	20	—	—	6	2	30	25	35	—	—
biscuit w/ bacon, egg & cheese 1 biscuit	440	25	40	—	80	11	—	51	—	20	15	—	—	10	*	25	20	10	—	—
w/ sausage 1 biscuit	420	20	43	—	15	11	—	43	—	8	10	—	—	*	*	30	10	20	—	—
w/ sausage & egg 1 biscuit	505	32	51	—	87	11	—	50	—	10	20	—	—	6	*	30	20	20	—	—
w/ spread 1 biscuit	260	8	20	—	*	11	—	30	—	8	8	—	—	*	*	15	6	8	—	—
breakfast burrito 1 burrito	280	20	26	—	45	7	—	24	—	10	8	—	—	10	10	20	15	10	—	—
cheeseburger 1 burger	305	25	20	25	17	10	—	30	—	20	15	—	—	8	4	20	15	20	—	—
chef salad 1 serving	170	28	14	20	37	3	—	17	—	15	8	—	—	100	35	20	15	20	—	—

	Calories	Protein	Fat	Sat. Fat	Cholesterol	Carbohydrates	Fiber	Sodium	Potassium	Calcium	Iron	Zinc	Magnesium	Vitamin A	Vitamin C	Thiamin	Riboflavin	Niacin	Vitamin B₁₂	Folic acid
FAST FOOD, MCDONALD'S (continued)																				
chicken fajita 1 sandwich	190	18	12	10	12	7	—	13	—	8	4	—	—	2	10	10	10	20	—	—
Chicken McNuggets large 1 serving	405	50	34	40	28	8	—	36	—	*	8	—	—	*	*	10	10	70	—	—
medium 1 serving	270	33	23	18	18	6	—	24	—	*	6	—	—	*	*	8	8	40	—	—
small 1 serving	180	22	15	10	12	4	—	16	—	*	2	—	—	*	*	4	4	30	—	—
chicken salad 1 serving	150	42	6	5	26	2	—	10	—	4	6	—	—	170	45	15	10	45	—	—
cookies chocolate chip 1 box	330	7	23	—	*	14	—	12	—	2	10	—	—	*	*	15	10	10	—	—
McDonaldland 1 box	290	7	14	—	*	16	—	12	—	*	10	—	—	*	*	10	10	10	—	—
danish apple 1 danish	390	5	26	—	8	17	—	15	—	*	8	—	—	*	25	20	10	10	—	—
cinnamon raisin 1 danish	440	10	32	—	11	19	—	18	—	4	10	—	—	*	6	20	15	15	—	—
iced cheese 1 danish	390	12	32	—	16	14	—	17	—	4	8	—	—	4	*	20	15	10	—	—
raspberry 1 danish	410	10	25	—	9	21	—	13	—	*	8	—	—	*	6	20	10	10	—	—
Egg McMuffin 1 sandwich	280	30	17	—	78	9	—	30	—	25	15	—	—	10	*	30	20	20	—	—
English muffin w/ spread 1 muffin	170	8	6	—	*	9	—	12	—	15	8	—	—	2	*	20	8	10	—	—
Filet-o-Fish 1 sandwich	370	23	28	20	17	13	—	30	—	15	10	—	—	2	*	20	8	45	—	—
french fries large 1 serving	400	10	34	25	*	15	—	8	—	*	6	—	—	*	25	15	*	15	—	—
medium 1 serving	320	7	26	18	*	12	—	6	—	*	4	—	—	*	20	15	*	15	—	—
small 1 serving	220	5	18	13	*	9	—	5	—	*	2	—	—	*	15	10	*	10	—	—
frozen yogurt cone vanilla 1 cone	105	7	2	—	*	7	—	3	—	10	*	—	—	2	*	20	10	2	—	—
frozen yogurt sundae hot caramel 1 sundae	270	12	5	—	4	20	—	7	—	20	*	—	—	6	*	6	20	*	—	—
hot fudge 1 sundae	240	12	5	—	2	17	—	7	—	25	2	—	—	4	*	4	20	*	—	—
strawberry 1 sundae	210	10	2	—	2	16	—	4	—	20	*	—	—	4	2	2	20	*	—	—
garden salad 1 serving	50	7	3	3	22	2	—	3	—	4	8	—	—	90	35	6	6	2	—	—
hamburger 1 burger	255	20	14	15	12	10	—	20	—	10	15	—	—	4	4	20	10	20	—	—
hash brown potatoes 1 serving	130	2	6	—	*	5	—	14	—	*	*	—	—	*	2	4	*	4	—	—
hotcake w/ margarine & syrup 1 serving	440	13	18	—	3	25	—	28	—	10	10	—	—	4	*	20	20	15	—	—
McChicken 1 order	415	32	31	20	17	13	—	35	—	15	15	—	—	2	4	60	10	45	—	—

	Calories	Protein	Fat	Sat. Fat	Cholesterol	Carbohydrates	Fiber	Sodium	Potassium	Calcium	Iron	Zinc	Magnesium	Vitamin A	Vitamin C	Thiamin	Riboflavin	Niacin	Vitamin B₁₂	Folic acid
FAST FOOD, MCDONALD'S (continued)																				
McLean deluxe																				
plain																				
1 sandwich	320	37	15	20	20	12	—	28	—	15	20	—	—	10	10	25	20	35	—	—
w/ cheese																				
1 sandwich	370	40	22	25	25	12	—	37	—	20	20	—	—	15	10	25	20	35	—	—
mustard sauce																				
1 serving	70	*	6	*	2	3	—	10	—	2	*	—	—	*	*	*	*	*	—	—
Quarter Pounder																				
regular																				
1 burger	410	38	31	40	28	11	—	27	—	15	20	—	—	4	6	25	15	35	—	—
w/ cheese																				
1 burger	510	47	43	55	38	11	—	46	—	30	20	—	—	15	6	25	20	35	—	—
sausage																				
1 serving	160	12	23	—	14	*	—	13	—	*	4	—	—	*	*	15	6	10	—	—
Sausage McMuffin																				
plain																				
1 sandwich	345	25	31	—	19	9	—	32	—	20	15	—	—	4	*	35	15	25	—	—
w/ egg																				
1 sandwich	430	35	38	—	90	9	—	38	—	25	20	—	—	10	*	35	25	25	—	—
scrambled eggs																				
1 serving	140	20	15	—	142	*	—	12	—	6	10	—	—	10	*	4	15	*	—	—
shake																				
chocolate																				
1 regular	320	18	3	—	3	22	—	10	—	35	*	—	—	6	*	8	30	2	—	—
strawberry																				
1 regular	320	18	2	—	3	22	—	7	—	35	*	—	—	6	*	8	30	2	—	—
vanilla																				
1 regular	290	18	2	—	3	20	—	7	—	35	*	—	—	6	*	10	30	*	—	—
side salad																				
1 serving	30	3	2	*	11	*	—	*	—	2	4	—	—	80	20	4	4	*	—	—
sweet 'n' sour sauce																				
1 serving	60	*	*	*	*	5	—	8	—	*	*	—	—	6	*	*	*	*	—	—
FAST FOOD, PIZZA HUT																				
beef																				
hand tossed																				
1 slice medium pizza	261	25	15	15	8	9	8	33	—	18	11	—	—	6	—	—	—	—	—	—
pan																				
1 slice medium pizza	288	17	28	15	8	9	12	28	—	18	11	—	—	8	—	—	—	—	—	—
thin 'n' crispy																				
1 slice medium pizza	231	22	17	15	8	7	8	29	—	17	9	—	—	8	—	—	—	—	—	—
cheese																				
bigfoot																				
1 slice Bigfoot pizza	179	15	8	15	5	8	8	40	—	2	9	—	—	6	—	—	—	—	—	—
hand tossed																				
1 slice medium pizza	253	25	14	20	8	9	8	25	—	24	9	—	—	9	—	—	—	—	—	—
pan																				
1 slice medium pizza	279	23	20	25	8	9	8	20	—	24	9	—	—	9	—	—	—	—	—	—
thin 'n' crispy																				
1 slice medium pizza	223	22	15	25	8	6	8	21	—	23	6	—	—	9	—	—	—	—	—	—
chunky combo																				
hand tossed																				
1 slice medium pizza	280	25	18	24	10	9	10	34	—	17	10	—	—	10	—	—	—	—	—	—
pan																				
1 slice medium pizza	306	23	24	26	10	9	10	29	—	17	12	—	—	10	—	—	—	—	—	—
thin 'n' crispy																				
1 slice medium pizza	250	21	20	25	10	7	8	31	—	17	11	—	—	10	—	—	—	—	—	—
chunky meat																				
hand tossed																				
1 slice medium pizza	325	28	25	30	13	9	10	40	—	17	11	—	—	10	—	—	—	—	—	—

FAST FOOD, PIZZA HUT (continued)

	Calories	Protein	Fat	Sat. Fat	Cholesterol	Carbohydrates	Fiber	Sodium	Potassium	Calcium	Iron	Zinc	Magnesium	Vitamin A	Vitamin C	Thiamin	Riboflavin	Niacin	Vitamin B12	Folic acid
pan 1 slice medium pizza	352	26	31	35	13	9	10	35	—	17	15	—	—	10	—	—	—	—	—	—
thin 'n' crispy 1 slice medium pizza	295	24	26	30	13	7	9	37	—	17	8	—	—	10	—	—	—	—	—	—
chunky veggie hand tossed 1 slice medium pizza	224	21	9	10	6	10	12	26	—	19	10	—	—	10	—	—	—	—	—	—
pan 1 slice medium pizza	251	20	15	15	6	7	12	21	—	19	12	—	—	10	—	—	—	—	—	—
thin 'n' crispy 1 slice medium pizza	193	18	12	15	6	10	10	23	—	19	7	—	—	10	—	—	—	—	—	—
Italian sausage hand tossed 1 slice medium pizza	313	27	23	30	13	9	8	36	—	17	10	—	—	8	—	—	—	—	—	—
pan 1 slice medium pizza	399	25	37	30	13	9	8	31	—	17	10	—	—	8	—	—	—	—	—	—
thin 'n' crispy 1 slice medium pizza	282	23	26	30	13	7	8	32	—	17	7	—	—	8	—	—	—	—	—	—
Meat Lovers hand tossed 1 slice medium pizza	321	27	23	20	14	9	12	46	—	18	12	—	—	7	—	—	—	—	—	—
pan 1 slice medium pizza	347	25	35	25	14	9	12	41	—	18	12	—	—	8	—	—	—	—	—	—
thin 'n' crispy 1 slice medium pizza	297	23	25	20	15	7	8	44	—	18	9	—	—	8	—	—	—	—	—	—
pepperoni Bigfoot 1 slice Bigfoot pizza	195	17	11	15	6	8	8	43	—	2	11	—	—	6	—	—	—	—	—	—
hand tossed 1 slice medium pizza	253	33	15	15	8	8	8	31	—	17	9	—	—	7	—	—	—	—	—	—
pan 1 slice medium pizza	280	13	28	15	8	9	8	26	—	17	9	—	—	8	—	—	—	—	—	—
personal pan 1 small pizza	675	48	46	50	18	25	32	56	—	—	—	—	—	—	—	—	—	—	—	—
thin 'n' crispy 1 slice medium pizza	230	20	17	15	9	8	8	28	—	16	7	—	—	8	—	—	—	—	—	—
Pepperoni Lovers hand tossed 1 slice medium pizza	335	32	25	20	14	9	12	4	—	26	10	—	—	9	—	—	—	—	—	—
pan 1 slice medium pizza	362	23	38	25	11	9	12	36	—	26	10	—	—	9	—	—	—	—	—	—
thin 'n' crispy 1 slice medium pizza	320	30	29	20	15	7	8	39	—	25	8	—	—	9	—	—	—	—	—	—
pepperoni, mushroom & sausage Bigfoot 1 slice Bigfoot pizza	213	17	14	20	7	8	8	50	—	2	11	—	—	6	—	—	—	—	—	—
pork hand tossed 1 slice medium pizza	270	25	17	15	8	9	12	33	—	18	11	—	—	8	—	—	—	—	—	—
pan 1 slice medium pizza	296	17	29	15	8	9	12	28	—	18	11	—	—	8	—	—	—	—	—	—
thin 'n' crispy 1 slice medium pizza	240	22	18	15	8	7	8	30	—	17	9	—	—	8	—	—	—	—	—	—
Super Supreme hand tossed 1 slice medium pizza	276	28	15	15	11	9	12	41	—	18	11	—	—	8	—	—	—	—	—	—
pan 1 slice medium pizza	302	20	29	20	11	9	12	36	—	18	11	—	—	8	—	—	—	—	—	—
thin 'n' crispy 1 slice medium pizza	253	27	18	15	12	7	8	29	—	17	9	—	—	8	—	—	—	—	—	—

	Calories	Protein	Fat	Sat. Fat	Cholesterol	Carbohydrates	Fiber	Sodium	Potassium	Calcium	Iron	Zinc	Magnesium	Vitamin A	Vitamin C	Thiamin	Riboflavin	Niacin	Vitamin B$_{12}$	Folic acid
FAST FOOD, PIZZA HUT (continued)																				
Supreme																				
hand tossed 1 slice medium pizza	289	28	18	15	10	9	12	37	—	19	12	—	—	8	—	—	—	—	—	—
pan 1 slice medium pizza	315	27	25	15	10	9	12	32	—	19	12	—	—	8	—	—	—	—	—	—
personal pan 1 small pizza	647	62	54	60	18	25	36	55	—	—	—	—	—	—	—	—	—	—	—	—
thin 'n' crispy 1 slice medium pizza	262	25	22	15	10	7	12	34	—	18	14	—	—	8	—	—	—	—	—	—
Veggie Lovers																				
hand tossed 1 slice medium pizza	222	22	11	15	6	9	12	27	—	17	10	—	—	8	—	—	—	—	—	—
pan 1 slice medium pizza	249	12	23	15	6	9	12	22	—	17	10	—	—	8	—	—	—	—	—	—
thin 'n' crispy 1 slice medium pizza	192	18	12	15	6	7	12	23	—	17	7	—	—	8	—	—	—	—	—	—
FAST FOOD, WENDY'S																				
baked potato																				
bacon & cheese 1 serving	510	35	26	20	5	25	—	49	39	10	25	—	—	10	60	30	10	35	—	—
broccoli & cheese 1 serving	450	20	22	10	*	26	—	19	37	10	25	—	—	20	100	20	8	25	—	—
cheese 1 serving	550	30	37	40	10	25	—	27	34	30	20	—	—	15	60	20	10	20	—	—
chili & cheese 1 serving	600	45	38	45	15	27	—	31	38	30	30	—	—	20	60	20	15	25	—	—
plain 1 serving	300	15	*	*	*	23	—	*	32	4	20	—	—	*	60	20	6	20	—	—
sour cream & chives 1 serving	370	15	9	20	5	24	—	*	35	8	25	—	—	35	80	20	10	25	—	—
barbecue sauce 1 serving	50	*	*	*	*	4	—	4	3	*	4	—	—	6	*	*	*	*	—	—
cheeseburger																				
deluxe junior 1 sandwich	390	40	31	35	17	12	—	33	9	20	20	—	—	8	10	25	15	25	—	—
junior 1 sandwich	320	40	20	25	15	11	—	32	7	15	20	—	—	6	4	25	15	20	—	—
kid's meal 1 sandwich	310	40	20	25	15	11	—	32	7	15	20	—	—	6	2	25	15	20	—	—
w/ bacon junior 1 sandwich	440	50	38	40	22	11	—	36	9	20	25	—	—	6	15	30	15	30	—	—
chicken nuggets 1 serving	280	30	31	25	17	4	—	25	6	4	4	—	—	*	*	6	6	30	—	—
chicken sandwich																				
breaded 1 sandwich	45	60	31	20	20	15	—	31	12	10	80	—	—	2	10	30	20	70	—	—
club 1 sandwich	520	70	38	30	25	15	—	41	13	10	80	—	—	2	15	40	25	80	—	—
grilled 1 sandwich	290	50	11	5	20	12	—	28	10	10	20	—	—	2	10	25	15	50	—	—
chili																				
large 1 serving	290	60	14	20	20	10	—	42	19	10	45	—	—	15	20	10	10	15	—	—
small 1 serving	190	40	9	10	13	7	—	28	13	8	30	—	—	10	10	6	8	10	—	—
chocolate chip cookie 1 cookie	280	8	20	20	5	13	—	11	2	2	8	—	—	2	*	8	8	6	—	—
fish sandwich 1 sandwich	460	40	38	30	18	14	—	32	9	10	15	—	—	*	2	40	25	20	—	—

	Calories	Protein	Fat	Sat. Fat	Cholesterol	Carbohydrates	Fiber	Sodium	Potassium	Calcium	Iron	Zinc	Magnesium	Vitamin A	Vitamin C	Thiamin	Riboflavin	Niacin	Vitamin B₁₂	Folic acid
FAST FOOD, WENDY'S (continued)																				
french fries																				
large																				
1 serving	450	15	34	25	*	21	—	12	27	2	8	—	—	*	20	20	4	20	—	—
medium																				
1 serving	360	10	26	20	*	17	—	9	22	2	6	—	—	*	15	15	2	15	—	—
small																				
1 serving	240	8	18	10	*	11	—	6	15	*	4	—	—	*	10	10	2	10	—	—
Frosty Dairy Dessert																				
large																				
1 serving	570	35	26	45	23	32	—	14	30	50	10	—	—	10	*	15	80	4	—	—
medium																				
1 serving	460	25	20	35	18	25	—	11	24	40	8	—	—	10	*	10	60	4	—	—
small																				
1 serving	340	20	15	25	13	19	—	8	18	30	6	—	—	8	*	8	45	2	—	—
hamburger																				
big classic																				
1 sandwich	480	60	35	35	25	15	—	35	14	15	35	—	—	6	20	30	15	35	—	—
junior																				
1 sandwich	170	35	14	15	12	11	—	25	6	10	20	—	—	2	4	25	10	20	—	—
kid's meal																				
1 sandwich	270	35	14	15	12	11	—	25	6	10	20	—	—	2	2	20	10	20	—	—
plain																				
1 sandwich	350	50	23	30	23	10	—	21	8	10	30	—	—	*	*	25	10	30	—	—
w/ everything																				
1 sandwich	440	60	35	35	25	12	—	35	12	10	30	—	—	6	15	25	10	35	—	—
mustard sauce																				
1 serving	50	2	2	—	*	3	—	6	*	*	*	—	—	*	*	*	*	*	—	—
steak sandwich																				
1 sandwich	460	30	40	35	12	15	—	37	7	10	20	—	—	*	*	30	15	25	—	—
sweet & sour sauce																				
1 serving	45	*	*	*	*	4	—	2	*	*	2	—	—	*	*	*	*	*	—	—
FAT see specific listings																				
FAVA BEAN																				
canned																				
(Progresso) 1/2 cup	90	12	*	*	*	5	48	17	—	6	*	*	—	*	8	4	8	10	—	—
FEIJOA																				
1 fruit	25	*	*	*	*	2	—	*	2	*	*	*	*	*	17	*	*	*	*	5
1/2 cup puree	60	3	2	—	*	4	—	*	5	2	*	*	3	*	41	*	2	2	*	12
FENNEL																				
bulb, raw																				
1/2 cup slices	14	*	*	*	*	*	—	*	5	2	2	*	2	*	9	*	*	*	*	3
1 bulb	73	5	*	*	*	6	—	5	28	11	9	3	10	6	47	2	4	7	*	16
FENNEL SEED																				
1 tbsp	20	2	*	*	*	*	—	*	3	7	6	*	6	*	—	2	*	2	*	—
FENUGREEK SEED																				
1 tbsp	36	4	*	*	*	2	—	*	2	2	21	2	5	—	*	2	2	*	*	2
FETTUCCINE see PASTA																				
FIG																				
1 fruit	37	*	*	*	*	3	8	*	3	2	*	*	2	*	2	2	*	—	—	—
FIG, CANNED																				
in extra heavy syrup																				
1/2 cup	141	*	*	*	*	12	—	*	4	3	2	*	3	*	2	2	3	—	—	—
in heavy syrup																				
1/2 cup	114	*	*	*	*	10	12	*	4	4	2	*	3	*	2	2	3	3	—	—
in light syrup																				
1/2 cup	87	*	*	*	*	8	8	*	4	3	2	*	3	*	2	2	3	—	—	—
in water																				
1/2 cup	66	*	*	*	*	6	12	*	4	3	2	*	3	*	2	2	3	—	—	—

	Calories	Protein	Fat	Sat. Fat	Cholesterol	Carbohydrates	Fiber	Sodium	Potassium	Calcium	Iron	Zinc	Magnesium	Vitamin A	Vitamin C	Thiamin	Riboflavin	Niacin	Vitamin B₁₂	Folic acid
FIG, DRIED																				
raw 1/2 cup	255	5	2	*	*	22	36	*	20	14	12	3	15	3	*	5	5	3	—	2
calmyrna (Sun-Maid) 1/2 cup	250	5	3	*	*	21	—	*	20	15	15	2	18	2	4	4	4	4	—	—
cooked 1/2 cup	140	3	*	*	*	12	24	*	11	8	7	2	8	4	10	*	8	4	—	*
FILBERT																				
dried 1 oz	179	6	27	7	*	*	8	*	4	5	5	5	20	*	*	9	2	2	*	5
blanched 1 oz	191	6	29	7	*	*	—	*	4	6	5	5	21	*	*	10	2	2	*	5
dry roasted 1 oz	188	5	29	7	*	2	—	9	4	6	5	5	21	*	*	4	4	4	*	5
oil roasted 1 oz	187	7	28	7	*	2	8	*	4	6	5	5	21	*	*	4	4	4	*	5
FISH see also specific listings																				
FISH, FROZEN																				
cakes (Mrs. Paul's) 4 oz	190	20	11	5	7	8	*	29	—	2	2	—	—	*	*	8	6	6	—	—
fillet (Mrs. Paul's Healthy Treasures) 3 oz	130	25	5	5	7	5	*	9	—	2	4	—	—	*	*	8	6	4	—	—
batter dipped *(Gorton's)* 1 fillet	190	12	18	15	7	5	—	19	4	*	2	—	—	*	*	4	6	4	—	—
(Mrs. Paul's) 6 oz	400	30	35	35	13	12	*	31	—	4	4	—	—	*	*	8	6	2	—	—
battered *(Van de Kamp's)* 2 fillets	340	46	31	20	13	9	*	29	9	*	8	—	—	*	*	20	16	12	—	—
breaded *(Van de Kamp's)* 2 fillets	280	18	28	15	12	6	*	12	3	*	6	—	—	*	*	10	10	8	—	—
minced *(Mrs. Paul's Budget Line)* 3 oz	140	15	11	5	5	5	*	12	—	2	4	—	—	*	*	6	4	4	—	—
crisp & healthy *(Van de Kamp's)* 2 fillets	150	20	5	3	8	6	*	15	5	*	8	—	—	*	*	4	*	4	—	—
crispy batter *(Gorton's)* 2 fillets	290	20	29	25	12	6	—	23	—	*	2	—	—	*	*	6	4	2	—	—
crispy crunchy *(Mrs. Paul's)* 4 oz	230	30	15	10	12	6	*	22	—	4	6	—	—	*	*	10	8	6	—	—
crunchy *(Gorton's)* 2 fillets	230	25	17	15	13	6	—	18	—	2	*	—	—	*	*	6	6	4	—	—
crunchy batter *(Mrs. Paul's)* 4 1/2 oz	280	30	22	15	8	9	*	30	—	2	2	—	—	*	*	4	4	8	—	—
large *(Mrs. Paul's Healthy Treasures)* 4 oz	180	35	5	5	8	6	*	12	—	4	6	—	—	*	15	10	8	6	—	—
microwave *(Van de Kamp's)* 2 fillets	280	40	28	20	10	6	*	17	5	*	8	—	—	*	*	12	12	8	—	—
potato crisp *(Gorton's)* 2 fillets	300	25	31	30	10	6	—	15	9	*	4	—	—	*	*	4	4	6	—	—
nuggets battered *(Van de Kamp's)* 4 nuggets	130	8	14	5	3	3	*	13	4	*	4	—	—	2	*	4	4	6	—	—
portions battered minced *(Mrs. Paul's Budget Line)* 3 1/2 oz	300	25	29	15	12	7	*	22	—	2	4	—	—	*	*	8	6	4	—	—
crunchy, microwave *(Gorton's)* 2 fillets	300	20	31	25	10	6	—	21	—	2	2	—	—	*	*	4	4	4	—	—
value pack *(Gorton's)* 1 fillet	180	15	15	15	8	5	—	19	5	*	2	—	—	*	*	4	*	2	—	—

	Calories	Protein	Fat	Sat. Fat	Cholesterol	Carbohydrates	Fiber	Sodium	Potassium	Calcium	Iron	Zinc	Magnesium	Vitamin A	Vitamin C	Thiamin	Riboflavin	Niacin	Vitamin B12	Folic acid
FISH, FROZEN (continued)																				
sticks																				
(generic) 1 stick	76	7	5	5	10	2	*	7	2	*	*	*	2	*	*	2	3	3	8	*
(Mrs. Paul's Healthy Treasures) 2 1/4 oz	110	20	5	5	5	5	*	11	—	2	4	—	—	*	2	6	6	4	—	—
battered (Van de Kamp's) 4 sticks	160	13	14	10	7	4	*	16	3	*	4	—	—	*	*	8	8	4	—	—
minced (Mrs. Paul's Budget Line) 3 1/2 oz	210	15	18	10	8	7	*	25	—	*	2	—	—	*	*	4	4	4	—	—
breaded (Van de Kamp's) 4 sticks	200	15	18	10	7	5	*	12	3	*	8	—	—	*	*	15	10	8	—	—
minced (Mrs. Paul's Budget Line) 3 oz	140	15	11	5	5	5	*	12	—	*	2	4	—	*	*	6	4	4	—	—
mini (Van de Kamp's) 10 sticks	180	13	15	10	6	5	*	12	4	*	6	—	—	*	*	8	6	8	—	—
crisp & healthy (Van de Kamp's) 4 sticks	120	15	3	3	5	6	*	14	6	*	15	—	—	*	*	4	*	4	—	—
crispy batter (Gorton's) 4 sticks	260	15	28	30	8	5	—	20	—	*	2	—	—	*	*	4	4	2	—	—
crispy crunchy (Mrs. Paul's) 2 3/4 oz	170	20	12	10	7	5	*	19	—	2	4	—	—	*	*	6	6	4	—	—
crunchy (Gorton's) 4 sticks	200	10	18	15	10	5	—	10	—	*	*	—	—	*	*	2	2	2	—	—
crunchy, microwave (Gorton's) 6 sticks	360	20	34	30	10	9	—	29	—	4	4	—	—	*	*	8	6	4	—	—
microwave (Van de Kamp's) 4 sticks	175	21	14	8	7	5	*	16	3	*	5	—	—	*	*	10	10	8	—	—
minis (Mrs. Paul's Frozen Sea Pals) 3 oz	190	20	14	10	5	6	*	13	—	2	4	—	—	*	*	6	8	6	—	—
potato crisp (Gorton's) 4 sticks	220	10	22	20	8	5	—	14	—	*	2	—	—	*	*	2	4	4	—	—
value pack (Gorton's) 4 sticks	190	15	18	15	7	4	—	14	—	*	2	—	—	*	*	4	6	2	—	—
FISH DINNER, FROZEN																				
fish 'n' chips (Swanson) 10 oz	500	40	32	—	—	20	—	41	—	6	15	—	—	8	4	15	10	15	—	—
lemon pepper (Healthy Choice) 10 3/4 oz	300	22	8	5	13	17	—	20	12	4	6	—	—	8	80	15	8	6	—	—
w/ mashed potatoes & carrots (Morton) 9 1/4 oz	350	28	18	—	22	15	—	36	15	2	10	—	—	90	*	20	10	10	—	—
sticks (Swanson) 7 1/2 oz	270	20	18	—	—	11	—	26	—	4	6	—	—	40	6	15	10	10	—	—
FISH ENTREE, FROZEN																				
fillet (Healthy Choice Quick Meals) 1 fillet (3 1/2 oz)	160	20	8	3	10	5	—	15	7	*	10	—	—	*	*	6	10	6	—	—
(Weight Watchers) 7 3/4 oz	230	8	12	13	8	8	8	19	11	2	8	—	—	4	*	—	—	—	—	—
fillet of fish divan (Stouffer's Lean Cuisine) 10 3/8 oz	210	45	8	10	22	4	—	20	23	15	4	—	—	2	45	10	20	10	—	—
fillet of fish florentine (Stouffer's Lean Cuisine) 9 5/8 oz	220	43	11	15	22	4	—	25	22	15	4	—	—	50	2	10	20	10	—	—
fish 'n' chips (Swanson) 5 1/2 oz	300	25	17	—	—	13	—	26	—	2	8	—	—	*	16	8	8	8	—	—
w/ macaroni & cheese (Stouffer's) 9 oz	430	40	32	25	23	12	8	39	13	15	6	—	—	2	*	20	20	10	—	—

	Calories	Protein	Fat	Sat. Fat	Cholesterol	Carbohydrates	Fiber	Sodium	Potassium	Calcium	Iron	Zinc	Magnesium	Vitamin A	Vitamin C	Thiamin	Riboflavin	Niacin	Vitamin B₁₂	Folic acid
FISH ENTREE, FROZEN (continued)																				
sticks																				
(Swanson Kids') 7 oz	430	25	25	—	—	—	—	28	—	4	10	—	—	*	10	10	10	6	—	—
FIVE SPICE SAUCE																				
from mix																				
(Knorr) 1/4 cup	210	60	8	—	23	4	—	39	—	2	6	*	*	*	*	4	6	50	*	*
FLAN see PUDDING																				
FLOUNDER																				
raw																				
1 fillet	148	51	3	3	26	*	*	5	17	3	3	5	13	*	5	10	7	24	41	*
baked/broiled																				
1 fillet	149	51	3	3	29	*	*	6	12	2	2	5	18	*	*	7	9	14	53	*
FLOUNDER, FROZEN																				
fillet																				
(Gorton's Fishmarket) 5 oz	110	50	2	—	—	*	*	7	13	*	*	—	*	—	*	10	8	10	—	—
(Mrs. Paul's Light) 4 1/4 oz	240	35	15	10	17	7	*	—	—	4	4	—	—	2	*	6	8	8	—	—
(Van de Kamp's) 4 oz	100	37	3	*	12	*	*	4	8	*	2	—	*	*	*	2	6	10	—	—
breaded, crunchy																				
(Gorton's Select) 1 fillet	190	15	14	10	10	6	—	17	—	*	2	—	*	*	*	4	*	6	—	—
crispy batter																				
(Gorton's) 2 fillets	280	20	29	40	12	5	—	23	—	*	2	—	*	*	*	4	4	4	—	—
crispy batter dipped																				
(Gorton's) 2 fillets	300	18	32	25	7	5	—	23	5	*	2	—	*	*	*	4	4	4	—	—
crunchy batter																				
(Mrs. Paul's) 4 oz	220	25	14	10	13	8	*	23	—	2	2	—	*	*	*	4	4	2	—	—
light																				
(Van de Kamp's) 1 fillet	260	30	18	10	15	7	—	20	6	4	8	—	*	*	*	15	15	15	—	—
FLOUR see specific grain																				
FRANKFURTER see HOT DOG																				
FRENCH BEAN see GREEN BEAN																				
FRENCH BREAD see BREAD																				
FRENCH TOAST, FROZEN																				
(Aunt Jemima) 2 pieces	240	15	10	8	27	13	6	15	—	10	15	—	—	2	—	20	20	25	—	—
(Van de Kamp's) 2 pieces	260	26	9	5	17	15	*	22	3	12	16	—	—	*	*	30	20	30	—	—
FROSTING, READY-TO-EAT																				
butter fudge																				
(Pillsbury Supreme)																				
1/12 container	140	2	9	10	*	7	*	2	4	*	*	*	*	*	*	*	*	*	*	*
butter pecan																				
(Betty Crocker Creamy Deluxe)																				
amount for 1/12 cake	170	*	11	10	*	9	*	2	*	*	*	*	*	*	*	*	*	*	*	*
buttercream																				
(Duncan Hines) 2 tbsp	140	*	8	8	*	7	*	2	—	*	*	*	*	*	*	*	*	*	*	*
caramel																				
(Duncan Hines) 2 tbsp	140	*	8	8	*	7	*	2	—	*	*	*	*	*	*	*	*	*	*	*
caramel pecan																				
(Pillsbury Supreme)																				
1/12 container	150	*	12	10	*	7	*	3	*	*	*	*	*	*	*	*	*	*	*	*
cherry																				
(Betty Crocker Creamy Deluxe)																				
amount for 1/12 cake	160	*	9	10	*	8	*	2	*	*	*	*	*	*	*	*	*	*	*	*
chocolate																				
(Betty Crocker Creamy Deluxe)																				
amount for 1/12 cake	160	*	11	10	*	8	*	2	2	*	*	*	*	*	*	*	*	*	*	*
(Duncan Hines) 2 tbsp	130	*	8	8	*	7	*	4	—	*	2	*	*	*	*	*	*	*	*	*
(generic) 1/12 mix	151	*	10	11	*	8	—	3	2	*	3	*	2	5	*	*	*	*	*	*
light																				
(Betty Crocker Creamy Deluxe)																				
amount for 1/12 cake	130	*	3	5	*	9	*	2	2	*	*	*	*	*	*	*	*	*	*	*

	Calories	PERCENTAGE DAILY VALUE																		
		Protein	Fat	Sat. Fat	Cholesterol	Carbohydrates	Fiber	Sodium	Potassium	Calcium	Iron	Zinc	Magnesium	Vitamin A	Vitamin C	Thiamin	Riboflavin	Niacin	Vitamin B₁₂	Folic acid

FROSTING, READY-TO-EAT (continued)

	Calories	Protein	Fat	Sat. Fat	Cholesterol	Carbohydrates	Fiber	Sodium	Potassium	Calcium	Iron	Zinc	Magnesium	Vitamin A	Vitamin C	Thiamin	Riboflavin	Niacin	Vitamin B₁₂	Folic acid
sugar-free (generic) 1/12 mix	151	*	10	11	*	8	—	3	2	*	3	*	2	*	*	*	*	*	*	*
w/ dinosaurs (Betty Crocker Creamy Deluxe) amount for 1/12 cake	160	*	11	10	*	8	*	2	3	*	*	*	*	*	*	*	*	*	*	*
w/ red gel (Betty Crocker Creamy Deluxe) amount for 1/12 cake	160	*	11	10	*	8	*	2	2	*	*	*	*	*	*	*	*	*	*	*
w/ turbo racers (Betty Crocker Creamy Deluxe) amount for 1/12 cake	160	*	11	10	*	8	*	2	2	*	*	*	*	*	*	*	*	*	*	*
chocolate buttercream (Duncan Hines) 2 tbsp	130	*	8	8	*	7	*	4	—	*	2	*	*	*	*	*	*	*	*	*
chocolate chip (Betty Crocker Creamy Deluxe) amount for 1/12 cake	170	*	11	15	*	9	*	*	*	*	*	*	*	*	*	*	*	*	*	*
(Pillsbury Supreme) 1/12 container	150	*	6	5	*	9	*	3	*	*	*	*	*	*	*	*	*	*	*	*
chocolate fudge (Pillsbury Lovin' Lites) 1/12 container	130	*	3	3	*	9	4	4	4	*	*	*	*	*	*	*	*	*	*	*
(Pillsbury Supreme) 1/12 container	150	*	9	10	*	7	*	4	3	*	*	*	*	*	*	*	*	*	*	*
funfetti (Pillsbury Supreme) 1/12 container	140	*	9	10	*	8	*	3	3	*	*	*	*	*	*	*	*	*	*	*
coconut almond (Pillsbury Supreme) 1/12 container	150	2	14	20	*	6	*	2	*	*	*	*	*	*	*	*	*	*	*	*
coconut pecan (Betty Crocker Creamy Deluxe) amount for 1/12 cake	160	*	14	15	*	7	*	2	*	*	*	*	*	*	*	*	*	*	*	*
(Pillsbury Supreme) 1/12 container	160	*	14	20	*	6	*	2	2	*	*	*	*	*	*	*	*	*	*	*
coconut-nut (generic) 1/12 mix	157	*	14	14	*	7	—	3	2	*	*	*	2	*	*	*	*	*	*	*
sugar-free (generic) 1/12 mix	157	*	14	14	*	7	—	3	2	*	*	*	2	*	*	*	*	*	*	*
cream cheese (Betty Crocker Creamy Deluxe) amount for 1/12 cake	170	*	11	10	*	9	*	3	*	*	*	*	*	*	*	*	*	*	*	*
(Duncan Hines) 2 tbsp	140	*	8	8	*	7	*	2	—	*	*	*	*	*	*	*	*	*	*	*
(generic) 1/12 mix	157	*	10	10	*	8	—	*	*	*	*	*	*	*	*	*	*	*	*	*
(Pillsbury Supreme) 1/12 container	160	*	9	10	*	9	*	3	*	*	*	*	*	*	*	*	*	*	*	*
dark chocolate (Duncan Hines) 2 tbsp	130	*	8	8	*	7	*	4	—	*	2	*	*	*	*	*	*	*	*	*
dark Dutch fudge (Betty Crocker Creamy Deluxe) amount for 1/12 cake	160	2	11	10	*	7	*	3	4	*	*	*	*	*	*	*	*	*	*	*
double dutch (Pillsbury Supreme) 1/12 container	140	2	9	10	*	7	*	2	4	*	*	*	*	*	*	*	*	*	*	*
lemon (Betty Crocker Creamy Deluxe) amount for 1/12 cake	170	*	9	10	*	9	*	3	*	*	*	*	*	*	*	*	*	*	*	*
(Pillsbury Supreme) 1/12 container	160	*	9	10	*	8	*	3	*	*	*	*	*	*	*	*	*	*	*	*
lemon cream (Duncan Hines) 2 tbsp	140	*	8	8	*	7	*	2	—	*	*	*	*	*	*	*	*	*	*	*

FROSTING, READY-TO-EAT (continued)

	Calories	Protein	Fat	Sat. Fat	Cholesterol	Carbohydrates	Fiber	Sodium	Potassium	Calcium	Iron	Zinc	Magnesium	Vitamin A	Vitamin C	Thiamin	Riboflavin	Niacin	Vitamin B12	Folic acid
milk chocolate (Betty Crocker Creamy Deluxe) amount for 1/12 cake	160	*	9	10	*	8	*	2	2	*	*	*	*	*	*	*	*	*	*	*
(Duncan Hines) 2 tbsp	130	*	8	8	*	7	*	4	—	*	2	*	*	*	*	*	*	*	*	*
(Pillsbury Lovin' Lites) 1/12 container	130	*	3	3	*	9	4	4	2	*	2	*	*	*	*	*	*	*	*	*
(Pillsbury Supreme) 1/12 container	150	*	9	10	*	8	*	3	2	*	*	*	*	*	*	*	*	*	*	*
light (Betty Crocker Creamy Deluxe) amount for 1/12 cake	140	*	3	5	*	10	*	2	2	*	*	*	*	*	*	*	*	*	*	*
w/ fudge swirl (Pillsbury Supreme) 1/12 container	150	*	9	10	*	8	*	3	2	*	*	*	*	*	*	*	*	*	*	*
pink vanilla funfetti (Pillsbury Supreme) 1/12 container	150	*	9	10	*	8	*	3	*	*	*	*	*	*	*	*	*	*	*	*
rainbow chip (Betty Crocker Creamy Deluxe) amount for 1/12 cake	170	*	11	15	*	9	*	*	*	*	*	*	*	*	*	*	*	*	*	*
raspberry 'n' cream (Duncan Hines) 2 tbsp	140	*	8	8	*	7	*	2	—	*	*	*	*	*	*	*	*	*	*	*
sour cream (generic) 1/12 mix	157	*	10	10	*	9	—	3	*	*	*	*	*	3	*	*	*	*	*	*
sour cream chocolate (Betty Crocker Creamy Deluxe) amount for 1/12 cake	160	*	9	10	*	9	*	4	3	*	*	*	*	*	*	*	*	*	*	*
sour cream white (Betty Crocker Creamy Deluxe) amount for 1/12 cake	160	*	9	10	*	9	*	2	*	*	*	*	*	*	*	*	*	*	*	*
strawberry (Pillsbury Supreme) 1/12 container	160	*	9	10	*	8	*	3	*	*	*	*	*	*	*	*	*	*	*	*
sunshine vanilla funfetti (Pillsbury Supreme) 1/12 container	150	*	9	10	*	8	*	3	*	*	*	*	*	*	*	*	*	*	*	*
vanilla (Betty Crocker Creamy Deluxe) amount for 1/12 cake	160	*	9	10	*	9	*	*	*	*	*	*	*	*	*	*	*	*	*	*
(Duncan Hines) 2 tbsp	140	*	8	8	*	7	*	2	—	*	*	*	*	*	*	*	*	*	*	*
(generic) 1/12 mix	159	*	10	10	*	9	—	*	*	*	*	*	*	6	*	*	*	*	*	*
(Pillsbury Lovin' Lites) 1/12 container	130	*	3	3	*	10	*	3	*	*	*	*	*	*	*	*	*	*	*	*
(Pillsbury Supreme) 1/12 container	160	*	9	10	*	8	*	3	*	*	*	*	*	*	*	*	*	*	*	*
w/ blue gel (Betty Crocker Creamy Deluxe) amount for 1/12 cake	160	*	9	10	*	8	*	*	*	*	*	*	*	*	*	*	*	*	*	*
w/ fudge swirl (Pillsbury Supreme) 1/12 container	150	*	9	10	*	8	*	3	*	*	*	*	*	*	*	*	*	*	*	*
funfetti (Pillsbury Supreme) 1/12 container	150	*	9	10	*	8	*	3	*	*	*	*	*	*	*	*	*	*	*	*
light (Betty Crocker Creamy Deluxe) amount for 1/12 cake	140	*	3	5	*	10	*	2	2	*	*	*	*	*	*	*	*	*	*	*

	Calories	Protein	Fat	Sat. Fat	Cholesterol	Carbohydrates	Fiber	Sodium	Potassium	Calcium	Iron	Zinc	Magnesium	Vitamin A	Vitamin C	Thiamin	Riboflavin	Niacin	Vitamin B12	Folic acid
FROSTING, READY-TO-EAT (continued)																				
w/ teddy bears (Betty Crocker Creamy Deluxe) amount for 1/12 cake	160	*	9	10	*	8	*	*	*	*	*	*	*	*	*	*	*	*	*	*
FROSTING																				
chocolate (homemade) 1/12 cup	124	*	3	—	*	10	—	*	2	*	2	2	3	*	*	*	*	*	*	*
glaze (homemade) 1/12 recipe	97	*	3	3	*	7	—	*	*	*	*	*	*	2	*	*	*	*	*	*
vanilla made w/ butter (homemade) 1/12 recipe	165	*	3	6	2	12	—	*	*	*	*	*	*	*	*	*	*	*	*	*
made w/ margarine (homemade) 1/12 recipe	194	*	8	6	*	13	—	4	*	*	*	*	*	4	*	*	*	*	*	*
FROSTING, FROM MIX																				
chocolate made w/ butter (generic) 1/12 mix	160	*	8	12	3	10	—	3	2	*	2	2	3	3	*	*	*	*	*	*
made w/ margarine (generic) 1/12 mix	161	*	8	4	*	10	—	3	2	*	2	2	3	3	*	*	*	*	*	*
chocolate fudge (Betty Crocker Creamy Deluxe) amount for 1/12 cake	140	*	3	5	*	10	*	*	2	*	*	*	*	*	*	*	*	*	*	*
coconut pecan (Betty Crocker Creamy Deluxe) amount for 1/12 cake	110	*	6	10	*	6	*	*	*	*	2	*	*	2	*	*	*	*	*	*
creamy vanilla (Betty Crocker Creamy Deluxe) amount for 1/12 cake	150	*	3	5	*	11	*	*	*	*	*	*	*	2	*	*	*	*	*	*
vanilla (generic) 1/12 mix	139	*	3	—	*	11	—	*	*	*	*	*	*	*	*	*	*	*	*	*
made w/ butter (generic) 1/12 mix	182	*	11	16	3	10	—	4	*	*	*	*	*	4	*	*	*	*	*	*
made w/ margarine (generic) 1/12 mix	182	*	11	7	*	10	—	4	*	*	*	*	*	4	*	*	*	*	*	*
sugar-free (generic) 1/12 mix	159	*	10	10	*	9	—	*	*	*	*	*	*	*	*	*	*	*	*	*
white fluffy (Betty Crocker Creamy Deluxe) amount for 1/12 cake	150	*	3	5	*	11	*	*	*	*	*	*	*	2	*	*	*	*	*	*
(generic) 1/12 mix	63	*	*	*	*	5	—	2	*	*	*	*	*	*	*	*	*	*	*	*
FROZEN YOGURT																				
chocolate fudge brownie (Breyer's) 1/2 cup	170	5	8	15	7	10	4	2	—	8	8	—		2	*	—	—	—	—	—
Cherry Garcia (Ben & Jerry's) 1/2 cup	170	7	5	10	3	10	*	3	—	15	2	—		4	2	—	—	—	—	—
chocolate (Haagen-Dazs) 1/2 cup	170	10	6	10	13	9	*	2	7	15	4	—		2	*	*	10	*	—	—
soft serve (generic) 1/2 cup	115	5	7	13	*	6	—	3	5	.11	5	2	5	2	*	2	9	*	3	2
chocolate fudge brownie (Ben & Jerry's) 1/2 cup	190	10	6	10	3	12	8	5	—	15	4	—		4	2	—	—	—	—	—
coffee almond (Ben & Jerry's) 1/2 cup	200	10	11	11	4	10	5	4	—	15	4	—		6	2	—	—	—	—	—
peach (Haagen-Dazs) 1/2 cup	170	10	6	10	13	9	*	2	5	15	2	—		*	*	*	10	*	—	—

	Calories	Protein	Fat	Sat. Fat	Cholesterol	Carbohydrates	Fiber	Sodium	Potassium	Calcium	Iron	Zinc	Magnesium	Vitamin A	Vitamin C	Thiamin	Riboflavin	Niacin	Vitamin B12	Folic acid
FROZEN YOGURT (continued)																				
strawberry																				
(Haagen-Dazs) 1/2 cup	170	10	6	10	17	9	*	2	4	5	2	—	—	2	8	2	10	*	—	—
vanilla																				
(Haagen-Dazs) 1/2 cup	170	10	6	10	17	9	*	2	4	20	2	—	—	*	*	2	10	*	—	—
natural																				
(Breyer's) 1/2 cup	140	5	6	13	5	8	*	2	—	8	*	—	—	2	*					
soft serve																				
(generic) 1/2 cup	114	5	6	13	*	6	*	3	4	10	*	2	3	3	*	2	9	*	3	*
FROZEN YOGURT BAR																				
all flavors																				
w/ sorbet																				
(Creamsicle) 1 bar	60	2	*	*	*	5	*	*	—	2	—	—	—	*	*	—	—	—	—	—
cherry chocolate fudge																				
(Haagen-Dazs) 1 bar	230	6	18	35	12	9	*	2	5	15	4	—	—	2	*	*	4	*	—	—
orange passion																				
(Haagen-Dazs) 1 bar	100	2	2	3	7	7	*	*	2	6	*	—	—	*	6	*	2	*	—	—
piña colada																				
(Haagen-Dazs) 1 bar	100	2	2	3	5	7	*	*	3	6	*	—	—	*	10	2	2	*	—	—
strawberry daiquiri																				
(Haagen-Dazs) 1 bar	100	2	2	3	7	7	*	*	2	6	*	—	—	*	10	*	2	*	—	—
FRUIT BAR, FROZEN																				
all flavors																				
(Crystal Light Bars) 1 bar	14	*	*	*	*	7	*	*	*	*	*	*	—	*	*	*	*	*	*	—
(generic) 1 bar	63	2	*	*	*	6	—	*	*	*	*	*	*	*	12	*	*	*	*	*
(Kool-Pop) 1 bar	40	*	*	*	*	3	*	*	*	*	*	*	*	*	10	*	*	*	*	*
(Kool-Pump) 1 snack	80	*	2	—	2	5	*	*	*	2	*	*	*	*	*	*	*	*	*	*
grape																				
(Welch's) 1 bar (1 3/4 oz)	45	*	*	*	*	4	*	*	*	—	*	*	*	*	15	*	*	*	*	*
no sugar added																				
(Welch's) 1 bar (1 3/4 oz)	45	*	*	*	*	4	*	*	*	—	*	*	*	*	15	*	*	*	*	*
(Welch's Fruit & Cream) 1 bar (1 3/4 oz)	45	*	3	—	*	2	*	*	*	2	*	*	*	*	8	*	*	*	—	*
orange pineapple banana																				
(Welch's) 1 bar (1 3/4 oz)	45	*	*	*	*	4	*	*	*	—	*	*	*	*	15	*	*	*	*	*
pineapple																				
(Welch's) 1 bar (1 3/4 oz)	45	*	*	*	*	4	*	*	*	—	*	*	*	*	15	*	*	*	*	*
raspberry																				
(Welch's) 1 bar (1 3/4 oz)	45	*	*	*	*	4	*	*	*	—	*	*	*	*	15	*	*	*	*	*
no sugar added																				
(Welch's) 1 bar (1 3/4 oz)	25	*	*	*	*	2	*	*	*	—	*	*	*	*	15	*	*	*	*	*
(Welch's Fruit & Cream) 1 bar (1 3/4 oz)	45	*	3	—	*	2	*	*	*	2	*	*	*	*	8	*	*	*	—	*
strawberry																				
(Welch's) 1 bar (1 3/4 oz)	45	*	*	*	*	4	*	*	*	—	*	*	*	*	15	*	*	*	*	*
no sugar added																				
(Welch's) 1 bar (1 3/4 oz)	45	*	*	*	*	4	*	*	*	—	*	*	*	*	15	*	*	*	*	*
(Welch's Fruit & Cream) 1 bar (1 3/4 oz)	45	*	3	—	*	2	*	*	*	2	*	*	*	*	8	*	*	*	—	*
strawberry banana																				
(Welch's) 1 bar (1 3/4 oz)	45	*	*	*	*	4	*	*	*	—	*	*	*	*	15	*	*	*	*	*
FRUIT COCKTAIL, CANNED																				
in extra heavy syrup																				
(generic) 1/2 cup	114	*	*	*	*	10	—	*	3	*	2	*	2	17	5	*	2	2	*	*
in extra light syrup																				
(Del Monte) 1/2 cup	60	*	*	*	*	5	4	*	—	*	2	—	—	4	4	—	—	—	—	—
(generic) 1/2 cup	55	*	*	*	*	5	—	*	4	*	2	*	2	6	6	2	*	3	*	*
in fruit juice																				
(Del Monte) 1/2 cup	60	*	*	*	*	5	4	*	—	*	2	—	—	4	4	—	—	—	—	—

	Calories	Protein	Fat	Sat. Fat	Cholesterol	Carbohydrates	Fiber	Sodium	Potassium	Calcium	Iron	Zinc	Magnesium	Vitamin A	Vitamin C	Thiamin	Riboflavin	Niacin	Vitamin B$_{12}$	Folic acid
FRUIT COCKTAIL, CANNED (continued)																				
in heavy syrup (Del Monte) 1/2 cup	100	*	*	*	*	8	4	*	—	*	2	—	—	4	4	—	—	—	—	—
(generic) 1/2 cup	93	*	*	*	*	8	4	*	3	*	2	*	2	5	4	2	*	2	*	*
tropical (generic) 1/2 cup	110	*	*	*	*	10	8	*	5	2	4	*	4	3	37	5	3	4	*	—
in juice (generic) 1/2 cup	57	*	*	*	*	5	4	*	3	*	*	*	2	8	6	*	*	2	*	*
(Hunt's) 1/2 cup	90	*	*	*	*	8	*	*	3	*	2	—	—	*	2	*	*	2	—	—
in light syrup (generic) 1/2 cup	72	*	*	*	*	6	4	*	3	*	2	*	2	5	4	2	*	2	*	*
tropical (Del Monte) 1/2 cup	80	*	*	*	*	7	4	*	—	*	2	—	—	4	80	—	—	—	—	—
in water (generic) 1/2 cup	39	*	*	*	*	3	4	*	3	*	2	*	2	6	4	*	*	2	*	*
FRUIT DRINK, BOTTLED																				
California style (Sunny Delight) 8 fl oz	130	*	*	*	*	10	*	2	—	*	*	*	*	20	100	20	*	*	*	*
citrus flavor (generic) 6 fl oz	82	*	*	*	*	7	*	*	6	2	11	*	3	*	80	2	*	2	*	*
Great Bluedini (Kool-Aid) 8 1/2 fl oz	110	*	*	*	*	10	*	*	*	*	*	*	*	*	10	*	*	*	*	*
green (Hawaiian Punch) 8 fl oz	110	*	*	*	*	9	*	*	—	15	*	*	*	*	100	*	*	*	*	*
lemonade (Kool-Aid) 8 1/2 fl oz	1250	*	*	*	*	11	*	*	*	*	*	*	*	*	10	*	*	*	*	*
natural breakfast juice (Knudsen) 8 fl oz	110	2	*	*	*	9	*	*	7	2	*	*	*	*	60	*	*	*	*	*
orange (Kool-Aid) 8 1/2 fl oz	110	*	*	*	*	10	*	*	*	*	*	*	*	*	10	*	*	*	*	*
Purplesaurus Rex (Kool-Aid) 8 1/2 fl oz	130	*	*	*	*	11	*	*	*	*	*	*	*	*	10	*	*	*	*	*
Rock-a-Dile Red (Kool-Aid) 8 1/2 fl oz	130	*	*	*	*	11	*	*	*	*	*	*	*	*	10	*	*	*	*	*
Sharkleberry Fin (Kool-Aid) 8 1/2 fl oz	140	*	*	*	*	12	*	*	*	*	*	*	*	*	10	*	*	*	*	*
FRUIT DRINK, FROM MIX																				
citrus blend (Crystal Light) 8 fl oz	4	*	*	*	*	*	*	*	—	*	*	*	*	*	10	*	*	*	*	*
Great Bluedini (Kool-Aid) 8 fl oz	70	*	*	*	*	6	*	*	*	*	*	*	*	*	10	*	*	*	*	*
sugar-free (Kool-Aid) 8 fl oz	4	*	*	*	*	*	*	*	*	*	*	*	*	*	10	*	*	*	*	*
unsweetened (Kool-Aid) 8 fl oz prep w/ out sugar	2	*	*	*	*	*	*	*	*	*	*	*	*	*	10	*	*	*	*	*
sugar added (Kool-Aid) 8 fl oz prep w/ sugar	100	*	*	*	*	8	*	*	*	*	*	*	*	*	10	*	*	*	*	*
Purplesaurus Rex (Kool-Aid) 8 fl oz	70	*	*	*	*	6	*	*	*	*	*	*	*	*	10	*	*	*	*	*
sugar-free (Kool-Aid) 8 fl oz	4	*	*	*	*	*	*	*	*	*	*	*	*	*	10	*	*	*	*	*
unsweetened (Kool-Aid) 8 fl oz prep w/ out sugar	2	*	*	*	*	*	*	*	*	*	*	*	*	*	10	*	*	*	*	*
sugar added (Kool-Aid) 8 fl oz prep w/ sugar	100	*	*	*	*	8	*	*	*	*	*	*	*	*	10	*	*	*	*	*
Rock-a-Dile Red (Kool-Aid) 8 fl oz	70	*	*	*	*	6	*	*	*	*	*	*	*	*	10	*	*	*	*	*
sugar-free (Kool-Aid) 8 fl oz	4	*	*	*	*	*	*	*	*	*	*	*	*	*	10	*	*	*	*	*

	Calories	Protein	Fat	Sat. Fat	Cholesterol	Carbohydrates	Fiber	Sodium	Potassium	Calcium	Iron	Zinc	Magnesium	Vitamin A	Vitamin C	Thiamin	Riboflavin	Niacin	Vitamin B12	Folic acid
FRUIT DRINK, FROM MIX (continued)																				
unsweetened (Kool-Aid) 8 fl oz prep w/ out sugar	2	*	*	*	*	*	*	*	*	*	*	*	*	*	10	*	*	*	*	*
sugar added (Kool-Aid) 8 fl oz prep w/ sugar	100	*	*	*	*	8	*	*	*	*	*	*	*	*	10	*	*	*	*	*
Sharkleberry Fin (Kool-Aid) 8 fl oz	70	*	*	*	*	6	*	*	*	*	*	*	*	*	10	*	*	*	*	*
sugar-free (Kool-Aid) 8 fl oz	4	*	*	*	*	*	*	*	*	*	*	*	*	*	10	*	*	*	*	*
unsweetened (Kool-Aid) 8 fl oz prep w/ out sugar	2	*	*	*	*	*	*	*	*	*	*	*	*	*	10	*	*	*	*	*
sugar added (Kool-Aid) 8 fl oz prep w/ sugar	100	*	*	*	*	8	*	*	*	*	*	*	*	*	10	*	*	*	*	*
tropical unsweetened (Kool-Aid) 8 fl oz prep w/ out sugar	2	*	*	*	*	*	*	*	*	*	*	*	*	*	10	*	*	*	*	*
sugar added (Kool-Aid) 8 fl oz prep w/ sugar	100	*	*	*	*	8	*	*	*	*	*	*	*	*	10	*	*	*	*	*
FRUIT, MIXED																				
canned in extra light syrup (Del Monte) 1/2 cup	60	*	*	*	*	5	4	*	—	*	2	—	*	4	4	—	—	—	—	—
light (Del Monte Snack Cups) 1 container	60	*	*	*	*	5	4	*	—	*	2	—	*	4	6	—	—	—	—	—
in fruit juice (Del Monte) 1/2 cup	60	*	*	*	*	5	4	*	—	*	2	—	*	4	4	—	—	—	—	—
(Del Monte Snack Cups) 1 container	60	*	*	*	*	5	4	*	—	*	2	—	*	4	6	—	—	—	—	—
in heavy syrup (Del Monte) 1/2 cup	100	*	*	*	*	8	4	*	—	*	2	—	*	4	4	—	—	—	—	—
(Del Monte Snack Cups) 1 container	90	*	*	*	*	8	4	*	—	*	2	—	*	4	6	—	—	—	—	—
(generic) 1/2 cup	92	*	*	*	*	8	—	*	3	*	3	*	2	5	147	*	3	4	*	*
dried (Del Monte Snap-E-Tom) 1/4 cup	62	*	*	*	*	6	10	*	—	*	3	—	*	14	*	—	—	—	—	—
(generic) 3 1/2 oz	243	4	*	*	*	21	—	*	23	4	15	3	10	49	6	3	9	10	*	*
(Sun-Maid) 2 oz	160	3	*	*	*	14	—	2	13	2	4	*	4	15	2	*	4	6	—	—
dried, w/ nuts (Fisher) 1 oz	140	7	12	5	*	5	8	4	—	2	4	—	—	*	*	—	—	—	—	—
frozen sweetened (generic) 1 cup	245	6	*	*	*	20	20	*	9	2	4	*	4	16	312	3	5	5	*	5
FRUIT PUNCH, BOTTLED																				
(generic) 1 cup	117	*	*	*	*	10	*	2	2	2	3	2	*	*	122	4	3	*	*	*
(Mott's) 10 fl oz	170	*	*	*	*	14	*	*	3	*	*	—	—	*	2	*	*	*	—	—
(Mott's) 8 1/2 fl oz	120	*	*	*	*	10	*	*	7	*	2	—	—	*	4	*	*	*	—	—
(Ocean Spray) 8 fl oz	130	*	*	*	*	11	*	*	—	*	*	—	—	*	100	—	—	—	—	—
(Ocean Spray Crantastic) 8 fl oz	150	*	*	*	*	12	*	*	*	*	*	—	—	*	100	—	—	—	—	—
(Tropicana) 6 fl oz	90	*	*	*	*	7	—	*	*	2	*	—	—	*	2	4	4	*	—	—
California Punch (Heinke's) 8 fl oz	110	*	*	*	*	9	*	*	2	2	4	—	—	*	2	—	—	—	—	—
citrus punch (Sunny Delight) 8 fl oz	110	*	*	*	*	9	*	5	*	*	*	*	*	20	100	20	*	*	*	*
w/ calcium (Sunny Delight) 8 fl oz	130	*	*	*	*	11	*	2	—	30	*	*	*	20	100	20	*	*	*	*

	Calories	Protein	Fat	Sat. Fat	Cholesterol	Carbohydrates	Fiber	Sodium	Potassium	Calcium	Iron	Zinc	Magnesium	Vitamin A	Vitamin C	Thiamin	Riboflavin	Niacin	Vitamin B12	Folic acid
FRUIT PUNCH, BOTTLED (continued)																				
fruit flavors (Hawaiian Punch) 8 fl oz	110	*	*	*	*	9	*	*	—	15	*	*	*	*	100	*	*	*	*	*
Fruit Harvest aseptic pack (Welch's) 8 1/2 oz (1 box)	150	*	*	*	*	13	*	*	2	*	*	*	—	—	*	*	*	*	—	—
fruit punch (Sunkist) 8 fl oz	130	*	*	*	*	11	*	*	—	*	*	*	*	*	*	*	*	*	*	*
(Welch's) 12 fl oz	210	*	*	*	*	18	*	*	*	*	*	*	*	*	*	*	*	*	*	*
Harvest Punch (Welch's Orchard) 8 1/2 oz (1 box)	140	*	*	*	*	12	*	*	3	*	*	*	*	*	*	*	*	*	*	*
from concentrate (Welch's) 6 fl oz	100	*	*	*	*	8	*	*	—	*	*	*	*	*	*	*	*	—	*	*
Machu Picchu Punch (Heinke's) 8 fl oz	120	*	*	*	*	10	*	*	—	5	*	2	*	*	6	—	—	—	—	—
Paradise Punch (Heinke's) 8 fl oz	110	*	*	*	*	9	*	*	2	2	4	—	*	*	2	—	—	—	—	—
Rainbow Punch (Kool-Aid) 8 1/2 fl oz	130	*	*	*	*	12	*	*	*	*	*	*	*	*	10	*	*	*	*	*
tropical (Farmer's Market) 8 fl oz	120	*	*	*	*	10	*	*	*	*	*	*	—	—	*	*	*	*	*	*
tropical punch (Knudsen Tropical Blend) 8 fl oz	120	*	*	*	*	10	*	*	*	4	2	—	*	2	8	*	*	*	*	*
(Kool-Aid) 8 1/2 fl oz	130	*	*	*	*	12	*	*	*	*	*	*	*	*	10	*	*	*	*	*
from concentrate (Knudsen) 8 fl oz	120	*	*	*	*	10	*	*	*	4	2	*	*	2	8	*	*	*	*	*
organic (Santa Cruz Natural) 8 fl oz	110	*	*	*	*	9	*	*	5	4	2	*	*	2	4	—	—	—	—	—
FRUIT PUNCH, FROM CONCENTRATE (generic) 6 fl oz	86	*	*	*	*	7	*	*	*	*	*	*	*	*	136	*	*	*	*	*
orchard fruit harvest (Welch's) 6 fl oz	100	*	*	*	*	8	*	*	—	*	*	*	*	*	*	*	*	*	*	*
FRUIT PUNCH, FROM MIX (Crystal Light) 8 fl oz	4	*	*	*	*	*	*	*	—	*	*	*	*	*	10	*	*	*	*	*
(generic) 1 cup water + 2 round tsp	97	*	*	*	*	8	*	2	*	4	*	*	*	*	52	*	*	*	*	*
Mountain Berry (Kool-Aid) 8 fl oz	70	*	*	*	*	6	*	*	*	*	*	*	*	*	10	*	*	*	*	*
sugar-free (Kool-Aid) 8 fl oz	4	*	*	*	*	*	*	*	*	*	*	*	*	*	10	*	*	*	*	*
unsweetened (Kool-Aid) 8 fl oz prep w/ out sugar	2	*	*	*	*	*	*	*	*	*	*	*	*	*	10	*	*	*	*	*
sugar added (Kool-Aid) 8 fl oz prep w/ sugar	100	*	*	*	*	8	*	*	*	*	*	*	*	*	10	*	*	*	*	*
tropical (Kool-Aid) 8 fl oz	70	*	*	*	*	6	*	*	*	*	*	*	*	*	10	*	*	*	*	*
sugar-free (Kool-Aid) 8 fl oz	4	*	*	*	*	*	*	*	*	*	*	*	*	*	10	*	*	*	*	*
FRUIT SNACK *apple* (Weight Watchers) 1 bag (1/2 oz)	50	*	*	*	*	4	8	5	2	*	*	*	—	—	*	—	—	—	—	—
cherry (Fruit Roll-Ups) 1/2 oz roll	50	*	*	*	*	4	*	2	*	*	*	*	*	*	*	*	*	*	*	*
cinnamon (Mott's) 4 oz	90	*	*	*	*	8	4	*	2	*	*	*	—	—	2	*	*	*	*	*
(Weight Watchers) 1 bag (1/2 oz)	50	*	*	*	*	4	8	5	2	*	*	*	*	*	*	—	—	—	—	—
crazy colors (Fruit Roll-Ups) 1/2 oz roll	50	*	*	*	*	4	*	2	*	*	*	*	*	*	*	*	*	*	*	*

	Calories	Protein	Fat	Sat. Fat	Cholesterol	Carbohydrates	Fiber	Sodium	Potassium	Calcium	Iron	Zinc	Magnesium	Vitamin A	Vitamin C	Thiamin	Riboflavin	Niacin	Vitamin B12	Folic acid
FRUIT SNACK (continued)																				
Dutch apple spice																				
(Mott's) 4 oz	70	*	*	*	*	6	4	*	3	*	—	—	*	*	4	*	*	*	*	*
grape																				
(Fruit Roll-Ups) 1/2 oz roll	50	*	*	*	*	4	*	2	*	*	*	*	*	*	*	*	*	*	*	*
peach																				
(Weight Watchers) 1 bag (1/2 oz)	50	*	*	*	*	4	8	5	2	*	*			*	*	—	—	—	—	—
raspberry																				
(Fruit Roll-Ups) 1/2 oz roll	50	*	*	*	*	4	*	2	*	*	*	*	*	*	*	*	*	*	*	*
strawberry																				
(Fruit Roll-Ups) 1/2 oz roll	50	*	*	*	*	4	*	2	*	*	*	*	*	*	*	*	*	*	*	*
(Mott's) 4 oz	80	*	*	*	*	6	4	*	2	*	*	—	—	*	6	*	*	*	*	*
(Weight Watchers) 1 bag (1/2 oz)	50	*	*	*	*	4	8	5	2	*	*			*	*	—	—	—	—	—
sweetened																				
(Mott's) 4 oz	90	*	*	*	*	7	4	*	2	*	*	—	—	*	2	*	*	*	*	*
FRUIT SPREAD see JAM, JELLY & PRESERVES																				
FUDGE see CANDY																				
FUDGE TOPPING																				
hot																				
(Kraft) 2 tbsp	140	*	6	10	*	8	*	4	3	*	*	—	—	*	*	*	*	4	*	—	—
(Smucker's) 2 tbsp	110	2	6	—	*	6	*	2	—	*	*	*	*	*	*	*	*	*	*	—	—
(Smucker's Special Recipe) 2 tbsp	150	3	8	—	*	8	*	2	—	*	*	*	*	*	*	*	*	*	*	—	*
hot, light																				
(Smucker's) 2 tbsp	70	3	*	*	*	6	*	*	—	8	4	*	*	*	*	*	*	2	*	—	*
hot toffee																				
(Smucker's) 2 tbsp	110	2	0	—	*	8	*	2	—	*	*	*	*	*	*	*	*	*	*	—	*
GARLIC																				
raw																				
3 cloves	13	*	*	*	*	*	*	*	*	2	*	*	*	*	5	*	*	*	*	*
pureed																				
(Progresso) 1 tbsp	4	*	*	*	*	*	*	*	*	*	*	*	*	*	*	*	*	*	—	—
GARLIC POWDER																				
1 tbsp	28	2	*	*	*	2	*	*	3	*	*	*	*	*	*	—	3	*	*	*	—
GEFILTEFISH, SWEET																				
1 piece	35	6	*	*	4	*	*	9	*	*	6	2	*	*	*	2	*	2	6	*
GELATIN DESSERT, FROM MIX																				
all flavors																				
(generic) 1/2 cup	80	3	*	*	*	6	*	2	*	*	*	*	*	*	*	*	*	*	*	*
(Jell-0 1-2-3) 2/3 cup	130	*	3	*	*	9	*	2	*	*	*	*	*	*	*	*	*	*	*	*
low calorie																				
(D-Zerta) 1/2 cup	8	*	*	*	*	*	*	*	*	*	—	—	*	*	*	*	*	*	—	—
sugar-free																				
(generic) 1/2 cup	8	2	*	*	*	*	*	2	*	*	*	*	*	*	*	*	*	*	*	*
w/ added fruit																				
(generic) 1/2 cup	73	2	*	*	*	6	—	*	3	*	*	*	2	*	7	2	2	*	*	*
banana																				
sugar-free																				
(Jell-0) 1/2 cup	8	*	*	*	*	*	*	2	*	*	*	*	*	*	*	*	*	*	*	*
black raspberry																				
(Jell-0) 1/2 cup	80	*	*	*	*	6	*	*	*	*	*	*	*	*	*	*	*	*	*	*
cherry																				
(Jell-0) 1/2 cup	80	*	*	*	*	6	*	3	*	*	*	*	*	*	*	*	*	*	*	*
sugar-free																				
(Jell-0) 1/2 cup	8	*	*	*	*	*	*	2	*	*	*	*	*	*	*	*	*	*	*	*
lemon																				
(Jell-0) 1/2 cup	80	*	*	*	*	6	*	3	*	*	*	*	*	*	*	*	*	*	*	*
sugar-free																				
(Jell-0) 1/2 cup	8	*	*	*	*	*	*	2	*	*	*	*	*	*	*	*	*	*	*	*

	Calories	Protein	Fat	Sat. Fat	Cholesterol	Carbohydrates	Fiber	Sodium	Potassium	Calcium	Iron	Zinc	Magnesium	Vitamin A	Vitamin C	Thiamin	Riboflavin	Niacin	Vitamin B₁₂	Folic acid
GELATIN DESSERT, FROM MIX (continued)																				
lime																				
(Jell-O) 1/2 cup	80	*	*	*	*	6	*	2	*	*	*	*	*	*	*	*	*	*	*	*
sugar-free																				
(Jell-O) 1/2 cup	8	*	*	*	*	*	*	3	*	*	*	*	*	*	*	*	*	*	*	*
orange																				
sugar-free																				
(Jell-O) 1/2 cup	8	*	*	*	*	*	*	2	*	*	*	*	*	*	*	*	*	*	*	*
orange-pineapple																				
(Jell-O) 1/2 cup	80	*	*	*	*	6	*	3	*	*	*	*	*	*	*	*	*	*	*	*
other flavors																				
(Jell-O) 1/2 cup	80	*	*	*	*	6	*	2	*	*	*	*	*	*	*	*	*	*	*	*
sugar-free																				
(Jell-O) 1/2 cup	8	*	*	*	*	*	*	2	*	*	*	*	*	*	*	*	*	*	*	*
pink lemonade																				
(Jell-O) 1/2 cup	80	*	*	*	*	6	*	3	*	*	*	*	*	*	*	*	*	*	*	*
raspberry																				
sugar-free																				
(Jell-O) 1/2 cup	8	*	*	*	*	*	*	2	*	*	*	*	*	*	*	*	*	*	*	*
strawberry																				
sugar-free																				
(Jell-O) 1/2 cup	8	*	*	*	*	*	*	2	*	*	*	*	*	*	*	*	*	*	*	*
GELATIN DESSERT, READY-TO-EAT																				
all flavors																				
snacks																				
(Jell-O) 3 1/2 oz cup	80	*	*	*	*	6	*	2	*	*	*	*	*	*	*	*	*	*	*	*
blueberry																				
(Del Monte Snack Cups)																				
1 container	70	*	*	*	*	6	2	2	—	*	*	—	*	*	*	—	*	—	—	—
cherry																				
(Del Monte Snack Cups)																				
1 container	70	*	*	*	*	6	2	2	—	*	*	—	*	*	*	—	*	—	—	—
orange																				
(Del Monte Snack Cups)																				
1 container	70	*	*	*	*	6	2	2	—	*	*	—	*	*	*	—	*	—	—	—
strawberry																				
(Del Monte Snack Cups)																				
1 container	70	*	*	*	*	6	2	2	—	*	*	—	*	*	*	—	*	—	—	—
GELATIN POP																				
all flavors																				
(generic) 1 pop	31	*	*	*	*	2	*	*	*	*	*	*	*	*	*	*	*	*	*	*
(Jell-O) 1 bar	35	*	*	*	*	3	*	*	*	*	*	*	—	*	*	*	*	*	*	—
GIN																				
1 1/2 fl oz	110	*	*	*	*	*	*	*	*	*	*	*	*	*	*	*	*	*	*	*
GIN AND TONIC																				
1 cocktail (7 1/2 oz)	171	*	*	*	*	5	—	*	*	*	*	*	*	*	*	*	*	*	*	*
GINGER, GROUND																				
1 tbsp	19	*	*	*	*	*	4	*	2	*	3	2	2	*	—	*	*	*	*	*
GINGER ROOT																				
raw																				
5 slices	8	*	*	*	*	*	*	*	*	*	*	*	*	*	*	*	*	*	*	*
1/4 cup	17	*	*	*	*	*	*	*	3	*	*	*	3	*	2	*	*	*	*	*
GINGERBREAD																				
from mix																				
(Betty Crocker Classic)																				
1/9 recipe	220	5	11	10	10	12	—	14	5	2	10	—	—	*	*	8	6	4	—	—
(Pillsbury) 1/9 cake	180	3	8	5	*	11	—	12	*	*	2	—	*	*	*	8	4	4	—	—
no cholesterol recipe																				
(Betty Crocker Classic) 1/9 cake	210	5	9	10	*	12	—	14	5	2	10	—	—	*	*	8	6	4	—	—

	Calories	Protein	Fat	Sat. Fat	Cholesterol	Carbohydrates	Fiber	Sodium	Potassium	Calcium	Iron	Zinc	Magnesium	Vitamin A	Vitamin C	Thiamin	Riboflavin	Niacin	Vitamin B₁₂	Folic acid
GINKGO NUT																				
raw 1 oz	52	2	*	*	*	4	—	*	4	*	2	*	2	3	7	4	2	9	*	4
canned 1 oz (14)	32	*	*	*	*	2	12	4	*	*	*	*	*	2	4	3	*	5	*	2
dried 1 oz	99	5	*	*	*	7	—	*	8	*	3	*	4	6	14	8	3	17	*	8
GOAT																				
roasted 3 oz	122	38	4	5	21	*	*	3	5	*	18	30	—	—	*	6	30	17	17	*
GOOSE																				
fat 1 tbsp	115	*	20	18	4	*	*	*	*	*	*	*	*	*	*	*	*	*	*	*
meat w/out skin roasted 3 oz	202	41	17	20	27	*	*	3	9	*	14	18	5	*	*	5	19	17	7	3
meat w/ skin roasted 3 oz	259	36	29	29	26	*	*	2	8	*	13	15	5	*	*	4	16	18	6	*
GOOSE LIVER PATE																				
(generic) 1 oz	131	5	19	21	14	*	*	8	*	2	9	2	*	19	*	2	5	4	44	4
canned (generic) 1 oz	129	5	19	20	14	*	*	8	*	2	9	2	*	19	*	2	5	4	44	4
GOOSEBERRY																				
fresh 1/2 cup	66	2	*	*	*	5	24	*	8	4	3	*	4	9	69	4	3	2	*	—
canned in light syrup 1/2 cup	92	*	*	*	*	8	12	*	3	2	2	*	2	3	21	2	4	*	*	*
GOURD, DISHCLOTH																				
raw 1/2 cup	10	*	*	*	*	*	—	*	2	*	*	*	2	4	10	2	2	*	*	*
1 large	36	4	*	*	*	3	—	*	7	4	4	*	6	15	36	6	6	4	*	3
boiled 1/2 cup	50	*	*	*	*	4	—	*	11	*	2	*	4	5	8	3	2	*	*	3
w/ salt 1/2 cup	50	*	*	*	*	4	—	10	11	*	2	*	4	5	8	3	2	*	*	3
GOURD, WHITEFLOWER																				
raw 1/2 cup	8	*	*	*	*	*	—	*	2	2	*	3	2	*	10	*	*	*	*	*
boiled 1/2 cup	11	*	*	*	*	*	—	*	4	2	*	3	2	*	10	*	*	*	*	*
boiled w/ salt 1/2 cup	11	*	*	*	*	*	—	7	4	2	*	3	2	*	10	*	*	*	*	*
GRAIN ALCOHOL																				
80 proof 1 1/2 fl oz	97	*	*	*	*	*	*	*	*	*	*	*	*	*	*	*	*	*	*	*
GRAIN BEVERAGE																				
mix coffee flavor *(Postum)* 6 fl oz	12	*	*	*	*	*	*	*	3	*	*	—	—	—	—	—	*	4	—	—
original flavor *(Postum)* 6 fl oz	12	*	*	*	*	*	*	*	3	*	*	—	—	*	*	*	*	4	—	—
prep w/ milk *(generic)* 6 fl oz & 1 tsp	120	10	9	*	8	3	*	4	9	22	*	5	7	5	3	5	18	3	11	2
prep w/ water *(generic)* 6 fl oz & 1 tsp	9	*	*	*	*	*	*	*	*	*	*	*	2	*	*	*	2	*	*	*
GRANOLA see CEREAL, COLD																				
GRANOLA BAR																				
almond (generic) 1 bar	117	3	9	15	*	5	—	2	2	*	3	2	5	*	*	4	*	*	*	*

	Calories	Protein	Fat	Sat. Fat	Cholesterol	Carbohydrates	Fiber	Sodium	Potassium	Calcium	Iron	Zinc	Magnesium	Vitamin A	Vitamin C	Thiamin	Riboflavin	Niacin	Vitamin B$_{12}$	Folic acid
GRANOLA BAR (continued)																				
apple																				
(Nutri-Grain) 1 bar	150	3	8	5	*	8	4	3	2	*	10	10	2	15	*	25	25	25	—	25
blueberry																				
(Nutri-Grain) 1 bar	150	3	8	5	*	8	4	3	2	*	10	10	2	15	*	25	25	25	—	25
blueberry apple																				
(Health Valley) 1 bar	140	6	*	*	*	11	12	*	3	2	20	6	10	*	*	2	4	2	—	—
chocolate																				
chewy																				
(generic) 1 bar	119	3	7	15	*	7	4	3	3	3	4	3	6	*	*	4	2	*	*	2
chocolate chip																				
(generic) 1 bar	103	3	6	14	*	6	4	3	2	2	4	3	4	*	*	3	*	*	*	*
chewy w/ coating																				
(generic) 1 bar	132	3	11	20	*	6	4	2	3	3	4	2	5	*	*	2	4	*	3	2
fat free																				
(Health Valley) 1 bar	140	8	*	*	*	13	12	*	3	2	20	8	10	*	*	2	4	2	—	—
cinnamon																				
(Nature Valley) 1 bar	120	3	8	5	*	6	—	3	2	*	4	—	—	*	*	4	*	*	—	—
date almond																				
(Health Valley) 1 bar	140	6	*	*	*	11	15	*	8	2	20	6	10	*	*	2	4	2	—	—
honey graham																				
(Nature Valley) 1 bar	110	3	6	3	*	5	—	4	2	*	4	—	—	*	*	6	*	*	—	—
nuts & raisins chewy																				
(generic) 1 bar	129	4	9	14	*	6	8	3	3	2	3	3	6	*	*	4	3	4	*	2
oat bran																				
(Nature Valley) 1 bar	110	3	6	3	*	5	—	4	2	*	4	—	—	*	*	6	*	*	—	—
oats 'n' honey																				
(Nature Valley) 1 bar	120	3	8	5	*	6	—	3	2	*	4	—	—	*	*	6	*	*	—	—
peanut																				
(generic) 1 bar	113	4	8	3	*	5	—	3	2	*	3	3	6	*	*	3	*	2	*	*
peanut butter																				
(generic) 1 bar	114	4	9	4	*	5	—	3	2	*	3	2	3	*	*	3	*	2	*	*
(Nature Valley) 1 bar	120	3	9	5	*	5	—	3	2	*	2	—	—	*	*	2	*	2	—	—
chewy																				
(generic) 1 oz bar	121	5	7	5	*	6	4	5	2	3	3	4	6	*	*	4	2	4	*	2
chewy w/ coating																				
(generic) 1 bar	187	6	18	31	*	7	—	3	4	4	3	4	6	*	*	2	5	6	*	2
peanut butter chocolate chip																				
chewy																				
(generic) 1 bar	122	5	9	8	*	6	4	4	3	2	3	3	6	*	*	2	2	4	2	2
plain																				
(generic) 1 bar	134	5	9	4	*	6	8	3	3	2	5	4	7	*	*	5	2	2	*	2
chewy																				
(generic) 1 bar	126	3	8	11	*	6	4	3	3	3	4	3	5	*	*	6	3	*	2	2
raisin																				
(Health Valley) 1 bar	140	6	*	*	*	11	12	*	3	2	20	6	10	*	*	2	4	2	—	—
chewy																				
(generic) 1 bar	127	4	8	14	*	6	4	3	3	3	4	2	5	*	*	4	3	2	*	2
fat free																				
(Health Valley) 1 bar	140	8	*	*	*	11	12	*	3	2	20	8	10	*	*	2	4	2	—	—
raspberry																				
(Health Valley) 1 bar	140	6	*	*	*	11	15	*	8	2	20	6	10	*	*	2	4	2	—	—
(Nutri-Grain) 1 bar	150	3	8	5	*	8	4	3	2	*	10	10	2	15	*	25	25	25	—	25
strawberry																				
(Nutri-Grain) 1 bar	150	3	8	5	*	8	4	3	2	*	10	10	2	15	*	25	25	25	—	25
GRAPE																				
adherent skin (European)																				
1/2 cup	57	*	*	*	*	5	4	*	4	*	*	*	*	*	*	14	5	3	*	—	*
10 grapes	36	*	*	*	*	3	4	*	3	*	*	*	*	*	*	9	3	2	*	—	*

	Calories	Protein	Fat	Sat. Fat	Cholesterol	Carbohydrates	Fiber	Sodium	Potassium	Calcium	Iron	Zinc	Magnesium	Vitamin A	Vitamin C	Thiamin	Riboflavin	Niacin	Vitamin B$_{12}$	Folic acid
GRAPE																				
slipskin (American)																				
1/2 cup	29	*	*	*	*	3	*	*	3	*	*	*	*	*	3	3	2	*	—	*
10 grapes	15	*	*	*	*	*	*	*	*	*	*	*	*	*	2	*	*	*	—	*
GRAPE, CANNED																				
Thompson																				
in heavy syrup 1/2 cup	93	*	*	*	*	8	4	*	4	*	7	*	2	2	2	3	2	*	—	*
in water 1/2 cup	49	*	*	*	*	4	4	*	4	*	7	*	2	2	2	3	2	*	—	*
GRAPE DRINK, BOTTLED/CANNED																				
(generic) 6 fl oz	94	*	*	*	*	8	*	*	2	*	*	*	*	2	*	50	*	*	*	*	*
(Kool-Aid) 8 1/2 fl oz	140	*	*	*	*	12	*	*	*	*	*	*	*	*	10	*	*	*	*	*
(Mott's) 10 fl oz	170	*	*	*	*	14	*	2	*	*	*	—	—	*	*	*	*	*	—	—
(Tang) 8 1/2 fl oz	130	*	*	*	*	11	*	*	*	*	*	—	—	*	100	*	10	10	*	20
(Tropicana) 6 fl oz	90	*	*	*	*	7	—	*	—	*	*	—	—	*	*	2	2	4	2	*	*
(Welch's) 6 fl oz	110	*	*	*	*	9	*	*	4	*	*	*	*	*	*	*	*	*	*	*
(Welch's Orchard) 8 1/2 oz (1 box)	150	*	*	*	*	13	*	*	*	*	*	*	*	*	*	*	*	*	*	*
(Welchade) 6 fl oz	100	*	*	*	*	8	*	*	*	*	*	—	—	*	*	*	*	*	*	*
GRAPE DRINK, FROM CONCENTRATE																				
(Mott's Fruit Basket) 8 fl oz	130	2	*	*	*	11	*	*	5	2	2	—	—	*	25	*	*	*	*	—	—
GRAPE DRINK, FROM MIX																				
(Kool-Aid) 8 fl oz	70	*	*	*	*	6	*	*	*	*	*	*	*	*	*	10	*	*	*	*	*
sugar-free (Kool-Aid) 8 fl oz	4	*	*	*	*	*	*	*	*	*	*	*	*	*	*	10	*	*	*	*	*
unsweetened (Kool-Aid) 8 fl oz prep w/ out sugar	2	*	*	*	*	*	*	*	*	*	*	*	*	*	*	10	*	*	*	*	*
w/ sugar added (Kool-Aid) 8 fl oz prep w/ sugar	100	*	*	*	*	8	*	*	*	*	*	*	*	*	*	10	*	*	*	*	*
GRAPE JUICE, BOTTLED/CANNED																				
concord (Knudsen) 8 fl oz	160	*	*	*	*	13	*	*	7	2	2	—	—	*	8	—	—	—	—	—
(Welch's) 6 fl oz	120	*	*	*	*	10	*	*	4	*	*	—	—	*	45	2	2	2	—	—
red (generic) 8 fl oz	154	2	*	*	*	13	*	*	10	2	3	*	6	*	*	4	6	3	—	2
(Knudsen) 8 fl oz	150	2	*	*	*	12	*	*	4	2	*	—	—	*	4	—	—	—	—	—
(Welch's) 6 fl oz	120	*	*	*	*	10	*	*	4	*	*	—	—	*	45	2	2	2	—	—
aseptic pack (Welch's) 8 1/2 oz (1 box)	150	*	*	*	*	13	*	*	*	*	*	*	*	*	*	*	*	*	*	*
organic (Knudsen) 8 fl oz	160	*	*	*	*	13	*	*	7	2	2	—	—	*	8	—	—	—	—	—
sparkling (Welch's) 6 fl oz	130	*	*	*	*	11	*	*	5	*	*	—	—	*	*	*	*	*	*	*
white (Welch's) 6 fl oz	110	*	*	*	*	9	*	*	3	*	*	—	—	*	45	*	*	*	*	*
aseptic pack (Welch's) 8 1/2 oz (1 box)	140	*	*	*	*	11	*	*	5	*	*	—	—	*	*	*	*	*	*	*
(Welch's Orchard) 8 1/2 oz (1 box)	160	*	*	*	*	13	*	*	5	*	*	*	*	*	60	*	*	*	*	*
sparkling (Welch's) 6 fl oz	110	*	*	*	*	9	*	*	3	*	*	—	—	*	*	*	*	*	*	*
GRAPE JUICE, FROM CONCENTRATE																				
red *sweetened* (generic) 6 fl oz	96	*	*	*	*	8	*	*	*	*	*	*	2	*	75	2	3	*	—	*
(Welch's) 6 fl oz	100	*	*	*	*	8	*	*	*	*	*	*	*	*	45	*	*	*	*	*

	Calories	Protein	Fat	Sat. Fat	Cholesterol	Carbohydrates	Fiber	Sodium	Potassium	Calcium	Iron	Zinc	Magnesium	Vitamin A	Vitamin C	Thiamin	Riboflavin	Niacin	Vitamin B₁₂	Folic acid
GRAPE JUICE, FROM CONCENTRATE (continued)																				
white (Welch's) 6 fl oz	100	*	*	*	*	8	*	*	—	*	*	*	*	*	45	*	*	—	*	*
sweetened (Welch's) 6 fl oz	100	*	*	*	*	8	*	*	—	*	*	*	—	*	45	*	*	*	*	—
GRAPE JUICE BLEND from concentrate organic (Knudsen) 8 fl oz	150	2	*	*	*	12	*	*	4	2	*	—	—	*	4	—	—	—	—	—
GRAPE JUICE COCKTAIL from concentrate (Welch's) 6 fl oz	120	*	*	*	*	10	*	*	2	*	*	*	*	*	100	*	*	—	*	*
light (Welch's) 6 fl oz	40	*	*	*	*	3	*	*	*	*	*	*	*	*	*	*	*	*	*	*
GRAPE-APPLE DRINK (Mott's) 10 fl oz	170	*	*	*	*	14	*	*	2	*	*	—	—	*	*	*	*	*	—	*
(Welch's) 6 fl oz	110	*	*	*	*	9	*	*	3	*	*	*	*	*	*	*	*	*	*	*
(Welch's Orchard) 8 1/2 oz (1 box)	150	*	*	*	*	13	*	*	2	*	*	*	*	*	*	*	*	*	*	*
from concentrate (Welch's) 6 fl oz	110	*	*	*	*	9	*	*	2	*	*	*	*	*	*	*	*	*	*	*
GRAPE-APPLE JUICE (Welch's) 6 fl oz	100	*	*	*	*	9	*	*	5	*	*	—	—	*	*	*	*	*	—	—
GRAPE-CRANBERRY DRINK (Ocean Spray Cran-Grape) 8 fl oz	170	—	*	*	*	14	*	*	—	*	*	*	*	*	100	—	—	—	—	—
low calorie (Lightstyle) 8 fl oz	40	—	*	*	*	3	*	*	—	*	*	*	*	*	100	—	—	—	—	—
GRAPE-CRANBERRY JUICE (Welch's) 6 fl oz	110	*	*	*	*	9	*	*	5	*	*	*	*	*	*	*	*	*	*	*
GRAPE-PEACH JUICE (Welch's) 6 fl oz	120	*	*	*	*	10	*	*	5	*	*	—	—	*	*	*	*	*	—	—
GRAPEFRUIT pink/red 1/2 fruit	37	*	*	*	*	3	4	*	4	2	*	*	2	6	76	3	*	*	*	3
all types 1/2 fruit	37	*	*	*	*	3	—	*	5	*	*	*	2	6	78	3	*	*	*	4
1/2 cup sections	35	*	*	*	*	3	—	*	4	*	*	*	2	6	73	3	*	*	*	3
California 1/2 fruit	46	*	*	*	*	4	*	*	5	*	*	*	3	6	78	3	*	*	*	4
white all types 1/2 fruit	39	*	*	*	*	3	4	*	5	*	*	*	3	*	65	3	*	2	*	3
California 1/2 fruit	44	2	*	*	*	4	—	*	5	*	*	*	3	*	65	3	*	2	*	3
Florida 1/2 fruit	38	*	*	*	*	3	—	*	5	2	*	*	3	*	73	3	*	*	*	3
1/2 cup sections	37	*	*	*	*	3	—	*	5	2	*	*	3	*	71	3	*	*	*	3
GRAPEFRUIT, CANNED in juice 1/2 cup	46	*	*	*	*	4	*	*	6	2	*	*	3	*	70	2	*	2	*	3
in light syrup 1/2 cup	76	*	*	*	*	7	4	*	5	2	3	*	3	*	45	3	*	2	*	3
in water 1/2 cup	44	*	*	*	*	4	*	*	5	2	3	*	3	*	44	3	2	2	*	3
GRAPEFRUIT JUICE, FRESH pink/red 6 fl oz	73	2	*	*	*	6	—	*	9	2	2	*	6	16	118	5	2	2	*	5
white 6 fl oz	73	2	*	*	*	6	*	*	9	2	2	*	6	*	118	5	2	2	*	5

	Calories	Protein	Fat	Sat. Fat	Cholesterol	Carbohydrates	Fiber	Sodium	Potassium	Calcium	Iron	Zinc	Magnesium	Vitamin A	Vitamin C	Thiamin	Riboflavin	Niacin	Vitamin B12	Folic acid
GRAPEFRUIT JUICE, BOTTLED/CANNED																				
(Del Monte) 8 fl oz	100	3	*	*	*	8	5	*	—	4	2	—	—	6	120	—	—	—	—	—
pink																				
(Knudsen) 8 fl oz	100	3	*	*	*	8	*	*	9	4	2	—	—	*	90	—	—	—	—	—
red																				
(Tropicana) 6 fl oz	70	2	*	*	*	5	—	*	—	2	2	—	—	6	70	15	2	10	—	—
yellow																				
(Ocean Spray) 8 fl oz	100	—	*	*	*	8	2	*	7	*	*	—	—	*	100	—	—	—	—	—
(Knudsen) 8 fl oz	100	3	*	*	*	8	*	*	9	4	2	—	—	*	90	—	—	—	—	—
(Mott's) 10 fl oz	120	3	*	*	*	9	*	*	13	*	4	—	—	*	130	*	*	*	—	—
(Tropicana) 6 fl oz	70	2	*	*	*	5	—	*	—	2	2	—	—	*	60	10	2	*	—	—
organic																				
(Knudsen) 8 fl oz	100	3	*	*	*	8	*	*	9	4	2	—	—	*	90	—	—	—	—	—
sweetened																				
(generic) 8 fl oz	115	2	*	*	*	9	*	*	12	2	5	*	6	*	112	7	3	4	*	6
unsweetened																				
(generic) 8 fl oz	94	2	*	*	*	7	*	*	11	2	3	*	6	*	120	7	3	3	*	6
GRAPEFRUIT JUICE, FROM CONCENTRATE																				
organic																				
(Knudsen) 8 fl oz	100	3	*	*	*	8	*	*	9	4	2	—	—	*	90	—	—	—	—	—
GRAPEFRUIT JUICE COCKTAIL																				
pink																				
(Ocean Spray) 8 fl oz	110	—	*	*	*	9	*	*	4	*	*	—	—	*	100	—	—	—	—	—
(Tropicana Twister) 6 fl oz	80	*	*	*	*	6	—	*	—	2	2	—	—	*	*	*	*	*	—	—
light																				
(Tropicana Twister) 6 fl oz	30	*	*	*	*	2	—	*	—	2	8	—	—	2	100	2	6	*	—	—
low calorie																				
(Lightstyle) 8 fl oz	40	—	*	*	*	3	*	*	3	*	*	—	—	*	100	—	—	—	—	—
red																				
(Ocean Spray) 8 fl oz	130	—	*	*	*	11	*	*	*	*	*	—	—	*	100	—	—	—	—	—
GRAPEFRUIT-TANGERINE DRINK																				
(Ocean Spray) 8 fl oz	130	—	*	*	*	11	*	*	2	*	*	—	—	*	100	—	—	—	—	—
GREAT NORTHERN BEAN																				
cooked																				
1/2 cup	104	12	*	*	*	6	24	*	10	6	10	5	11	*	2	9	3	3	*	22
cooked w/ salt																				
1/2 cup	104	12	*	*	*	6	—	9	10	6	10	5	11	*	2	9	3	3	*	22
GREAT NORTHERN BEAN, CANNED																				
(Bush Bros) 1/2 cup	110	12	*	*	*	6	28	17	—	4	8	—	—	*	*	—	—	—	—	—
(generic) 1/2 cup	149	16	*	*	*	9	24	*	13	7	11	6	17	*	3	12	5	3	*	27
(Hain) 1/2 cup	80	10	2	*	*	6	28	9	12	6	10	—	—	*	*	6	*	2	—	—
dry, canned in brine																				
(Green Giant/Joan of Arc) 1/2 cup	20	20	*	*	*	6	20	12	4	10	10	—	—	*	*	2	*	2	—	—
w/ pork																				
(Bush Bros) 1/2 cup	110	10	2	3	—	6	24	19	—	4	6	—	—	*	*	—	—	—	—	—
GREEN BEAN																				
raw																				
1/2 cup	123	12	*	*	*	2	2	*	5	3	8	4	4	*	7	6	8	4	*	14
boiled w/ salt																				
1/2 cup	22	2	*	*	*	2	—	6	5	3	4	*	4	8	10	3	4	2	*	5
cooked																				
1/2 cup	111	10	*	*	*	7	—	*	9	5	5	4	12	*	2	7	3	2	*	16
cooked w/ salt																				
1/2 cup	111	10	*	*	*	7	—	9	9	5	5	4	12	*	2	7	3	2	*	16
GREEN BEAN, CANNED																				
(generic) 1/2 cup	18	2	*	*	*	*	4	*	3	3	6	2	4	2	8	2	4	*	*	5
cut																				
(Bush Bros) 1/2 cup	25	2	*	*	*	2	8	18	—	2	6	—	—	10	2	—	—	—	—	—

	Calories	Protein	Fat	Sat. Fat	Cholesterol	Carbohydrates	Fiber	Sodium	Potassium	Calcium	Iron	Zinc	Magnesium	Vitamin A	Vitamin C	Thiamin	Riboflavin	Niacin	Vitamin B$_{12}$	Folic acid
GREEN BEAN, CANNED (continued)																				
(Del Monte) 1/2 cup	20	*	*	*	*	*	6	15	—	2	4	—	—	6	8	—	—	—	—	—
(Green Giant) 1/2 cup	16	*	*	*	*	*	4	16	3	2	4	—	—	6	4	*	2	2	—	—
50% less salt (Green Giant) 1/2 cup	16	*	*	*	*	*	4	8	3	2	4	—	—	8	2	*	2	2	—	—
no salt added (Del Monte) 1/2 cup	20	*	*	*	*	*	6	*	—	2	4	—	—	6	8	—	—	—	—	—
reduced salt (Del Monte) 1/2 cup	20	*	*	*	*	*	6	8	—	2	4	—	—	6	8	—	—	—	—	—
drained (generic) 1/2 cup	14	*	*	*	*	*	4	7	2	2	3	*	2	5	5	*	2	*	*	5
French cut (Del Monte) 1/2 cup	20	*	*	*	*	*	6	15	—	2	4	—	—	6	8	—	—	—	—	—
(Green Giant) 1/2 cup	16	*	*	*	*	*	4	16	3	2	2	—	—	6	4	*	2	2	—	—
no salt added (Del Monte) 1/2 cup	20	2	*	*	*	*	6	*	—	2	4	—	—	6	8	—	—	—	—	—
reduced salt (Del Monte) 1/2 cup	20	*	*	*	*	*	6	8	—	2	4	—	—	6	8	—	—	—	—	—
seasoned (Del Monte) 1/2 cup	20	2	*	*	*	*	6	15	—	2	4	—	—	6	8	—	—	—	—	—
w/ ham flavor (Bush Bros) 1/2 cup	35	3	*	*	*	*	2	8	21	—	2	6	—	—	10	2	—	—	—	—
Italian (Del Monte) 1/2 cup	30	2	*	*	*	*	2	12	15	—	2	4	—	—	4	15	—	—	—	—
kitchen sliced (Green Giant) 1/2 cup	16	*	*	*	*	*	4	16	3	2	4	—	—	4	4	*	4	*	—	—
seasoned (generic) 1/2 cup	18	2	*	*	*	*	—	18	3	3	3	*	4	12	6	2	3	*	*	5
solid & liquid (generic) 1/2 cup	18	2	*	*	*	*	4	*	3	3	6	2	4	8	8	2	4	*	*	5
whole (Del Monte) 1/2 cup	20	*	*	*	*	*	6	15	—	2	4	—	—	6	8	—	—	—	—	—
GREEN BEAN, FROZEN																				
(Bird's Eye Deluxe) 3 oz	25	2	*	*	*	2	—	*	—	4	4	*	4	10	15	4	4	*	*	2
boiled (generic) 1/2 cup	19	2	*	*	*	*	8	*	2	3	3	2	4	5	5	2	4	*	*	4
boiled w/ salt (generic) 1/2 cup	18	2	*	*	*	*	—	7	2	3	3	3	4	7	9	2	3	*	*	*
in butter sauce (Green Giant One Serving) 5 1/2 oz	60	3	3	5	2	3	12	15	5	4	4	—	—	6	8	2	4	2	—	—
cut (Green Giant) 1/2 cup	14	2	*	*	*	*	4	*	3	2	2	—	—	2	4	*	2	*	—	—
(Green Giant Harvest Fresh) 1/2 cup	16	2	*	*	*	*	4	4	3	2	4	—	—	2	6	*	2	*	—	—
microwave (Green Giant) 1/2 cup	12	*	*	*	*	*	4	11	2	2	2	—	—	10	*	*	*	*	—	—
cut, in butter sauce (Green Giant) 1/2 cup	30	2	2	3	2	*	6	10	3	2	2	—	—	4	4	*	2	2	—	—
French cut (Bird's Eye) 3 oz	25	2	*	*	*	2	4	*	—	4	4	—	4	8	15	4	4	*	—	2
GREEN BEAN COMBINATION																				
almondine (Green Giant) 1/2 cup	45	3	5	*	*	2	8	15	4	2	4	—	—	6	*	*	4	2	—	—
green beans w/ ham flavor & potatoes (Bush Bros) 1/2 cup	40	3	*	*	*	2	12	23	—	2	2	—	—	8	10	—	—	—	—	—
green & shelley beans (Bush Bros) 1/2 cup	45	5	*	*	*	2	12	17	—	4	4	—	—	4	*	—	—	—	—	—
GREENS see specific green																				

	Calories	Protein	Fat	Sat. Fat	Cholesterol	Carbohydrates	Fiber	Sodium	Potassium	Calcium	Iron	Zinc	Magnesium	Vitamin A	Vitamin C	Thiamin	Riboflavin	Niacin	Vitamin B₁₂	Folic acid
GROUNDCHERRY 1/2 cup	37	2	*	*	*	3	—	—		*	4	—	—	10	13	5	2	10	*	—
GROUPER raw 1 fillet	238	84	4	3	32	*	*	6	36	7	13	8	20	7	*	12	*	4	26	*
baked/broiled 1 fillet	238	84	4	3	32	*	*	4	27	4	13	7	19	7	*	11	*	4	23	*
GUACAMOLE (Kraft) 2 tbsp	50	*	6	10	*	*	*	9	*	*	*	*	—	—	*	*	*	*	*	—
GUACAMOLE SEASONING MIX (Old El Paso) 1/7 pkg	7	*	*	*	*	*	*	10	*	*	*		—	—	2	15	*	*	*	—
GUAVA 1 fruit	46	*	*	*	*	4	20	*	7	2	2	*	2	14	275	3	3	—	—	—
1/2 cup	42	*	*	*	*	3	16	*	7	2	*	*	2	13	254	3	2	—	—	—
strawberry 1 fruit	4	*	*	*	*	—	*	*	*	*	—	*	*	4	*	*	—	—	—	
1/2 cup	84	*	*	*	*	7	—	2	10	3	x	—	5	2	75	2	2	x	—	—
GUAVA DRINK (Mauna La'i) 8 fl oz	130	—	*	*	*	11	*	*	*	*	*	*	*	*	100	—	—	—	—	—
from concentrate (Welch's) 6 fl oz	100	*	*	*	*	8	*	*	3	*	*	*	*	*	*	*	*	*	*	*
GUAVA SAUCE 1/2 cup	43	*	*	*	*	4	16	*	8	*	*	*	2	7	290	2	*	2	—	—
GUAVA-PASSIONFRUIT DRINK (Mauna La'i) 8 fl oz	130	—	*	*	*	11	*	*	2	*	*	*	*	10	100	—	—	—	—	—
GUINEA HEN meat w/out skin raw 3 oz	94	29	3	3	18	*	*	2	5	*	4	7	5	*	2	4	6	37	5	x
meat w/ skin raw 3 oz	134	33	8	8	21	*	*	2	5	*	4	6	5	2	*	3	5	33	5	*
HADDOCK raw 1 fillet	168	61	2	*	37	*	*	5	17	6	11	5	19	2	*	4	4	37	39	*
baked/broiled 1 fillet	168	61	2	*	37	*	*	5	17	6	11	5	19	2	*	4	4	35	35	*
smoked 3 oz	99	36	*	*	22	*	*	27	10	4	7	3	11	*	*	3	2	22	23	*
HADDOCK, FROZEN battered (Van de Kamp's) 2 fillets	250	20	23	15	10	6	*	24	6	4	6	—	—	*	*	10	10	10	—	—
breaded (Van de Kamp's) 2 fillets	270	20	25	15	8	6	*	12	6	*	8	—	—	*	*	15	10	20	—	—
crispy batter dipped (Gorton's) 2 fillets	300	18	32	25	7	5	—	24	5	*	2	—	—	*	*	4	2	8		
crunchy batter (Mrs. Paul's) 4 1/2 oz	190	30	8	5	8	7	*	24	—	*	4	—	—	*	*	8	6	10	—	—
light (Mrs. Paul's Light) 4 1/4 oz	220	40	14	5	15	5	*	15	—	2	2	—	—	*	*	8	8	10	—	—
(Van de Kamp's) 1 fillet	240	25	17	10	12	7	—	25	7	2	15	—	—	*	*	15	15	15	—	—
HALIBUT raw 1/2 fillet	224	71	7	4	22	*	*	5	26	10	10	6	42	6	*	8	9	60	40	*
baked/broiled 1/2 fillet	223	71	7	4	22	*	*	5	26	10	9	6	43	6	*	7	9	57	36	*
HALIBUT, GREENLAND broiled/baked 1/2 fillet	380	49	43	25	31	*	*	7	16	*	8	5	13	2	*	8	10	15	25	*

	Calories	Protein	Fat	Sat. Fat	Cholesterol	Carbohydrates	Fiber	Sodium	Potassium	Calcium	Iron	Zinc	Magnesium	Vitamin A	Vitamin C	Thiamin	Riboflavin	Niacin	Vitamin B₁₂	Folic acid
HALIBUT, FROZEN																				
battered (Van de Kamp's) 2 fillets	150	13	9	5	3	5	*	17	5	2	6	—	—	*	*	10	8	20	—	—
HAM, FRESH																				
center slice lean & fat unheated 3 oz	173	29	17	20	15	*	*	49	8	*	4	11	4	*	*	48	10	20	11	*
lean only raw 3 oz	166	39	11	12	20	*	*	95	12	*	5	16	5	*	*	32	12	17	12	*
chopped 1 oz	65	8	8	8	5	*	*	16	3	*	*	4	*	*	9	12	3	5	4	*
minced 3 oz	224	23	27	31	20	*	*	44	8	*	4	11	4	*	42	40	10	18	13	*
patty 1	205	14	28	33	15	*	*	29	4	*	4	7	4	*	*	20	6	10	12	*
rump lean & fat roasted 3 oz	214	41	19	23	27	*	*	2	9	*	5	16	5	*	*	42	16	20	10	*
lean only roasted 3 oz	175	44	11	12	27	*	*	2	9	*	5	17	5	*	*	45	18	21	11	*
shank lean & fat roasted 3 oz	246	36	26	32	26	*	*	2	8	*	5	17	5	*	*	33	15	19	9	*
lean only roasted 3 oz	183	40	14	16	26	*	*	2	9	*	5	20	5	*	*	36	17	21	10	*
steak (Oscar Mayer) 1 slice	55	16	3	4	10	*	*	31	4	*	3	7	3	*	*	—	—	—	—	—
extra lean unheated 3 oz	104	28	6	6	13	*	*	45	8	*	5	11	5	*	46	45	10	22	11	*
w/natural juices (Oscar Mayer) 1 slice	35	8	2	3	5	*	*	13	2	*	*	3	*	*	—	—	—	—	—	—
whole leg lean & fat roasted 3 oz	232	38	23	28	27	*	*	2	9	*	5	17	5	*	*	36	16	19	10	2
lean only roasted 3 oz	179	42	12	14	27	*	*	2	9	*	5	18	5	*	*	39	17	21	10	3
HAM, CURED																				
boneless roasted 3 oz	151	32	12	14	17	*	*	53	10	*	6	14	6	*	32	41	17	26	10	*
unheated 3 oz	155	25	14	15	16	*	*	47	8	*	5	12	5	*	39	49	13	22	12	*
extra lean roasted 3 oz	123	30	7	8	15	*	*	43	7	*	7	16	7	*	30	43	10	17	9	*
unheated 3 oz	111	27	6	7	13	*	*	51	8	*	4	11	4	*	37	53	11	21	11	*
lean & fat roasted 3 oz	207	31	22	*	2	*	*	42	7	*	4	13	4	*	*	13	14	2	3	*
unheated 3 oz	209	26	24	*	2	*	*	45	8	*	3	10	3	*	*	11	14	2	3	*

	Calories	Protein	Fat	Sat. Fat	Cholesterol	Carbohydrates	Fiber	Sodium	Potassium	Calcium	Iron	Zinc	Magnesium	Vitamin A	Vitamin C	Thiamin	Riboflavin	Niacin	Vitamin B₁₂	Folic acid
HAM, CURED (continued)																				
lean only																				
roasted																				
3 oz	134	35	7	*	*	*	*	47	8	*	4	15	4	*	*	14	16	2	4	*
unheated																				
3 oz	125	32	8	*	*	*	*	54	9	*	4	12	4	*	*	13	18	2	4	*
HAM, CANNED																				
(Hormel Cure 81) 3 oz	96	33	6	9	15	*	*	36	12	*	6	12	*	*	27	45	12	24	—	
boneless																				
(Bryan Centerpiece) 3 oz	120	20	14	—	15	*	*	45	—	—	—	—	—							
(Bryan Classic) 3 oz	90	25	5	—	15	*	*	49	—	—	—	—	—							
(Bryan Southern Supreme) 3 oz	90	25	5	—	15	*	*	50	—	—	—	—	—							
baked																				
(Bryan Southern Supreme) 3 oz	120	25	5	—	15	*	*	47	—	—	—	—	—							
honey																				
(Bryan Southern Supreme) 3 oz	90	25	9	—	15	*	*	52	—	—	—	—	—							
chopped																				
(Black Label) 3 oz	210	21	27	30	15	*	*	42	9	*	4	9	4	*	30	24	9	15	—	
(generic) 3 oz	203	23	25	27	14	*	*	48	7	*	4	10	4	*	3	30	8	14	10	*
chunk																				
(Hormel) 3 oz	132	22	13	15	15	*	*	36	11	*	4	10	—	*	32	17	10	19	—	
extra lean																				
roasted																				
(generic) 3 oz	116	30	6	7	8	*	*	40	8	*	4	13	4	*	39	59	12	21	10	*
unheated																				
(generic) 3 oz	102	26	6	7	11	*	*	44	9	*	4	11	4	*	38	47	12	23	12	*
pre-sliced																				
(Bryan) 3 oz	90	25	5	—	15	*	*	49												
jubilee																				
(Oscar Mayer) 1 slice	31	9	2	2	5	*	*	12	3	*	*	4	*	*	*	15	4	8	3	—
boneless																				
(Oscar Mayer) 1 slice	43	8	4	4	5	*	*	15	3	*	2	4	*	*	*	15	4	7	4	*
roasted																				
(generic) 1 cup diced	316	48	33	36	29	*	*	55	14	*	11	23	11	*	33	76	21	37	25	2
unheated																				
(generic) 1 cup diced	266	40	28	30	18	*	*	72	13	*	6	15	6	*	51	90	19	23	18	2
HAM, COLD CUTS																				
(Oscar Mayer Healthy Favorites) 1 slice	14	4	*	*	2	*	*	5	2	*	*	2	*	*	*	—	—	—	—	—
baked																				
(Bryan Thin Sliced) 1 slice	30	10	2	—	5	—	*	4	—	—	—	—	—							
w/ natural juices																				
(Oscar Mayer) 1 slice	21	6	*	*	4	*	*	10	2	*	*	3	*	*	*	—	—	—	—	—
boiled																				
w/ natural juices																				
(Oscar Mayer) 1 slice	22	6	*	*	4	*	*	12	2	*	*	3	*	*	*	—	—	—	—	—
(Oscar Mayer Healthy Favorites) 1 slice	13	4	*	*	2	*	*	5	2	*	*	*	*	*	*	—	—	—	—	—
breakfast																				
(Oscar Mayer Healthy Favorites) 1 slice	30	8	*	2	5	*	*	14	2	*	*	2	*	*	*	—	—	—	—	—
chopped																				
(Bryan) 1 slice	50	7	5	—	5	*	*	14	—	—	—	—	—							
(generic) 1 slice	65	8	8	8	4	*	*	8	*	*	*	3	*	*	*	9	12	3	16	6
w/ natural juices																				
(Oscar Mayer) 1 slice	35	5	4	4	4	*	*	9	*	*	*	3	*	*	*	—	—	—	—	—
cooked																				
(Bryan) 1 slice	30	5	2	—	5	*	*	16	—	—	—	—	—							
(Bryan Thin Sliced) 1 slice	30	10	2	—	5	—	*	4	—	—	—	—	—							
(Hormel) 1 slice	29	7	2	3	4	*	*	14	3	*	1	3	1	*	13	10	3	5	—	

	Calories	Protein	Fat	Sat. Fat	Cholesterol	Carbohydrates	Fiber	Sodium	Potassium	Calcium	Iron	Zinc	Magnesium	Vitamin A	Vitamin C	Thiamin	Riboflavin	Niacin	Vitamin B₁₂	Folic acid
HAM, COLD CUTS (continued)																				
dinner (Oscar Mayer) 1 slice	28	8	2	2	5	*	*	14	2	*	2	3	*	*	*	13	4	7	2	—
extra lean (generic) 1 slice	37	9	2	3	4	*	*	17	3	*	4	*	*	*	12	18	4	7	4	*
ham & cheese loaf (Bryan) 1 slice	80	8	9	—	7	*	*	7	—	—	—	—	—	—	—	—	—	—	—	—
(generic) 1 slice	73	8	9	11	5	*	*	16	2	2	*	4	*	*	12	11	3	5	4	*
(Oscar Mayer) 1 slice	66	6	8	11	6	*	*	14	2	2	*	3	*	*	*	11	3	5	3	*
honey (Bryan) 1 slice	30	8	2	—	5	*	*	17	—	—	—	—	—	—	—	—	—	—	—	—
(Bryan Thin Sliced) 1 slice	30	10	2	—	5	—	*	4	—	—	—	—	—	—	—	—	—	—	—	—
(Thorn Apple Valley) 1 slice	35	7	2	—	*	*	*	14	—	—	—	—	—	*	*	—	—	—	—	—
w/ natural juices (Oscar Mayer) 1 slice	14	4	*	*	2	*	*	6	*	*	*	*	*	*	*	—	—	—	—	—
lower salt (Bryan) 1 slice	30	8	2	—	5	*	*	12	—	—	—	—	—	—	—	—	—	—	—	—
mesquite (Bryan) 1 slice	30	8	2	—	5	*	*	17	—	—	—	—	—	—	—	—	—	—	—	—
regular (generic) 1 slice	52	8	5	5	5	*	*	16	3	*	2	4	*	*	13	16	4	7	4	*
sliced (Thorn Apple Valley) 1 slice	35	7	2	—	5	*	*	15	—	—	—	—	—	*	*	—	—	—	—	—
smoked (Bryan Thin Sliced) 1 slice	30	10	2	—	5	—	*	4	—	—	—	—	—	—	—	—	—	—	—	—
(Oscar Mayer) 1 slice	27	8	*	*	5	*	*	15	2	*	2	4	2	*	*	—	—	—	—	—
(Oscar Mayer Healthy Favorites) 1 slice	22	6	*	*	3	*	*	7	5	*	*	3	*	—	—	—	—	—	—	—
HAM SALAD (generic) 2 oz	61	4	7	7	3	*	*	11	*	*	2	*	*	3	8	2	3	4	*	
canned (Libby's) 2 oz	70	10	5	5	3	2	*	16	3	*	2	*	*	*	*	8	*	6	2	*
HAM SPREAD w/ cheese (generic) 2 tbsp	69	8	8	12	6	*	*	14	*	6	*	4	*	2	3	6	4	3	3	*
deviled (Underwood) 2 1/8 oz	220	13	29	30	17	*	*	18	4	*	6	—	—	*	*	4	4	8	—	—
deviled, light (Underwood) 2 1/8 oz	120	18	12	5	12	*	*	10	5	*	5	—	—	*	15	5	8	20	—	—
HAM, TURKEY see TURKEY, COLD CUTS																				
HAM ENTREE, FROZEN																				
w/ asparagus au gratin (Budget Gourmet Light & Healthy) 8 3/4 oz	300	25	22	35	17	9	—	36	17	15	4	—	—	2	25	40	15	30	—	—
w/ asparagus bake (Stouffer's) 9 1/2 oz	520	30	55	70	25	11	8	43	11	20	8	—	—	6	40	35	30	15	—	—
w/ cheddar pretzel sandwich (Weight Watchers) 4 oz	260	25	12	15	3	11	12	24	11	10	8	—	—	2	2	—	—	—	—	—
w/ cheese sandwich (Weight Watchers) 5 oz	240	23	11	13	3	11	20	20	7	10	6	—	—	4	6	—	—	—	—	—
glazed (Morton) 8 oz	230	20	5	—	12	13	—	47	11	2	8	—	—	50	100	35	10	8	—	—
HAMBURGER ENTREE, FROM MIX																				
beef noodle (Hamburger Helper) 1 cup	330	33	23	—	—	10	—	40	7	*	15	—	—	*	*	20	15	25	—	—
cheddar 'n' bacon (Hamburger Helper) 1 cup	400	40	31	—	—	10	—	42	12	10	15	—	—	2	*	20	20	25	—	—
cheeseburger macaroni (Hamburger Helper) 1 cup	370	35	29	—	—	9	—	43	11	6	15	—	—	4	*	20	20	25	—	—

	Calories	Protein	Fat	Sat. Fat	Cholesterol	Carbohydrates	Fiber	Sodium	Potassium	Calcium	Iron	Zinc	Magnesium	Vitamin A	Vitamin C	Thiamin	Riboflavin	Niacin	Vitamin B₁₂	Folic acid
HAMBURGER ENTREE, FROM MIX (continued)																				
cheesy Italian (Hamburger Helper) 1 cup	360	35	26	—	—	10	—	40	11	10	15	—	—	6	*	20	20	25	—	—
chili macaroni (Hamburger Helper) 1 cup	330	32	22	—	—	11	—	40	12	2	15	—	—	6	*	20	15	25	—	—
hamburger pizza (Hamburger Helper) 1 cup	360	35	22	—	—	12	—	42	14	2	20	—	—	10	2	30	15	35	—	—
hamburger stew (Hamburger Helper) 1 cup	300	32	20	—	—	9	—	43	15	4	15	—	—	15	*	6	10	25	—	—
hash (Hamburger Helper) 1 cup	320	30	23	—	—	9	—	42	16	2	15	—	—	*	2	4	10	25	—	—
mushroom & wild rice (Hamburger Helper) 1 cup	380	35	25	—	—	12	—	40	13	8	15	—	—	6	*	15	15	25	—	—
pizzabake (Hamburger Helper) 1 cup	300	32	22	—	—	10	—	35	10	4	15	—	—	4	*	15	10	25	—	—
potatoes au gratin (Hamburger Helper) 1 cup	350	33	28	—	—	9	—	37	17	2	15	—	—	2	*	6	10	25	—	—
rice oriental (Hamburger Helper) 1 cup	340	32	22	—	—	13	—	47	9	2	15	—	—	*	*	15	10	25	—	—
romanoff (Hamburger Helper) 1 cup	350	37	23	—	—	10	—	45	11	6	20	—	—	*	*	25	20	25	—	—
stroganoff (Hamburger Helper) 1 cup	390	37	29	—	—	11	—	36	11	10	15	—	—	6	*	20	20	25	—	—
taco (Hamburger Helper) 1 cup	330	32	22	—	—	11	—	40	9	2	15	—	—	6	*	20	15	25	—	—
tacobake (Hamburger Helper) 1 cup	320	28	22	—	—	10	—	39	9	4	20	—	—	6	*	20	15	25	—	—
teriyaki (Hamburger Helper) 1 cup	360	33	22	—	—	13	—	48	11	2	20	—	—	8	*	10	10	20	—	—
zesty Italian (Hamburger Helper) 1 cup	350	33	22	—	—	12	—	36	12	2	20	—	—	2	*	20	15	25	—	—
HAMBURGER ENTREE, FROZEN																				
bacon cheeseburger (Hormel Quickmeal) 5 oz	440	40	37	45	27	11	—	33	10	10	15	26	8	4	2	30	25	25	—	—
beef patty sandwich (Swanson Kids') 8 oz	440	50	29	—	—	14	—	30	—	4	25	—	—	*	10	15	15	15	—	—
w/ cheese (Kid Cuisine) 6 1/4 oz	430	22	34	—	12	15	—	23	—	10	15	—	—	*	4	20	10	10	—	—
beef patty w/ gravy, charbroiled (Morton) 9 oz	270	20	18	—	10	9	—	54	13	4	12	—	—	2	*	8	8	6	—	—
cheeseburger chili (Hormel Quickmeal) 6 oz	450	38	34	50	30	13	—	29	12	10	15	26	9	10	*	20	20	25	—	—
double (Hormel Quickmeal) 7 1/2 oz	590	58	45	—	40	16	—	32	—	10	20	—	—	4	2	30	30	35	—	—
regular (Hormel Quickmeal) 4 3/4 oz	400	35	31	40	25	12	—	25	9	10	15	24	8	4	*	30	25	25	—	—
hamburger (Hormel Quickmeal) 4 1/4 oz	350	30	25	30	20	11	—	15	8	4	10	20	6	*	*	20	20	20	—	—
HAMBURGER ROLL see ROLL																				
HAZELNUT OIL 1 tbsp	120	*	22	5	*	*	*	*	*	*	*	*	*	*	*	*	*	*	*	*
HEAD CHEESE *pork* (generic) 1 1 oz slice	60	8	7	7	8	*	*	15	*	*	2	2	*	*	10	*	3	2	5	*
(Oscar Mayer) 1 slice	53	7	6	7	8	*	*	15	*	*	2	2	*	*	*	*	3	*	4	*
HEART OF PALM see PALM																				
HERB PEPPERCORN SAUCE *from mix* (Knorr) 1/4 cup	210	60	11	—	23	3	—	32	—	2	6	*	*	*	*	4	6	50	*	*

Encyclopedia of Daily Values

	Calories	Protein	Fat	Sat. Fat	Cholesterol	Carbohydrates	Fiber	Sodium	Potassium	Calcium	Iron	Zinc	Magnesium	Vitamin A	Vitamin C	Thiamin	Riboflavin	Niacin	Vitamin B₁₂	Folic acid
HERBS see specific listings																				
HERRING, ATLANTIC																				
raw 1 fillet	291	55	26	19	37	*	*	7	17	10	11	12	15	3	2	11	25	30	417	*
baked/broiled 1 fillet	290	55	26	19	37	*	*	7	17	11	11	12	15	3	2	11	25	29	312	*
kippered 1 fillet	87	16	8	6	11	*	*	15	5	3	3	4	5	*	*	3	8	9	124	*
pickled 1 piece	39	4	4	2	*	*	*	5	*	*	*	*	*	*	*	3	*	*	2	11	*
HERRING, PACIFIC																				
broiled/baked 1 fillet	360	50	39	30	47	*	*	6	22	15	12	7	15	3	*	7	22	20	230	*
HERRING, CANNED see SARDINE																				
HERRING, LAKE see CISCO																				
HIBISCUS-CRANBERRY JUICE																				
(Heinke's) 8 fl oz	120	*	*	*	*	10	*	*	3	2	2	—	—	*	*	—	—	—	—	—
(Knudsen Exotic Blends) 8 fl oz	120	*	*	*	*	10	*	*	3	2	2	—	—	*	*	—	—	—	—	—
HICKORY NUT																				
dried (generic) 1 oz	187	6	28	10	*	2	8	*	4	2	3	8	12	*	*	16	2	*	*	3
HOLLANDAISE SAUCE																				
microwave (Knorr) 1/4 cup	120	4	16	—	6	*	—	18	—	4	4	*	*	50	60	4	4	*	*	*
from mix (Knorr) 1/4 oz	180	2	26	—	2	2	—	13	—	4	*	*	*	10	*	*	2	*	*	*
prep w/ butter (generic) 1/4 cup	63	2	8	—	*	*	*	17	*	3	*	*	*	4	*	*	3	*	3	2
HOMESTYLE GRAVY																				
from mix (Pillsbury) 1/4 cup	16	*	*	*	*	*	*	10	*	*	*	*	*	*	*	*	*	*	*	*
HOMINY, CANNED																				
golden (Bush Bros) 1/2 cup	60	2	*	*	*	4	12	23	—	*	2	—	—	4	*	—	—	—	—	
w/ peppers (Bush Bros) 1/2 cup	70	3	2	*	*	5	12	24	—	*	2	—	—	4	*	—	—	*	—	
white (Bush Bros) 1/2 cup	70	7	2	*	*	5	18	*	*	*	*	—	—	*	*	—	—	*	—	
w/ peppers (Bush Bros) 1/2 cup	80	3	2	*	*	5	16	21	—	*	2	—	—	*	*	—	—	*	—	
HONEY																				
(generic) 1 tbsp	64	*	*	*	*	6	*	*	*	*	*	*	*	*	*	*	*	*	*	*
HONEY BUN																				
glazed (Hostess) 1 bun	30	3	32	50	5	13	3	10	3	15	10	—	—	*	*	15	10	8	—	
iced (Hostess) 1 bun	430	8	34	50	7	18	7	10	3	10	10	—	—	*	*	15	10	10	—	
plain (Rich's) 1 bun	270	5	25	20	2	10	4	2	*	6	9	*	*	*	*	7	59	*	—	
HONEY LOAF LUNCHEON MEAT																				
pork (generic) 1 1 oz slice	52	9	5	6	5	*	*	16	2	*	3	6	*	*	8	2	3	6	11	*
pork & beef (generic) 1 1 oz slice	36	7	2	2	3	*	*	16	3	*	2	5	*	*	10	9	4	4	5	*
(Oscar Mayer) 1 slice	33	9	2	2	5	*	*	16	3	*	2	5	*	*	17	13	5	5	4	*
HONEYDEW MELON																				
1 cup cubed	60	*	*	*	*	5	4	*	13	*	*	—	3	*	70	9	2	5	*	—
1/10 fruit	45	*	*	*	*	4	4	*	10	*	*	—	2	*	53	7	*	4	*	—

	Calories	Protein	Fat	Sat Fat	Cholesterol	Carbohydrates	Fiber	Sodium	Potassium	Calcium	Iron	Zinc	Magnesium	Vitamin A	Vitamin C	Thiamin	Riboflavin	Niacin	Vitamin B₁₂	Folic acid
HORSERADISH LEAF																				
raw																				
1/2 cup chopped	6	2	*	*	*	*	*	*	*	2	2	*	4	15	9	2	4	*	*	*
boiled																				
1/2 cup chopped	13	2	*	*	*	*	*	*	2	3	3	*	8	29	11	3	6	2	*	*
boiled w/ salt																				
1/2 cup chopped	13	2	*	*	*	*	—	2	2	3	3	*	8	29	11	3	6	2	*	*
HORSERADISH POD																				
raw																				
1/2 cup slices	19	2	*	*	*	*	8	*	7	*	*	*	6	*	117	2	2	2	*	6
2 pods	8	*	*	*	*	*	4	*	3	*	*	*	2	*	52	*	*	*	*	2
boiled																				
1/2 cup slices	21	2	*	*	*	2	8	*	8	*	*	2	6	*	95	2	2	2	*	5
HORSERADISH, PREPARED																				
(Kraft) 1 tbsp	10	*	*	*	*	*	*	6	*	*	*	—	—	*	2	*	*	*	—	—
HORSERADISH SAUCE																				
(Kraft) 1 tbsp	12	*	2	*	*	*	*	4	*	*	*	*	*	*	*	*	*	*	*	*
(Sauceworks) 1 tbsp	50	*	8	5	2	*	*	4	*	*	*	*	*	*	*	*	*	*	*	*
HOT CHOCOLATE see COCOA DRINK																				
HOT DOG																				
beef																				
(Armour) 1 hot dog	150	8	20	25	8	*	*	18	—	*	2	—	*	*	—	—	—	—	—	—
(Bryan) 1 hot dog	110	7	8	—	7	*	*	16	—	—	—	—	—	—	—	—	—	—	—	—
(generic) 1 hot dog	142	9	20	27	9	*	*	19	2	*	4	7	*	*	18	2	3	5	12	*
(Hebrew National) 1 hot dog	150	10	20	25	10	*	*	15	—	*	4	—	*	*	—	—	—	—	—	—
(Hormel Wranglers) 1 hot dog	170	12	23	30	13	*	—	22	4	*	6	9	2	*	24	2	5	7	—	—
(Hygrade) 1 hot dog	180	10	26	34	11	*	*	25	—	*	4	—	*	*	—	—	—	—	—	—
(Kahn's) 1 hot dog	150	8	21	32	10	*	*	19	—	4	2	—	*	*	—	—	—	—	—	—
(Nathan's) 1 hot dog	160	12	23	30	10	*	*	20	—	*	4	—	*	*	—	—	—	—	—	—
bun size																				
(Bryan) 1 hot dog	180	10	26	—	10	*	*	26	—	—	—	—	—	—	—	—	—	—	—	—
(Healthy Choice) 1 hot dog	70	2	2	3	7	2	*	25	—	2	4	—	*	6	—	—	—	—	—	—
jumbo																				
(Bryan) 1 hot dog	180	10	25	—	10	*	*	26	—	—	—	—	—	—	—	—	—	—	—	—
lowfat																				
(Hebrew National) 1 hot dog	120	8	15	20	8	*	*	15	—	*	5	—	*	*	—	—	—	—	—	—
beef & pork																				
(generic) 1 hot dog	182	11	26	31	9	*	*	27	3	*	4	7	*	*	25	8	4	8	12	*
(Hormel Wranglers) 1 2 oz hot dog	180	12	25	30	13	*	—	21	4	*	5	9	2	*	25	6	5	8	—	—
cheese																				
jumbo																				
(Bryan) 1 hot dog	190	12	26	—	12	*	*	26	—	—	—	—	—	—	—	—	—	—	—	—
pork & beef																				
(generic) 1 hot dog	93	7	13	15	6	*	*	13	2	2	2	4	*	*	9	5	3	4	8	*
chicken																				
(generic) 1 hot dog	116	10	14	13	15	*	*	26	*	4	5	3	*	*	*	2	3	7	2	*
(Wampler-Longacre) 1 hot dog	120	12	17	15	20	*	4	20	—	8	6	—	*	*	—	—	—	—	—	—
hot dinner frank																				
(Bryan) 1 hot dog	180	10	26	—	10	*	*	25	—	—	—	—	—	—	—	—	—	—	—	—
juicy jumbo																				
(Bryan) 1 hot dog	180	10	25	—	10	*	*	25	—	—	—	—	—	—	—	—	—	—	—	—
light																				
(Bryan) 1 hot dog	110	10	14	—	13	*	*	26	—	—	—	—	—	—	—	—	—	—	—	—
light weiner																				
lower sodium																				
(Bryan) 1 hot dog	70	7	8	—	7	*	*	10	—	—	—	—	—	—	—	—	—	—	—	—

	Calories	Protein	Fat	Sat. Fat	Cholesterol	Carbohydrates	Fiber	Sodium	Potassium	Calcium	Iron	Zinc	Magnesium	Vitamin A	Vitamin C	Thiamin	Riboflavin	Niacin	Vitamin B₁₂	Folic acid
HOT DOG (continued)																				
meat frank																				
bun size																				
(Bryan) 1 hot dog	180	10	26	—	10	*	*	25	—	—	—	—	—	—	—	—	—	—	—	—
meat weiner																				
(Bryan) 1 hot dog	110	7	8	—	7	*	*	15	—	—	—	—	—	—	—	—	—	—	—	—
smoked																				
jumbo																				
(Bryan) 1 hot dog	180	10	26	—	10	7	*	24	—	—	—	—	—	—	—	—	—	—	—	—
turkey																				
(generic) 1 hot dog	102	11	12	14	16	*	*	27	2	5	5	9	2	*	*	*	5	9	2	*
(Oscar Mayer) 1 hot dog	85	9	10	10	11	*	*	21	2	5	5	6	2	*	*	—	—	—	—	—
(Wampler-Longacre) 1 hot dog	90	10	12	13	12	*	8	18	—	4	4	—	—	*	*	—	—	—	—	—
turkey cheese																				
(Oscar Mayer) 1 hot dog	89	10	10	11	13	*	*	21	2	6	4	7	2	2	*	—	—	—	—	—
HOT DOG ENTREE, FROZEN																				
(Kid Cuisine) 6 3/4 oz	450	22	29	—	13	19	—	37	12	10	25	—	—	*	6	30	15	15	—	—
(Swanson Kids') 7 2/3 oz	330	25	15	—	—	—	—	31	—	10	10	—	—	20	10	15	15	15	—	—
chili dog w/ cheese																				
(Hormel Quickmeal) 4 1/2 oz	340	23	31	40	27	8	—	22	8	10	10	12	6	10	10	30	20	15	—	—
corn dog																				
(Hormel) 2 3/4 oz	210	10	15	20	12	8	—	21	5	2	4	5	3	*	10	10	8	8	—	—
HOT DOG ROLL see ROLL																				
HOT DOG SAUCE																				
(Gebhardt) 3 tbsp	25	2	2	2	*	*	*	7	2	*	—	—	—	*	*	*	*	*	—	—
(Just Rite) 1/4 cup	60	3	5	6	2	2	*	9	5	*	4	—	—	*	2	3	2	2	—	—
HOT SAUCE																				
(Gebhardt) 1/4 tsp	0	*	*	*	*	*	*	*	*	*	*	*	*	*	*	*	*	*	*	*
hot pepper																				
(generic) 1/4 tsp	0	*	*	*	*	*	*	*	*	*	*	*	*	*	*	*	*	*	*	*
Tabasco																				
(generic) 1/4 tsp	0	*	*	*	*	*	*	*	*	*	*	*	*	*	*	*	*	*	*	*
HUBBARD SQUASH see SQUASH																				
HUMMUS																				
(generic) 1/3 cup	140	7	11	5	*	5	16	8	4	4	7	6	6	*	11	5	3	2	*	12
HUNTER SAUCE																				
from mix																				
(Knorr) 1/4 oz	25	*	2	—	*	*	—	13	—	*	*	*	*	*	*	*	*	*	*	*
HYACINTH BEAN																				
cooked																				
1/2 cup	113	13	*	*	*	7	—	*	9	4	25	18	20	*	*	17	2	2	*	*
cooked w/ salt																				
1/2 cup	113	13	*	*	*	7	—	10	9	4	25	18	20	*	*	17	2	2	*	*
ICE CREAM																				
chocolate																				
(generic) 1/2 cup	143	4	11	23	7	6	—	2	5	7	3	3	5	5	*	2	8	*	3	3
(Haagen-Dazs) 1/2 cup	270	6	26	40	40	8	*	2	7	10	2	—	—	10	*	*	10	4	—	—
coffee																				
(Haagen-Dazs) 1/2 cup	270	6	26	40	40	8	*	2	5	10	2	—	—	10	*	2	15	4	—	—
cookie dough																				
(Weight Watchers) 1/2 cup	140	5	5	10	8	4	4	4	—	20	—	—	—	*	*	—	—	—	—	—
deep dark chocolate																				
(Ben & Jerry's) 1/2 cup	250	7	23	45	18	10	8	2	—	10	6	—	—	10	*	—	—	—	—	—
French vanilla																				
soft serve																				
(generic) 1/2 cup	185	6	17	32	26	6	—	2	4	11	*	3	3	9	*	3	9	*	7	2
mint cookies in cream																				
reduced fat																				
(Breyer's) 1/2 cup	140	7	8	12	10	7	2	3	—	10	4	—	—	4	*	—	—	—	—	—

ICE CREAM (continued)

	Calories	Protein	Fat	Sat. Fat	Cholesterol	Carbohydrates	Fiber	Sodium	Potassium	Calcium	Iron	Zinc	Magnesium	Vitamin A	Vitamin C	Thiamin	Riboflavin	Niacin	Vitamin B12	Folic acid
praline crunch (Weight Watchers) 1/2 cup	140	5	5	8	2	8	*	4	3	20	8	—	—	2	*	—	—	—	—	—
rocky road (Weight Watchers) 1/2 cup	140	7	5	8	2	8	4	3	5	20	4	—	—	2	*	—	—	—	—	—
strawberry (generic) 1/2 cup	127	4	8	—	6	6	—	2	4	8	*	*	2	4	8	2	10	*	3	2
(Haagen-Dazs) 1/2 cup	250	6	23	40	32	8	*	2	5	10	4	—	—	10	*		2	10	2	—
triple chocolate (Weight Watchers) 1/2 cup	150	7	5	8	2	9	4	3	6	20	6	—	—	2	*	—	—	—	—	—
vanilla																				
(Ben & Jerry's) 1/2 cup	230	7	26	50	32	7	*	2	—	10	2	—	—	15	*	—	—	—	—	—
(Haagen-Dazs) 1/2 cup	260	6	26	40	40	8	*	2	4	10	*	—	—	10	*		2	10	4	—
(Sealtest) 1/2 cup	140	3	11	25	10	5	*	2	—	8	*	—	—	4	*	—	—	—	—	—
(Weight Watchers) 1/2 cup	120	7	4	8	2	7	4	3	5	20	*	—	—	2	*	—	—	—	—	—
fat free (Sealtest) 1/2 cup	100	3	*	*	*	7	*	2	—	8	*	—	—	8	*	—	—	—	—	—
light (Breyer's) 1/2 cup	130	7	7	15	12	6	*	2	—	10	*	—	—	4	*	—	—	—	—	—
natural (Breyer's) 1/2 cup	150	5	12	30	12	5	*	2	—	10	*	—	—	6	*	—	—	—	—	—
regular (generic) 1/2 cup	133	4	11	23	10	5	*	2	4	8	*	3	2	5	*	2	9	*	4	*
rich (generic) 1/2 cup	178	4	18	37	15	6	*	2	3	9	*	2	2	10	*	2	7	*	4	*
vienetta (Breyer's) 1/2 cup	190	5	18	35	13	6	*	2	—	11	*	—	—	6	*	—	—	—	—	—
vanilla/chocolate/strawberry (Breyer's) 1/2 cup	150	5	12	25	10	5	*	*	—	8	*	—	—	6	*	—	—	—	—	—

ICE CREAM, IMITATION

	Calories	Protein	Fat	Sat. Fat	Cholesterol	Carbohydrates	Fiber	Sodium	Potassium	Calcium	Iron	Zinc	Magnesium	Vitamin A	Vitamin C	Thiamin	Riboflavin	Niacin	Vitamin B12	Folic acid
brownie parfait (Weight Watchers) 5 1/3 fl oz	190	10	4	10	2	13	8	7	6	20	6	—	—	*	*	—	—	—	—	—
butter pecan crunch (Healthy Choice) 1/2 cup	140	5	3	5	2	9	—	3	4	10	*	—	—	*	2		4	10	*	—
cherry chocolate chip (Healthy Choice) 1/2 cup	130	5	3	5	2	8	—	3	4	10	*	—	—	*	*		2	10	*	—
chocolate caramel mousse (Weight Watchers) 2 3/4 oz	190	7	6	5	2	10	8	5	5	4	4	—	—	*	2	—	—	—	—	—
chocolate chip (Healthy Choice) 1/2 cup	130	5	3	5	2	8	—	3	5	10	2	—	—	*	2		4	8	*	—
chocolate mousse (Weight Watchers) 2 3/4 oz	190	10	6	8	2	11	12	6	9	6	10	—	—	*	*	—	—	—	—	—
coffee toffee (Healthy Choice) 1/2 cup	130	5	3	5	2	8	—	3	5	10	*	—	—	*	2		4	10	*	—
cookies 'n' cream (Healthy Choice) 1/2 cup	130	4	3	5	2		—	3	5	15	*	—	—	*	*		2	10	*	—
double fudge swirl (Healthy Choice) 1/2 cup	130	5	3	5	2	8	—	3	6	10	4	—	—	*	*		4	8	*	—
fudge brownie (Healthy Choice) 1/2 cup	140	5	3	5	2	9	—	3	5	10	2	—	—	*	*		2	8	*	—
mint chocolate chip (Healthy Choice) 1/2 cup	140	5	3	10	2	8	—	3	5	10	2	—	—	*	*		4	8	*	—
neapolitan (Healthy Choice) 1/2 cup	120	5	3	5	2	7	—	2	5	10	*	—	—	*	*		2	10	*	—
peanut butter cookie dough 'n' fudge (Healthy Choice) 1/2 cup	130	7	3	3	2	8	—	3	4	10	*	—	—	*	*		2	10	*	—

	Calories	Protein	Fat	Sat. Fat	Cholesterol	Carbohydrates	Fiber	Sodium	Potassium	Calcium	Iron	Zinc	Magnesium	Vitamin A	Vitamin C	Thiamin	Riboflavin	Niacin	Vitamin B$_{12}$	Folic acid
ICE CREAM, IMITATION (continued)																				
praline & caramel (Healthy Choice) 1/2 cup	130	5	3	*	2	9	—	3	5	10	*	—	—	*	*	2	10	*	—	—
praline pecan mousse (Weight Watchers) 2 3/4 oz	170	7	5	5	*	10	*	6	4	8	10	—	—	*	2	*	*	*	—	—
praline toffee crunch parfait (Weight Watchers) 5 oz	190	8	5	10	2	13	8	6	5	20	*	—	—	*	*	*	*	*	—	—
rocky road (Healthy Choice) 1/2 cup	160	5	3	5	2	11	—	3	5	10	*	—	—	*	*	2	10	*	—	—
vanilla (Healthy Choice) 1/2 cup	120	7	3	5	2	7	—	2	5	15	*	—	—	*	*	4	15	*	—	—
ICE CREAM BAR																				
almond (Dove) 3 2/3 oz	335	10	34	58	12	10	*	3	6	10	2	—	—	8	*	2	10	*	6	—
(Mars) 1 3/4 oz	210	8	21	30	5	7	*	2	4	8	2	—	—	4	*	*	10	*	4	—
caramel almond crunch (Haagen-Dazs) 1 bar	240	4	28	35	13	6	*	3	4	8	2	—	—	6	*	*	6	*	*	—
caramel/pecan (Dove) 3 2/3 oz	350	10	35	60	12	12	*	4	6	10	2	—	—	8	*	2	10	*	6	—
cherry w/ dark choclolate (Bounty) 3/4 oz	70	*	7	15	2	3	*	*	*	*	*	—	—	*	*	*	*	*	*	—
chocolate (Milky Way) 2 oz	210	6	17	33	7	8	*	2	4	8	*	—	—	4	*	*	6	*	*	—
(3 Musketeers) 2 oz	160	6	15	30	7	5	*	*	3	6	*	—	—	4	*	*	6	*	4	—
w/ dark chocolate coating (Dove) 3 3/4 oz	340	8	34	65	15	11	*	3	6	10	6	—	—	10	*	2	8	*	4	—
w/ milk chocolate coating (Dove) 3 3/4 oz	340	10	32	63	13	12	*	3	6	10	2	—	—	8	*	2	10	*	6	—
chocolate eclair (Good Humor) 1 bar	170	3	14	13	3	7	5	3	—	4	4	—	—	6	*	—	—	—	—	—
chocolate fudge (Fudgsicle) 1 bar	35	3	2	—	—	2	—	2	—	6	*	—	—	*	*	2	4	*	—	—
chocolate peanut butter crunch (Haagen-Dazs) 1 bar	270	8	32	35	12	5	*	2	5	8	4	—	—	4	*	4	2	10	—	—
chocolate/dark chocolate (Haagen-Dazs) 1 bar	380	8	42	75	28	13	*	2	7	10	10	—	—	10	*	*	6	*	6	—
coconut w/ dark choclolate coating (Bounty) 3/4 oz	70	*	7	15	2	*	*	*	*	*	*	—	—	*	*	*	*	*	*	—
w/ milk chocolate coating (Bounty) 3/4 oz	70	2	8	15	2	*	*	*	*	2	*	—	—	*	*	*	2	*	*	—
coffee almond crunch (Haagen-Dazs) 1 bar	360	8	40	75	33	9	*	4	6	15	2	—	—	15	*	6	10	10	*	—
coffee/cashew (Dove) 3 2/3 oz	335	10	34	63	12	10	*	2	7	8	6	—	—	8	*	4	8	4	4	—
crunchy cookie (Dove) 3 3/4 oz	340	10	32	63	13	12	*	3	6	15	*	—	—	8	*	4	10	*	6	—
fudge (Haagen-Dazs) 1 bar	210	2	22	35	25	6	*	2	5	10	2	—	—	10	*	*	6	*	*	—
orange & cream (Haagen-Dazs) 1 bar	130	2	9	15	13	6	*	*	2	6	4	—	—	6	10	*	2	*	—	—
peanut (Dove) 3 3/4 oz	380	15	38	65	13	12	*	4	8	15	2	—	—	8	*	4	10	*	6	—
Snickers (Snickers) 2 oz	220	10	20	30	5	7	*	3	5	8	*	—	—	4	*	2	6	6	4	—
vanilla (3 Musketeers) 2 oz	160	4	15	30	5	5	*	*	3	6	*	—	—	44	*	*	6	*	4	—
(Milky Way) 2 oz	200	6	18	33	7	8	*	2	4	6	2	—	—	44	*	*	6	*	*	—

	Calories	Protein	Fat	Sat. Fat	Cholesterol	Carbohydrates	Fiber	Sodium	Potassium	Calcium	Iron	Zinc	Magnesium	Vitamin A	Vitamin C	Thiamin	Riboflavin	Niacin	Vitamin B₁₂	Folic acid
ICE CREAM BAR (continued)																				
w/ chocolate coating (Klondike) 1 bar	290	5	31	70	5	8	0	3	—	10	*	—	—	6	*	—	—	—	—	—
w/ dark chocolate coating (Dove) 3 3/4 oz	340	8	34	65	15	11	*	2	6	10	4	—	—	10	*	2	8	*	4	—
(Haagen-Dazs) 1 bar	380	8	42	75	30	13	*	3	7	10	8	—	—	10	*	*	8	*	—	—
w/ milk chocolate coating (Dove) 3 3/4 oz	340	10	32	63	13	11	*	2	6	15	*	—	—	8	*	2	10	*	6	—
(Haagen-Dazs) 1 bar	330	6	37	70	30	8	*	3	6	15	2	—	—	10	*	*	8	*	—	—
vanilla & almonds (Haagen-Dazs) 1 bar	370	8	42	70	30	9	*	4	6	15	*	—	—	15	*	*	10	*	—	—
vanilla caramel brittle (Haagen-Dazs) 1 bar	370	8	38	70	28	11	*	7	6	15	*	—	—	10	*	*	10	2	—	—
vanilla crisp (Haagen-Dazs) 1 bar	220	4	25	30	13	5	*	2	4	8	2	—	—	6	*	*	4	*	—	—
ICE CREAM BAR, IMITATION																				
Arctic d'lites (Weight Watchers) 1 bar	130	3	11	10	2	4	*	2	7	15	*	—	—	*	*	—	—	—	—	—
berries & creme mousse (Weight Watchers) 1 bar	70	5	2	*	*	2	4	3	3	15	*	—	—	**	*	—	—	—	—	—
caramel nut (Weight Watchers) 1 bar	130	3	12	20	2	4	4	2	2	8	*	—	—	*	*	—	—	—	—	—
chcocolate mousse (Weight Watchers) 1 bar	70	7	2	3	2	6	16	3	6	15	*	—	—	2	*	—	—	—	—	—
chocolate almond crunch (Weight Watchers) 1 bar	130	3	11	10	2	4	4	2	*	8	*	—	—	*	*	—	—	—	—	—
chocolate fudge (Crystal Light) 1 bar	50	2	3	—	*	2	*	2	2	2	*	—	2	*	*	*	2	*	*	—
chocolate mousse (Light 'N' Lively) 1 bar	50	4	*	*	*	4	*	2	3	4	*	—	2	*	*	*	4	*	2	—
chocolate treat (Weight Watchers) 1 bar	100	5	2	*	3	7	4	6	6	15	*	—	—	*	*	—	—	—	—	—
chocolate w/ fudge (Sealtest) 1 bar	80	6	*	*	*	6	*	2	5	6	*	—	4	*	*	*	6	*	4	—
cool 'n' creamy bars orange vanilla (Crystal Light) 1 bar	50	2	3	—	*	2	*	2	2	2	*	—	2	*	*	*	2	*	*	—
double chocolate fudge (Light 'N' Lively) 1 bar	50	4	*	*	*	4	*	2	3	4	*	—	2	*	*	*	4	*	2	—
orange vanilla (Light 'N' Lively) 1 bar	40	*	*	*	*	3	*	*	*	*	*	—	*	*	*	*	*	*	*	—
(Weight Watchers) 1 bar	70	7	2	3	*	6	12	3	2	10	2	—	—	*	2	—	—	—	—	—
pralines & creme (Weight Watchers) 1 bar	120	3	9	10	2	4	*	2	2	8	*	—	—	*	*	—	—	—	—	—
strawberry (Light 'N' Lively) 1 bar	80	2	*	*	*	4	*	*	2	4	*	—	*	*	*	*	4	*	2	—
toffee crunch (Weight Watchers) 1 bar	120	3	11	15	2	4	4	2	2	8	*	—	—	*	*	—	—	—	—	—
vanilla w/ chocolate coating (Klondike Lite) 1 bar	110	5	8	20	2	5	3	2	—	10	*	—	—	4	*	—	—	—	—	—
(Light 'N' Lively) 1 bar	110	4	9	*	*	5	*	*	3	4	*	—	2	*	*	*	4	*	2	—
vanilla sandwich (Weight Watchers) 1 bar	160	7	5	10	2	10	4	7	3	10	4	—	—	*	*	—	—	—	—	—
vanilla w/ fudge (Sealtest) 1 bar	80	6	*	*	*	6	*	2	3	6	*	—	2	*	*	*	6	*	4	—
vanilla w/ strawberry (Sealtest) 1 bar	70	4	*	*	*	6	*	2	3	4	*	—	*	*	4	*	4	*	4	—

	Calories	Protein	Fat	Sat. Fat	Cholesterol	Carbohydrates	Fiber	Sodium	Potassium	Calcium	Iron	Zinc	Magnesium	Vitamin A	Vitamin C	Thiamin	Riboflavin	Niacin	Vitamin B₁₂	Folic acid
ICE CREAM CONE																				
cups																				
(Comet) 1 cone	18	*	*	*	*	*	—	*	*	*	*	—	—	*	*	*	*	*	—	—
rainbow cups																				
(Comet) 1 cone	16	*	*	*	*	*	—	*	*	*	*	—	—	*	*	*	*	*	—	—
sugar																				
(Comet) 1 cone	50	2	*	*	*	4	—	2	*	*	*	—	—	*	*	*	*	*	—	—
waffle																				
(Comet) 1 cone	70	2	*	*	*	5	*	*	*	*	*	—	*	*	*	*	*	*	—	—
ICE CREAM SHAKE																				
chocolate yogurt																				
(Weight Watchers) 7 1/2 fl oz	220	13	2	*	2	15	12	6	11	25	8	—	—	*	*	—	—	—	—	—
Milky Way																				
(Milky Way) 10 fl oz	390	20	25	50	20	18	*	10	11	25	4	—	—	10	*	6	20	2	15	—
ICE CREAM SNACK																				
almond praline																				
(Dove) 3/4 oz	80	*	8	13	2	3	*	*	*	2	*	—	—	*	*	*	2	*	*	—
cherry royale																				
(Dove) 3/4 oz	70	*	7	15	3	3	*	*	*	*	*	—	—	*	*	*	*	*	*	—
chocolate																				
(Milky Way) 3/4 oz	70	2	6	10	2	3	*	*	*	2	*	—	—	*	*	*	2	*	*	—
chocolate																				
(3 Musketeers) 3/4 oz	60	*	5	10	2	2	*	*	*	2	*	—	—	*	*	*	*	*	*	—
mint supreme																				
(Dove) 3/4 oz	80	*	7	13	2	3	*	*	*	2	*	—	—	*	*	*	*	*	*	—
Snickers																				
(Snickers) 1 oz	110	4	10	15	2	4	*	*	2	4	*	—	—	**	*	*	2	2	*	—
vanilla																				
(Milky Way) 3/4 oz	70	*	6	13	2	3	*	*	*	2	*	—	—	*	*	*	*	*	*	—
(3 Musketeers) 3/4 oz	60	*	5	10	2	2	*	*	*	2	*	—	—	*	*	*	*	*	*	—
vanilla classic																				
(Dove) 3/4 oz	70	*	7	13	3	2	*	*	*	*	*	—	—	*	*	*	*	*	*	—
ICE CREAM SUNDAE, IMITATION																				
chocolate chip cookie dough																				
(Weight Watchers) 1 sundae	180	5	6	8	2	11	8	5	5	8	4	—	—	*	*	—	—	—	—	—
hot caramel fudge																				
(Weight Watchers) 1 sundae	160	8	6	10	5	9	4	6	4	20	*	—	—	2	*	—	—	—	—	—
hot chocolate fudge																				
(Weight Watchers) 1 sundae	160	10	6	10	5	9	88	5	4	20	*	—	—	*	*	—	—	—	—	—
ICE DESSERT																				
lime																				
(generic) 1/2 cup	75	*	*	*	*	10	*	*	*	*	*	*	*	*	2	*	*	*	*	*
pineapple-coconut																				
(generic) 1/2 cup	108	*	4	—	*	8	—	*	*	*	19	*	*	*	21	*	*	*	*	*
ICE MILK																				
vanilla																				
(generic) 1/2 cup	92	4	4	9	3	5	*	2	4	9	*	2	2	2	*	3	10	*	7	*
soft serve																				
(generic) 1/2 cup	111	7	4	7	4	6	*	3	6	14	*	3	3	2	*	3	10	*	7	*
ICE POP																				
all flavors																				
(generic) 1 bar	37	*	*	*	*	3	*	*	*	*	*	*	*	*	*	*	*	*	*	*
(Kool-Aid) 1 bar	50	*	3	—	2	3	*	*	*	2	*	—	*	*	10	*	*	*	*	*
(Popsicle) 1 pop	45	*	*	*	*	4	*	*	—	*	*	—	—	*	*	—	—	—	—	—
juice jets																				
(Popsicle) 1 pop	45	*	*	*	*	4	*	*	*	*	*	—	—	*	*	—	—	—	—	—
sugar-free																				
(Popsicle) 1 pop	15	*	*	*	*	*	*	*	*	*	*	—	—	*	*	—	—	—	—	—
w/ added vitamin C																				
(generic) 1 bar	37	*	*	*	*	3	—	*	*	*	*	*	*	*	9	*	*	*	*	*

	Calories	Protein	Fat	Sat. Fat	Cholesterol	Carbohydrates	Fiber	Sodium	Potassium	Calcium	Iron	Zinc	Magnesium	Vitamin A	Vitamin C	Thiamin	Riboflavin	Niacin	Vitamin B₁₂	Folic acid
ICE POP (continued)																				
fruit flavors																				
reduced calorie																				
(generic) 1 bar	12	*	*	*	*	*	—	*	*	*	*	*	*	*	*	*	*	*	*	*
ICING see FROSTING																				
ITALIAN BREAD see BREAD																				
ITALIAN SAUSAGE																				
raw																				
mild																				
(generic) 1 link	315	22	44	52	23	*	*	28	7	2	6	11	3	*	3	34	9	15	14	2
cooked																				
mild																				
(generic) 1 link	220	23	27	31	18	*	*	26	6	2	6	11	3	*	2	28	9	14	15	*
spicy																				
(generic) 1 link	220	23	27	31	18	*	*	30	6	2	6	11	3	*	2	28	9	14	15	*
sliced																				
(Oscar Mayer) 1 slice	249	19	34	38	19	*	*	22	5	2	7	12	3	*	*	—	—	—	—	—
JACKFRUIT																				
3 1/2 oz	94	2	*	*	*	8	8	*	9	3	3	9	6	11	2	6	2	*	—	
JALAPENO DIP																				
(Kraft) 2 tbsp	50	*	6	10	*	*	*	7	*	*	*	—	—	*	4	*	*	*	—	—
JAM, JELLY & PRESERVES																				
all-fruit spread																				
all flavors																				
(Polaner) 1 tbsp	42	*	*	*	*	4	—	*	*	*	*	*	*	*	*	*	*	*	*	*
(Smucker's Extra) 1 tbsp	15	*	*	*	*	*	*	*	*	*	*	*	*	*	*	*	*	*	*	*
(Smucker's Simply Fruit) 1 tbsp	16	*	*	*	*	*	*	*	*	*	*	*	*	*	*	*	*	*	*	*
apricot																				
(Sorrell Ridge) 1 tbsp	35	*	*	*	*	3	*	*	*	*	*	*	*	*	*	*	*	*	*	*
(Welch's Totally Fruit) 1 tbsp	21	*	*	*	*	2	*	*	*	*	*	*	*	*	*	*	*	*	*	—
blackberry																				
(Welch's Totally Fruit) 1 tbsp	21	*	*	*	*	2	*	*	*	*	*	*	*	*	*	*	*	*	*	—
blueberry																				
(Welch's Totally Fruit) 1 tbsp	21	*	*	*	*	2	*	*	*	*	*	*	*	*	*	*	*	*	*	—
grape																				
(Welch's Totally Fruit) 1 tbsp	42	*	*	*	*	4	*	*	*	*	*	*	*	*	*	*	*	*	*	—
orange marmalade																				
(Welch's Totally Fruit) 1 tbsp	21	*	*	*	*	2	*	*	*	*	*	*	*	*	*	*	*	*	*	—
raspberry																				
(Sorrell Ridge) 1 tbsp	35	*	*	*	*	3	*	*	*	*	*	*	*	*	*	*	*	*	*	*
(Welch's) 1 tbsp	52	*	*	*	*	5	*	*	*	*	*	*	*	*	*	*	*	*	*	—
(Welch's Totally Fruit) 1 tbsp	21	*	*	*	*	2	*	*	*	*	*	*	*	*	*	*	*	*	*	—
strawberry																				
(Welch's) 1 tbsp	52	*	*	*	*	5	*	*	*	*	*	*	*	*	*	*	*	*	*	—
(Welch's Totally Fruit) 1 tbsp	21	*	*	*	*	2	*	*	*	*	*	*	*	*	*	*	*	*	*	—
diet spread																				
all flavors low sugar																				
(Slenderella) 1 tbsp	8	*	*	*	*	*	*	*	*	*	*	*	*	*	*	*	*	*	*	*
reduced calorie																				
(Slenderella) 1 tbsp	7	*	*	*	*	*	*	*	*	*	*	*	*	*	*	*	*	*	*	*
(Smucker's) 1 tbsp	7	*	*	*	*	*	*	*	*	*	*	*	*	*	*	*	*	*	*	*
grape																				
(Weight Watchers) 1 tsp	8	—	*	*	*	*	*	*	*	*	*	*	*	*	*	—	—	—	*	—
raspberry																				
(Weight Watchers) 1 tsp	8	3	*	*	*	*	*	*	*	*	*	*	*	*	*	—	—	—	*	—
strawberry																				
(Weight Watchers) 1 tsp	8	3	*	*	*	*	*	—	*	*	*	*	*	*	*	—	—	—	*	—

	Calories	Protein	Fat	Sat. Fat	Cholesterol	Carbohydrates	Fiber	Sodium	Potassium	Calcium	Iron	Zinc	Magnesium	Vitamin A	Vitamin C	Thiamin	Riboflavin	Niacin	Vitamin B₁₂	Folic acid
JAM, JELLY, & PRESERVES (continued)																				
jam																				
all flavors																				
(generic) 1 tbsp	48	*	*	*	*	4	*	*	*	*	*	*	*	*	3	*	*	*	*	2
(Kraft) 1 tsp	17	*	*	*	*	*	*	*	*	*	*	*	*	*	*	*	*	*	*	—
(Smucker's) 1 tbsp	18	*	*	*	*	*	*	*	*	*	*	*	*	*	*	*	*	*	*	*
apricot																				
(generic) 1 tbsp	48	*	*	*	*	4	*	*	*	*	*	*	*	*	3	*	*	*	*	2
grape																				
(Welch's) 1 tbsp	52	*	*	*	*	5	*	*	*	*	*	*	*	*	*	*	*	*	*	—
jelly																				
all flavors																				
(Kraft) 1 tsp	17	*	*	*	*	*	*	*	*	*	*	*	*	*	*	*	*	*	*	—
(Smucker's) 1 tbsp	18	*	*	*	*	*	*	*	*	*	*	*	*	*	*	*	*	*	*	*
grape																				
(Welch's) 1 tbsp	52	*	*	*	*	5	*	*	*	*	*	*	*	*	*	*	*	*	*	*
reduced calorie																				
(Kraft) 1 tsp	6	*	*	*	*	*	*	*	*	*	*	*	*	*	*	*	*	*	*	—
marmalade																				
orange																				
(generic) 1 tbsp	49	*	*	*	*	4	*	*	*	*	*	*	*	*	2	*	*	*	*	2
(Smucker's) 1 tbsp	18	*	*	*	*	*	*	*	*	*	*	*	*	*	*	*	*	*	*	*
preserves																				
all flavors																				
(generic) 1 tbsp	48	*	*	*	*	4	*	*	*	*	*	*	*	*	3	*	*	*	*	2
(Kraft) 1 tsp	17	*	*	*	*	*	*	*	*	*	*	*	*	*	*	*	*	*	*	—
(Smucker's) 1 tbsp	18	*	*	*	*	*	*	*	*	*	*	*	*	*	*	*	*	*	*	*
apricot																				
(generic) 1 tbsp	48	*	*	*	*	4	*	*	*	*	*	*	*	*	3	*	*	*	*	2
strawberry reduced calorie																				
(Kraft) 1 tsp	6	*	*	*	*	*	*	*	*	*	*	*	*	*	*	*	*	*	*	—
JAVA-PLUM																				
1/2 cup	41	*	*	*	*	4	—	*	2	*	*	—	3	*	16	*	*	*	*	*
6 fruits	11	*	*	*	*	*	—	*	*	*	*	—	*	*	4	*	*	*	*	*
JELLY see JAM, JELLY & PRESERVES																				
JERUSALEM ARTICHOKE																				
raw																				
1/2 cup slices	57	2	*	*	*	4	4	*	9	*	14	*	3	*	5	10	3	5	*	3
JUICE DRINK																				
Ambrosia																				
(Knudsen Tropical Blend) 8 fl oz	130	*	*	*	*	11	*	2	6	4	2	*	*	8	6	*	*	*	*	*
Calamansi																				
(Knudsen Tropical Blend) 8 fl oz	120	*	*	*	*	10	*	*	4	2	2	*	*	2	8	*	*	*	*	*
Cupuassu																				
(Knudsen Tropical Blend) 8 fl oz	120	*	*	*	*	10	*	*	4	2	2	*	*	2	8	*	*	*	*	*
Guanabana																				
(Knudsen Tropical Blend) 8 fl oz	120	*	*	*	*	10	*	*	4	2	2	*	*	2	8	*	*	*	*	*
Harvest blend																				
(Welch's Orchard) 8 1/2 oz (1 box)	150	*	*	*	*	13	*	*	3	*	*	*	*	*	*	*	*	*	*	*
mixed fruit																				
(Tang) 8 1/2 fl oz	140	*	*	*	*	12	*	*	*	*	*	*	*	*	100	*	10	10	*	20
Razzleberry																				
(Knudsen Exotic Blends) 8 fl oz	130	*	*	*	*	11	*	*	7	2	4	*	*	*	2	*	*	*	*	*
Tropical Cruz, organic																				
(Santa Cruz Natural) 8 fl oz	110	*	*	*	*	9	*	*	5	4	2	*	*	2	4	*	*	*	*	*
vitamin fortified																				
(Knudsen Vita Juice) 8 fl oz	110	2	*	*	*	10	*	2	5	6	15	*	*	100	100	*	*	*	*	*
JUICE DRINK, FROM CONCENTRATE																				
guanabana																				
(Knudsen) 8 fl oz	120	*	*	*	*	10	*	*	4	2	2	*	*	2	8	*	*	*	*	*

	Calories	Protein	Fat	Sat. Fat	Cholesterol	Carbohydrates	Fiber	Sodium	Potassium	Calcium	Iron	Zinc	Magnesium	Vitamin A	Vitamin C	Thiamin	Riboflavin	Niacin	Vitamin B₁₂	Folic acid
JUICE DRINK, FROM CONCENTRATE (continued)																				
harvest juice blend (Welch's) 6 fl oz	110	*	*	*	*	9	*	*	3	*	*	*	*	*	*	*	*	*	*	*
natural breakfast juice (Knudsen) 8 fl oz	110	2	*	*	*	9	*	*	7	2	4	*	*	*	60	*	*	*	*	*
tropical (Mott's Fruit Basket) 8 fl oz	120	*	*	*	*	10	*	*	5	2	2	*	*	*	25	*	*	*	*	*
JUJUBE FRUIT																				
fresh 3 1/2 oz	79	2	*	*	*	7	—	*	7	2	3	*	3	*	115	*	2	5	*	—
dried 3 1/2 oz	287	6	2	*	*	25	—	*	15	8	10	*	9	—	22	14	21	3	*	—
JUTE, POTHERB																				
raw 1/2 cup	5	*	*	*	*	*	—	*	2	3	4	*	2	16	9	*	4	*	*	4
boiled 1/2 cup	16	3	*	*	*	*	4	*	7	9	7	2	7	45	24	3	5	2	*	11
boiled w/ salt 1/2 cup	16	3	*	*	*	*	—	4	7	9	7	2	7	45	24	3	5	2	*	11
KALE																				
raw 1/2 cup chopped	17	2	*	*	*	*	4	*	4	5	3	*	3	61	68	2	3	2	*	3
boiled 1/2 cup chopped	21	2	*	*	*	*	4	*	4	5	3	*	3	96	44	2	3	2	*	2
boiled w/ salt 1/2 cup chopped	21	2	*	*	*	*	*	7	4	5	3	*	3	96	44	2	3	2	*	2
canned (Bush Bros) 1/2 cup	30	3	*	*	*	*	8	14	—	10	6	—	—	70	15	—	—	—	—	—
frozen																				
boiled 1/2 cup chopped	20	3	*	*	*	*	*	*	6	9	3	*	3	83	27	2	4	2	*	2
w/ salt 1/2 cup chopped	20	3	*	*	*	*	—	7	6	9	3	*	3	83	27	2	4	2	*	2
KALE, SCOTCH																				
raw 1/2 cup chopped	14	2	*	*	*	*	*	*	4	7	6	*	7	21	74	2	*	2	*	2
boiled 1/2 cup chopped	18	2	*	*	*	*	—	*	5	9	7	*	9	26	57	2	*	3	*	2
boiled w/ salt 1/2 cup chopped	18	2	*	*	*	*	—	8	5	9	7	*	9	26	57	2	*	3	*	2
KANPYO (generic) 1/2 cup	70	4	*	*	*	6	—	*	12	8	8	11	8	*	*	*	*	4	*	4
KELP see SEAWEED																				
KETCHUP																				
(Del Monte) 1 tbsp	15	*	*	*	*	*	*	8	—	*	*	—	—	2	2	—	—	—	—	—
(generic) 1 tbsp	16	*	*	*	*	*	*	7	2	*	*	*	*	3	4	*	*	*	*	*
(Heinz) 1 tbsp	15	*	*	*	*	*	*	8	—	*	*	—	—	*	*	—	—	—	—	—
(Hunt's) 1 tbsp	15	*	*	*	*	*	*	7	*	*	*	—	—	*	2	*	—	—	—	—
(Smucker's) 1 tbsp	8	*	*	*	*	*	*	2	*	*	*	*	*	*	*	—	—	—	—	—
(Weight Watchers) 1 tbsp	8	*	*	*	*	*	*	5	—	*	*	*	*	*	*	—	—	—	—	—
low salt (generic) 1 tbsp	16	*	*	*	*	*	*	*	2	*	*	*	*	3	4	*	*	*	*	*
no salt added (Hunt's) 1 tbsp	20	*	*	*	*	2	*	*	2	*	*	—	—	*	2	*	*	*	—	*
natural (Hain) 1 tbsp	16	*	*	*	*	*	*	*	—	*	*	*	*	*	*	*	*	*	*	*
KIDNEY see specific meats																				

Food	Calories	Protein	Fat	Sat. Fat	Cholesterol	Carbohydrates	Fiber	Sodium	Potassium	Calcium	Iron	Zinc	Magnesium	Vitamin A	Vitamin C	Thiamin	Riboflavin	Niacin	Vitamin B12	Folic acid
KIDNEY BEAN																				
all types cooked 1/2 cup	112	13	*	*	*	7	24	*	10	2	14	6	10	*	2	9	3	3	*	29
cooked w/ salt 1/2 cup	112	13	*	*	*	7	—	9	10	2	14	6	10	*	2	9	3	3	*	29
red cooked 1/2 cup	112	13	*	*	*	7	28	*	10	2	14	6	10	*	2	9	3	3	*	29
cooked w/ salt 1/2 cup	112	13	*	*	*	7	—	9	10	2	14	6	10	*	2	9	3	3	*	29
red California cooked 1/2 cup	109	13	*	*	*	7	—	*	11	6	15	5	11	*	2	8	3	2	*	16
cooked w/ salt 1/2 cup	109	13	*	*	*	7	—	9	11	6	15	5	11	*	2	8	3	2	*	16
red royal cooked w/ salt 1/2 cup	108	14	*	*	*	6	—	9	9	4	14	5	9	*	2	6	3	2	*	16
KIDNEY BEAN, CANNED																				
dark red (Bush Bros) 1/2 cup	130	13	2	3		7	28	11	—	8	10	—	—	*	*	—	—	—	—	—
(Hain) 1/2 cup	60	12	*	*		5	28	11	11	2	10	—	—	*	*	4	2	2	—	—
dry, canned in brine (Green Giant/Joan of Arc) 1/2 cup	45	12	*	*		4	10	7	5	3	5	—	—	*	*	2	*	*	—	—
50% less salt (Green Giant/Joan of Arc) 1/2 cup	45	12	*	*		4	10	4	5	3	5	—	—	*	*	2	*	*	—	—
light red (Bush Bros) 1/2 cup	110	12	*	*		7	28	11	—	8	10	—	—	*	*	—	—	—	—	—
dry, canned in brine (Green Giant/Joan of Arc) 1/2 cup	45	12	*	*		4	10	7	5	3	5	—	—	*	*	2	*	*	—	—
50% less salt (Green Giant/Joan of Arc) 1/2 cup	45	12	*	*		4	10	4	5	3	5	—	—	*	*	2	*	*	—	—
red (generic) 1/2 cup	109	11	*	*	*	7	32	18	9	3	9	5	9	*	2	9	7	3	*	16
(Hunt's) 1/2 cup	100	10	*	*	*	7	20	17	10	3	10	—	—	*	1	6	4	4	—	—
(Progresso) 1/2 cup	100	15	*	*	*	7	28	9	6	4	10	—	—	*	*	8	2	*	—	—
baked (B & M) 4 oz	150	10	3	3	*	9	20	16	11	4	15	—	—	*	*	4	4	4	—	—
w/ pork (Friends) 4 oz	140	10	2	3	*	9	20	18	11	4	15	—	—	*	*	4	4	4	—	—
KIELBASA																				
(Bryan) 1 oz	90	5	12	—	7	*	*	12	—	—	—	—	—	—	—	—	—	—	—	—
(generic) 1 oz	88	6	12	14	6	*	*	13	2	*	2	4	*	*	10	4	4	4	8	*
(Oscar Mayer) 1 slice	290	21	40	50	18	*	*	40	5	2	8	14	4	*	*	—	—	—	—	—
bun size (Bryan) 2 oz	180	12	26	—	13	*	*	25	—	—	—	—	—	—	—	—	—	—	—	—
KIWIFRUIT																				
1 fruit	46	*	*	*	*	4	12	*	7	2	2	—	6	3	124	*	2	2	*	—
KNOCKWURST																				
beef (Hebrew National) 1 hot dog	260	17	38	45	18	*	*	15	—	—	6	—	—	*	*	—	—	—	—	—
pork & beef (generic) 1 oz	87	6	12	15	5	*	*	12	2	*	*	3	*	*	13	6	2	4	6	*

	Calories	Protein	Fat	Sat Fat	Cholesterol	Carbohydrates	Fiber	Sodium	Potassium	Calcium	Iron	Zinc	Magnesium	Vitamin A	Vitamin C	Thiamin	Riboflavin	Niacin	Vitamin B12	Folic acid
KOHLRABI																				
raw																				
1/2 cup slices	19	2	*	*	*	*	12	*	7	2	2	*	3	*	72	2	*	*	*	3
boiled																				
1/2 cup slices	24	2	*	*	*	2	4	*	8	2	2	2	4	*	74	2	*	2	*	2
boiled w/ salt																				
1/2 cup slices	24	2	*	*	*	2	4	9	8	2	2	2	4	*	74	2	*	2	*	2
KUMQUAT																				
1 fruit	12	*	*	*	*	*	4	*	*	*	*	*	*	*	*	12	*	*	*	—
LAMB, DOMESTIC																				
blade																				
lean & fat																				
braised																				
3 oz	293	41	32	44	33	*	*	3	6	2	11	39	5	*	*	4	11	26	40	4
broiled																				
3 oz	236	32	26	35	27	*	*	3	8	2	8	32	5	*	*	5	13	27	38	4
roasted																				
3 oz	239	32	27	37	26	*	*	2	6	2	9	32	5	*	*	5	11	25	38	5
lean only																				
broiled																				
3 oz	179	36	15	17	26	*	*	3	9	2	8	37	5	*	*	6	13	26	40	5
roasted																				
3 oz	177	35	15	19	25	*	*	2	6	2	10	37	5	*	*	5	13	23	38	5
brain																				
braised																				
3 oz	123	18	14	11	577	*	*	5	5	*	8	8	3	*	17	6	12	11	131	*
fried																				
3 oz	231	24	29	24	707	*	*	5	9	2	10	11	5	*	32	10	19	20	339	2
cubed																				
broiled																				
3 oz	158	40	10	11	26	*	*	3	8	*	11	32	7	*	*	6	15	28	43	5
ground																				
broiled																				
3 oz	240	35	26	35	27	*	*	3	8	2	8	26	5	*	*	6	13	29	37	4
kidney																				
braised																				
3 oz	116	34	5	5	160	*	*	5	5	2	59	22	5	8	17	20	104	26	1110	17
leg																				
lean & fat																				
cooked																				
3 oz	219	36	22	29	26	*	*	2	8	*	9	25	5	*	*	6	14	28	37	5
lean only																				
cooked																				
3 oz	173	40	12	14	26	*	*	2	8	*	11	28	5	*	*	7	16	26	36	5
liver																				
braised																				
3 oz	187	44	11	15	142	*	*	2	5	*	39	44	5	423	6	13	201	52	1076	16
fried																				
3 oz	202	36	17	21	140	*	*	5	8	*	48	32	5	441	18	20	229	71	1206	85
loin																				
lean & fat																				
broiled																				
3 oz	268	35	30	42	29	*	*	3	8	2	8	20	5	*	*	6	13	30	35	4
roasted																				
3 oz	262	32	31	44	27	*	*	2	6	2	10	20	5	*	*	6	12	30	31	4
lean only																				
broiled																				
3 oz	183	42	13	15	27	*	*	3	9	2	10	23	6	*	*	6	14	29	35	5
roasted																				
3 oz	171	38	13	16	25	*	*	2	7	2	11	23	6	*	*	6	14	29	31	5

	Calories	Protein	Fat	Sat. Fat	Cholesterol	Carbohydrates	Fiber	Sodium	Potassium	Calcium	Iron	Zinc	Magnesium	Vitamin A	Vitamin C	Thiamin	Riboflavin	Niacin	Vitamin B₁₂	Folic acid

LAMB, DOMESTIC (continued)

rib

lean & fat

broiled

| 3 oz | 306 | 32 | 38 | 54 | 28 | * | * | 3 | 7 | 2 | 9 | 23 | 5 | * | * | 5 | 11 | 30 | 36 | 3 |

roasted

| 3 oz | 305 | 30 | 39 | 54 | 27 | * | * | 2 | 7 | 2 | 8 | 20 | 5 | * | * | 5 | 11 | 29 | 32 | 3 |

lean only

broiled

| 3 oz | 200 | 39 | 17 | 20 | 26 | * | * | 3 | 8 | 2 | 11 | 30 | 6 | * | * | 6 | 13 | 28 | 38 | 5 |

roasted

| 3 oz | 197 | 37 | 17 | 20 | 25 | * | * | 3 | 8 | 2 | 8 | 26 | 5 | * | * | 5 | 11 | 26 | 31 | 5 |

shank

lean & fat

cooked

| 3 oz | 191 | 38 | 17 | 22 | 26 | * | * | 2 | 8 | * | 9 | 26 | 5 | * | * | 6 | 14 | 28 | 38 | 5 |

lean only

cooked

| 3 oz | 152 | 40 | 9 | 11 | 25 | * | * | 2 | 8 | * | 10 | 29 | 5 | * | * | 6 | 14 | 27 | 38 | 5 |

shoulder

lean & fat

braised

| 3 oz | 292 | 41 | 32 | 44 | 33 | * | * | 3 | 6 | 2 | 11 | 36 | 5 | * | * | 4 | 11 | 27 | 40 | 4 |

broiled

| 3 oz | 236 | 35 | 26 | 35 | 27 | * | * | 3 | 8 | 2 | 10 | 32 | 5 | * | * | 5 | 13 | 27 | 42 | 4 |

roasted

| 3 oz | 234 | 32 | 26 | 36 | 26 | * | * | 2 | 6 | 2 | 9 | 29 | 5 | * | * | 5 | 12 | 26 | 38 | 5 |

lean only

braised

| 3 oz | 240 | 47 | 21 | 26 | 33 | * | * | 3 | 6 | 2 | 13 | 43 | 6 | * | * | 4 | 11 | 26 | 41 | 5 |

broiled

| 3 oz | 178 | 38 | 14 | 17 | 26 | * | * | 3 | 8 | 2 | 11 | 38 | 6 | * | * | 6 | 14 | 26 | 44 | 5 |

roasted

| 3 oz | 173 | 35 | 14 | 17 | 25 | * | * | 2 | 7 | 2 | 10 | 34 | 5 | * | * | 5 | 13 | 25 | 38 | 5 |

sirloin

lean & fat

cooked

| 3 oz | 248 | 35 | 27 | 38 | 27 | * | * | 2 | 8 | * | 10 | 23 | 5 | * | * | 6 | 14 | 28 | 35 | 4 |

sweetbreads

pancreas

braised

| 3 oz | 198 | 32 | 20 | 29 | 113 | * | * | 2 | 7 | * | 10 | 15 | 4 | * | 29 | 2 | 11 | 11 | 78 | 3 |

spleen

braised

| 3 oz | 132 | 38 | 6 | 7 | 109 | * | * | 2 | 6 | * | 182 | 23 | 5 | * | 37 | 3 | 16 | 25 | 74 | * |

tongue

braised

| 3 oz | 233 | 31 | 26 | 33 | 53 | * | * | 2 | 4 | * | 12 | 17 | 4 | * | 10 | 5 | 21 | 16 | 89 | * |

LAMB, NEW ZEALAND

brain

braised

| 3 oz | 123 | 18 | 14 | 11 | 577 | * | * | 5 | 5 | * | 8 | 8 | 3 | * | 17 | 6 | 12 | 11 | 131 | * |

fried

| 3 oz | 231 | 24 | 29 | 24 | 707 | * | * | 5 | 9 | 2 | 10 | 11 | 5 | * | 32 | 10 | 19 | 20 | 339 | 2 |

kidney

braised

| 3 oz | 116 | 34 | 5 | 5 | 160 | * | * | 5 | 5 | 2 | 59 | 22 | 5 | 8 | 17 | 20 | 104 | 26 | 1110 | 17 |

leg

lean & fat

| 3 oz | 209 | 35 | 20 | 32 | 29 | * | * | 2 | 4 | * | 10 | 20 | 5 | * | * | 7 | 23 | 32 | 37 | * |

lean only

| 3 oz | 154 | 39 | 9 | 13 | 29 | * | * | 2 | 5 | * | 11 | 23 | 5 | * | * | 7 | 25 | 32 | 37 | * |

	Calories	Protein	Fat	Sat. Fat	Cholesterol	Carbohydrates	Fiber	Sodium	Potassium	Calcium	Iron	Zinc	Magnesium	Vitamin A	Vitamin C	Thiamin	Riboflavin	Niacin	Vitamin B₁₂	Folic acid
LAMB, NEW ZEALAND (continued)																				
liver																				
braised 3 oz	187	44	11	15	142	*	*	2	5	*	39	44	5	423	6	13	201	52	1076	16
fried 3 oz	202	36	17	21	140	*	*	5	8	*	48	32	5	441	18	20	229	71	1206	85
loin																				
lean & fat 3 oz	267	33	32	51	32	*	*	2	4	2	10	15	4	*	*	7	18	34	35	*
lean only 3 oz	169	41	11	15	32	*	*	2	5	2	11	19	5	*	*	8	22	34	36	*
rib																				
lean & fat 3 oz	288	27	38	62	29	*	*	2	3	2	8	15	3	*	*	5	14	29	33	*
lean only roasted 3 oz	166	35	14	19	26	*	*	2	4	2	9	20	4	*	*	6	17	26	32	*
shoulder																				
lean & fat roasted 3 oz	302	40	35	54	35	*	*	2	4	2	10	26	4	*	*	5	16	27	48	*
lean only braised 3 oz	242	48	20	29	36	*	*	2	4	2	11	32	5	*	*	5	18	25	53	*
sweetbreads																				
pancreas braised 3 oz	198	32	20	29	113	*	*	2	7	*	10	15	4	*	29	2	11	11	78	3
spleen braised 3 oz	132	38	6	7	109	*	*	2	6	*	182	23	5	*	37	3	16	25	74	*
tongue																				
braised 3 oz	233	31	26	33	53	x	x	2	4	*	12	17	4	*	10	5	21	16	89	*
LAMBSQUARTER																				
raw 3 oz	37	6	*	*	*	2	12	2	11	26	6	2	7	197	113	9	22	5	*	6
boiled 1/2 cup chopped	29	5	*	*	*	*	8	*	7	23	3	2	5	175	55	6	14	4	*	3
boiled w/ salt 1/2 cup chopped	29	5	*	*	*	*	—	10	7	23	3	2	5	175	55	6	14	4	*	3
LARD see PORK																				
LASAGNA see PASTA ENTREE																				
LEBANON BOLOGNA see BOLOGNA																				
LEEK																				
raw																				
1/2 cup chopped	32	*	*	*	*	2	4	*	3	3	6	*	4	*	10	2	*	*	*	8
1 medium	76	3	*	*	*	6	8	*	6	7	14	*	9	2	25	5	2	2	*	20
boiled																				
1/2 cup chopped	16	*	*	*	*	*	—	*	*	2	3	*	2	*	4	*	*	*	*	3
1 medium	38	2	*	*	*	3	—	*	3	4	8	*	4	*	9	2	*	*	*	8
boiled w/ salt																				
1/2 cup chopped	16	*	*	*	*	*	—	5	*	2	3	*	2	*	4	*	*	*	*	3
freeze-dried 1 tbsp	1	*	*	*	*	*	*	*	*	*	*	*	*	*	*	*	*	*	*	*
LEMON																				
w/out peel 1 fruit	17	*	*	*	*	2	8	*	2	2	2	*	*	*	51	2	*	*	*	2
w/peel 1 fruit	22	2	*	*	*	4	—	*	4	7	4	*	3	*	139	4	3	*	*	—
LEMON PEEL 1 tsp	0	*	*	*	*	*	*	*	*	*	*	*	*	*	4	*	*	*	*	*
LEMON DRINK																				
lemon ginger, organic (Santa Cruz Natural) 8 fl oz	110	*	*	*	*	9	*	*	3	4	4	*	*	*	4	—	—	*	*	*

	Calories	Protein	Fat	Sat. Fat	Cholesterol	Carbohydrates	Fiber	Sodium	Potassium	Calcium	Iron	Zinc	Magnesium	Vitamin A	Vitamin C	Thiamin	Riboflavin	Niacin	Vitamin B$_{12}$	Folic acid
LEMON DRINK (continued)																				
old fashioned																				
(Heinke's) 8 fl oz	120	*	*	*	*	10	*	*	2	*	*	*	*	*	8	—	—	*	*	*
LEMON JUICE																				
fresh																				
1 tbsp	4	*	*	*	*	*	*	*	*	*	*	*	*	*	12	*	*	*	*	*
bottled																				
1 tbsp	3	*	*	*	*	*	*	*	*	*	*	*	*	*	6	*	*	*	*	*
LEMONADE																				
bottled																				
w/ cranberry juice																				
(Ocean Spray) 8 fl oz	110	*	*	*	*	9	*	*	—	*	*	*	*	*	100	—	—	*	*	*
w/ raspberry juice																				
(Ocean Spray) 8 fl oz	110	*	*	*	*	9	*	*	—	*	*	*	*	*	100	—	—	*	*	*
raspberry																				
(Knudsen) 8 fl oz	120	*	*	*	*	10	*	*	2	*	*	*	*	*	8	—	—	*	*	*
strawberry																				
(Knudsen) 8 fl oz	120	*	*	*	*	10	*	*	2	*	*	*	*	*	8	—	—	*	*	*
cherry																				
(Knudsen) 8 fl oz	120	*	*	*	*	10	*	*	2	*	*	*	*	*	8	—	—	*	*	*
organic																				
(Santa Cruz Natural) 8 fl oz	120	*	*	*	*	10	*	*	2	*	*	*	*	*	8	—	—	*	*	*
cranberry																				
(Heinke's) 8 fl oz	120	*	*	*	*	10	*	*	2	*	*	*	*	*	8	—	—	*	*	*
(Knudsen) 8 fl oz	120	*	*	*	*	10	*	*	2	*	*	*	*	*	8	—	—	*	*	*
from concentrate																				
natural																				
(Knudsen) 8 fl oz	120	*	*	*	*	10	*	*	2	*	*	*	*	*	8	—	—	*	*	*
organic																				
(Knudsen) 8 fl oz	120	*	*	*	*	10	*	*	2	*	*	*	*	*	8	—	—	*	*	*
pink																				
(generic) 8 fl oz	99	*	*	*	*	9	*	*	*	*	2	*	*	*	16	*	3	*	*	*
white																				
(generic) 6 fl oz	75	*	*	*	*	7	*	*	*	*	2	*	*	*	12	*	2	*	*	*
(Mott's) 10 fl oz	160	*	*	*	*	14	*	*	*	2	2	*	*	*	12	*	*	*	*	*
from mix																				
pink																				
(Country Time) 8 fl oz	70	*	*	*	*	6	*	*	—	*	*	*	*	*	10	*	*	*	*	*
(generic)																				
1 cup water + 2 tsp powder	103	*	*	*	*	9	*	*	*	7	*	*	*	*	14	*	*	*	*	*
sugar-free																				
(Country Time) 8 fl oz	4	*	*	*	*	*	*	*	—	*	*	*	*	*	10	*	*	*	*	*
sugar-free																				
(Crystal Light) 8 fl oz	4	*	*	*	*	*	*	*	—	*	*	*	*	*	10	*	*	*	*	*
punch																				
(Country Time) 8 fl oz	70	*	*	*	*	6	*	*	—	*	*	*	*	*	10	*	*	*	*	*
yellow																				
(Country Time) 8 fl oz	70	*	*	*	*	6	*	*	—	*	*	*	*	*	10	*	*	*	*	*
(Kool-Aid) 8 fl oz	70	*	*	*	*	6	*	*	*	*	*	*	*	*	10	*	*	*	*	*
sugar-free																				
(Country Time) 8 fl oz	4	*	*	*	*	*	*	*	—	*	*	*	*	*	10	*	*	*	*	*
(Crystal Light) 8 fl oz	4	*	*	*	*	*	*	*	—	*	*	*	*	*	10	*	*	*	*	*
(Kool-Aid) 8 fl oz	4	*	*	*	*	*	*	*	*	*	*	*	*	*	10	*	*	*	*	*
unsweetened, sugar-added																				
(Kool-Aid) 8 fl oz prep w/ sugar	100	*	*	*	*	8	*	*	*	*	*	*	*	*	10	*	*	*	*	*
natural																				
(Knudsen) 8 fl oz	120	*	*	*	*	10	*	*	2	*	*	*	*	*	8	—	—	*	*	*

	Calories	Protein	Fat	Sat. Fat	Cholesterol	Carbohydrates	Fiber	Sodium	Potassium	Calcium	Iron	Zinc	Magnesium	Vitamin A	Vitamin C	Thiamin	Riboflavin	Niacin	Vitamin B12	Folic acid
LEMONADE (continued)																				
organic (Santa Cruz Natural) 8 fl oz	120	*	*	*	*	10		*	2	*	*	*	*	*	8	—	—	*	*	*
unsweetened pink (Kool-Aid) 8 fl oz prep w/ out sugar	2	*	*	*	*	*	*	*	*	*	*	*	*	*	10	*	*	*	*	*
white (Ocean Spray) 8 fl oz	110	*	*	*	*	10	*	*	—	*	*	*	*	*	100	—	—	*	*	*
(Tropicana) 6 fl oz	100	*	*	*	*	7	*	*	—	2	2	*	*	*	4	2	4	*	*	*
LEMON BUTTER SAUCE (Weight Watchers) 1 tbsp	7	2	*	*	—	*	—	4	—	*	*	—	*	*	*	—	—	—	—	—
LEMON DILL SAUCE *from mix* (Knorr) 1/4 oz	120	2	14	—	2	2	—	14	—	4	*	*	*	6	*	2	4	*	*	*
LEMON-LIME DRINK *from mix* sugar-free (Crystal Light) 8 fl oz	4	*	*	*	*	*	*	*	—	*	*	*	*	*	10	*	*	*	*	*
unsweetened (Kool-Aid) 8 fl oz prep w/ out sugar	2	*	*	*	*	*	*	*	*	*	*	*	*	*	10	*	*	*	*	*
(Kool-Aid) 8 fl oz prep w/ sugar	100	*	*	*	*	8	*	*	*	*	*	*	*	*	10	*	*	*	*	*
LENTIL *cooked* 1/2 cup	115	15	*	*	*	7	32	*	10	2	18	8	9	*	2	11	4	5	*	45
cooked w/ salt 1/2 cup	115	15	*	*	*	7	32	10	10	2	18	8	9	*	2	11	4	5	*	45
LENTIL SPROUT *raw* 1/2 cup	40	6	*	*	*	3	—	*	3	*	7	4	4	*	10	6	3	2	*	10
stir-fried 3 oz	86	12	*	*	*	6	—	*	7	*	15	9	7	*	18	12	4	5	*	14
stir-fried, salted 3 oz	86	12	*	*	*	6	—	9	7	*	15	9	7	*	18	12	—	—	—	—
LETTUCE *butterhead* raw 2 leaves	2	*	*	*	*	*	*	*	*	*	*	*	*	3	2	*	*	*	*	3
cos raw 1/2 cup shredded	4	*	*	*	*	*	*	4	*	2	*	2	*	15	11	2	2	*	*	10
iceberg raw 1 leaf	3	*	*	*	*	*	*	*	*	*	*	*	*	*	*	*	*	*	*	3
looseleaf raw 1/2 cup shredded	5	*	*	*	*	*	*	4	*	2	2	*	*	11	8	*	*	*	*	3
romaine raw 1/2 cup shredded	4	*	*	*	*	*	*	4	*	2	*	2	*	15	11	2	2	*	*	10
LICORICE see CANDY																				
LIMA BEAN *baby* raw 1/2 cup	338	35	*	*	*	21	—	*	40	8	35	17	47	*	*	39	13	9	*	101
cooked 1/2 cup	115	12	*	*	*	7	28	*	10	3	12	6	12	*	*	10	3	3	*	34
cooked w/ salt 1/2 cup	115	12	*	*	*	7	—	9	10	3	12	6	12	*	*	10	3	3	*	34

	Calories	Protein	Fat	Sat. Fat	Cholesterol	Carbohydrates	Fiber	Sodium	Potassium	Calcium	Iron	Zinc	Magnesium	Vitamin A	Vitamin C	Thiamin	Riboflavin	Niacin	Vitamin B₁₂	Folic acid
LIMA BEAN (continued)																				
large																				
raw																				
1/2 cup	301	32	*	*	*	19	68	*	44	7	37	17	50	*	*	30	11	7	*	88
cooked																				
1/2 cup	108	12	*	*	*	7	28	*	14	2	12	6	10	*	*	10	3	2	*	20
cooked w/ salt																				
1/2 cup	108	12	*	*	*	7	—	9	14	2	12	6	10	*	*	10	3	2	*	20
LIMA BEAN, CANNED																				
raw																				
(generic) 1/2 cup	88	9	*	*	*	5	16	*	10	3	14	4	11	5	30	11	5	6	*	7
green																				
(Del Monte) 1/2 cup	80	7	*	*	*	5	16	15	—	2	8	—	—	2	15	—	—	—	*	—
medium																				
(Bush Bros) 1/2 cup	110	10	2	*	*	6	20	13	—	2	8	—	—	*	2	—	—	—	*	—
small																				
(Bush Bros) 1/2 cup	100	8	2	*	*	5	20	13	—	2	10	—	—	2	10	—	—	—	*	—
green & white																				
(Bush Bros) 1/2 cup	110	10	*	*	*	7	20	15	—	4	10	—	—	*	*	—	—	—	*	—
large																				
(generic) 1/2 cup	95	10	*	*	*	6	24	17	8	3	12	5	12	*	*	4	2	2	*	15
low salt																				
(generic) 1/2 cup	93	9	*	*	*	6	16	*	10	3	11	5	11	4	18	2	3	3	*	5
solid & liquid																				
(generic) 1/2 cup	93	9	*	*	*	6	16	13	10	3	11	5	11	4	18	2	3	3	*	5
LIMA BEAN, FROZEN																				
baby																				
(Green Giant Harvest Fresh)																				
1/2 cup	80	10	*	*	*	6	16	7	10	2	8	—	—	*	4	6	*	*	*	—
in butter sauce																				
(Green Giant) 1/2 cup	100	10	5	5	2	6	18	16	11	*	10	—	—	2	6	4	*	*	*	—
LIME																				
1 fruit	20	*	*	*	*	2	8	*	2	2	2	*	*	*	32	*	*	*	*	*
LIME DRINK																				
Lime Cactus Cooler																				
(Knudsen Exotic Blends) 8 fl oz	120	*	*	*	*	10	*	*	2	*	*	*	*	*	8	*	*	*	*	*
Lime Cruz, organic																				
(Santa Cruz Natural) 8 fl oz	110	*	*	*	*	9	*	*	3	4	4	*	*	*	4	*	*	*	*	*
Tropical Lime Cooler																				
(Knudsen Tropical Blend) 8 fl oz	110	*	*	*	*	9	*	*	3	4	4	*	*	*	4	*	*	*	*	*
LIME JUICE																				
fresh																				
1 tbsp	4	*	*	*	*	*	*	*	*	*	*	*	*	*	8	*	*	*	*	*
bottled																				
1 tbsp	3	*	*	*	*	*	*	*	*	*	*	*	*	*	2	*	*	*	*	*
LIMEADE																				
from concentrate																				
(generic) 1 cup	101	*	*	*	*	9	*	*	*	*	*	*	*	*	11	*	*	*	*	*
LING																				
raw																				
1 fillet	168	61	2	*	26	*	*	11	21	7	7	10	30	4	*	14	22	22	18	*
broiled/baked																				
1 fillet	168	61	2	—	26	*	*	11	21	7	7	10	31	3	*	13	21	21	16	*
LINGUINE see PASTA																				
LIVER see specific meats																				
LIVER CHEESE																				
pork																				
(generic) 1 1 oz slice	86	7	11	13	16	*	*	14	2	*	17	7	*	99	*	4	37	17	116	7
pork fat wrapped																				
(Oscar Mayer) 1 slice	116	10	15	18	27	*	*	17	2	*	24	10	*	172	2	5	49	23	153	11

	Calories	Protein	Fat	Sat. Fat	Cholesterol	Carbohydrates	Fiber	Sodium	Potassium	Calcium	Iron	Zinc	Magnesium	Vitamin A	Vitamin C	Thiamin	Riboflavin	Niacin	Vitamin B12	Folic acid
LIVER LOAF																				
(Bryan) 1 1/2 oz	150	10	20	—	23	*	*	22	—	—	—	—	—	—	—	—	—	—	—	—
LIVER PATE																				
(generic) 1 oz	90	7	12	14	24	*	*	8	*	2	9	5	*	19	*	*	10	5	15	4
LIVERWURST																				
sausage (generic) 1 1 oz slice	92	7	12	15	15	*	*	10	*	*	10	4	*	157	*	5	17	6	63	2
spread (Underwood) 2 1/8 oz	190	13	25	—	—	*	*	19	5	*	35	—	—	180	*	20	50	30	—	—
LOBSTER, NORTHERN																				
raw 1 lobster	135	47	2	*	47	*	*	18	12	7	2	30	10	2	*	*	4	11	23	*
steamed/poached 1/2 cup	71	12	*	*	9	*	*	6	4	2	*	7	3	*	*	*		2	37	*
LOBSTER, SPINY																				
raw 1 lobster	234	72	5	3	49	2	*	15	11	10	14	79	21	*	7	*	8	44	121	*
steamed/poached 1 lobster	233	72	5	3	49	2	*	15	10	10	13	79	21	*	6	*	5	40	109	*
LOGANBERRY																				
frozen 1/2 cup	81	4	*	*	*	6	28	*	6	4	5	3	8	*	37	5	3	6	*	10
LOLLIPOP see CANDY																				
LONGAN																				
fresh 3 1/2 oz	60	2	*	*	*	5	4	*	8	*	*	*	3	*	140	2	8	*	—	—
dried 3 1/2 oz	286	8	*	*	*	25	—	2	19	5	30	*	12	*	47	3	29	5	—	—
LOQUAT																				
1 fruit	5	*	*	*	*	*	*	*	*	*	*	*	—	*	3	*	*	*	—	—
LOTUS ROOT																				
raw 10 slices	45	4	*	*	*	5	16	*	13	4	5	2	5	*	59	9	10	2	*	3
boiled 10 slices	59	2	*	*	*	5	12	2	9	2	4	2	5	*	41	8	*	*	*	2
boiled w/ salt 10 slices	59	2	*	*	*	5	12	10	9	2	4	2	5	*	41	8	*	*	*	2
LOTUS SEED																				
raw 1 oz	25	2	*	*	*	2	—	*	3	*	*	*	4	*	*	3	*	*	*	2
dried 1 oz	94	7	*	*	*	6	—	*	11	5	6	2	15	*	*	12	3	2	*	7
LUNCHEON LOAF																				
plain (Bryan) 3/4 oz	60	5	8	—	5	*	*	14	—	—	—	—	—	—	—	—	—	—	—	—
spiced (Oscar Mayer) 1 slice	66	6	7	8	6	*	*	14	2	3	2	4	2	*	*	—	—	—	—	—
LUNCHEON MEAT (see also **specific meats**)																				
beef (generic) 1 1 oz slice	50	13	2	3	4	*	*	17	3	*	4	8	*	*	7	2	3	7	12	*
jellied (generic) 1 1 oz slice	63	18	3	4	6	*	*	31	6	*	11	13	3	*	16	5	10	14	48	*
pork (generic) 1 1 oz slice	95	6	13	16	6	*	*	15	2	*	3	*	*	*	*	7	3	4	4	*
pork & beef (generic) 1 1 oz slice	100	6	14	17	5	*	*	15	2	*	3	*	*	*	6	6	3	4	6	*
LUNCHEON SAUSAGE																				
(generic) 1 1 oz slice	74	7	9	11	6	*	*	14	2	*	2	5	*	*	9	4	3	5	9	*
LUPIN																				
cooked 1/2 cup	99	22	4	*	*	3	8	*	6	4	6	8	11	*	2	7	3	2	*	12

	Calories	Protein	Fat	Sat Fat	Cholesterol	Carbohydrates	Fiber	Sodium	Potassium	Calcium	Iron	Zinc	Magnesium	Vitamin A	Vitamin C	Thiamin	Riboflavin	Niacin	Vitamin B₂	Folic acid
LUPIN (continued)																				
cooked w/ salt																				
1/2 cup	99	22	4	*	*	3	8	8	6	4	6	8	11	*	2	7	3	2	*	12
LUXURY LOAF																				
pork																				
1 1 oz slice	40	9	2	2	3	*	*	14	3	*	2	6	*	*	10	13	5	5	6	*
LYCHEE																				
fresh																				
1 fruit	6	*	*	*	*	*	*	*	*	*	*	*	*	*	11	*	*	*	*	—
dried																				
1/2 cup	249	6	2	*	*	21	16	*	28	3	8	2	9	*	274	*	30	14	*	—
LYONNAISE SAUCE																				
from mix																				
(Knorr) 1/4 oz	25	*	2	—	*	2	—	15	—	*	*	*	*	*	*	*	*	*	*	*
MACADAMIA NUT																				
dried																				
(generic) 1 oz	199	4	32	16	*	*	12	*	3	2	4	3	8	*	*	*	7	2	3	*
oil roasted																				
(generic) 1 oz	204	3	33	17	*	*	12	*	3	*	3	2	8	*	*	*	4	2	3	*
w/ salt																				
(generic) 1 oz	204	3	33	17	*	*	12	3	3	*	3	2	8	*	*	*	4	2	3	*
salted																				
(Blue Diamond) 1 oz	190	10	28	10	*	*	12	6	3	2	2	2	8	*	*	*	*	*	2	*
MACARONI see PASTA																				
MACE, GROUND																				
1 tbsp	25	*	3	3	*	*	4	*	*	*	4	*	2	*	*	*	*	*	*	*
MACKEREL, ATLANTIC																				
raw																				
1 fillet	164	35	24	18	26	*	*	4	10	*	10	5	21	4	*	13	21	51	162	*
baked/broiled																				
1 fillet	230	35	24	19	22	*	*	3	10	*	8	6	21	3	*	9	21	30	278	*
MACKEREL, JACK																				
raw																				
1 fillet	208	75	27	26	35	*	*	8	26	5	14	10	16	2	7	17	56	94	164	*
canned																				
1/2 can	231	35	9	9	24	*	*	14	5	22	10	6	8	8	*	2	11	28	207	*
MACKEREL, KING																				
raw																				
1/2 fillet	281	67	6	4	35	*	*	13	25	6	20	7	16	29	5	13	55	85	513	*
broiled/baked																				
1/2 fillet	206	67	6	4	35	*	*	13	24	6	19	7	16	26	4	12	53	81	460	*
MACKEREL, PACIFIC																				
raw																				
1 fillet	356	75	27	26	35	*	*	8	26	5	14	10	16	2	7	17	56	94	164	*
MACKEREL, PACIFIC & JACK																				
broiled/baked																				
1 fillet	354	75	27	26	35	*	*	8	26	5	15	10	16	2	6	16	56	94	124	*
MACKEREL, SPANISH																				
raw																				
1 fillet	260	60	18	17	47	*	*	5	24	2	5	6	15	4	5	16	19	22	75	*
baked/broiled																				
1 fillet	231	57	14	13	35	*	*	4	23	2	6	6	14	3	4	13	18	37	170	*
MALT SYRUP																				
(generic) 1 tbsp	76	2	*	*	*	6	*	*	2	*	*	*	*	4	*	*	*	6	10	*
MALTED MILK																				
chocolate																				
(generic) 1 cup milk																				
w/ 3/4 oz powder	228	15	14	28	11	10	*	7	14	30	3	7	12	7	4	9	*	3	15	4
(Kraft) 3 tsp + 1 cup milk	211	16	9	—	—	10	*	7	—	31	2	—	*	*	4	8	2	2	—	—
fortified																				
(Ovaltine) 3/4 oz + 1 cup milk	216	19	8	15	6	10	*	9	—	43	15	—	9	49	50	52	45	45	16	22

	Calories	Protein	Fat	Sat. Fat	Cholesterol	Carbohydrates	Fiber	Sodium	Potassium	Calcium	Iron	Zinc	Magnesium	Vitamin A	Vitamin C	Thiamin	Riboflavin	Niacin	Vitamin B12	Folic acid
MALTED MILK (continued)																				
natural (generic) 1 cup milk w/ 3/4 oz powder	236	17	15	30	12	9	*	9	15	36	*	8	13	7	5	13	*	7	17	5
natural (Kraft) 3 tsp + 1 cup milk	211	20	10	—	—	9	*	9	—	36	*	—	—	*	6	14	10	4	—	—
fortified (generic) 1 cup milk + 4–5 heaping tsp	231	16	13	*	11	9	*	8	16	37	20	7	12	51	49	47	67	52	17	5
unfortified (generic) 1 cup milk + 3 heaping tsp	236	17	15	*	12	9	*	9	15	36	*	8	13	7	5	13	35	7	17	5
MAMMY-APPLE 1 fruit	431	7	6	—	*	35	100	5	11	9	33	—	—	39	197	11	20	17	*	—
MANDARIN GINGER SAUCE *microwave* (Knorr) 1 1/2 oz	190	60	9	—	*	2	—	24	—	*	6	*	*	2	4	4	6	60	*	*
MANDARIN ORANGE-PAPAYA JUICE (Tropicana Twister) 6 fl oz	90	*	*	*	*	7	—	2	—	2	2	*	*	*	20	*	*	*	*	*
MANGO 1 fruit	135	2	*	*	*	12	16	*	9	2	*	*	5	161	96	8	7	6	—	—
1/2 cup slices	54	*	*	*	*	5	4	*	4	*	*	*	2	65	38	3	3	2	—	—
MANGO DRINK (Sunny Delight) 8 fl oz	110	*	*	*	*	9	*	5	—	*	*	*	*	20	100	20	*	*	*	*
from mix (Tang) 6 fl oz	80	*	*	*	*	7	*	*	*	*	*	—	—	10	100	*	10	10	*	20
MANGO-GUAVA DRINK (Mauna La'i) 8 fl oz	130	*	*	*	*	11	*	*	—	*	*	*	*	*	100	—	—	—	—	—
MANGO-PEACH JUICE (Knudsen Tropical Blend) 8 fl oz	120	*	*	*	*	10	*	2	4	2	4	*	*	50	4	*	*	*	*	*
MANHATTAN 1 cocktail (2 fl oz)	128	*	*	*	*	*	—	*	*	*	*	*	*	*	*	*	*	*	*	*
MAPLE SUGAR see SUGAR																				
MAPLE SYRUP 1 tbsp	52	*	*	*	*	4	*	*	*	*	*	6	*	*	*	*	*	*	*	*
MARGARINE (Mazola) 1 tbsp	100	*	17	10	*	*	*	4	*	*	*	*	*	10	*	*	*	*	*	*
extra light (Mazola) 1 tbsp	50	*	9	5	*	*	*	5	*	*	*	*	*	10	*	*	*	*	*	*
spread (Weight Watchers) 1 tbsp	45	*	6	5	*	*	*	*	*	*	*	*	*	10	*	*	—	—	*	*
unsalted (Weight Watchers) 1 tbsp	45	*	6	5	*	*	*	5	*	*	*	*	*	10	*	*	—	—	*	*
imitation 17% vegetable oil spread (Smartbeat) 1 tbsp	20	*	5	*	*	*	*	5	*	*	*	*	*	10	*	*	*	*	*	*
unsalted (Smartbeat) 1 tbsp	20	*	5	*	*	*	*	*	*	*	*	*	*	10	*	*	*	*	*	*
nucanola spread soft (Smartbeat) 1 tbsp	70	*	11	3	*	*	*	4	*	*	*	*	*	10	*	*	*	*	*	*
nucanola spread stick (Smartbeat) 1 tbsp	80	*	14	5	*	*	*	4	*	*	*	*	*	10	*	*	*	*	*	*
reduced calorie (Mazola) 1 tbsp	50	*	9	5	*	*	*	4	*	*	*	*	*	10	*	*	*	*	*	*
safflower (Hollywood) 1 tbsp	100	*	17	10	*	*	*	5	*	*	*	*	*	10	*	*	*	*	*	*
(Hollywood) 1 tbsp	100	*	17	10	*	*	*	5	*	*	*	*	*	*	10	*	*	*	*	*
regular (Hain) 1 tbsp	100	*	17	10	*	*	*	7	*	*	*	*	*	10	*	*	*	*	*	*

	Calories	Protein	Fat	Sat. Fat	Cholesterol	Carbohydrates	Fiber	Sodium	Potassium	Calcium	Iron	Zinc	Magnesium	Vitamin A	Vitamin C	Thiamin	Riboflavin	Niacin	Vitamin B12	Folic acid
MARGARINE (continued)																				
soft																				
(Hain) 1 tbsp	100	*	17	10	*	*	*	7	*	*	*	*	*	10	*	*	*	*	*	*
unsalted																				
(Hain) 1 tbsp	100	*	17	10	*	*	*	*	*	*	*	*	*	10	*	*	*	*	*	*
(Hollywood) 1 tbsp	100	*	17	10	*	*	*	*	*	*	*	*	*	10	*	*	*	*	*	*
(Hollywood) 1 tbsp	100	*	17	10	*	*	*	*	*	*	*	*	*	*	10	*	*	*	*	*
soft																				
(Chiffon) 1 tbsp	90	*	15	5	*	*	*	4	*	*	*	*	*	6	*	*	*	*	*	*
(Parkay) 1 tbsp	100	*	17	10	*	*	*	4	*	*	*	*	*	10	*	*	*	*	*	*
reduced calorie																				
(Parkay) 1 tbsp	50	*	9	5	*	*	*	5	*	*	*	*	*	10	*	*	*	*	*	*
stick																				
(Chiffon) 1 tbsp	100	*	17	10	*	*	*	4	*	*	*	*	*	8	*	*	*	*	*	*
unsalted																				
(Chiffon) 1 tbsp	90	*	15	10	*	*	*	*	*	*	*	*	*	6	*	*	*	*	*	*
whipped																				
(Chiffon) 1 tbsp	70	*	12	5	*	*	*	3	*	*	*	*	*	4	*	*	*	*	*	*
soft spread																				
(Hollywood) 1 tbsp	90	*	15	5	*	*	*	6	*	*	*	*	*	*	10	*	*	*	*	*
spread																				
50 % fat																				
(Parkay) 1 tbsp	60	*	11	5	*	*	*	5	*	*	*	*	*	10	*	*	*	*	*	*
squeeze																				
(Parkay) 1 tbsp	90	*	15	10	*	*	*	5	*	*	*	*	*	10	*	*	*	*	*	*
Touch of Butter																				
40 % fat																				
(Kraft) 1 tbsp	50	*	9	5	*	*	*	5	*	*	*	*	*	10	*	*	*	*	*	*
70 % fat																				
(Kraft) 1 tbsp	90	*	15	10	*	*	*	5	*	*	*	*	*	10	*	*	*	*	*	*
whipped																				
cup																				
(Miracle) 1 tbsp	60	*	11	5	*	*	*	3	*	*	*	*	*	6	*	*	*	*	*	*
cup																				
(Parkay) 1 tbsp	70	*	11	5	*	*	*	3	*	*	*	*	*	6	*	*	*	*	*	*
stick																				
(Miracle) 1 tbsp	70	*	11	5	*	*	*	3	*	*	*	*	*	6	*	*	*	*	*	*
stick																				
(Parkay) 1 tbsp	70	*	11	5	*	*	*	3	*	*	*	*	*	6	*	*	*	*	*	*
stick																				
(Land O'Lakes) 1 tbsp	100	*	17	10	*	*	*	4	*	*	*	*	*	10	*	*	*	*	*	*
(Parkay) 1 tbsp	100	*	17	10	*	*	*	4	*	*	*	*	*	10	*	*	*	*	*	*
light																				
(Weight Watchers) 1 tbsp	60	*	11	5	*	*	*	19	*	*	*	*	*	10	*	*	*	*	*	*
tub																				
(Land O'Lakes) 1 tbsp	100	*	17	10	*	*	*	4	*	*	*	*	*	10	*	*	*	*	*	*
unsalted																				
(Mazola) 1 tbsp	100	*	17	10	*	*	*	*	*	*	*	*	*	10	*	*	*	*	*	*
MARINARA SAUCE see PASTA SAUCE																				
MARJORAM, DRIED																				
1 tbsp	5	*	*	5	*	*	*	*	*	3	8	*	*	3	*	*	*	*	*	*
MARMALADE see JAM, JELLY & PRESERVES																				
MARSHMALLOW																				
(Funmallows) 1 piece	30	*	*	*	*	2	*	*	*	*	*	*	*	*	*	*	*	*	*	*
(generic) 1 piece	23	*	*	*	*	2	*	*	*	*	*	*	*	*	*	*	*	*	*	*
(Kraft) 1 piece	25	*	*	*	*	2	*	*	*	*	*	*	*	*	*	*	*	*	*	*
creme																				
(Kraft) 1 oz	90	*	*	*	*	8	*	*	*	*	*	*	*	*	*	*	*	*	*	*

	Calories	Protein	Fat	Sat. Fat	Cholesterol	Carbohydrates	Fiber	Sodium	Potassium	Calcium	Iron	Zinc	Magnesium	Vitamin A	Vitamin C	Thiamin	Riboflavin	Niacin	Vitamin B₁₂	Folic acid
MARSHMALLOW (continued)																				
miniature																				
(Funmallows) 10 pieces	18	*	*	*	*	2	*	*	*	*	*	*	*	*	*	*	*	*	*	*
(Kraft) 10 pieces	18	*	*	*	*	2	*	*	*	*	*	*	*	*	*	*	*	*	*	*
MARSHMALLOW CREAM TOPPING																				
(generic) 1 oz	88	*	*	*	*	7	—	*	*	*	*	*	*	*	*	*	*	*	*	*
MARSHMALLOW TOPPING																				
(Smucker's) 2 tbsp	120	*	*	*	*	10	*	*	—	*	*	*	*	*	*	*	*	*	*	*
MARTINI																				
1 cocktail (2 1/2 oz)	156	*	*	*	*	*	—	*	*	*	*	*	*	*	*	*	*	*	*	*
MAYONNAISE																				
(Best) 1 tbsp	100	*	17	10	2	*	*	3	*	*	*	*	*	35	*	*	*	*	*	*
(Hain) 1 tbsp	110	*	18	10	2	*	*	3	*	*	*	*	*	35	*	*	*	*	*	*
(Kraft) 1 tbsp	100	*	18	10	2	*	*	3	*	*	*	*	*	*	*	*	*	*	*	*
canola																				
(Hain) 1 tbsp	100	*	17	5	2	*	*	4	*	*	*	*	*	35	*	*	*	*	*	*
(Hollywood) 1 tbsp	100	*	17	5	2	*	*	4	*	*	*	*	*	*	*	*	*	*	*	*
reduced calorie																				
(Hain) 1 tbsp	60	*	8	*	*	*	*	7	*	*	*	*	*	35	*	2	*	*	*	*
eggless, no salt added																				
(Hain) 1 tbsp	110	*	18	10	*	*	*	*	*	*	*	*	*	35	*	*	*	*	*	*
fat free																				
(Smartbeat) 1 tbsp	10	*	*	*	*	*	*	5	*	*	*	*	*	*	*	*	*	*	*	*
light																				
(Kraft Light) 1 tbsp	50	*	8	5	*	*	*	5	*	*	*	*	*	*	*	*	*	*	*	*
(Weight Watchers) 1 tbsp	25	*	3	*	2	*	*	5	*	*	*	*	*	*	*	—	*	*	*	*
low sodium																				
(Hain) 1 tbsp	60	*	9	5	3	*	*	4	*	*	*	*	*	35	*	*	*	*	*	*
(Weight Watchers) 1 tbsp	25	*	3	*	2	*	*	2	*	*	*	*	*	*	*	—	*	*	*	*
w/ canola oil																				
(Smartbeat) 1 tbsp	40	*	6	3	*	*	*	5	*	*	*	*	*	*	*	*	*	*	*	*
w/ corn oil																				
(Smartbeat) 1 tbsp	40	*	6	3	*	*	*	5	*	*	*	*	*	*	*	*	*	*	*	*
w/ soybean oil																				
(Smartbeat) 1 tbsp	40	*	6	3	*	*	*	5	*	*	*	*	*	*	*	*	*	*	*	*
reduced calorie																				
(Best) 1 tbsp	50	*	8	5	2	*	*	5	*	*	*	*	*	*	*	*	*	*	*	*
safflower																				
(Hain) 1 tbsp	110	*	18	5	2	*	*	3	*	*	*	*	*	35	*	*	*	*	*	*
(Hollywood) 1 tbsp	110	*	18	5	2	*	*	3	*	*	*	*	*	*	*	*	*	*	*	*
safflower & soybean																				
(generic) 1 tbsp	99	*	17	6	3	*	*	3	*	*	*	*	*	*	*	*	*	*	*	*
sandwich spread																				
(Best) 1 tbsp	50	*	8	5	2	*	*	7	*	*	*	*	*	*	*	*	*	*	*	*
(Hellman's) 1 tbsp	50	*	8	5	2	*	*	7	*	*	*	*	*	*	*	*	*	*	*	*
MAYONNAISE, IMITATION																				
cholesterol free																				
(Best) 1 tbsp	40	*	5	5	*	*	*	7	*	*	*	*	*	*	*	*	*	*	*	*
(generic) 1 tbsp	67	*	10	6	*	*	*	2	*	*	*	*	*	*	*	*	*	*	*	*
(Hellman's) 1 tbsp	40	*	5	5	*	*	*	7	*	*	*	*	*	*	*	*	*	*	*	*
coleslaw dressing																				
(Miracle Whip) 1 tbsp	70	*	9	5	2	*	*	4	*	*	*	*	*	*	*	*	*	*	*	*
mayonnaise dressing																				
(Weight Watchers) 1 tbsp	10	*	*	*	*	*	*	4	*	*	*	*	*	*	*	—	*	*	*	*
milkcream																				
(generic) 1 tbsp	14	*	*	2	2	*	*	3	*	*	*	*	*	*	*	*	*	*	*	*
nonfat																				
(Kraft Free) 1 tbsp	12	*	*	*	*	*	*	8	*	*	*	*	*	*	*	*	*	*	*	*
(Miracle Whip Free) 1 tbsp	20	*	*	*	*	2	*	9	*	*	*	*	*	*	*	*	*	*	*	*

	Calories	Protein	Fat	Sat. Fat	Cholesterol	Carbohydrates	Fiber	Sodium	Potassium	Calcium	Iron	Zinc	Magnesium	Vitamin A	Vitamin C	Thiamin	Riboflavin	Niacin	Vitamin B12	Folic acid
MAYONNAISE, IMITATION (continued)																				
reduced calorie																				
(Hellman's) 1 tbsp	50	*	8	5	2	*	*	5	*	*	*	*	*	*	*	*	*	*	*	*
(Miracle Whip Light) 1 tbsp	45	*	6	5	*	*	*	5	*	*	*	*	*	*	*	*	*	*	*	*
salad dressing																				
(Miracle Whip) 1 tbsp	70	*	11	5	2	*	*	4	*	*	*	*	*	*	*	*	*	*	*	*
sandwich spread																				
(Kraft) 1 tbsp	50	*	8	5	2	*	*	4	*	*	*	*	*	*	*	*	*	*	*	*
soybean																				
(generic) 1 tbsp	35	*	4	3	*	*	*	3	*	*	*	*	*	*	*	*	*	*	*	*
whipped dressing																				
(Weight Watchers) 1 tbsp	15	*	*	*	*	*	*	4	*	**	*	*	*	*	*	*	—	*	*	*
MEAT EXTENDER																				
(generic) 3 oz	266	54	4	2	*	11	—	*	46	17	57	13	46	*	*	40	45	94	85	42
MEAT LOAF DINNER, FROZEN																				
(Armour Classics) 11 1/4 oz	360	33	26	—	22	11	—	49	17	6	20	—		6	15	20	15	15	—	—
(Healthy Choice) 12 oz	340	28	12	15	13	16	—	23	20	4	6	—		15	20	6	4	6	—	—
(Swanson Hungry-Man) 16 1/2 oz	660	60	102	—	—	20	—	77	—	15	35	—		10	30	15	10	30	—	—
large																				
(Swanson) 10 oz	270	35	28	—	—	13	—	39	—	8	20	—		15	20	8	10	10	—	—
regular																				
(Swanson) 9 1/4 oz	320	25	26	—	—	10	—	44	—	4	15	—		4	80	8	10	20	—	—
MEAT LOAF ENTREE, FROM MIX																				
(Hamburger Helper) 1 cup	360	45	34	—	—	5	—	31	13	4	20	—		2	*	10	15	30	—	—
MEAT LOAF ENTREE, FROZEN																				
w/ macaroni & cheese (Stouffer's Lean Cuisine) 9 3/8 oz	280	43	12	15	18	9	—	22	16	15	20	—		6	15	15	25	20	—	—
w/ tomato sauce (Morton) 9 oz	280	17	25	—	15	8	—	57	16	4	10	—		80	*	10	8	6	—	—
w/ whipped potatoes (Stouffer's) 9 7/8 oz	380	33	37	40	27	8	12	38	13	4	15	—		2	2	10	15	20	—	—
MEAT & POULTRY COATINGS																				
country mild (Shake & Bake) 1/4 pouch	80	*	6	—	*	3	—	21	*	*	*	—		8	*	*	*	*	—	—
for chicken (Shake & Bake) 1/4 pouch	80	2	3	—	*	5	—	19	*	*	2	—		6	*	4	4	*	—	—
barbecue (Shake & Bake) 1/4 pouch	90	*	3	—	*	6	—	35	2	*	2	—		8	4	*	*	*	—	—
extra crispy (oven fry) 1/4 pouch	120	6	3	—	*	7	—	35	2	2	6	—		4	*	*	*	*	—	—
homestyle (oven fry) 1/4 pouch	90	*	3	—	*	5	—	41	*	*	*	—		4	*	*	*	*	—	—
hot & spicy (Shake & Bake) 1/4 pouch	80	2	3	—	*	5	—	16	*	4	*	—		4	*	2	2	2	—	—
for fish (Shake & Bake) 1/4 pouch	70	*	2	—	*	5	—	17	*	*	*	—		2	*	*	*	*	—	—
for pork (Shake & Bake) 1/8 pouch	40	*	2	—	*	3	—	13	*	*	*	—		*	*	*	*	4	—	—
barbecue (Shake & Bake) 1/8 pouch	35	*	*	*	*	3	—	11	*	*	*	—		4	*	*	*	*	—	—
extra crispy (oven fry) 1/4 pouch	60	2	2	—	*	3	—	15	*	*	*	—		*	*	*	*	*	—	—
hot & spicy (Shake & Bake) 1/8 pouch	45	*	2	—	*	3	—	9	*	*	*	—		*	*	*	*	*	—	—
Italian herb (Shake & Bake) 1/4 pouch	80	4	2	—	*	5	—	25	*	4	4	—		2	*	2	*	2	—	—
MEAT see specific listings																				

	Calories	Protein	Fat	Sat. Fat	Cholesterol	Carbohydrates	Fiber	Sodium	Potassium	Calcium	Iron	Zinc	Magnesium	Vitamin A	Vitamin C	Thiamin	Riboflavin	Niacin	Vitamin B12	Folic acid
MEAT SPREAD																				
deviled																				
(Libby's) 1 can	160	18	20	25	30	*	*	26	—	4	8	—	—	*	*	—	—	—	—	—
potted meat																				
(Hormel) 2 oz	53	13	6	10	8	*	—	12	2	1	3	2	1	*	*	*	4	4	—	—
(Libby's) 1 can	160	18	20	25	30	*	*	26	—	4	8	—	—	*	*	—	—	—	—	—
MEATBALL DINNER, FROZEN																				
Swedish meatballs																				
(Armour Classics) 11 1/4 oz	330	32	28	—	27	8	—	47	13	10	15			50	15	20	15	10		
MEATBALL ENTREE, CANNED																				
stew																				
(Chef Boyardee) 8 oz	330	17	35	—	13	7	—	61	—	2	10	—		25	6	10	15	2		
(Dinty Moore) 8 oz	240	18	25	35	10	5	—	41	15	3	11	16	7	25	2	4	8	15	—	—
microwave																				
(Dinty Moore) 7 1/2 oz	240	18	25	35	10	5	—	41	14	3	10	15	6	23	2	3	7	14	—	—
MEATBALL ENTREE, FROZEN																				
Swedish meatballs																				
(Light & Elegant) 9 oz	280	23	15	—	18	11	—	27	8	8	10			*	*	20	15	10		
(Weight Watchers) 9 oz	280	30	12	15	10	12	12	21	14	10	20	—		15	6	—	—	—	—	—
in cream sauce																				
(Swanson) 8 1/2 oz	350	35	29	—	—	9	—	31	—	8	15			6	*	10	8	15		
in gravy w/ pasta																				
(Stouffer's Lean Cuisine) 9 1/8 oz	290	38	12	15	18	10	—	23	13	6	15			2	*	15	20	20		
in gravy w/ parsley noodles																				
(Stouffer's) 9 1/4 oz	440	37	35	40	28	12	12	35	9	4	15			2	*	10	15	15		
w/ noodles																				
(Budget Gourmet) 10 oz	590	35	58	—	48	12	—	38	10	10	15			20	6	30	25	30		
w/ pasta																				
(Stouffer's Lunch Express) 10 1/4 oz	280	—	49	55	22	14	12	42	9	6	15			*	2	—	—	—		
MELON BALLS																				
frozen																				
canteloupe & honeydew 1 cup	57	2	*	*	*	5	4	2	14	2	3	2	6	61	18	19	2	6	*	11
MENHADEN OIL																				
1 tbsp	123	*	22	21	24	*	*	*	*	*	*	*	*	*	*	*	*	*	*	*
MENUDO MIX																				
(Gebhardt) 1 tsp	5	*	*	*	*	*	*	13	*	*	2	—	—	*	*	*	*	*		
MEXICAN STYLE DINNER, FROZEN																				
(Banquet Extra Helping) 19 oz	680	42	38	—	2	34	—	163	19	30	45			2	25	60	40	50	—	—
(Kid Cuisine) 5 3/4 oz	290	17	12	—	7	15	—	25	9	8	10			2	10	6	10	15		
(Patio) 13 1/4 oz	650	25	38	—	15	21	—	81	19	15	20			30	6	20	15	30		
combination																				
(Swanson Hungry-Man) 20 oz	820	45	63	—	—	29	—	87	—	30	25			40	10	20	20	25		
large																				
(Swanson) 13 1/4 oz	490	30	28	—	—	20	—	70	—	20	20			25	*	10	15	15		
regular																				
(Swanson) 11 oz	410	15	29	—	—	17	—	64	—	15	15			30	20	15	15	15		
MEXICAN STYLE ENTREE, FROZEN																				
chili gravy w/ beef enchilada & tamale																				
(Morton) 10 oz	300	15	15	—	7	15	—	58	14	8	15			30	6	100	10	6		
fiesta																				
(Patio) 12 oz	460	27	31	—	10	18	—	83	17	20	20			10	*	15	10	4		
rice & chicken																				
(Stouffer's Lean Cuisine) 9 oz	70	—	12	8	7	13	12	25	9	4	4	—		30	20	—	—	—	—	—
MILK																				
lowfat, 1%																				
1 cup	102	13	4	8	3	4	*	5	11	30	*	6	8	10	4	6	*	*	15	3

	Calories	Protein	Fat	Sat. Fat	Cholesterol	Carbohydrates	Fiber	Sodium	Potassium	Calcium	Iron	Zinc	Magnesium	Vitamin A	Vitamin C	Thiamin	Riboflavin	Niacin	Vitamin B12	Folic acid
MILK (continued)																				
protein fortified 1 cup	119	16	4	9	3	5	*	6	13	35	*	7	10	10	5	7	*	*	17	4
lowfat, 2%																				
no vitamin A added 1 cup	136	16	8	15	6	4	*	6	13	35	*	7	9	4	5	7	*	*	16	3
w/ nonfat dry milk 1 cup	125	14	7	15	6	4	*	5	11	31	*	7	9	10	4	7	*	*	16	3
protein fortified 1 cup	137	16	8	15	6	4	*	6	13	35	*	7	10	10	5	7	*	*	17	4
w/ vitamin A 1 cup	121	14	7	15	6	4	*	5	11	30	*	6	8	10	4	6	*	*	15	3
skim																				
no vitamin A added 1 cup	86	14	*	*	*	4		5	12	30	*	7	7	*	4	6	*	*	15	3
w/ nonfat dry milk 1 cup	90	15	*	2	2	4	*	5	12	32	*	7	9	10	4	7	*	*	16	3
protein fortified 1 cup	100	16	*	2	2	5	*	6	13	35	*	7	10	10	5	7	*	*	17	4
w/ vitamin A 1 cup	86	14	*	*	*	4	*	5	12	30	*	7	7	10	4	6	*	*	15	3
whole																				
low sodium 1 cup	149	13	13	27	11	4	*	*	18	25	*	6	3	6	4	3	*	*	15	3
whole, 3.3% 1 cup	150	13	12	26	11	4	*	5	11	29	*	6	8	6	4	6	*	*	14	3
whole, 3.7% 1 cup	157	13	14	28	12	4	*	5	10	29	*	6	8	7	6	6	*	*	14	3
MILK, BUTTER see BUTTERMILK																				
MILK DRINK see specific listings																				
MILK, DRY																				
nonfat																				
w/ vitamin A added 1 cup	244	40	*	*	4	12	*	16	33	84	*	20	20	*	6	19	*	3	45	8
skim																				
no vitamin A added 1 cup	435	72	*	3	8	21	*	27	61	151	2	33	33	53	14	33	*	6	80	15
MILK, EVAPORATED																				
(Carnation) 2 tbsp	40	3	4	8	12	*	*	*	—	8	*	—	—	*	*	—	—	—	—	—
(Dairymate) 1/4 cup	85	3.5	8	*	6	2	*	3	*	15	*	—	—	2	*	1	10	*	—	—
(Pet) 1/4 cup	85	3.5	8	*	6	2	*	3	*	15	*	—	—	2	*	1	10	*	—	—
filled																				
(Dairymate) 1/4 cup	75	3.5	6	*	*	2	*	3	5	15	*	—	—	10	*	1	10	*	—	—
(Pet) 1/4 cup	75	3.5	6	*	*	2	*	3	5	15	*	—	—	10	*	1	10	*	—	—
light skimmed																				
(Dairymate) 1/4 cup	50	3.5	*	*	*	2	*	3	*	18	*	—	—	5	*	1	10	*	—	—
(Pet) 1/4 cup	50	3.5	*	*	*	2	*	3	*	18	*	—	—	5	*	1	10	*	—	—
lowfat																				
(Carnation) 1/4 cup	50	6	*	*	6	*	*	4	—	16	*	—	—	4	*	—	—	—	—	—
skim																				
(Carnation) 1/4 cup	50	6	*	*	6	*	*	4	—	16	*	—	—	4	*	—	—	—	—	—
(generic) 1/4 cup	50	8	*	*	*	3	*	3	6	19	*	4	5	5	2	2	*	*	3	2
whole																				
(generic) 1/4 cup	85	7	8	15	6	2	*	3	6	17	*	3	4	5	2	2	*	*	2	2
w/ vitamin A (generic) 1/4 cup	85	7	8	15	6	2	*	3	6	17	*	3	4	5	2	2	*	*	2	2
MILK, FILLED																				
w/ vegetable oil 1 cup	154	14	13	10	*	4	*	6	10	31	*	6	8	*	4	5	*	*	14	3

Food	Calories	Protein	Fat	Sat. Fat	Cholesterol	Carbohydrates	Fiber	Sodium	Potassium	Calcium	Iron	Zinc	Magnesium	Vitamin A	Vitamin C	Thiamin	Riboflavin	Niacin	Vitamin B$_{12}$	Folic acid
MILK, GOAT *whole* 1 cup	168	14	16	33	9	4	*	5	14	33	*	5	9	9	5	8	*	3	3	*
MILK, HUMAN *whole* 1 fl oz	21	*	2	3	*	*	*	*	*	*	*	*	*	*	3	*	*	*	*	*
MILK, IMITATION *w/ vegetable oil* 1 cup	150	7	13	10	*	5	*	8	8	8	5	19	4	*	*	*	2	4	*	*
w/ lauric oil 1 cup	150	7	13	37	*	5	*	8	8	8	5	19	4	*	*	*	2	*	*	*
MILK, INDIAN BUFFALO *whole* 1 cup	236	15	26	56	15	4	*	5	12	41	2	*	19	9	9	8	*	*	15	3
MILK, INSTANT *nonfat* (Carnation) 1/3 cup dry	80	13	*	*	2	4	*	5	—	30	*	—	—	10	2	6	25	*	15	2
(Weight Watchers) 1 packet	10	2	*	*	—	*	*	*	*	*	—	—	—	*	*	—	—	—	—	—
MILK, LOW-CALCIUM *w/ nonfat dry milk* 1 cup	863	144	*	*	2	42	*	231	47	68	4	65	37	*	27	26	*	8	161	30
MILK PRODUCT *dry* nonfat (Sanalac) 1 cup	80	13	*	*	*	4	*	5	11	30	*	—	—	*	1	6	25	*	—	—
MILK, SHEEP *whole* 1 cup	264	24	26	57	22	4	*	4	10	47	*	9	11	7	17	11	*	5	29	4
MILK, SWEETENED CONDENSED (Carnation) 1/4 cup	260	10	10	20	16	14	*	4	—	20	*	—	—	4	*	—	—	—	6	4
(generic) 1/4 cup	246	10	10	22	8	14	*	4	8	22	*	4	4	6	4	4	*	*	6	*
MILKSHAKE *chocolate* (generic) 11 oz	356	15	12	25	10	21	4	14	19	40	5	10	12	5	*	9	*	2	16	4
vanilla (generic) 11 oz	350	20	15	30	12	19	*	12	16	46	2	8	9	7	*	6	18	2	27	5
MILKFISH *raw* 3 oz	126	29	9	7	15	*	*	3	7	4	2	5	6	2	*	*	3	27	48	*
broiled/baked 3 oz	162	37	11	—	19	*	*	3	9	6	2	6	8	2	*	*	3	35	46	*
MISO (generic) 2 tbsp	71	6	3	2	*	3	7	52	2	2	5	7	3	*	*	2	5	2	*	3
MOLASSES *blackstrap* (generic) 1 tbsp	47	*	*	*	*	4	—	*	14	17	19	*	11	*	*	*	*	*	*	*
medium (generic) 1 tbsp	53	*	*	*	*	5	*	*	8	4	5	*	12	*	*	*	*	*	*	*
(La Choy) 1 tbsp	21	*	*	*	*	6	*	*	4	2	2	—	6	*	*	*	*	*	—	—
MONKFISH *raw* 3 oz	65	21	2	*	7	*	*	*	10	*	2	2	4	*	*	*	3	9	13	*
broiled/baked 3 oz	82	26	3	—	9	*	*	*	12	*	2	3	6	*	*	2	4	11	15	*
MOOSE *roasted* 4 oz	151	55	2	*	29	*	*	3	11	*	26	28	7	*	9	4	23	30	—	—
MORTADELLA *beef & pork* (generic) 1 1 oz slice	88	8	11	14	5	*	*	15	*	*	2	4	*	*	12	2	3	4	7	*

MINTS see CANDY

	Calories	Protein	Fat	Sat. Fat	Cholesterol	Carbohydrates	Fiber	Sodium	Potassium	Calcium	Iron	Zinc	Magnesium	Vitamin A	Vitamin C	Thiamin	Riboflavin	Niacin	Vitamin B₁₂	Folic acid
MOTHBEAN																				
cooked 1/2 cup	103	11	*	*	*	6	—	*	8	*	15	3	23	*	*	7	*	3	*	32
cooked w/ salt 1/2 cup	103	11	*	*	*	6	—	9	8	*	15	3	23	*	*	7	*	3	*	32
MOTHERS LOAF																				
pork 1 1 oz slice	80	6	10	12	4	*	*	13	2	*	2	3	*	*	*	10	3	4	5	*
MOUSSE																				
chocolate (generic) 1/2 cup	446	14	51	93	100	11	—	4	8	20	7	10	11	23	2	6	24	*	15	8
dark chocolate from mix (Knorr) 1/2 cup	90	4	8	20	2	3	—	2	—	4	2	*	*	*	*	*	2	*	*	*
milk chocolate from mix (Knorr) 1/2 cup	90	4	8	—	2	4	—	2	—	4	2	*	*	*	*	*	2	*	*	*
white chocolate from mix (Knorr) 1/2 cup	80	4	15	—	2	3	—	2	—	6	*	*	*	*	*	*	2	*	*	*
MUFFIN																				
apple oatmeal (Pepperidge Farm Wholesome Choice) 1 muffin	120	6	6	5	*	9	12	8	—	2	10	—	—	*	*	6	6	6	—	—
apple spice (Health Valley) 1 muffin	130	6	*	*	*	10	20	5	7	2	8	6	15	10	2	15	8	8	—	—
apple streusel 97% fat free (Hostess) 1 muffin	100	2	2	3	*	8	4	7	*	12	2	—	—	*	*	2	4	2	—	—
banana (Health Valley) 1 muffin	130	6	*	*	*	10	18	5	15	2	8	6	15	10	2	15	8	8	—	—
banana nut (Weight Watchers) 1 muffin	170	5	8	5	3	11	16	10	3	2	4	—	—	2	2	—	—	—	—	—
banana walnut mini (Hostess) 1 muffin	260	5	25	10	13	9	2	7	3	2	4	—	—	*	*	6	8	4	—	—
blueberry (Pepperidge Farm Wholesome Choice) 1 muffin	130	4	3	—	*	9	8	8	—	*	4	—	—	*	2	*	2	*	—	—
(Weight Watchers) 1 muffin	170	5	8	5	3	11	20	9	2	4	4	—	—	4	2	—	—	—	—	—
97% fat free (Hostess) 1 muffin	100	3	2	3	*	7	4	7	*	12	4	—	—	*	*	4	4	2	—	—
mini (Hostess) 1 muffin	240	5	20	10	13	10	3	7	2	2	4	—	—	*	*	4	8	4	—	—
Bran'nola (Arnold) 1 muffin	160	8	2	*	*	10	8	9	—	6	10	—	—	*	*	10	10	8	—	—
chocolate chocolate chip (Weight Watchers) 1 muffin	200	7	6	8	2	13	4	10	7	4	10	—	—	*	4	—	—	—	—	—
cinnamon apple mini (Hostess) 1 muffin	260	5	25	10	15	9	2	7	2	2	4	—	—	*	*	4	6	6	—	—
cinnamon raisin (Pepperidge Farm) 1 muffin	150	6	*	*	*	10	—	8	—	2	8	—	—	*	*	15	10	8	—	—
corn (Pepperidge Farm Wholesome Choice) 1 muffin	150	6	5	—	*	9	4	7	—	*	4	—	—	*	*	4	6	4	—	—
English bran nut (Thomas') 1 muffin	140	8	5	*	*	8	16	8	—	6	6	—	—	*	*	10	8	4	—	—
cinnamon raisin (Oatmeal Goodness) 1 muffin	140	10	3	3	*	9	8	8	3	8	15	—	—	*	*	20	10	10	—	—

MUFFIN (continued)	Calories	Protein	Fat	Sat. Fat	Cholesterol	Carbohydrates	Fiber	Sodium	Potassium	Calcium	Iron	Zinc	Magnesium	Vitamin A	Vitamin C	Thiamin	Riboflavin	Niacin	Vitamin B$_{12}$	Folic acid
honey & oatmeal (Oatmeal Goodness) 1 muffin	140	10	3	3	*	8	6	9	2	10	15	—	—	*	*	25	15	15	—	—
honey wheat (Thomas') 1 muffin	120	8	2	*	*	7	12	8	3	6	6	—	—	*	*	20	6	10	—	—
oat bran (Thomas') 1 muffin	120	6	2	*	*	9	12	9	2	6	6	—	—	*	*	10	6	6	—	—
onion (Thomas') 1 muffin	130	6	2	—	*	9	8	8	—	8	8	—	—	*	*	10	6	6	—	—
plain (Thomas') 1 muffin	130	6	2	*	*	8	4	9	2	8	6	—	—	*	*	15	8	10	—	—
raisin (Thomas') 1 muffin	150	6	2	*	*	10	8	8	4	*	6	—	—	*	*	20	8	6	—	—
(Wonder) 1 muffin	140	7	3	3	*	9	6	9	3	10	10	—	—	*	*	15	10	10	—	—
regular (Wonder) 1 muffin	120	8	2	3	*	8	6	12	2	20	10	—	—	*	*	20	10	10	—	—
rye (Thomas') 1 muffin	120	8	2	5	*	8	12	9	—	6	6	—	—	*	*	8	6	4	—	—
sandwich size (Thomas') 1 muffin	210	10	2	3	*	14	8	14	—	15	15	—	—	*	*	15	10	10	—	—
seven grain (Pepperidge Farm) 1 muffin	150	8	2	*	*	10	8	7	—	6	6	—	—	*	*	20	10	10	—	—
sourdough (Thomas') 1 muffin	130	6	2	*	*	9	8	9	3	8	10	—	—	*	*	10	8	6	—	—
(Wonder) 1 muffin	120	8	2	3	*	8	6	10	2	20	10	—	—	*	*	15	10	10	—	—
extra crisp (Arnold) 1 muffin	130	6	2	*	*	9	4	10	—	*	8	—	—	*	*	20	10	8	—	—
honey bran (Weight Watchers) 1 muffin	160	5	6	5	2	11	40	6	3	2	6	—	—	*	*	—	—	—	—	—
oat bran (Hostess) 1 muffin	160	3	11	5	*	7	6	6	*	2	4	—	—	*	*	2	4	4	—	—
w/ almonds & dates (Health Valley) 1 muffin	150	8	*	*	*	10	33	5	7	2	8	4	10	10	8	10	4	6	—	—
banana nut (Hostess) 1 muffin	140	3	8	5	*	7	4	7	2	*	4	—	—	*	*	4	4	*	—	—
w/ blueberries (Health Valley) 1 muffin	140	6	*	*	*	11	30	4	6	6	25	8	15	*	6	15	8	2	—	—
w/ raisins (Health Valley) 1 muffin	150	8	*	*	*	10	24	5	7	2	8	4	10	10	8	10	4	6	—	—
plain (Pepperidge Farm) 1 muffin	140	8	3	*	*	9	—	9	—	2	8	—	—	*	*	20	10	10	—	—
raisin (Arnold) 1 muffin	160	8	2	*	*	11	8	9	—	4	8	—	—	*	*	15	8	8	—	—
raisin bran (Pepperidge Farm Wholesome Choice) 1 muffin	140	6	3	—	*	10	16	11	—	4	10	—	—	*	2	6	8	10	—	—
raisin spice (Health Valley) 1 muffin	140	6	*	*	*	11	20	4	7	2	8	6	15	10	2	15	8	4	—	—
sourdough (Arnold) 1 muffin	130	6	2	*	*	8	4	10	—	*	10	—	—	*	*	10	8	6	—	—
MUFFIN, FROM MIX																				
apple cinnamon (Betty Crocker) 1 muffin	120	3	6	5	8	6	—	6	*	2	2	—	—	*	*	4	4	2	—	—
(Robin Hood) 1 muffin	170	5	11	10	12	8	—	9	2	2	4	—	—	*	*	8	6	4	—	—
no cholesterol recipe (Betty Crocker) 1 muffin	110	3	5	5	*	6	—	6	*	2	2	—	—	*	*	4	4	2	—	—
banana (Robin Hood) 1 muffin	170	5	12	10	12	7	—	8	2	2	4	—	—	*	*	8	6	4	—	—
banana nut (Betty Crocker) 1 muffin	120	3	6	5	7	6	—	6	2	2	2	—	—	*	*	6	4	2	—	—

	Calories	Protein	Fat	Sat. Fat	Cholesterol	Carbohydrates	Fiber	Sodium	Potassium	Calcium	Iron	Zinc	Magnesium	Vitamin A	Vitamin C	Thiamin	Riboflavin	Niacin	Vitamin B₁₂	Folic acid

MUFFIN, FROM MIX (continued)

	Calories	Protein	Fat	Sat. Fat	Cholesterol	Carbohydrates	Fiber	Sodium	Potassium	Calcium	Iron	Zinc	Magnesium	Vitamin A	Vitamin C	Thiamin	Riboflavin	Niacin	Vitamin B12	Folic acid
no cholesterol recipe (Betty Crocker) 1 muffin	120	3	6	5	*	6	—	6	2	2	2	—	—	*	*	6	4	2	—	—
blueberry (Betty Crocker) 1 muffin	120	3	6	5	7	6	—	6	*	*	2	—	—	*	*	4	2	2	—	—
(Pillsbury Lovin Lites) 1 muffin	100	3	2	*	7	7	—	7	2	4	2	—	—	*	*	4	6	2	—	—
(Robin Hood) 1 muffin	170	5	9	—	—	8	—	10	*	2	2	—	—	*	*	4	6	2	—	—
bakery style (Duncan Hines) 1 muffin	190	3	9	8	5	11	2	11	—	*	4	—	—	*	*	—	—	—	—	—
no cholesterol recipe (Duncan Hines) 1 muffin	180	3	8	8	*	11	2	11	—	*	4	—	—	*	*	—	—	—	—	—
basic recipe (Duncan Hines) 1 muffin	110	3	5	3	7	6	2	7	—	*	2	—	—	*	*	—	—	—	—	—
no cholesterol recipe (Betty Crocker) 1 muffin	110	3	5	5	*	6	—	6	*	*	2	—	—	*	*	4	2	2	—	—
(Duncan Hines) 1 muffin	100	3	4	3	*	6	2	7	—	*	2	—	—	*	*	—	—	—	—	—
(Pillsbury Lovin Lites) 1 muffin	100	3	2	*	*	7	—	7	2	4	*	—	—	*	*	4	6	2	—	—
caramel (Robin Hood) 1 muffin	170	5	11	5	12	8	—	10	*	2	2	—	—	*	*	6	6	4	—	—
cinnamon streusel (Betty Crocker) 1 muffin	200	5	14	10	8	9	—	10	2	6	6	—	—	*	*	8	6	4	—	—
cinnamon swirl bakery style (Duncan Hines) 1 muffin	200	5	9	8	7	11	2	10	—	*	4	—	—	*	*	—	—	—	—	—
no cholesterol recipe (Duncan Hines) 1 muffin	200	3	9	8	*	11	2	10	—	*	4	—	—	*	*	—	—	—	—	—
corn (Robin Hood) 1 muffin	180	5	11	—	—	9	—	13	2	2	2	—	—	4	*	8	8	4	—	—
honey bran (Robin Hood) 1 muffin	170	8	8	—	—	8	—	10	4	4	6	—	—	*	*	8	8	8	—	—
oat bran (Betty Crocker) 1 muffin	180	7	11	10	12	9	—	10	4	8	8	—	—	*	*	8	6	2	—	—
no cholesterol recipe (Betty Crocker) 1 muffin	170	7	9	5	*	9	—	11	5	8	8	—	—	*	*	8	6	2	—	—
wild blueberry (Betty Crocker) 1 muffin	120	3	6	5	7	6	—	6	*	*	2	—	—	*	*	4	4	2	—	—
light (Betty Crocker) 1 muffin	90	3	2	3	7	7	—	6	*	*	2	—	—	*	*	4	4	2	—	—
no cholesterol recipe (Betty Crocker) 1 muffin	110	3	5	3	*	6	—	6	*	*	2	—	—	*	*	4	4	2	—	—

MUFFIN, FROZEN

	Calories	Protein	Fat	Sat. Fat	Cholesterol	Carbohydrates	Fiber	Sodium	Potassium	Calcium	Iron	Zinc	Magnesium	Vitamin A	Vitamin C	Thiamin	Riboflavin	Niacin	Vitamin B12	Folic acid
apple spice (Healthy Choice) 1 muffin	190	5	6	5	*	13	—	4	5	10	10	—	—	*	8	10	8	4	—	—
banana nut (Healthy Choice) 1 muffin	180	5	9	5	*	11	—	3	7	10	10	—	—	*	*	10	8	4	—	—
blueberry (Healthy Choice) 1 muffin	190	5	6	5	*	13	—	5	6	10	8	—	—	*	6	10	10	4	—	—

MULBERRY

	Calories	Protein	Fat	Sat. Fat	Cholesterol	Carbohydrates	Fiber	Sodium	Potassium	Calcium	Iron	Zinc	Magnesium	Vitamin A	Vitamin C	Thiamin	Riboflavin	Niacin	Vitamin B12	Folic acid
1/2 cup	30	2	*	*	*	2	4	*	4	3	7	—	3	*	42	*	4	2	*	—
20 berries	13	*	*	*	*	*	4	*	2	*	3	—	*	*	18	*	2	*	*	—

MULLET, STRIPED

	Calories	Protein	Fat	Sat. Fat	Cholesterol	Carbohydrates	Fiber	Sodium	Potassium	Calcium	Iron	Zinc	Magnesium	Vitamin A	Vitamin C	Thiamin	Riboflavin	Niacin	Vitamin B12	Folic acid
raw 1 fillet	139	38	7	7	19	*	*	3	12	5	7	4	9	3	2	7	6	31	4	*
baked/broiled 1 fillet	140	38	7	7	20	*	*	3	12	3	7	5	8	3	2	6	5	29	4	*

MUNG BEAN

	Calories	Protein	Fat	Sat. Fat	Cholesterol	Carbohydrates	Fiber	Sodium	Potassium	Calcium	Iron	Zinc	Magnesium	Vitamin A	Vitamin C	Thiamin	Riboflavin	Niacin	Vitamin B12	Folic acid
cooked 1/2 cup	106	12	*	*	*	6	32	*	8	3	8	6	12	*	2	11	4	3	*	40
cooked w/ salt 1/2 cup	106	12	*	*	*	6	32	10	8	3	8	6	12	*	2	11	4	3	*	40

PERCENTAGE DAILY VALUE (Protein through Folic acid)

	Calories	Protein	Fat	Sat. Fat	Cholesterol	Carbohydrates	Fiber	Sodium	Potassium	Calcium	Iron	Zinc	Magnesium	Vitamin A	Vitamin C	Thiamin	Riboflavin	Niacin	Vitamin B12	Folic acid
MUNGO BEAN																				
cooked 1/2 cup	95	11	*	*	*	5	24	*	6	5	9	5	14	*	*	9	4	7	*	21
cooked w/ salt 1/2 cup	95	11	*	*	*	5	24	9	6	5	9	5	14	*	*	9	4	7	*	21
MUSHROOM																				
enoki raw 5 large	9	*	*	*	*	*	—	*	3	*	*	*	*	*	5	*	2	5	*	2
shiitake boiled w/ salt 1/2 cup pieces	20	*	*	*	*	2	—	4	*	*	*	*	3	2	*	*	*	4	3	*
shiitake cooked 1/2 cup pieces	20	*	*	*	*	2	3	*	*	*	*	4	2	*	*	*	4	3	*	2
shiitake dried 4 mushrooms	44	2	*	*	*	4	8	*	7	*	8	5	*	*	*	3	11	11	*	6
white pieces & stems, sliced (Green Giant) 1/4 cup	12	2	*	*	*	*	4	9	2	*	*	—	—	*	*	*	6	4	—	—
pieces & stems, whole (B in B) 1/4 cup	12	2	*	*	*	*	4	10	2	*	2	—	—	*	*	*	6	4	—	—
raw 1/2 cup pieces	5	*	*	*	*	*	*	*	2	*	*	*	*	*	*	*	5	4	*	*
4 mushrooms	18	3	*	*	*	*	4	*	8	*	5	4	2	*	4	5	19	15	*	4
sliced w/ garlic (B in B) 1/4 cup	12	2	*	*	*	*	4	8	2	*	2	—	—	*	*	*	6	4	—	—
whole straw mushrooms (Green Giant) 1/4 cup	12	2	*	*	*	*	4	12	2	*	*	—	—	*	*	*	4	2	—	—
boiled 1/2 cup pieces	10	2	*	*	*	*	4	*	4	*	4	3	*	*	3	2	7	9	*	2
4 mushrooms	13	2	*	*	*	*	4	*	5	*	5	3	*	*	3	2	8	11	*	2
w/ salt 1/2 cup pieces	10	2	*	*	*	*	—	4	4	*	4	3	*	*	3	2	7	9	*	2
MUSHROOM, CANNED																				
white drained (generic) 1/2 cup pieces	10	*	*	*	*	*	4	7	*	*	2	2	2	*	*	2	*	3	*	*
(generic) 4 mushrooms	12	*	*	*	*	*	4	8	2	*	2	2	2	*	*	3	*	4	*	2
pieces & stems, sliced (B in B) 1/4 cup	12	2	*	*	*	*	4	10	2	*	2	—	—	*	*	*	6	4	—	—
MUSHROOM GRAVY																				
canned (Franco-American) 1/4 cup	25	*	2	—	—	*	*	12	—	*	*	—	—	*	*	*	*	*	—	—
(generic) 1/4 cup	32	*	3	—	—	*	4	15	2	*	2	2	3	*	*	*	2	3	2	2
w/ wine (Pepperidge Farm) 1/4 cup	30	*	2	—	—	*	—	11	—	*	*			*	*	2	6	2	*	*
from mix (generic) 1/4 cup	82	4	2	—	—	6	—	72	2	6	2	3	2	*	3	3	6	5	3	*
MUSHROOM SAUCE																				
from mix (generic) 1/4 cup	20	*	*	*	*	*	—	15	*	*	*	*	*	*	*	*	2	*	*	*
(Knorr) 1/4 oz	60	4	5	—	3	2	—	10	—	8	*	*	*	*	*	2	8	2	*	*
MUSHROOM & WINE SAUCE																				
from mix (Knorr) 1/2 cup	90	4	8	—	4	3	—	17	—	10	*	*	*	*	*	3	2	*	8	*
MUSSEL, BLUE																				
raw 1/2 cup	73	7	*	*	3	*	*	4	3	*	8	4	3	*	5	4	5	3	149	*

PERCENTAGE DAILY VALUE

	Calories	Protein	Fat	Sat. Fat	Cholesterol	Carbohydrates	Fiber	Sodium	Potassium	Calcium	Iron	Zinc	Magnesium	Vitamin A	Vitamin C	Thiamin	Riboflavin	Niacin	Vitamin B₁₂	Folic acid
MUSSEL, BLUE (continued)																				
steamed/poached 3 oz	146	34	6	4	16	2	*	13	6	3	32	15	8	5	19	17	21	13	339	*
MUSTARD																				
(Grey Poupon) 1 tbsp	15	*	*	*	*	*	*	18	—	*	*	*	*	*	*	*	*	*	*	*
(Kraft) 1 tbsp	11	*	2	*	*	*	*	7	*	*	—	—	*	*	*	*	*	*	—	—
brown (Gulden's) 1 tbsp	15	*	*	*	*	*	*	6	*	*	*	*	*	*	*	*	*	*	*	*
w/ horseradish (Kraft) 1 tbsp	14	*	2	*	*	*	*	6	*	*	*	—	—	*	*	*	*	*	—	—
no salt added (Hain) 1 tbsp	14	2	2	—	*	*	*	—	*	*	*	*	*	*	*	*	*	*	*	*
spicy (French's) 1 tbsp	18	*	*	*	*	*	*	18	*	*	*	*	*	*	*	*	*	*	*	*
yellow (French's) 1 tbsp	15	*	*	*	*	*	*	6	*	*	*	*	*	*	*	*	*	*	*	*
MUSTARD GREENS																				
fresh boiled w/ salt 1/2 cup chopped	11	3	*	*	*	*	—	7	4	5	3	*	3	42	30	2	3	2	*	13
raw 1/2 cup chopped	7	*	*	*	*	*	4	*	3	3	2	*	2	30	33	*	2	*	*	13
boiled 1/2 cup chopped	11	3	*	*	*	*	4	*	4	5	3	*	3	42	30	2	3	2	*	13
canned (Bush Bros) 1/2 cup	25	3	*	*	*	*	8	17	—	10	6	—	—	60	15	—	—	—	—	—
frozen 1/2 cup chopped	15	3	*	*	*	*	4	*	4	8	5	*	3	75	31	2	3	*	*	25
boiled 1/2 cup chopped	14	3	*	*	*	*	—	*	3	8	5	*	2	67	17	2	2	*	*	13
w/ salt 1/2 cup chopped	14	3	*	*	*	*	—	8	3	8	5	*	2	67	17	2	2	*	*	13
MUSTARD HERB SAUCE																				
from mix (Knorr) 1/4 oz	90	6	6	—	5	3	—	20	—	10	2	*	*	2	*	4	8	*	*	*
MUSTARD SEED																				
1 tbsp	53	5	5	*	*	*	4	*	2	6	6	4	8	*	—	4	3	4	*	—
MUSTARD SPINACH																				
raw 1/2 cup chopped	17	3	*	*	*	*	—	*	10	16	6	*	2	149	162	3	4	3	*	30
boiled 1/2 cup chopped	14	3	*	*	*	*	—	*	7	14	4	*	2	148	97	2	3	2	*	16
boiled w/ salt 1/2 cup chopped	14	3	*	*	*	*	—	9	7	14	4	*	2	148	97	2	3	2	*	16
MUSTARD SPREAD																				
Dijonnaise (Best) 1 tsp	12	*	2	*	*	*	*	3	—	*	*	*	*	*	*	*	*	*	*	*
(Hellman's) 1 tbsp	36	*	2	*	*	*	*	9	—	*	*	*	*	*	*	*	*	*	*	*
NAPOLI SAUCE																				
from mix (Knorr) 1/2 cup	100	4	5	—	—	6	—	40	—	4	8	*	*	35	70	6	4	10	*	*
NATTO																				
1/2 cup	187	26	15	7	*	4	20	*	18	19	42	18	25	*	19	9	10	*	*	2
NAVY BEAN																				
canned (Bush Bros) 1/2 cup	110	8	*	*	*	6	24	19	—	4	8	—	—	*	*	—	—	—	—	—
cooked w/ salt (generic) 1/2 cup	129	13	*	*	*	8	—	9	10	6	13	6	13	*	*	12	3	2	*	32
NECTARINE																				
1 fruit	67	2	*	*	*	5	8	*	8	*	*	*	3	20	12	2	3	7	*	*

418   THE HEALTH NUTRIENT BIBLE

	Calories	Protein	Fat	Sat. Fat	Cholesterol	Carbohydrates	Fiber	Sodium	Potassium	Calcium	Iron	Zinc	Magnesium	Vitamin A	Vitamin C	Thiamin	Riboflavin	Niacin	Vitamin B₁₂	Folic acid
NECTARINE (continued)																				
1/2 cup sections	34	*	*	*	*	3	4	*	4	*	*	*	*	10	6	*	2	3	*	*
NEWBURG SAUCE																				
from mix																				
(Knorr) 1/4 cup	100	2	14	—	2	*	—	11	—	4	*	*	*	6	*	*	2	*	*	*
NEW ZEALAND SPINACH																				
raw																				
1/2 cup chopped	4	*	*	*	*	*	—	*	*	2	*	*	3	25	14	*	2	*	*	*
boiled																				
1/2 cup chopped	11	2	*	*	*	*	—	4	3	4	3	2	7	65	24	2	6	2	*	2
boiled w/ salt																				
1/2 cup chopped	11	2	*	*	*	*	—	13	3	4	3	2	7	65	24	2	6	2	*	2
NON-DAIRY CREAMER see COFFEE CREAMER																				
NOPALES																				
raw																				
1/2 cup sliced	7	*	*	*	*	*	4	*	4	7	2	*	6	4	10	*	*	*	*	*
cooked																				
1 pad	4	*	*	*	*	*	4	*	2	5	*	*	3	3	3	*	*	*	*	*
NUTS, MIXED																				
(Planter's) 1 oz	170	10	24	11	*	2	9	5	5	4	6	—	15	*	*	*	*	10	—	10
glazed w/ cashews																				
honey																				
(Fisher) 1 oz	170	10	20	10	*	3	8	5	—	2	*	—	—	*	*	—	—	—	—	—
regular																				
(Fisher) 1 oz	170	8	18	10	*	4	2	4	—	*	4	—	—	*	*	—	—	—	—	—
toffee																				
(Fisher) 1 oz	170	8	17	10	*	4	8	4	—	—	—	—	—	*	*	—	—	—	—	—
w/ peanuts																				
dry roasted																				
(generic) 1 oz	169	8	22	10	*	2	12	*	5	2	6	7	16	*	*	4	3	7	*	4
w/ salt																				
(generic) 1 oz	169	8	22	10	*	2	12	8	5	2	6	7	16	*	*	4	3	7	*	4
oil roasted																				
(generic) 1 oz	175	8	25	13	*	2	12	*	5	3	5	10	17	*	*	9	4	7	*	6
w/ salt																				
(generic) 1 oz	175	8	25	13	*	2	12	8	5	3	5	10	17	*	*	9	4	7	*	6
w/ out peanuts																				
oil roasted w/ salt																				
(generic) 1 oz	175	7	25	13	*	2	8	8	4	3	4	9	18	*	*	10	8	3	*	4
roasted																				
(generic) 1 oz	175	7	25	13	*	2	—	*	4	3	4	9	18	*	*	10	8	3	*	
peanuts & cashews																				
(Fisher) 1 oz	170	10	20	10	*	3	4	5	—	*	4	—	—	*	*	—	—	—	—	—
reduced salt																				
(Fisher) 1 oz	180	10	25	13	*	2	8	2	—	2	4	—	—	*	*	—	—	—	—	—
NUT TOPPING																				
(Fisher) 1 oz	170	10	23	13	*	2	8	3	—	2	4	—	—	*	*	—	—	—	—	—
(generic) 2 tbsp	167	3	14	4	*	7	4	*	2	2	2	3	6	*	*	5	3	*	*	2
NUTMEG, GROUND																				
1 tbsp	37	*	4	9	*	4	*	*	*	*	*	*	3	*	—	2	*	*	*	*
NUTMEG BUTTER OIL																				
1 tbsp	120	*	20	61	*	*	*	*	*	*	*	*	*	*	*	*	*	*	*	*
OATS see CEREAL, HOT																				
OAT OIL																				
1 tbsp	120	*	21	14	*	*	*	*	*	*	*	*	*	*	*	*	*	*	*	*
OATMEAL BREAD see BREAD																				
OCTOPUS																				
raw																				
3 oz	70	21	*	*	14	*	*	8	8	5	25	10	6	3	7	2	2	9	282	*

	Calories	Protein	Fat	Sat. Fat	Cholesterol	Carbohydrates	Fiber	Sodium	Potassium	Calcium	Iron	Zinc	Magnesium	Vitamin A	Vitamin C	Thiamin	Riboflavin	Niacin	Vitamin B12	Folic acid
OCTOPUS (continued)																				
steamed/poached																				
3 oz	139	42	3	2	27	*	*	16	15	9	45	19	13	5	11	3	4	16	508	*
OHELOBERRY																				
1/2 cup	20	*	*	*	*	2	—	*	*	*	*	—	*	12	7	*	*	*	*	—
20 berries	6	*	*	*	*	*	—	*	*	*	*	—	*	4	2	*	*	*	*	—
OKARA																				
nigari																				
(generic) 1/2 cup	47	3	2	*	*	3	—	*	4	5	4	2	4	*	*	*	*	*	*	4
OKRA																				
raw																				
1/2 cup slices	19	2	*	*	*	*	4	*	4	4	2	2	7	7	18	7	2	3	*	11
8 pods	36	3	*	*	*	2	8	*	8	8	4	4	14	13	33	13	3	5	*	21
boiled																				
1/2 cup slices	26	2	*	*	*	2	8	*	7	5	2	3	11	9	22	7	3	3	*	9
8 pods	27	3	*	*	*	2	8	*	8	5	2	3	12	10	23	7	3	4	*	10
boiled w/ salt																				
1/2 cup slices	26	2	*	*	*	2	—	8	7	5	2	3	11	9	22	7	3	3	*	9
OKRA, CANNED																				
cut																				
(Bush Bros) 1/2 cup	25	2	*	*	*	*	12	32	—	6	2	*	*	2	*	—	—	—	—	—
OKRA, FROZEN																				
boiled																				
1/2 cup slices	34	3	*	*	*	2	12	*	6	9	3	4	12	9	19	6	7	4	*	34
boiled w/ salt																				
1/2 cup slices	34	3	*	*	*	2	12	9	6	9	3	4	12	9	19	6	7	4	*	34
OKRA COMBINATION, CANNED																				
cut okra & tomatoes																				
(Bush Bros) 1/2 cup	25	3	*	*	*	*	12	27	—	6	4	—	*	15	*	—	—	—	—	—
OLD FASHIONED LOAF																				
(Oscar Mayer) 1 slice	64	6	7	8	6	*	*	14	2	3	2	3	*	*	*	—	—	—	—	—
OLIVE																				
Early California																				
chopped ripe																				
(Vlasic) 1/2 oz	18	*	3	*	*	*	—	5	—	*	2	*	*	*	*	*	*	*	—	—
w/ jalapeños																				
(Vlasic) 1/2 oz	18	*	3	*	*	*	—	5	—	*	2	*	*	*	*	*	*	*	—	—
pitted ripe																				
(Vlasic) 1/2 oz	16	*	3	*	*	*	*	5	—	*	2	*	*	*	*	*	*	*	—	—
sliced ripe																				
(Vlasic) 1/2 oz	18	*	3	*	*	*	*	5	—	*	2	—	*	*	*	*	*	*	—	—
whole ripe																				
(Vlasic) 1/2 oz	18	*	3	*	*	*	*	5	—	*	2	*	*	*	*	*	*	*	—	—
Early California Enticing																				
chopped ripe																				
(Vlasic) 1/2 oz	18	*	3	*	*	*	*	5	—	*	2	—	*	*	*	*	*	*	—	—
pitted ripe																				
(Vlasic) 1/2 oz	18	*	3	*	*	*	*	5	—	*	2	—	*	*	*	*	*	*	—	—
sliced ripe																				
(Vlasic) 1/2 oz	18	*	3	*	*	*	*	5	—	*	2	—	*	*	*	*	*	*	—	—
whole ripe																				
(Vlasic) 1/2 oz	18	*	3	*	*	*	*	5	—	*	2	—	*	*	*	*	*	*	—	—
Manzanilla																				
pitted																				
(Vlasic) 1/2 oz	14	*	*	*	*	*	*	12	—	*	*	—	*	*	*	*	*	*	—	—
stuffed																				
(Vlasic) 1/2 oz	14	*	*	*	*	*	*	12	—	*	*	—	*	*	*	*	*	*	—	—

	Calories	Protein	Fat	Sat. Fat	Cholesterol	Carbohydrates	Fiber	Sodium	Potassium	Calcium	Iron	Zinc	Magnesium	Vitamin A	Vitamin C	Thiamin	Riboflavin	Niacin	Vitamin B12	Folic acid
OLIVE (continued)																				
oil cured																				
(Progresso) 5 olives	60	*	8	*	*	*	2	12	3	*	—			*	*	*	4	*	—	
ripe																				
chopped																				
(Vlasic) 1/2 oz	18	*	3	*	*	*	*	5	—	*	2	—		*	*	*	*	*	—	
w/ jalapeños																				
(Vlasic) 1/2 oz	18	*	3	*	*	*	*	5	—	*	2	—		*	*	*	*	*	—	
extra small																				
(generic) 1 olive	4	*	*	*	*	*	—	*	*	*	*	*	*	*	*	*	*	*	—	*
jumbo																				
(generic) 1 olive	7	*	*	*	*	*	—	3	*	*	2	*	*	*	*	*	*	*	—	*
pitted																				
(Vlasic) 1/2 oz	18	*	3	*	*	*	*	5	—	*	2	—		*	*	*	*	*	—	
sliced																				
(Vlasic) 1/2 oz	18	*	3	*	*	*	*	5	—	*	2	—		*	*	*	*	*	—	
w/ jalapeños																				
(Vlasic) 1/2 oz	18	*	3	*	*	*	*	5	—	*	2	—		*	*	*	*	*	—	
whole																				
(Vlasic) 1/2 oz	18	*	3	*	*	*	*	5	—	*	2	—		*	*	*	*	*	—	
Spanish																				
cocktail, petite																				
(Vlasic) 1/2 oz	14	*	*	*	*	*	*	12	—	*	*	—		*	*	*	*	*	—	
Plain Queens Thrown																				
(Vlasic) 1/2 oz	14	*	*	*	*	*	*	12	—	*	*	—		*	*	*	*	*	—	
Salad Chunky Style																				
(Vlasic) 1/2 oz	14	*	*	*	*	*	*	12	—	*	*	—		*	*	*	*	*	—	
Salad Sliced																				
(Vlasic) 1/2 oz	14	*	*	*	*	*	*	12	—	*	*	—		*	*	*	*	*	—	
Stuffed Queens Thrown																				
(Vlasic) 1/2 oz	14	*	*	*	*	*	*	12	—	*	*	—		*	*	*	*	*	—	
OLIVE LOAF																				
(Bryan) 1 1 oz slice	50	5	6	—	5	*	*	17	—	—	—			—	—	—	—	—	—	—
(generic) 1 1 oz slice	67	6	7	9	4	*	*	18	2	3	*	3	*	*	4	6	4	3	6	*
(Oscar Mayer) 1 slice	60	5	6	7	4	*	*	16	2	4	2	2	2	*	*	—	—	—	—	—
OLIVE OIL																				
(generic) 1 tbsp	119	*	22	9	*	*	*	*	*	*	*	*	*	*	*	*	*	*	*	*
(Wesson) 1 tbsp	120	*	22	10	*	*	*	*	*	*	*	—	*	*	*	*	*	*	*	—
OLIVE SALAD																				
bottled																				
(Progresso) 1/2 cup	130	*	22	10	*	2	8	36	4	2	6	—	—	2	35	*	*	*	—	—
ONION																				
raw																				
1/2 cup chopped	30	2	*	*	*	2	4	*	4	2	*	*	2	*	9	2	*	*	*	4
boiled																				
1/2 cup chopped	46	2	*	*	*	4	4	*	5	2	*	*	3	*	9	3	*	*	*	4
boiled w/ salt																				
1/2 cup chopped	46	2	*	*	*	4	8	10	5	2	*	*	3	*	9	3	*	*	*	4
ONION, CANNED																				
cocktail																				
lightly spiced																				
(Vlasic) 1 oz	4	*	*	*	*	*	*	17	—	*	*	—		*	*	*	*	*	*	—
plain																				
(Vlasic) 1 oz	4	*	*	*	*	*	*	17	—	*	*	—	—	*	*	*	*	*	*	—
solid & liquid																				
1/2 cup chopped	21	2	*	*	*	4	17	4	5	*	2	2	*	8	2	*	*	*	3	
ONION, FROZEN																				
chopped																				
boiled																				
1/2 cup	29	*	*	*	*	2	8	*	3	2	2	*	2	*	5	2	2	*	*	3

	Calories	Protein	Fat	Sat. Fat	Cholesterol	Carbohydrates	Fiber	Sodium	Potassium	Calcium	Iron	Zinc	Magnesium	Vitamin A	Vitamin C	Thiamin	Riboflavin	Niacin	Vitamin B₁₂	Folic acid
ONION, FROZEN (continued)																				
boiled w/ salt 1/2 cup	29	*	*	*	*	2	—	11	3	2	2	*	2	*	5	2	2	*	*	—
in cream sauce (Bird's Eye) 1/2 cup	60	3	3	5	2	3	8	13	—	6	*	—	—	*	8	2	4	*	*	—
whole boiled 3 oz	24	*	*	*	*	2	8	*	2	2	2	*	2	*	7	*	*	*	*	3
boiled w/ salt 3 oz	24	*	*	*	*	2	—	9	2	2	2	*	2	*	7	*	*	*	*	3
ONION DIP																				
creamy premium (Kraft) 2 tbsp	45	2	6	10	3	*	*	7	*	2	*	—	—	2	*	*	2	*	—	—
French (Frito-Lay) 2 tbsp	60	2	8	15	5	*	*	10			—	—	—		*	*			—	—
(Kraft) 2 tbsp	60	2	6	10	*	*	*	10	*	*	*	—		4	*	*			—	—
premium (Kraft) 2 tbsp	45	2	6	10	3	*	*	6	*	2	*	—		*	*	*	2	*	—	—
green onion (Kraft) 2 tbsp	60	*	6	10	*	*	*	7	*	*	*	—		*	*	*			—	—
w/ chives (Knorr) 1 tbsp	50	*	8	—	3	*	*	4	—	*	*	*	*	*	*	*	*	*		—
ONION FLAKES 1 tbsp	16	*	*	*	*	*	*	*	2	*	*	*	*	*	6	2	*	*	*	2
ONION GRAVY from mix 1/4 cup	193	9	3	—	—	18	18	105	5	17	3	3	5	*	7	8	14	11	14	2
ONION POWDER 1 tbsp	23	*	*	*	*	2	*	*	2	2	*	*	2	*	2	2	*	*	*	—
ONION RING frozen (Mrs. Paul's) 2 oz	150	2	15	5	*	5	*	7	—	*	2	*	*	*	*	2	2	2	*	—
oven heated (generic) 4 rings	326	7	33	35	*	10	—	12	3	2	8	2	4	4	2	15	7	14	*	3
ONION, SPRING (SCALLION) raw 1/2 cup chopped	16	2	*	*	*	*	4	*	4	4	4	*	3	4	16	2	2	*	*	8
OPOSSUM roasted 4 oz	250	57	18	—	—	*	*	—		—	—	—	—	*	*	—	25	—	—	—
ORANGE all types 1 fruit	62	2	*	*	*	5	12	*	7	5	*	*	3	5	116	8	3	2	*	10
1/2 cup sections	42	*	*	*	*	4	8	*	5	4	*	*	2	4	80	5	2	*	*	7
California navel 1 fruit	64	2	*	*	*	5	—	*	7	6	*	*	4	5	134	8	3	2	*	12
1/2 cup sections	38	*	*	*	*	3	—	*	4	3	*	*	2	3	79	5	2	*	*	7
Valencia 1 fruit	59	2	*	*	*	5	—	*	6	5	*	*	3	6	98	7	3	2	*	12
1/2 cup sections	44	2	*	*	*	4	—	*	5	4	*	*	2	4	73	5	2	*	*	9
Florida 1 fruit	69	2	*	*	*	6	16	*	7	6	*	*	4	6	113	10	4	3	*	6
1/2 cup sections	38	*	*	*	*	3	8	*	4	4	*	*	2	3	62	6	2	2	*	4
ORANGE, CANNED in light syrup Mandarin (Del Monte) 1/2 cup	80	*	*	*	*	6	2	*	—	*	4	*		*	20	—	—	—	*	—
ORANGE DRINK (generic) 8 fl oz	122	*	*	*	*	10	*	2	2	2	4	2	2	*	140	*	*	*	*	2
(Hawaiian Punch) 8 fl oz	110	*	*	*	*	9	*	*	—	15	*	*	*	*	100	*	*	*	*	*

	Calories	Protein	Fat	Sat. Fat	Cholesterol	Carbohydrates	Fiber	Sodium	Potassium	Calcium	Iron	Zinc	Magnesium	Vitamin A	Vitamin C	Thiamin	Riboflavin	Niacin	Vitamin B12	Folic acid
ORANGE DRINK (continued)																				
(Tropicana) 6 fl oz	90	*	*	*	*	*	—	*	—	2	*	—	—	*	4	*	4	*	*	—
aseptic pack (Tang) 8 1/2 fl oz (1 box)	130	*	*	*	*	11	*	*	6	*	*	—	—	*	100	*	10	10	*	20
from mix (generic) 6 fl oz (1 box)	86	*	*	*	*	7	*	*	*	5	*	*	*	28	151	*	2	*	*	27
(Kool-Aid) 8 fl oz	70	*	*	*	*	6	*	*	*	*	*	*	*	*	10	*	*	*	*	*
(Tang) 6 fl oz	70	*	*	*	*	6	*	*	*	*	*	—	—	10	100	*	10	10	*	20
sugar-free (Tang) 6 fl oz	6	*	*	*	*	*	*	*	*	*	*	—	—	10	100	*	10	10	*	20
unsweetened (Kool-Aid) 8 fl oz prep w/ out sugar	2	*	*	*	*	*	*	*	*	*	*	*	*	*	10	*	*	*	*	*
(Kool-Aid) 8 fl oz prep w/ sugar	100	*	*	*	*	8	*	*	*	*	*	*	*	*	10	*	*	*	*	*
orange float (Knudsen) 8 fl oz	140	2	*	*	*	11	*	2	3	4	4	—	—	25	40	—	—	—	*	—
ORANGE JUICE																				
from concentrate (Tropicana) 6 fl oz	80	2	*	*	*	5	—	*	—	2	2	—	—	2	110	8	4	2	*	—
organic (Knudsen) 8 fl oz	100	3	*	*	*	8	*	*	9	4	2	—	—	*	150	—	—	—	*	—
(Del Monte) 8 fl oz	110	3	*	*	*	9	3	*	—	4	2	—	—	4	120	—	—	—	*	—
(generic) 8 fl oz	105	2	*	*	*	8	*	*	12	2	6	*	7	9	143	10	4	4	*	11
(Knudsen) 8 fl oz	100	3	*	*	*	8	*	*	9	4	2	—	—	*	150	—	—	—	*	—
(Mott's) 10 fl oz	130	3	*	*	*	10	*	*	18	2	6	—	—	8	140	*	*	*	*	—
(Ocean Spray) 8 fl oz	120	*	*	*	*	10	*	*	9	*	*	—	—	*	130	—	—	—	*	—
(Tropicana) 6 fl oz	80	2	*	*	*	6	—	—	—	2	2	—	—	2	100	2	2	2	*	—
tropical (Farmer's Market) 8 fl oz	120	*	*	*	*	10	*	*	2	*	*	—	—	*	2	—	—	—	*	—
ORANGE PEEL 1 tsp	0	*	*	*	*	*	*	*	*	*	*	—	*	*	*	5	*	*	*	*
ORANGE-APRICOT DRINK (generic) 6 fl oz	95	*	*	*	*	8	*	*	4	*	*	*	2	22	62	2	*	2	*	3
ORANGE-CRANBERRY DRINK (Ocean Spray Refreshers) 8 fl oz	130	*	*	*	*	11	*	*	2	*	*	—	—	*	100	—	—	—	*	—
(Tropicana) 6 fl oz	100	*	*	*	*	8	—	*	—	2	*	—	—	*	2	*	2	4	*	—
light (Tropicana Twister) 6 fl oz	25	*	*	*	*	*	—	*	—	2	2	—	—	*	100	2	*	*	*	—
ORANGE-CRANBERRY JUICE (Tropicana Twister) 6 fl oz	100	*	*	*	*	8	—	*	—	2	2	—	—	*	*	*	2	*	*	—
organic (Santa Cruz Natural) 8 fl oz	110	*	*	*	*	9	*	*	2	4	2	—	—	*	4	—	—	—	*	—
ORANGE-GRAPEFRUIT JUICE (generic) 8 fl oz	106	2	*	*	*	8	*	*	11	2	6	*	6	6	120	9	4	4	*	9
ORANGE-KIWI-PASSION JUICE (Tropicana) 6 fl oz	80	2	*	*	*	6	—	*	—	2	2	—	—	2	40	4	2	2	*	—
ORANGE-MANGO JUICE (Knudsen Tropical Blend) 8 fl oz	120	*	*	*	*	10	*	2	4	2	4	—	—	10	4	—	—	—	*	—
(Tropicana Twister) 6 fl oz	90	*	*	*	*	7	—	2	—	2	2	—	—	6	20	*	*	*	*	—
ORANGE-PASSIONFRUIT JUICE (Tropicana Twister) 6 fl oz	80	*	*	*	*	6	—	*	—	2	2	—	—	*	15	*	*	*	*	—
ORANGE-PEACH JUICE (Tropicana Twister) 6 fl oz	90	*	*	*	*	7	—	*	—	2	2	—	—	*	4	*	2	*	*	—
ORANGE-PEACH-MANGO JUICE (Tropicana) 6 fl oz	80	2	*	*	*	6	—	*	—	2	4	—	—	10	10	4	2	*	*	—

	Calories	Protein	Fat	Sat. Fat	Cholesterol	Carbohydrates	Fiber	Sodium	Potassium	Calcium	Iron	Zinc	Magnesium	Vitamin A	Vitamin C	Thiamin	Riboflavin	Niacin	Vitamin B12	Folic acid
ORANGE-PINEAPPLE JUICE																				
(Tropicana) 6 fl oz	80	2	*	*	*	6	—	*	—	2	2	—	—	2	60	2	4	2	*	—
ORANGE-PINEAPPLE-APPLE DRINK																				
(Welch's) 6 fl oz	110	*	*	*	*	9	*	*	3	*	*	*	*	*	15	*	*	*	*	*
(Welch's Orchard) 8 1/2 oz (1 box)	150	*	*	*	*	13	*	*	5	*	*	*	*	*	*	*	*	*	*	*
aseptic pack (Welch's) 8 1/2 oz (1 box)	140	*	*	*	*	12	*	*	3	*	*	*	*	*	*	*	*	*	*	—
from concentrate (Welch's) 6 fl oz	110	*	*	*	*	9	*	*	4	*	*	*	*	*	15	*	*	*	*	*
ORANGE-RASPBERRY JUICE																				
(Tropicana Twister) 6 fl oz	80	*	*	*	*	7	—	*	—	2	2	—	*	*	*	2	*	*	*	—
light (Tropicana Twister) 6 fl oz	30	*	*	*	*	2	—	*	—	2	2	—	*	*	100	2	*	*	*	—
ORANGE-STRAWBERRY BANANA JUICE																				
(Tropicana) 6 fl oz	80	2	*	*	*	6	—	*	—	2	2	—	*	*	60	2	4	2	*	—
(Tropicana Twister) 6 fl oz	80	*	*	*	*	7	—	2	—	2	2	—	*	*	*	*	2	*	*	—
ORANGE-STRAWBERRY-BANANA DRINK																				
light (Tropicana Twister) 6 fl oz	25	*	*	*	*	2	—	*	—	2	2	—	*	*	100	2	*	*	*	—
ORANGE-STRAWBERRY-GUAVA JUICE																				
(Tropicana Twister) 6 fl oz	80	*	*	*	*	7	—	2	—	2	2	—	—	*	10	10	*	*	*	—
OREGANO, GROUND																				
1 tbsp	14	*	*	*	*	*	4	*	2	7	11	*	3	6	—	*	*	16	*	*	—
ORGAN MEATS see specific meat																				
OYSTER, EASTERN																				
breaded & fried 6 medium oysters	173	13	17	14	24	3	—	15	6	5	34	511	13	5	6	9	10	7	228	*
canned 1/2 cup	86	7	2	2	11	*	*	3	4	3	23	376	8	4	5	6	6	4	394	*
farmed broiled/baked 6 medium oysters	47	7	2	2	7	*	*	4	3	*	—	177	5	*	6	5	2	5	238	*
raw 6 medium oysters	50	7	2	2	7	2	*	6	3	*	—	212	7	*	7	6	3	5	226	*
wild broiled/baked 6 medium oysters	42	8	2	*	10	*	*	6	3	*	—	289	7	*	4	3	3	5	272	*
raw 6 medium oysters	57	10	3	3	15	*	*	7	4	4	31	508	10	2	5	6	5	6	271	*
steamed/poached 6 medium oysters	116	10	3	3	15	*	*	7	3	4	28	508	10	2	4	5	4	5	244	*
OYSTER, PACIFIC																				
raw 6 medium oysters	246	48	12	*	48	*	*	12	12	*	84	330	18	18	42	12	42	30	798	*
steamed/poached 6 medium oysters	246	48	12	*	48	*	*	12	12	*	78	330	18	12	30	12	42	30	720	*
OYSTER STEW see SOUP																				
PALM HEART, CANNED																				
1 heart	9	*	*	*	*	*	4	6	2	2	6	3	3	*	4	*	*	*	*	3
PALM OIL																				
1 tbsp	120	*	3	34	*	*	*	*	*	*	*	*	*	*	*	*	*	*	*	—
PANCAKE																				
frozen (Aunt Jemima) 2 pancakes	200	10	5	3	6	13	8	29	4	2	2	—	—	—	—	15	10	10	—	—
buttermilk (Downyflake) 3 pancakes	280	8	14	—	—	15	—	38	3	6	25	—	—	*	*	35	25	25	—	—
regular (Downyflake) 3 pancakes	280	8	14	—	—	15	—	38	3	6	25	—	—	*	*	35	25	25	—	—

	Calories	Protein	Fat	Sat. Fat	Cholesterol	Carbohydrates	Fiber	Sodium	Potassium	Calcium	Iron	Zinc	Magnesium	Vitamin A	Vitamin C	Thiamin	Riboflavin	Niacin	Vitamin B₁₂	Folic acid
PANCAKE (continued)																				
pourable batter																				
apple cinnamon																				
(Bisquick Shake 'N' Pour)																				
3 4" pancakes	240	10	5	—	*	16	—	37	3	10	10	—	—	*	*	20	15	10	—	—
PANCAKE SYRUP																				
(Country Kitchen) 1/4 cup	200	*	*	*	*	20	*	*	*	*	*	*	*	*	*	*	*	*	*	*
(generic) 1/4 cup	228	*	*	*	*	20	*	*	*	*	*	*	*	*	*	*	*	*	*	*
(Golden Griddle) 1/4 cup	200	*	*	*	*	20	*	*	*	*	*	*	*	*	*	*	*	*	*	*
(Hungry Jack) 1/4 cup	200	*	*	*	*	20	*	*	*	*	*	*	*	*	*	*	*	*	*	*
(Karo) 1/4 cup	240	*	*	*	*	20	*	*	*	*	*	*	*	*	*	*	*	*	*	*
(Log Cabin) 1/4 cup	200	*	*	*	*	20	*	*	*	*	*	*	*	*	*	*	*	*	*	*
butter flavored																				
(Country Kitchen) 1/4 cup	200	*	*	*	*	20	*	2	*	*	*	*	*	*	*	*	*	*	*	*
lite																				
(Aunt Jemima) 1/4 cup	100	*	*	*	*	8	*	2	*	*	*	*	*	*	*	*	*	*	*	*
(Country Kitchen Lite) 1/4 cup	100	*	*	*	*	8	*	2	*	*	*	*	*	*	*	*	*	*	*	*
(generic) 1/4 cup	132	*	*	*	*	12	*	2	*	*	*	*	*	*	*	*	*	*	*	*
(Hungry Jack) 1/4 cup	100	*	*	*	*	12	*	2	*	*	*	*	*	*	*	*	*	*	*	*
(Log Cabin Lite) 1/4 cup	100	*	*	*	*	8	*	2	*	*	*	*	*	*	*	*	*	*	*	*
butter flavor																				
(Aunt Jemima) 1/4 cup	100	*	*	*	*	9	2	6	*	*	*	*	*	*	*	*	*	*	*	*
reduced calorie																				
(Weight Watchers) 1/4 cup	110	*	*	*	*	9	*	6	*	*	*	*	*	*	*	*	*	*	*	*
w/ butter																				
(generic) 1/4 cup	236	*	*	*	*	20	*	*	*	*	*	*	*	*	*	*	*	*	*	*
w/ 15% maple syrup																				
(generic) 1/4 cup	224	*	*	*	*	20	*	*	*	*	*	*	*	*	*	*	*	*	*	*
w/ 2% maple syrup																				
(generic) 1/4 cup	212	*	*	*	*	20	*	*	*	*	*	*	*	*	*	*	*	*	*	*
PANCAKE & WAFFLE MIX																				
buttermilk																				
(Betty Crocker) 3 4" pancakes	280	13	15	—	—	13	—	34	5	—	—	—	—	—	—	—	—	—	—	—
(Hungry Jack) 3 4" pancakes	210	10	14	10	18	9	2	23	3	6	6	—	—	2	*	10	15	8	—	—
(Robin Hood) 1/8 mix	110	8	5	—	—	5	—	11	2	6	4	—	—	2	*	8	8	4	—	—
no cholesterol recipe																				
(Hungry Jack) 3 4" pancakes	200	10	11	5	*	9	2	24	4	6	4	—	—	*	*	10	10	8	—	—
buttermilk, complete																				
(Betty Crocker) 3 4" pancakes	210	8	5	—	—	14	—	21	4	—	—	—	—	—	—	—	—	—	—	—
(Hungry Jack) 3 4" pancakes	180	8	2	3	2	13	4	30	2	15	6	—	—	*	*	15	10	10	—	—
extra lights																				
(Hungry Jack) 3 4" pancakes	190	8	9	5	18	9	2	20	3	15	6	—	—	4	*	10	15	6	—	—
no cholesterol recipe																				
(Hungry Jack) 3 4" pancakes	170	10	6	3	*	9	2	21	4	15	4	—	—	2	*	10	10	6	—	—
extra lights complete																				
(Hungry Jack) 3 4" pancakes	180	7	5	*	*	13	4	30	2	10	8	—	—	*	*	15	8	10	—	—
reduced fat																				
(Bisquick) 1 cup	210	17	6	5	*	13	—	27	2	6	10	—	—	*	*	20	10	10	—	—
regular																				
(Bisquick) 1 cup	240	13	12	10	*	12	—	29	2	8	8	—	—	*	*	20	15	10	—	—
wild blueberry																				
(Hungry Jack) 3 4" pancakes	320	10	22	15	15	14	—	34	5	10	6	—	—	4	*	15	15	10	—	—
PAPAYA																				
1 fruit	119	3	*	*	*	10	20	*	22	7	2	*	8	17	313	5	6	5	—	2
1/2 cup slices	27	*	*	*	*	2	4	*	5	2	*	*	2	4	72	*	*	*	—	*

PERCENTAGE DAILY VALUE

	Calories	Protein	Fat	Sat. Fat	Cholesterol	Carbohydrates	Fiber	Sodium	Potassium	Calcium	Iron	Zinc	Magnesium	Vitamin A	Vitamin C	Thiamin	Riboflavin	Niacin	Vitamin B₁₂	Folic acid
PAPAYA DRINK																				
organic (Santa Cruz Natural) 8 fl oz	110	*	*	*	*	9	*	*	5	4	2	—	—	2	4	—	—	—	—	—
PAPAYA JUICE																				
(Farmer's Market) 8 fl oz	130	2	*	*	*	11	*	*	4	*	*	—	—	*	30	—	—	—	—	—
creamed from concentrate (Knudsen Tropical Blend) 8 fl oz	40	*	*	*	*	3	*	*	3	*	*	—	—	40	60	—	—	—	—	—
PAPAYA NECTAR																				
(generic) 8 fl oz	143	*	*	*	*	12	8	*	2	3	5	2	2	6	12	*	*	2	*	*
(Knudsen Tropical Blend) 8 fl oz	130	*	*	*	*	11	*	*	7	2	*	—	—	10	45	—	—	—	—	—
from concentrate (Knudsen Tropical Blend) 8 fl oz	130	*	*	*	*	11	*	*	7	2	*	—	—	10	45	—	—	—	—	—
PAPAYA-LIME JUICE																				
(Knudsen Tropical Blend) 8 fl oz	130	*	*	*	*	11	*	*	7	2	*	—	—	10	45	—	—	—	—	—
PAPRIKA																				
1 tbsp	20	2	*	*	*	4	*	*	5	*	9	2	3	84	8	3	7	5	*	—
PARMA ROSA SAUCE																				
from mix (Knorr) 1/4 cup	90	4	9	—	4	3	—	14	—	10	*	*	*	8	15	2	8	*	*	*
PARMESANO SAUCE																				
microwave (Knorr) 1/4 cup	190	60	8	—	23	*	—	29	—	4	6	*	*	2	*	4	6	60	*	*
PARSLEY																				
raw 1/2 cup chopped	11	*	*	*	*	*	4	*	5	4	10	2	4	31	66	2	2	2	*	11
dried 1/4 cup	4	*	*	*	*	*	—	*	3	*	4	*	*	18	3	*	2	*	*	5
ground 1 tbsp	4	*	*	*	*	*	*	*	*	2	7	*	*	6	3	*	*	*	*	*
PARSNIP																				
raw 1/2 cup slices	50	*	*	*	*	4	12	*	7	2	2	3	5	*	19	4	2	2	*	11
boiled 1/2 cup slices	63	2	*	*	*	5	12	*	8	3	3	*	6	*	17	4	2	3	*	11
boiled w/ salt 1/2 cup slices	63	2	*	*	*	5	12	8	8	3	3	*	6	*	17	4	2	3	*	11
PASSIONFRUIT																				
purple 1 fruit	17	*	*	*	*	*	8	*	2	*	2	—	*	3	9	*	*	*	*	*
PASSIONFRUIT DRINK																				
(Sunny Delight) 8 fl oz	130	*	*	*	*	10	*	5	—	*	*	*	*	20	50	20	*	*	*	*
(Welch's Orchard) 8 1/2 oz (1 box)	140	*	*	*	*	12	*	*	5	*	*	*	*	*	*	*	*	*	*	*
aseptic pack (Welch's) 8 1/2 oz (1 box)	150	*	*	*	*	13	*	*	5	*	*	—	—	*	*	*	*	*	*	*
from concentrate (Welch's) 6 fl oz	100	*	*	*	*	8	*	*	3	*	*	*	*	*	*	*	*	*	*	*
PASSIONFRUIT JUICE																				
purple 8 fl oz	126	2	*	*	*	11	*	*	20	*	3	—	10	35	123	*	19	18	*	*
yellow 8 fl oz	148	3	*	*	*	12	*	*	20	*	5	—	10	119	75	*	15	28	*	*
PASSIONFRUIT-MANGO JUICE																				
(Heinke's) 8 fl oz	130	*	*	*	*	11	*	*	*	2	2	—	—	15	2	—	—	*	*	*
PASSIONFRUIT-RASPBERRY JUICE																				
(Knudsen Tropical Blend) 8 fl oz	130	*	*	*	*	11	*	*	7	2	4	—	—	*	2	—	—	—	*	*
PASTA																				
all shapes (Master Choice) 6 oz	210	12	2	*	*	14	7	*	—	*	10	—	—	*	*	30	20	15	—	—

	Calories	Protein	Fat	Sat. Fat	Cholesterol	Carbohydrates	Fiber	Sodium	Potassium	Calcium	Iron	Zinc	Magnesium	Vitamin A	Vitamin C	Thiamin	Riboflavin	Niacin	Vitamin B₁₂	Folic acid
PASTA (continued)																				
(Mueller's) 6 oz cooked	210	12	2	*	*	14	*	*	—	*	10	—	—	*	*	35	15	15	—	—
(Ronzoni) 6 oz	210	15	2	*	*	13	8	*	—	*	8	—	—	*	*	30	10	15	—	—
angel hair																				
(Contadina Fresh) 1 1/4 cups	240	17	5	4	30	14	9	*	—	2	15	—	—	*	*	—	—	—	—	—
cholesterol free																				
(Mueller's) 6 oz cooked	210	13	2	*	*	14	*	*	—	2	10	—	—	*	*	35	15	15	—	—
chow mein noodles																				
narrow																				
(La Choy) 1 cup	150	10	12	6	*	5	*	10	*	*	10	—	—	*	*	17	8	10	—	—
wide																				
(La Choy) 1 cup	150	10	12	6	*	5	*	12	*	*	10	—	—	*	*	15	8	10	—	—
egg noodles																				
(America's Choice) 6 oz	220	13	4	4	18	13	4	1	—	*	10	—	—	*	*	30	10	15	—	—
(Mueller's) 6 oz	220	7	5	2	20	13	4	*	—	*	10	—	—	*	*	30	10	15	—	—
(Pennsylvania Dutch) 6 oz	220	13	4	4	18	13	4	1	—	*	10	—	—	*	*	30	10	15	—	—
fettuccine																				
(Contadina Fresh) 1 1/4 cups	250	17	5	4	31	15	9	*	—	2	15	—	—	*	*	—	—	—	—	—
cholesterol free																				
(Contadina Fresh) 1 cup	240	15	3	2	*	15	9	1	—	*	10	—	—	*	*	—	—	—	—	—
linguine																				
(Contadina Fresh) 1 1/4 cups	260	17	5	4	32	15	10	*	—	2	15	—	—	*	*	—	—	—	—	—
cholesterol free																				
(Contadina Fresh) 1 1/4 cups	250	15	4	2	*	16	10	1	—	*	10	—	—	*	*	—	—	—	—	—
ravioli																				
beef & garlic																				
(Contadina Fresh) 1 1/4 cups	350	28	21	24	36	13	13	15	—	4	20	—	—	2	*	—	—	—	—	—
cheese																				
(Contadina Fresh) 1 cup	280	22	18	31	27	10	9	15	—	20	10	—	—	*	*	—	—	—	—	—
cheese, light																				
(Contadina Fresh) 1 cup	240	22	7	10	18	12	9	13	—	10	8	—	—	*	*	—	—	—	—	—
chicken & rosemary																				
(Contadina Fresh) 1 1/4 cups	330	22	19	16	27	14	12	17	—	6	15	—	—	*	*	—	—	—	—	—
vegetable																				
(Contadina Fresh) 1 1/4 cups	290	25	9	15	21	14	11	16	—	15	15	—	—	15	*	—	—	—	—	—
rice noodles																				
(La Choy) 1 cup	130	7	8	*	*	7	*	17	*	*	4	—	—	*	*	4	2	6	—	—
tagliatelle																				
spinach																				
(Contadina Fresh) 1 1/4 cups	270	20	6	5	34	15	14	4	—	6	15	—	—	4	*	—	—	—	—	—
tortellini																				
cheese																				
(Contadina Fresh) 3/4 cup	260	22	9	13	14	13	10	14	—	15	10	—	—	*	*	—	—	—	—	—
cheese & basil																				
(Contadina Fresh) 1 cup	360	27	16	20	21	16	14	15	—	20	15	—	—	4	*	—	—	—	—	—
chicken & prosciutto																				
(Contadina Fresh) 1 cup	360	25	20	19	23	15	11	18	—	8	15	—	—	2	*	—	—	—	—	—
chicken & vegetable																				
(Contadina Fresh) 3/4 cup	260	17	10	8	14	13	9	9	—	2	10	—	—	4	*	—	—	—	—	—
sausage & pepper																				
(Contadina Fresh) 1 cup	330	22	15	19	29	16	13	12	—	4	15	—	—	2	*	—	—	—	—	—
spinach three cheese																				
(Contadina Fresh) 3/4 cup	260	22	9	14	18	13	12	16	—	15	10	—	—	4	*	—	—	—	—	—
tri-color																				
(Mueller's) 6 oz cooked	210	12	2	*	*	14	*	*	—	*	10	—	—	*	*	35	15	15	—	—
PASTA DINNER, FROZEN																				
Cacciatore chicken																				
(Healthy Choice Homestyle) 12 1/2 oz	310	43	5	3	12	16	—	18	19	4	15	—	—	10	10	30	25	35	—	—

	Calories	Protein	Fat	Sat Fat	Cholesterol	Carbohydrates	Fiber	Sodium	Potassium	Calcium	Iron	Zinc	Magnesium	Vitamin A	Vitamin C	Thiamin	Riboflavin	Niacin	Vitamin B12	Folic acid
PASTA DINNER, FROZEN (continued)																				
Italiano (Healthy Choice Homestyle) 12 oz	350	27	8	10	10	20	—	22	15	6	20	—	—	6	*	35	30	15	—	—
meat sauce (Swanson) 11 oz	340	35	17	—	—	15	—	44	—	15	15	—	—	25	50	8	15	15	—	—
ribbed (Swanson Hungry-Man) 17 1/4 oz	550	60	38	—	—	17	—	66	—	20	50	—	—	40	60	20	25	35	—	—
rigatoni chicken & vegetable (Healthy Choice Homestyle) 12 1/2 oz	360	52	6	10	20	17	—	18	15	10	10	—	—	6	15	30	30	30	—	—
rings & meatballs (Swanson Kids') 12 oz	520	40	25	—	—	—	—	36	—	6	20	—	—	10	6	10	10	25	—	—
shells w/ tomato sauce (Healthy Choice Homestyle) 12 oz	330	40	5	10	12	18	—	20	18	40	15	—	—	10	*	35	25	15	—	—
shrimp & vegetables (Healthy Choice Homestyle) 12 1/2 oz	270	27	6	10	17	15	—	20	9	6	10	—	—	10	15	20	15	15	—	—
spaghetti meat sauce (Top Shelf) 10 oz	260	23	9	10	7	12	—	41	25	6	15	16	13	10	4	15	15	20	—	—
meatballs (Swanson) 12 1/2 oz	280	20	17	—	—	12	—	45	—	4	15	—	—	35	50	15	15	15	—	—
Teriyaki chicken (Healthy Choice Homestyle) 12 2/3 oz	350	40	5	5	15	19	—	15	11	6	15	—	—	10	10	20	20	20	—	—
turkey & vegetables (Swanson) 11 1/4 oz	310	45	14	—	—	12	—	28	—	20	10	—	—	150	60	15	30	50	—	—
vegetable Italiano (Healthy Choice Quick Meals) 10 oz	220	12	2	3	*	15	—	14	11	4	25	—	—	25	*	20	15	8	—	—
ziti in meat sauce (Swanson) 11 oz	340	35	17	—	—	15	—	44	—	15	15	—	—	25	50	8	15	15	—	—
(Swanson Hungry-Man) 17 1/4 oz	550	60	38	—	—	17	—	66	—	20	50	—	—	40	60	20	25	35	—	—
PASTA ENTREE																				
pasta i fagioli (Homemade) 1 cup	195	14	8	—	—	10	—	33	15	6	15	7	13	38	20	13	6	8	*	12
PASTA ENTREE, CANNED																				
ABC's & 123's (Chef Boyardee) 8 2/3 oz	200	10	2	3	*	14	—	42	—	2	8	—	—	6	*	10	15	20	—	—
in sauce (Chef Boyardee) 7 1/2 oz	160	8	2	3	*	10	12	35	—	2	10	—	—	4	*	10	10	20	—	—
mini meatballs (Chef Boyardee) 7 1/2 oz	240	13	14	—	6	11	—	38	—	*	10	—	—	8	*	10	15	10	—	—
beef ravioli in sauce (Libby's) 7 3/4 oz	230	18	14	18	5	10	28	43	—	10	10	—	—	*	*	—	—	—	—	—
Beef Raviolio's canned (Franco-American) 7 1/2 oz	250	15	12	—	—	12	—	39	—	2	10	—	—	10	10	15	10	15	—	—
Beef-o-ghetti (Chef Boyardee) 7 1/2 oz	220	12	14	—	7	9	—	52	—	*	10	—	—	6	*	10	10	10	—	—
Beefaroni (Chef Boyardee) 7 1/2 oz	220	13	12	—	6	10	—	45	—	*	10	—	—	6	*	10	15	8	—	—
Beefy macaroni microwave (Hormel Kid's Kitchen) 7 1/2 oz	200	18	9	10	8	8	—	32	11	4	12	15	8	18	*	7	12	13	—	—

	Calories	Protein	Fat	Sat. Fat	Cholesterol	Carbohydrates	Fiber	Sodium	Potassium	Calcium	Iron	Zinc	Magnesium	Vitamin A	Vitamin C	Thiamin	Riboflavin	Niacin	Vitamin B12	Folic acid
PASTA ENTREE, CANNED (continued)																				
cannelloni																				
mini																				
(Chef Boyardee) 7 1/2 oz	230	15	11	5	5	11	20	44	—	2	10	—	—	6	*	10	15	10	—	—
cheese ravioli																				
(Chef Boyardee Sir Chomps)																				
7 1/2 oz	170	10	2	3	2	13	24	31	—	4	15	—	—	4	6	15	15	10	—	—
chicken																				
(Chef Boyardee) 7 1/2 oz	180	17	3	3	5	10	4	35	—	2	8	—	—	22	*	10	30	10	—	—
chicken ravioli																				
mini																				
(Chef Boyardee) 7 1/2 oz	220	12	12	—	—	10	—	45	—	4	10	—	—	10	*	10	8	8	—	—
CircusOs																				
(Franco-American) 7 1/2 oz	160	6	3	—	—	10	—	36	—	2	8	—	—	10	*	10	8	10	—	—
meatballs																				
(Franco-American) 7 1/3 oz	210	15	12	—	—	9	—	40	—	2	10	—	—	8	2	10	8	10	—	—
dinosaurs																				
in sauce																				
(Chef Boyardee) 7 1/2 oz	160	7	2	3	*	11	12	33	—	2	6	—	—	6	*	10	10	20	—	—
meatballs																				
(Chef Boyardee) 8 2/3 oz	280	15	17	—	7	12	—	47	—	*	15	—	—	10	*	10	15	15	—	—
mini meatballs																				
(Chef Boyardee) 7 1/2 oz	230	12	12	—	6	11	—	40	—	*	10	—	—	10	*	8	15	10	—	—
lasagna																				
(Chef Boyardee) 7 1/2 oz	240	13	12	—	6	10	—	42	—	*	10	—	—	6	*	10	10	6	—	—
meat sauce																				
(Healthy Choice) 7 1/2 oz	220	25	8	—	8	10	—	22	15	8	10	—	—	30	8	10	15	15	—	—
(Libby's) 7 3/4 oz	200	15	11	18	5	8	12	36	—	10	10	—	—	4	2	—	—	—	—	—
microwave																				
(Healthy Choice) 7 1/2 oz	220	25	8	—	8	10	—	22	15	8	10	—	—	30	8	10	15	15	—	—
macaroni & beef in sauce																				
(Libby's) 7 3/4 oz	220	15	14	20	7	10	20	32	—	6	10	—	—	*	*	—	—	—	—	—
macaroni & cheese																				
(Chef Boyardee) 7 1/2 oz	170	12	3	3	8	11	8	40	—	6	6	—	—	8	*	10	15	15	—	—
(Libby's) 7 3/4 oz	320	20	31	35	10	8	8	58	—	25	6	—	—	10	*	—	—	—	—	—
canned																				
(Franco-American) 7 1/3 oz	160	15	9	—	—	8	—	37	—	10	8	—	—	10	8	15	10	8	—	—
microwave																				
(Hormel Kid's Kitchen) 7 1/2 oz	260	20	17	30	15	9	—	27	6	10	6	7	7	8	10	6	4	10	—	—
macaroni shells																				
(Chef Boyardee) 7 1/2 oz	150	10	2	3	—	10	—	39	—	*	8	—	—	2	*	8	15	10	—	—
mini bites																				
(Chef Boyardee) 7 1/2 oz	260	13	18	10	39	10	44	42	—	2	10	—	—	8	*	10	10	8	—	—
Pac man																				
in chicken sauce																				
(Chef Boyardee) 7 1/2 oz	170	10	11	—	—	7	—	38	—	*	8	—	—	2	*	10	10	10	—	—
in tomato sauce																				
(Chef Boyardee) 7 1/2 oz	150	10	2	3	*	10	—	35	—	2	6	—	—	6	*	10	10	10	—	—
meatballs																				
(Chef Boyardee) 7 1/2 oz	230	12	14	15	6	11	20	37	—	*	8	—	—	8	*	10	10	10	—	—
ravioli																				
(Chef Boyardee) 7 1/2 oz	180	12	6	—	4	10	—	46	—	6	10	—	—	2	*	10	8	10	—	—
mini																				
microwave																				
(Hormel Kid's Kitchen) 7 1/2 oz	230	17	9	15	5	11	—	36	10	6	6	9	8	13	21	12	19	14	—	—
rigatoni																				
(Chef Boyardee																				
Special Recipe) 7 1/2 oz	210	15	9	10	7	11	16	43	—	2	20	—	—	10	6	15	20	10	—	—
roller coasters																				
(Chef Boyardee) 7 1/2 oz	230	12	15	15	6	9	12	45	—	*	10	—	—	4	*	10	15	10	—	—

PASTA ENTREE, CANNED (continued)

	Calories	Protein	Fat	Sat. Fat	Cholesterol	Carbohydrates	Fiber	Sodium	Potassium	Calcium	Iron	Zinc	Magnesium	Vitamin A	Vitamin C	Thiamin	Riboflavin	Niacin	Vitamin B12	Folic acid
sharks in sauce (Chef Boyardee) 7 1/2 oz	170	8	2	3	*	11	—	32	—	2	6	—	—	4	*	10	10	20	—	—
meatballs (Chef Boyardee) 7 1/2 oz	230	13	12	—	5	10	—	37	—	*	10	—	—	8	*	10	15	10	—	—
shells in meat sauce (Chef Boyardee) 7 1/2 oz	190	12	9	5	2	10	16	34	—	2	10	—	—	15	6	10	20	15	—	—
Smurf beef ravioli in pasta & meat sauce (Chef Boyardee) 7 1/2 oz	230	15	8	—	4	13	—	48	—	*	15	—	—	8	*	10	10	8	—	—
Smurf pasta w/ meatballs (Chef Boyardee) 7 1/2 oz	240	13	14	10	6	10	—	37	—	*	6	—	—	8	*	10	10	8	—	—
Smurfs in sauce (Chef Boyardee) 7 1/2 oz	150	10	2	—	*	10	12	35	—	2	8	—	—	6	*	10	10	10	—	—
spaghetti (Bush Bros) 1 cup	180	12	5	5	*	10	8	60	—	2	10	—	—	40	*	—	—	—	—	—
spaghetti & beef in tomato sauce (Chef Boyardee) 7 1/2 oz	240	12	14	—	6	10	—	47	—	*	10	—	—	6	*	10	10	4	—	—
spaghetti & cheese (Franco-American) 7 1/3 oz	180	8	3	—	—	12	—	35	—	4	6	—	—	8	*	10	10	10	—	—
spaghetti & meat sauce (Healthy Choice) 7 1/2 oz	150	17	5	—	7	7	—	16	16	8	6	—	—	10	8	8	10	10	—	—
microwave (Healthy Choice) 7 1/2 oz	150	17	5	—	7	7	—	16	16	8	6	—	—	10	8	8	10	10	—	—
spaghetti & meatballs (Franco-American) 7 1/3 oz	220	15	12	—	—	9	—	36	—	2	10	—	—	10	*	10	6	10	—	—
(Libby's) 7 3/4 oz	190	17	8	10	7	9	8	39	—	6	10	—	—	4	*	—	—	—	—	—
in tomato sauce (Chef Boyardee) 7 1/2 oz	240	12	15	—	6	10	—	47	—	*	10	—	—	6	*	10	10	8	—	—
microwave (Hormel Kid's Kitchen) 7 1/2 oz	220	18	12	20	7	9	—	37	14	8	11	13	8	20	6	8	14	14	—	—
spaghetti rings (Healthy Choice) 7 1/2 oz	140	8	*	*	*	10	—	19	8	2	15	—	—	10	4	10	6	6	—	—
microwave (Healthy Choice) 7 1/2 oz	140	8	*	*	*	10	—	19	8	2	15	—	—	10	4	10	6	6	—	—
(Hormel Kid's Kitchen) 7 1/2 oz	180	13	2	5	3	12	—	39	10	8	8	6	8	10	4	6	10	8	—	—
SpaghettiOs franks (Franco-American) 7 1/3 oz	210	13	12	—	—	9	—	42	—	2	10	—	—	8	*	10	10	15	—	—
in tomato & cheese sauce (Franco-American) 7 1/2 oz	160	7	3	—	—	10	—	37	—	2	8	—	—	10	*	10	8	10	—	—
meatballs (Franco-American) 7 1/3 oz	210	15	12	—	—	8	—	39	—	2	10	—	—	8	2	10	8	10	—	—
spirals & chicken (Libby's) 7 3/4 oz	130	13	6	5	5	5	16	41	—	*	*	—	—	8	*	—	—	—	—	—
spirals in pizza sauce (Chef Boyardee 7 1/2 oz	180	8	5	3	2	12	12	45	—	2	8	—	—	6	2	10	15	10	—	—
TeddyOs in tomato & cheese sauce (Franco-American) 7 1/2 oz	160	8	3	—	—	10	—	36	—	2	10	—	—	10	*	10	8	10	—	—
meatballs (Franco-American) 7 1/3 oz	210	15	12	—	—	9	—	40	—	2	10	—	—	8	2	10	8	10	—	—
Tic tac toes meatballs (Chef Boyardee) 7 1/2 oz	240	13	14	—	6	10	—	42	—	*	10	—	—	8	*	15	15	10	—	—
in sauce (Chef Boyardee) 7 1/2 oz	160	8	2	3	*	10	12	36	—	*	6	—	—	4	*	10	10	10	—	—

	Calories	Protein	Fat	Sat. Fat	Cholesterol	Carbohydrates	Fiber	Sodium	Potassium	Calcium	Iron	Zinc	Magnesium	Vitamin A	Vitamin C	Thiamin	Riboflavin	Niacin	Vitamin B₁₂	Folic acid
PASTA ENTREE, CANNED (continued)																				
turtles																				
in sauce (Chef Boyardee) 7 1/2 oz	150	7	2	—	*	10	—	35	—	*	6	—	—	4	*	8	10	10	—	—
meatballs (Chef Boyardee) 7 1/2 oz	220	12	12	—	7	10	—	39	—	*	8	—	—	6	*	10	15	15	—	—
WaldOs																				
in tomato & cheese sauce (Franco-American) 7 1/2 oz	160	8	3	—	—	10	—	36	—	2	8	—	—	10	*	10	8	10	—	—
meatballs (Franco-American) 7 1/3 oz	210	15	12	—	—	9	—	40	—	2	10	—	—	8	2	10	8	10	—	—
Zooroni w/ meatballs in sauce (Chef Boyardee) 7 1/2 oz	240	13	12	—	6	11	—	40	—	*	10	—	—	8	*	10	15	10	—	—
PASTA ENTREE, FROM MIX																				
chicken w/ herbs (Kraft) 1/2 cup	170	8	11	10	8	7	—	23	3	4	6	—	—	4	*	10	8	6	—	—
fettuccine alfredo (Hain) 1 cup	190	20	15	15	3	7	6	18	3	4	6	—	—	8	*	2	6	4	—	—
(Chicken Helper) 7 1/2 oz	320	43	18	20	23	9	—	32	8	10	10	—	—	6	*	20	20	30	—	—
(Tuna Helper) 7 oz	300	25	22	—	—	9	—	39	7	10	8	—	—	10	*	20	15	25	—	—
(Kraft) 1/2 cup	180	10	14	15	10	6	—	25	2	10	4	—	—	4	*	10	8	6	—	—
lasagna (Hamburger Helper) 1 cup	340	33	22	—	—	11	—	39	12	2	15	—	—	4	*	20	15	25	—	—
macaroni & cheese (Kraft) 3/4 cup	290	15	20	15	2	11	—	22	5	8	10	—	—	10	—	15	20	8	—	—
deluxe (Kraft) 3/4 cup	260	15	12	20	7	12	—	25	3	10	10	—	—	8	—	15	15	8	—	—
Dinomac (Kraft) 3/4 cup	310	15	22	15	3	12	—	23	7	10	10	—	—	8	—	20	15	10	—	—
spirals (Kraft) 3/4 cup	340	15	28	20	3	12	—	25	8	10	10	—	—	10	—	20	15	10	—	—
teddy bears (Kraft) 3/4 cup	310	15	22	15	3	12	—	23	7	10	10	—	—	8	—	20	15	10	—	—
Wild Wheels (Kraft) 3/4 cup	310	15	22	15	3	12	—	23	7	10	10	—	—	8	—	20	15	10	—	—
parmesan (Kraft) 1/2 cup	180	10	12	10	10	6	—	26	3	10	6	—	—	4	*	10	8	6	—	—
ramen noodles beef flavor (La Choy) 1 cup	225	10	12	6	*	11	16	36	*	*	11	—	—	*	*	15	10	12	—	—
chicken flavor (La Choy) 1 cup	200	10	11	6	*	10	16	31	*	*	11	—	—	*	*	15	10	12	—	—
shells & cheese (Velveeta) 3/4 cup	315	20	18	30	10	12	—	36	4	20	10	—	—	8	—	15	15	10	—	—
bacon bits (Velveeta) 3/4 cup	360	20	23	35	12	13	—	43	3	20	15	—	—	10	—	30	15	15	—	—
Mexican style (Velveeta) 3/4 cup	315	20	18	30	10	13	—	39	5	20	10	—	—	8	—	30	20	15	—	—
spaghetti (Hamburger Helper) 1 cup	330	33	22	—	—	7	—	42	12	10	15	—	—	2	*	20	15	25	—	—
American (Kraft) 3/4 cup	225	12	8	8	*	13	—	20	10	5	12	—	—	15	8	15	8	12	—	—
Italian (Kraft) 3/4 cup	233	12	9	8	*	12	—	21	10	6	12	—	—	15	12	15	12	15	—	—
meat sauce (Kraft) 3/4 cup	270	15	17	15	4	12	—	27	8	8	12	—	—	8	3	12	12	12	—	—
three cheese w/ vegetables (Kraft) 1/2 cup	180	10	12	15	8	6	—	26	3	10	6	—	—	6	*	10	8	6	—	—

PASTA ENTREE, FROZEN

	Calories	Protein	Fat	Sat. Fat	Cholesterol	Carbohydrates	Fiber	Sodium	Potassium	Calcium	Iron	Zinc	Magnesium	Vitamin A	Vitamin C	Thiamin	Riboflavin	Niacin	Vitamin B₁₂	Folic acid
angel hair pasta																				
(Stouffer's Lean Cuisine) 10 oz	240	17	8	5	3	13	—	17	14	10	15	—	—	25	10	20	20	15	—	—
(Weight Watchers) 8 1/2 oz	150	13	2	*	*	9	20	13	15	10	15	—	—	10	15	—	—	—	—	—
beef cannelloni w/ tomato sauce (Stouffer's Lean Cuisine) 9 5/8 oz	200	23	5	5	8	9	—	20	23	15	15	—	—	35	10	8	10	15	—	—
cannelloni																				
cheese (Light & Elegant) 9 oz	310	32	14	—	23	13	—	27	15	35	15	—	—	15	8	25	20	10	—	—
tomato sauce (Stouffer's Lean Cuisine) 9 1/8 oz	270	38	12	20	8	9	—	25	11	30	4	—	—	6	35	8	15	8	—	—
fettuccine primavera (Green Giant Garden Meals) 1 pkg (9 1/2 oz)	230	22	12	15	8	9	24	25	7	15	10	—	—	15	20	10	30	6	—	—
fettuccine alfredo																				
(Healthy Choice Quick Meals) 8 oz	240	17	11	10	15	12	—	19	2	10	10	—	—	*	*	15	10	6	—	—
(Light & Elegant) 9 oz	290	20	18	—	12	11	—	42	7	20	15	—	—	6	35	15	20	8	—	—
(Stouffer's) 10 oz	480	—	45	85	33	13	12	35	5	40	8	—	—	2	*	—	—	—	—	—
(Stouffer's Lean Cuisine) 9 oz	280	23	11	15	5	14	—	24	8	25	8	—	—	*	*	20	25	8	—	—
w/ broccoli (Weight Watchers) 8 1/2 oz	220	25	9	13	5	8	24	22	15	25	15	—	—	6	2	—	—	—	—	—
beef & broccoli (Healthy Choice Homestyle) 12 oz	290	32	5	5	7	15	—	22	10	2	6	—	—	15	45	10	6	8	—	—
chicken (Weight Watchers) 8 1/4 oz	280	37	14	15	13	8	8	25	21	20	10	—	—	4	*	—	—	—	—	—
primavera (Stouffer's Lean Cuisine) 10 oz	260	23	11	10	7	12	—	24	11	30	8	—	—	50	20	20	20	6	—	—
(Stouffer's Lunch Express) 10 1/4 oz	220	—	38	60	32	11	16	29	8	25	10	—	—	50	15	—	—	—	—	—
lasagna																				
(Light & Elegant) 9 oz	240	22	8	—	8	12	—	33	18	10	20	—	—	25	10	15	10	10	—	—
(Top Shelf) 10 oz	350	38	25	40	20	10	—	35	21	30	15	21	14	10	4	20	30	20	—	—
cheese (Light & Elegant) 9 oz	260	23	9	—	10	12	—	33	22	30	15	—	—	40	10	15	15	8	—	—
florentine (Weight Watchers) 10 oz	190	27	2	3	3	12	20	17	14	35	10	—	—	20	25	—	—	—	—	—
four cheese (Stouffer's) 10 3/4 oz	410	—	29	50	18	12	12	35	13	50	8	—	—	20	20	—	—	—	—	—
garden (Weight Watchers) 11 oz	230	28	8	5	2	10	24	19	21	35	30	—	—	20	15	—	—	—	—	—
Italian cheese (Weight Watchers) 11 oz	300	32	12	15	8	9	28	23	21	65	15	—	—	35	25	—	—	—	—	—
Italian sausage (Budget Gourmet) 10 oz	430	30	35	—	15	11	—	35	11	30	10	—	—	100	20	25	20	25	—	—
meat sauce																				
(Budget Gourmet Light & Healthy) 9 1/2 oz	290	25	17	20	10	10	—	30	13	20	10	—	—	100	8	20	20	25	—	—
(Dinty Moore American Classics) 10 oz	320	27	22	35	12	11	—	36	13	16	13	19	12	13	1	9	19	16	—	—
(Healthy Choice) 10 oz	260	30	8	10	7	12	—	17	14	10	15	—	—	15	4	20	15	10	—	—
(Stouffer's) 10 1/2 oz	360	—	20	25	17	11	20	32	15	25	10	—	—	10	6	—	—	—	—	—
(Stouffer's Lean Cuisine) 10 1/4 oz	280	33	9	15	8	12	—	23	20	15	10	—	—	10	10	10	15	15	—	—
(Stouffer's Lean Cuisine Lunch Express) 9 1/2 oz	60	—	11	13	5	13	20	25	12	20	8	—	—	15	30	—	—	—	—	—

PERCENTAGE DAILY VALUE

	Calories	Protein	Fat	Sat. Fat	Cholesterol	Carbohydrates	Fiber	Sodium	Potassium	Calcium	Iron	Zinc	Magnesium	Vitamin A	Vitamin C	Thiamin	Riboflavin	Niacin	Vitamin B$_{12}$	Folic acid
PASTA ENTREE, FROZEN (continued)																				
(Stouffer's Lunch Express) 10 oz	90	—	18	23	13	14	16	39	16	15	15	—	—	15	20	—	—	—	—	—
(Swanson) 10 oz	410	45	23	—	—	15	—	45	—	45	15	—	—	10	10	20	20	15	—	—
(Weight Watchers) 10 1/4 oz	270	40	9	10	2	10	32	21	21	40	15	—	—	35	20	—	—	—	—	—
microwave (Hormel Micro Cup) 7 1/2 oz	250	13	20	30	8	8	—	39	9	5	8	7	7	10	3	8	12	10	—	—
vegetable (Stouffer's) 10 1/2 oz	370	33	29	25	12	10	12	34	12	45	6	—	—	30	2	15	30	6	—	—
zucchini (Healthy Choice Quick Meals) 11 1/2 oz	250	23	5	10	5	14	—	17	24	25	15	—	—	35	10	25	15	10	—	—
(Stouffer's Lean Cuisine) 11 oz	260	28	9	10	7	11	—	22	19	25	8	—	—	15	10	10	15	10	—	—
linguini																				
clam sauce (Stouffer's Lean Cuisine) 9 5/8 oz	280	28	12	10	22	12	—	23	3	4	15	—	—	*	*	20	10	10	—	—
scallops & clams (Budget Gourmet Light & Healthy) 9 1/2 oz	280	20	15	25	15	11	—	30	9	10	10	—	—	4	15	2	15	15	—	—
shrimp & clams (Budget Gourmet) 10 oz	270	20	14	—	17	12	—	48	11	8	2	—	—	90	10	20	10	15	—	—
macaroni & beef (Healthy Choice Quick Meals) 8 1/2 oz	200	20	5	5	5	11	—	17	15	4	10	—	—	20	25	20	15	*	—	—
(Weight Watchers) 9 1/2 oz	230	23	8	8	5	11	8	22	18	8	20	—	—	15	15	—	—	—	—	—
cheese (Swanson) 9 oz	260	40	14	—	—	9	—	43	—	15	15	—	—	8	40	20	20	20	—	—
in tomato sauce (Stouffer's Lean Cuisine) 10 oz	250	23	9	5	8	12	—	22	13	6	15	—	—	10	6	10	10	15	—	—
tomato (Stouffer's) 11 1/2 oz	340	35	18	25	17	13	16	64	19	4	15	—	—	8	20	4	6	10	—	—
macaroni & cheese (Budget Gourmet Side Dish) 5 3/4 oz	230	14	18	—	12	7	—	24	3	20	6	—	—	12	2	10	10	6	—	—
(Green Giant One Serving) 5 3/4 oz	220	17	12	25	8	9	—	20	4	15	6	—	—	10	*	8	8	10	—	—
(Healthy Choice Quick Meals) 9 oz	280	20	9	15	7	15	—	22	6	15	10	—	—	*	*	20	15	6	—	—
(Stouffer's) 12 oz	330	18	26	30	10	10	8	39	5	30	2	—	—	2	*	10	15	2	—	—
(Stouffer's Lean Cuisine) 9 oz	290	25	14	20	10	12	—	23	5	25	8	—	—	*	*	20	25	8	—	—
(Swanson) 7 oz	200	15	12	—	—	—	—	31	—	15	6	—	—	8	*	6	10	4	—	—
(Swanson) 12 1/4 oz	340	25	18	—	—	16	—	40	—	20	10	—	—	50	30	15	20	6	—	—
(Swanson) 9 oz	220	20	14	—	—	8	—	34	—	15	6	—	—	*	*	10	10	2	—	—
(Weight Watchers) 9 oz	260	25	9	10	7	14	28	23	12	25	10	—	—	10	*	—	—	—	—	—
broccoli (Stouffer's Lean Cuisine) 9 1/2 oz	60	—	11	15	7	10	20	19	9	10	6	—	—	25	20	—	—	—	—	—
(Stouffer's Lunch Express) 10 3/8 oz	170	—	29	25	10	11	12	37	11	30	6	—	—	20	50	—	—	—	—	—
casserole (Banquet) 6 1/2 oz	290	13	22	—	—	10	—	32	—	15	4	—	—	8	*	2	6	2	—	—
(Morton) 6 1/2 oz	290	13	22	—	—	10	—	32	—	15	4	—	—	8	*	2	6	2	—	—
cheddar & parmesan (Budget Gourmet Light & Healthy) 10 1/2 oz	330	30	12	20	10	16	—	32	7	35	8	—	—	6	2	30	30	15	—	—
microwave (Hormel Micro Cup) 7 1/2 oz	260	20	17	30	15	9	—	27	6	10	6	7	7	8	10	6	15	6	—	—

	Calories	Protein	Fat	Sat. Fat	Cholesterol	Carbohydrates	Fiber	Sodium	Potassium	Calcium	Iron	Zinc	Magnesium	Vitamin A	Vitamin C	Thiamin	Riboflavin	Niacin	Vitamin B12	Folic acid
PASTA ENTREE, FROZEN (continued)																				
mini-franks (Kid Cuisine) 9 oz	360	13	23	—	12	16	—	38	10	10	10	—	—	2	6	15	15	4	—	—
nacho (Healthy Choice Quick Meals) 9 oz	280	22	8	15	7	15	—	23	12	20	8	—	—	*	*	40	30	*	—	—
manicotti cheese (Budget Gourmet) 10 oz	440	30	37	—	25	12	—	31	17	35	15	—	—	190	10	30	25	25	—	—
(Healthy Choice) 9 1/4 oz	220	25	5	10	10	11	—	13	17	15	15	—	—	25	10	20	15	10	—	—
(Stouffer's) 9 oz	150	—	25	35	17	11	28	34	15	40	6	—	—	10	20	—	—	—	—	—
(Weight Watchers) 9 1/4 oz	260	28	12	13	8	10	16	21	21	35	10	—	—	30	15	—	—	—	—	—
noodles & chicken (Swanson) 10 1/2 oz	250	10	17	—	—	10	—	27	—	6	10	—	—	30	45	15	15	20	—	—
microwave (Hormel Micro Cup) 7 1/2 oz	174	12	11	10	10	6	—	42	7	4	7	5	6	27	14	5	7	9	—	—
noodles romanoff (Stouffer's) 12 oz	460	—	38	30	16	16	16	58	7	15	6	—	—	5	*	—	—	—	—	—
pasta dijon (Green Giant Garden Gourmet) 1 pkg (9 1/2 oz)	260	12	26	45	18	7	16	26	9	8	8	—	—	25	50	8	10	10	—	—
pasta florentine (Green Giant Garden Gourmet) 1 pkg (9 1/2 oz)	230	23	14	25	8	9	16	35	8	30	10	—	—	190	10	8	20	10	—	—
penne sun-dried tomatoes (Weight Watchers) 10 oz	290	22	14	13	5	16	32	23	11	15	20	—	—	4	4	—	—	—	—	—
Italian sausage (Budget Gourmet Light & Healthy) 10 oz	320	20	14	10	2	18	—	25	11	8	10	—	—	15	25	35	20	20	—	—
portafino (Weight Watchers) 9 1/2 oz	150	12	2	*	*	10	16	11	13	10	10	—	—	25	25	—	—	—	—	—
ravioli beef (Hormel Micro Cup) 7 1/2 oz	270	15	17	20	7	11	—	38	10	6	9	7	8	10	19	10	16	13	—	—
(Stouffer's) 9 1/2 oz	370	—	22	20	27	14	20	28	15	8	10	—	—	10	10	—	—	—	—	—
cheese (Budget Gourmet Light & Healthy) 9 1/2 oz	290	20	20	30	10	11	—	31	12	20	15	—	—	100	20	20	15	20	—	—
(Healthy Choice) 9 oz	250	23	3	5	7	15	—	17	17	25	15	—	—	50	8	20	15	10	—	—
(Stouffer's Lean Cuisine) 8 1/2 oz	240	22	11	15	18	10	—	18	11	15	6	—	—	10	10	*	10	6	—	—
(Stouffer's Lunch Express) 8 1/2 oz	90	—	18	20	20	13	8	26	12	20	10	—	—	10	20	—	—	—	—	—
(Weight Watchers) 9 oz	280	28	9	10	5	13	20	23	19	35	15	—	—	20	8	—	—	—	—	—
florentine (Weight Watchers) 8 1/2 oz	170	18	2	*	3	10	24	22	15	10	15	—	—	25	20	—	—	—	—	—
mini-cheese (Kid Cuisine) 8 3/4 oz	290	10	12	—	5	17	—	32	10	8	8	—	—	25	2	10	10	4	—	—
(Swanson Kids') 11 3/4 oz	530	30	20	—	—	—	—	25	—	10	20	—	—	10	35	20	20	10	—	—
tomato sauce (Stouffer's) 9 1/2 oz	360	—	22	25	28	14	16	30	12	25	8	—	—	8	10	—	—	—	—	—
rigatoni broccoli & chicken (Budget Gourmet Light & Healthy) 10 3/4 oz	290	30	11	15	15	—	—	30	9	25	10	—	—	8	2	25	25	15	—	—
meat sauce (Healthy Choice Quick Meals) 9 1/2 oz	260	25	9	10	10	11	—	22	20	15	15	—	—	20	4	20	15	15	—	—

	Calories	Protein	Fat	Sat. Fat	Cholesterol	Carbohydrates	Fiber	Sodium	Potassium	Calcium	Iron	Zinc	Magnesium	Vitamin A	Vitamin C	Thiamin	Riboflavin	Niacin	Vitamin B₁₂	Folic acid
PASTA ENTREE, FROZEN (continued)																				
(Stouffer's Lunch Express) 10 3/4 oz	90	—	18	13	10	15	12	30	13	6	10	—	—	15	20	—	—	—	—	—
meat sauce & cheese *(Stouffer's Lean Cuisine)* 9 oz	210	23	6	5	8	10	—	23	18	10	15	—	—	15	10	15	15	10	—	—
rotini three cheese *(Weight Watchers)* 9 1/2 oz	270	23	14	15	3	12	16	19	11	25	10	—	—	20	6	—	—	—	—	—
rotini cheddar (Green Giant Garden Gourmet) 1 pkg (9 1/2 oz)	230	15	15	25	7	11	18	24	15	15	6	—	—	220	50	10	20	10	—	—
shells tomato sauce *(Stouffer's)* 9 1/4 oz	340	—	25	35	17	10	20	38	13	45	8	—	—	15	10	—	—	—	—	—
spaghetti (Light & Elegant) 9 oz	220	20	12	—	7	8	—	18	16	8	15	—	—	20	20	15	10	10	—	—
chunky tomato & meat sauce *(Budget Gourmet Light & Healthy)* 10 oz	300	30	12	10	12	15	—	20	11	6	8	—	—	8	15	25	15	25	—	—
meat sauce *(Healthy Choice Quick Meals)* 10 oz	280	23	9	10	7	14	—	20	15	6	20	—	—	25	8	25	15	10	—	—
(Kid Cuisine) 9 1/4 oz	310	12	12	—	10	17	—	32	10	6	15	—	—	25	4	15	10	6	—	—
(Morton) 8 1/2 oz	170	8	3	—	3	11	—	39	8	*	8	—	—	60	15	8	4	4	—	—
(Stouffer's) 12 7/8 oz	430	27	20	23	13	19	24	32	228	18	8	15	—	—	10	10	10	10	20	—
(Stouffer's Lean Cuisine Lunch Express) 11 1/2 oz	290	25	9	10	7	15	—	21	14	6	20	—	—	10	10	20	20	20	—	—
(Stouffer's Lean Cuisine Lunch Express) 9 1/2 oz	290	33	11	10	10	12	—	23	14	8	20	—	—	8	*	20	20	20	—	—
(Stouffer's Lunch Express) 9 5/8 oz	90	—	15	18	10	14	20	24	14	6	10	—	—	10	10	—	—	—	—	—
(Weight Watchers) 10 oz	240	27	11	8	2	9	32	20	20	6	15	—	—	15	15	—	—	—	—	—
meatballs *(Hormel Micro Cup)* 7 1/2 oz	210	17	11	15	7	9	—	39	10	4	11	10	6	14	6	8	15	12	—	—
(Stouffer's) 12 5/8 oz	420	37	23	20	15	17	20	28	17	6	15	—	—	15	20	10	15	25	—	—
three cheese *(Budget Gourmet)* 10 oz	390	35	26	—	23	12	—	27	10	45	10	—	—	100	15	20	25	10	—	—
tortellini cheese *(Budget Gourmet Side Dish)* 5 1/2 oz	200	10	12	—	7	8	—	22	6	10	8	—	—	90	8	15	10	15	—	—
cheese w/ alfredo sauce *(Stouffer's)* 8 7/8 oz	550	—	51	90	53	13	20	30	8	40	15	—	—	2	6	—	—	—	—	—
cheese w/ tomato sauce *(Stouffer's)* 9 1/4 oz	290	—	9	25	35	13	16	31	13	30	20	—	—	10	10	—	—	—	—	—
(Weight Watchers) 9 oz	290	20	6	10	8	17	12	21	20	25	15	—	—	20	15	—	—	—	—	—
tortellini provencale (Green Giant Garden Gourmet) 1 pkg (9 1/2 oz)	260	17	9	10	5	11	12	35	15	20	15	—	—	150	2	10	10	20	—	—
vegetable (Budget Gourmet Light & Healthy) 10 1/2 oz	290	25	15	25	5	12	—	32	12	30	10	—	—	80	8	20	20	15	—	—
w/ chicken marinara *(Stouffer's Lean Cuisine Lunch Express)* 9 1/8 oz	50	—	9	8	7	13	16	22	11	4	4	—	—	20	20	—	—	—	—	—
w/ tuna casserole *(Stouffer's Lean Cuisine Lunch Express)* 9 5/8 oz	50	—	9	10	7	13	16	25	8	20	10	—	—	25	2	—	—	—	—	—

	Calories	Protein	Fat	Sat. Fat	Cholesterol	Carbohydrates	Fiber	Sodium	Potassium	Calcium	Iron	Zinc	Magnesium	Vitamin A	Vitamin C	Thiamin	Riboflavin	Niacin	Vitamin B12	Folic acid
PASTA ENTREE, FROZEN (continued)																				
w/ turkey dijon (Stouffer's Lean Cuisine Lunch Express) 9 7/8 oz	60	—	9	8	10	12	24	24	9	10	10	—	—	25	30	—	—	—	—	—
wheels & cheese sauce (Swanson Kids') 10 3/4 oz	390	25	22	—	—	—		32	—	25	10	—	—	30	20	4	15	50		
PASTA SAUCE (see also TOMATO SAUCE)																				
alfredo (Contadina Refrigerated) 1/2 cup	400	12	58	89	26	2	1	21	—	20	*	—	—	*	*	—	—	—	—	—
light (Contadina Refrigerated) 1/2 cup	190	13	20	35	14	3	1	23	—	25	*	—	—	*	*	—	—	—	—	—
mix (Knorr) 1/4 oz mix	80	2	8	—		3	3	—	20	—	6	*	*	*	2	*	*	4	*	*
chunky (Hunt's) 1/2 cup	50	2	*	*	*	4	8	20	13	3	6	—	—	*	9	5	4	5	—	
light (Contadina Refrigerated) 1/2 cup	45	3	*	*	*	2	9	19	—	6	4	—	—	35	*					
clam red (Progresso) 1/2 cup	70	8	5	—	—	2	—	23	6	2	—	—	—	8	*	*	12	8	—	
clam white (Progresso) 1/2 cup	110	15	12	—	—	*	*	12	2	*	—	—	—	—	4	*	4	2	—	—
four cheese w/ wine (Contadina Refrigerated) 1/2 cup	250	13	43	70	24	3	2	20	—	25	*	—	—	*	*	—	—	—	—	—
garden combination extra chunky (Prego) 1/2 cup	80	2	3	—	—	*		17	—	4	6	—	—	20	40	6	4	6		
garden vegetable light (Contadina Refrigerated) 1/2 cup	45	3	*	*	*	3	12	22	—	6	4	—	—	25	2					
garlic & onion (Del Monte) 1/2 cup	70	3	*	*	*	5	3	18	—	4	10	—	—	15	40	—	—	—	—	—
green pepper & mushroom (Del Monte) 1/2 cup	70	3	*	*	*	4	2	13	—	4	8	—	—	15	40					
homestyle plain (Hunt's) 1/2 cup	60	3	3	*	*	3	8	22	11	2	9	—	—	*	12	6	4	15		
homestyle w/ meat (Hunt's) 1/2 cup	60	5	3	*	*	3	8	24	11	2	9	—	—	*	18	6	4	15		
homestyle w/ mushrooms (Hunt's) 1/2 cup	50	3	2	*	*	3	8	22	10	2	9	—	—	*	18	6	4	14		
low sodium (Prego) 1/2 cup	100	2	8	—	—	4	*	*	—	4	6	—	—	30	30	4	4	8		
marinara (Contadina Refrigerated) 1/2 cup	80	3	5	2	—	2	8	19	—	4	8	—	—	15	*					
marinara (Hain) 1/2 cup	40	3	2	*	*	3	12	17	8	2	10	—	—	45	25	*	6	6		
marinara (Prego) 1/2 cup	100	2	9	—	—	3	*	26	—	4	4	—	—	20	30	4	2	6		
marinara (Progresso) 1/2 cup	90	7	8	5	*	3	—	22	16	2	—	—	—	10	*	*	2	6		
marinara canned 1/2 cup	85	3	6	3	*	4	—	33	15	2	6	2	8	24	27	4	4	10	*	4
meat flavor (Del Monte) 1/2 cup	70	5	3	*	*	4	3	16	—	4	6	—	—	15	35	—	—	—	—	—
meat flavor (Progresso) 1/2 cup	110	7	8	5	2	4	—	27	17	4	—	—	—	6	*	*	4	8	—	—
meat flavor (Weight Watchers) 1/2 cup	60	3	2	*	*	3	16	18	13	4	—	—	—	10	20	—	—	—	—	—

PASTA SAUCE (continued)

	Calories	Protein	Fat	Sat. Fat	Cholesterol	Carbohydrates	Fiber	Sodium	Potassium	Calcium	Iron	Zinc	Magnesium	Vitamin A	Vitamin C	Thiamin	Riboflavin	Niacin	Vitamin B$_{12}$	Folic acid
mushroom																				
(Contadina Pasta Ready) 1/2 cup	50	4	2	3	*	3	4	27	—	6	4	—	—	10	15	—	—	—	—	—
(Del Monte) 1/2 cup	80	3	2	*	*	5	3	21	—	4	6	—	—	10	30	—	—	—	—	—
(Hain) 1/2 cup	40	3	2	*	*	3	12	15	8	2	15	—	—	45	20	*	6	10	—	—
(Progresso) 1/2 cup	30	5	8	5	2	4	—	26	15	4	—	—	—	4	*	*	4	8	—	—
(Weight Watchers) 1/2 cup	60	3	*	*	*	4	16	17	16	6	—	—	—	10	25	—	—	—	—	—
mushroom & green pepper																				
extra chunky																				
(Prego) 1/2 cup	90	2	5	—	—		*	17	—	2	6	—	—	15	20	4	4	4	—	—
mushroom & onion																				
extra chunky																				
(Prego) 1/2 cup	100	2	6	—	—		*	20	—	2	6	—	—	10	20	4	2	6	—	—
mushroom & tomato																				
extra chunky																				
(Prego) 1/2 cup	100	2	5	—	—		*	20	—	2	6	—	—	20	15	2	6	6	—	—
mushroom w/ extra spice																				
extra chunky																				
(Prego) 1/2 cup	100	2	5	—	—		*	19	—	4	6	—	—	15	35	6	4	6	—	—
onion & garlic																				
(Prego) 1/2 cup	100	2	6	—	—	5	*	21	—	2	6	—	—	20	8	2	2	6	—	—
pesto																				
mix																				
(Knorr) 1 1/2 oz	130	*	22	—	—	*	—	10	—	2	2	*	*	20	6	*	*	*	*	*
w/ sun-dried tomatoes																				
(Contadina Refrigerated)																				
1/2 cup	250	5	37	18	1	2	13	20	—	4	6	—	—	3	*	—	—	—	—	—
w/ basil																				
(Contadina Refrigerated)																				
1/2 cup	310	10	48	23	4	2	*	18	—	15	4	—	—	8	*	—	—	—	—	—
plain																				
(Contadina Pasta Ready) 1/2 cup	50	4	3	*	*	2	4	23	—	6	4	—	—	10	25	—	—	—	—	—
(Del Monte) 1/2 cup	80	3	2	*	*	5	3	19	—	4	8	—	—	10	35	—	—	—	—	—
(Prego) 1/2 cup	120	2	6	—	—	7	*	22	—	4	6	—	—	20	30	2	2	4	—	—
(Progresso) 1/2 cup	110	5	8	5	*	4	—	27	13	4	—	—	—	15	4	*	2	8	—	—
no sugar added																				
(Del Monte) 1/2 cup	60	3	2	*	*	4	3	19	—	4	8	—	—	10	35	—	—	—	—	—
plum tomato w/ basil																				
(Contadina Refrigerated) 1/2 cup	70	3	4	4	*	3	12	19	—	4	6	—	—	15	*	—	—	—	—	—
primavera																				
(Contadina Pasta Ready) 1/2 cup	50	4	2	3	*	3	4	25	—	6	4	—	—	15	15	—	—	—	—	—
rock lobster																				
(Progresso) 1/2 cup	120	7	12	5	3	4	8	18	12	2	—	—	—	15	30	6	6	8	—	—
sausage & green pepper																				
extra chunky																				
(Prego) 1/2 cup	160	6	12	—	—		*	21	—	4	6	—	—	20	30	4	2	4	—	—
sausage & pepper																				
spicy																				
(Contadina Refrigerated)																				
1/2 cup	100	7	7	5	4	3	11	22	—	4	4	—	—	10	*	—	—	—	—	—
three cheese																				
(Contadina Pasta Ready) 1/2 cup	70	4	6	*	—	3	—	27	—	10	4	—	—	10	15	—	—	—	—	—
(Prego) 1/2 cup	100	4	3	—	—		*	17	—	4	8	—	—	15	35	6	4	8	—	—
tomato & basil																				
(Prego) 1/2 cup	100	2	3	—	—		*	15	—	4	6	—	—	20	35	6	4	8	—	—
tomato, onion & garlic																				
extra chunky																				
(Prego) 1/2 cup	100	2	8	—	—		*	20	—	2	6	—	—	10	20	2	2	4	—	—
traditional																				
(Hunt's) 1/2 cup	70	3	3	*	*	4	8	22	19	2	9	—	—	*	9	6	4	8	—	—

		PERCENTAGE DAILY VALUE																		
	Calories	Protein	Fat	Sat. Fat	Cholesterol	Carbohydrates	Fiber	Sodium	Potassium	Calcium	Iron	Zinc	Magnesium	Vitamin A	Vitamin C	Thiamin	Riboflavin	Niacin	Vitamin B_{12}	Folic acid
PASTA SAUCE (continued)																				
w/ crushed red pepper *(Contadina Pasta Ready)* 1/2 cup	60	4	5	3	*	3	4	29	—	8	6	—	—	10	15	—	—	—	—	—
w/ meat *(Hunt's)* 1/2 cup	70	3	3	*	*	4	8	24	19	2	10	—	—	*	18	7	4	9	—	—
w/ meat flavor *(Prego)* 1/2 cup	120	4	6	—	—	7	*	24	—	4	6	—	—	20	25	2	2	6	—	—
w/ mushrooms *(Hunt's)* 1/2 cup	70	3	3	*	*	4	8	23	19	2	11	—	—	*	9	7	4	9	—	—
(Prego) 1/2 cup	120	2	6	—	—	7	*	23	—	4	4	—	—	20	25	2	4	6	—	—
w/ olives *(Contadina Pasta Ready)* 1/2 cup	60	4	5	3	*	3	4	27	—	8	4	—	—	10	15	—	—	—	—	—
PASTA SIDE DISH, FROM MIX																				
alfredo *(Lipton Noodles & Sauce)* 1/2 cup	200	10	15	—	—	7	—	25	—	8	6	4	4	6	*	20	8	10	—	—
angel hair parmesan *(Uncle Ben's Country Inn)* 1/2 cup	245	16	8	—	4	13	12	39	4	6	11	—	2	5	3	40	22	22	—	—
broccoli & white cheddar *(Uncle Ben's Country Inn)* 1/2 cup	240	16	8	—	3	13	10	33	2	6	6	—	*	*	2	20	12	11	—	—
butter & herb *(Uncle Ben's Country Inn)* 1/2 cup	230	12	9	—	3	12	4	37	2	3	11	—	*	*	24	37	24	18	—	—
w/ cheddar broccoli *(Kraft)* 1/2 cup	180	10	12	15	10	6	—	26	3	10	6	—	—	6	*	10	8	6	—	—
cheese *(Lipton Noodles & Sauce)* 1/2 cup	190	8	12	—	—	8	—	22	—	4	6	4	4	6	*	20	10	10	—	—
cheesy noodles *(Tuna Helper)* 7 3/4 oz	240	23	12	—	—	9	—	40	7	8	8	—	—	4	*	15	15	20	—	—
chicken *(Lipton Noodles & Sauce)* 1/2 cup	180	8	12	—	—	7	—	19	—	*	6	4	2	4	*	15	10	10	—	—
chicken broccoli *(Lipton Noodles & Sauce)* 1/2 cup	190	10	14	—	—	8	—	21	—	6	6	4	4	6	4	15	10	10	—	—
creamy garlic *(Uncle Ben's Country Inn)* 1/2 cup	261	16	7	—	3	15	8	25	2	3	6	—	*	*	*	21	10	10	—	—
creamy parmesan *(Hain)* 1/2 cup	80	12	6	5	2	4	6	9	5	3	3	—	—	2	*	2	3	2	—	—
creamy Swiss *(Hain)* 1/2 cup	90	12	7	8	2	4	7	8	6	3	3	—	—	2	*	2	4	*	—	—
fettuccine alfredo *(Uncle Ben's Country Inn)* 1/2 cup	310	14	9	—	4	14	7	27	2	4	6	—	*	*	*	20	12	10	—	—
herb linguine *(Uncle Ben's Country Inn)* 1/2 cup	240	14	5	—	2	14	9	27	2	3	6	—	*	*	6	20	9	11	—	—
Italian herb *(Hain)* 1/2 cup	85	12	8	8	2	3	8	8	2	5	4	—	—	2	*	*	*	3	—	—
mushroom fettuccine *(Uncle Ben's Country Inn)* 1/2 cup	250	15	9	—	4	14	9	27	2	3	6	—	*	*	*	19	7	14	—	—
noodle & cheese *(Kraft)* 1/2 cup	226	10	18	14	12	8	—	18	4	7	7	—	—	10	—	10	14	6	—	—
noodle & chicken *(Kraft)* 1/2 cup	160	7	10	7	10	8	—	30	3	*	7	—	—	*	*	10	6	6	—	—

	Calories	Protein	Fat	Sat. Fat	Cholesterol	Carbohydrates	Fiber	Sodium	Potassium	Calcium	Iron	Zinc	Magnesium	Vitamin A	Vitamin C	Thiamin	Riboflavin	Niacin	Vitamin B₁₂	Folic acid
PASTA SIDE DISH, FROM MIX (continued)																				
parmesan (Lipton Noodles & Sauce) 1/2 cup	210	10	17	—	—	7	—	20	—	8	6	4	4	8	*	20	10	10	—	—
primavera (Hain) 1/2 cup	90	10	8	5	3	3	5	8	3	5	3	—	—	10	*	2	3	2	—	—
salad																				
broccoli & vegetables (Kraft) 1/2 cup	210	6	25	10	3	5	—	12	3	2	6	—	—	8	*	8	4	4	—	—
garden primavera (Kraft) 1/2 cup	170	8	11	10	*	7	—	19	2	6	4	—	—	4	2	10	6	6	—	—
homestyle (Kraft) 1/2 cup	240	6	25	10	3	7	—	12	3	*	8	—	—	2	*	10	6	6	—	—
Italian (Kraft Light) 1/2 cup	130	8	5	20	*	7	—	17	4	6	8	—	—	4	2	10	6	6	—	—
rancher's choice (Kraft) 1/2 cup	250	8	25	30	3	7	—	15	3	*	8	—	—	2	*	10	6	6	—	—
(Kraft Light) 1/2 cup	170	8	11	20	*	8	—	15	4	2	8	—	—	2	*	10	6	6	—	—
sour cream w/ chives (Kraft) 1/2 cup	180	8	12	10	8	7	—	15	2	4	4	—	—	4	*	10	6	6	—	—
stroganoff (Lipton Noodles & Sauce) 1/2 cup	180	8	12	—	—	7	—	20	—	4	6	4	4	8	*	20	8	10	—	—
tangy cheddar (Hain) 1/2 cup	95	12	9	8	3	3	7	7	4	5	2	—	—	4	*	5	3	3	—	—
vegetable alfredo (Uncle Ben's Country Inn) 1/2 cup	240	14	7	—	4	14	9	23	2	4	6	—	*	*	4	21	11	11	—	—
PASTA SIDE DISH, FROZEN																				
alfredo w/ broccoli (Budget Gourmet Side Dish) 5 1/2 oz	210	10	15	—	10	7	—	26	4	20	4	—	—	8	8	10	10	4	—	—
pasta parmesan with sweet peas (Green Giant One Serving) 1 pkg (5 1/2 oz)	160	16	8	16	4	8	10	18	5	16	8	—	—	4	*	8	8	8	—	—
ziti in marinara sauce (Budget Gourmet Side Dish) 6 1/4 oz	200	10	14	—	3	8	—	25	6	8	6	—	—	50	8	10	8	10	—	—
PASTRAMI																				
beef (generic) 2 slices	198	16	25	30	78	*	*	29	*	*	6	76	3	*	3	4	6	74	17	7
(Thorn Apple Valley) 2 slices	200	76	*	*	10	*	*	34	—	—	—	—	—	*	*	—	—	—	—	—
PASTRAMI, TURKEY see TURKEY, COLD CUTS																				
PASTRY see specific listing																				
PASTRY COATING																				
butterscotch (generic) 1 cup	884	6	76	204	*	38	*	7	9	6	*	*	*	*	*	9	*	*	3	*
peanut butter (generic) 1 cup	845	52	78	112	*	25	8	18	24	19	16	23	47	*	*	6	20	70	2	40
PEA, GREEN																				
raw (generic) 1/2 cup	58	7	*	*	*	3	16	*	5	2	6	6	6	9	48	13	6	8	*	12
boiled (generic) 1/2 cup	67	7	*	*	*	4	16	*	6	2	7	6	8	10	19	14	7	8	*	13
boiled w/ salt (generic) 1/2 cup	67	7	*	*	*	4	—	8	6	2	7	6	8	10	19	14	7	8	*	13
PEA, GREEN, CANNED																				
drained (generic) 1/2 cup	59	6	*	*	*	4	12	8	4	2	4	4	4	13	14	7	4	3	*	10
early June (Bush Bros) 1/2 cup	80	8	2	*	*	4	16	14	—	2	8	—	—	6	15	—	—	—	—	—

	Calories	Protein	Fat	Sat. Fat	Cholesterol	Carbohydrates	Fiber	Sodium	Potassium	Calcium	Iron	Zinc	Magnesium	Vitamin A	Vitamin C	Thiamin	Riboflavin	Niacin	Vitamin B₁₂	Folic acid
PEA, GREEN, CANNED (continued)																				
low salt																				
drained																				
(generic) 1/2 cup	59	6	*	*	*	4	—	*	4	2	4	4	4	13	14	7	4	3	*	10
solid & liquid																				
(generic) 1/2 cup	61	6	*	*	*	4	8	*	3	2	8	6	5	9	23	9	5	5	*	9
seasoned																				
(generic) 1/2 cup	57	6	*	*	*	3	—	12	4	2	8	5	4	10	22	7	4	4	*	8
small early																				
(Bush Bros) 1/2 cup	70	7	2	*	*	4	12	14	—	2	8	—	—	6	15	—	—	—	—	—
solid & liquid																				
(generic) 1/2 cup	61	6	*	*	*	4	8	14	3	2	8	6	5	9	23	9	5	5	*	9
sweet																				
(Bush Bros) 1/2 cup	90	8	2	*	*	5	20	16	—	2	8	—	—	6	6	—	—	—	—	—
(Del Monte) 1/2 cup	60	5	*	*	*	4	16	15	—	2	8	—	—	4	30	—	—	—	—	—
early																				
(Del Monte) 1/2 cup	60	5	*	*	*	3	16	15	—	*	8	—	—	6	40	—	—	—	—	—
low salt																				
(Green Giant) 1/2 cup	50	7	*	*	*	4	12	8	3	2	6	—	—	6	10	6	4	8	—	—
no salt added																				
(Del Monte) 1/2 cup	60	5	*	*	*	4	16	*	—	2	8	—	—	4	30	—	—	—	—	—
reduced salt																				
(Del Monte) 1/2 cup	60	5	*	*	*	4	16	8	2	2	8	—	—	4	30	—	—	—	—	—
very young small early																				
(Green Giant) 1/2 cup	50	5	*	*	*	4	12	16	3	2	8	—	—	6	10	8	4	4	—	—
very young small sweet																				
(Green Giant) 1/2 cup	50	7	*	*	*	4	16	16	3	2	8	—	—	6	15	10	4	6	—	—
very young tender sweet																				
(Green Giant) 1/2 cup	50	7	*	*	*	4	16	16	3	2	8	—	—	6	10	10	4	6	—	—
w/ pork																				
(Friends) 4 oz	140	12	2	3	*	9	24	14	12	6	20	—	—	*	*	*	4	4	—	—
PEA, GREEN, FROZEN																				
(Bird's Eye) 3 1/3 oz	80	8	*	*	*	4	16	5	—	2	8	6	6	15	30	20	6	10	—	15
(generic) 1/2 cup	55	6	*	*	*	3	12	3	3	2	6	4	5	10	22	12	4	6	*	10
baby early																				
in butter sauce																				
(Green Giant One Serving)																				
4 1/2 oz	90	8	3	10	2	6	20	17	*	4	8	—	—	10	10	10	4	8	—	—
baby early																				
plain																				
(Le Sueur Harvest Fresh) 1/2 cup	60	7	2	*	*	4	12	6	3	2	6	—	—	10	25	8	4	6	—	—
boiled																				
(generic) 1/2 cup	62	7	*	*	*	4	16	3	4	2	7	5	6	11	13	15	5	6	*	12
boiled w/ salt																				
(generic) 1/2 cup	62	7	*	*	*	4	—	11	4	2	7	5	6	11	13	15	5	6	*	12
early green																				
in butter sauce																				
(Le Sueur) 1/2 cup	80	8	3	3	2	5	12	18	3	2	6	—	—	10	15	10	4	6	—	—
Le Sueur																				
(Green Giant Select) 1/2 cup	60	7	*	*	*	4	16	5	3	2	6	—	—	10	20	10	10	6	—	—
sweet																				
(Green Giant) 1/2 cup	50	7	*	*	*	4	16	4	3	*	4	—	—	6	15	15	4	8	—	—
in butter sauce																				
(Green Giant) 1/2 cup	80	8	3	3	2	5	16	17	4	2	8	—	—	10	15	15	4	8	—	—
plain																				
(Green Giant Harvest Fresh)																				
1/2 cup	50	7	*	*	*	4	12	6	3	2	6	—	—	6	10	10	2	6	—	—
tender																				
(Bird's Eye Deluxe) 1/2 cup	60	8	*	*	*	4	22	5	—	*	6	—	—	15	30	—	—	—	—	—

	Calories	Protein	Fat	Sat. Fat	Cholesterol	Carbohydrates	Fiber	Sodium	Potassium	Calcium	Iron	Zinc	Magnesium	Vitamin A	Vitamin C	Thiamin	Riboflavin	Niacin	Vitamin B$_{12}$	Folic acid
PEA, POD																				
raw																				
1/2 cup	30	3	*	*	*	2	8	*	4	3	8	*	4	2	72	7	3	2	*	8
boiled																				
1/2 cup	34	4	*	*	*	2	8	*	5	3	9	2	5	2	64	7	4	2	*	6
boiled w/ salt																				
1/2 cup	34	4	*	*	*	2	—	8	5	3	9	2	5	2	64	7	4	2	*	6
PEA, POD, FROZEN																				
boiled																				
(generic) 1/2 cup	42	5	*	*	*	2	—	*	5	5	11	3	6	3	29	3	6	2	*	7
boiled w/salt																				
(generic) 1/2 cup	42	5	*	*	*	2	—	8	5	5	11	3	6	3	29	3	6	2	*	7
Chinese																				
(Chun King) 1 1/2 oz	20	2	*	*	*	*	—	*	*	*	2	—	—	2	15	4	2	*	—	—
snap peas																				
(Bird's Eye Deluxe) 2 1/2 oz	45	3	*	*	*	3	—	*	—	6	4	2	4	8	35	8	4	4	*	*
snow																				
(La Choy) 3 oz	35	3	*	*	*	2	—	*	—	4	10	*	—	4	30	4	6	2	*	—
sugar snap																				
(Green Giant Harvest Fresh)																				
1/2 cup	30	3	*	*	*	3	8	4	2	2	2	—	—	4	10	4	2	*	—
(Green Giant Select) 1/2 cup	30	3	*	*	*	3	8	*	2	4	2	—	—	4	15	6	2	*	—
PEA COMBINATION, CANNED																				
peas & carrots																				
(Bush Bros) 1/2 cup	60	5	2	*	*	3	12	15	—	2	10	—	—	100	10	—	—	—	*	—
(Del Monte) 1/2 cup	60	3	*	*	*	4	8	15	—	2	4	—	—	100	20	—	—	—	*	—
diet																				
(generic) 1/2 cup	49	5	*	*	*	4	16	*	4	3	5	5	4	148	14	6	4	4	*	6
solid & liquid																				
(generic) 1/2 cup	49	5	*	*	*	4	16	14	4	3	5	4	4	148	14	6	4	4	*	6
peas & onions																				
(Green Giant) 1/2 cup	50	7	*	*	*	4	16	21	4	2	6	—	—	6	10	6	4	8	*	—
PEA COMBINATION, FROZEN																				
Le Sueur peas & mushrooms																				
(Green Giant Select) 1/2 cup	30	7	*	*	*	4	16	4	4	2	6	—	—	8	20	10	10	8	*	—
Le Sueur style																				
(Green Giant Valley																				
Combinations) 1/2 cup	70	7	3	*	*	4	8	17	4	2	6	—	—	6	25	10	2	6	*	—
peas & carrots																				
(generic) 1/2 cup	37	4	*	*	*	3	8	2	4	2	4	2	3	133	13	9	3	5	*	6
boiled																				
(generic) 1/2 cup	38	4	*	*	*	3	12	2	4	2	4	2	3	124	11	12	3	5	*	5
peas & onions																				
boiled																				
(generic) 1/2 cup	41	4	*	*	*	3	12	*	3	*	5	2	3	6	10	9	4	5	*	5
boiled w/ salt																				
(generic) 1/2 cup	41	4	*	*	*	3	—	10	3	*	5	2	3	6	10	9	4	5	*	5
PEA, SPLIT see SPLIT PEA																				
PEA SPROUT																				
raw																				
1/2 cup	77	9	*	*	*	6	—	*	7	2	8	4	8	2	10	9	5	9	*	22
boiled																				
3 oz	100	10	*	*	*	6	—	*	6	2	8	4	9	2	9	12	14	5	*	8
boiled w/ salt																				
3 oz	100	10	*	*	*	6	—	8	6	2	8	4	9	2	9	12	14	5	*	8
PEACH																				
1 fruit	37	*	*	*	*	3	8	*	5	*	*	*	*	2	9	10	*	2	4	*	*
1/2 cup slices	37	*	*	*	*	3	8	*	5	*	*	*	*	9	9	*	2	4	*	*

	Calories	Protein	Fat	Sat. Fat	Cholesterol	Carbohydrates	Fiber	Sodium	Potassium	Calcium	Iron	Zinc	Magnesium	Vitamin A	Vitamin C	Thiamin	Riboflavin	Niacin	Vitamin B₁₂	Folic acid
PEACH, CANNED																				
in extra heavy syrup (generic) 1/2 cup	126	*	*	*	*	11	—	*	3	*			2	3	3	*	2	3	*	*
in extra light syrup (Del Monte Snack Cups) 1 container	60	*	*	*	*	5	4	*	—	*	2	—	—	6	8	—	—	—	*	*
(generic) 1/2 cup	52	*	*	*	*	5	—	*	3	*	2	*	2	7	6	2	*	5	*	*
freestone (Del Monte) 1/2 cup	60	*	*	*	*	5	4	*	—	*	2	—	—	2	2	—	—	—	*	*
slices cling (Del Monte) 1/2 cup	60	*	*	*	*	5	4	*	—	*	2	—	—	6	8	—	—	—	*	*
in fruit juice slices cling (Del Monte) 1/2 cup	60	*	*	*	*	5	4	*	—	*	2	—	—	6	8	—	—	—	*	*
in heavy syrup (Del Monte Snack Cups) 1 container	90	*	*	*	*	8	4	*	—	*	2	—	—	6	8	—	—	—	*	*
(generic) 1/2 cup	95	*	*	*	*	8	4	*	3	*	2	*	2	8	6	*	2	4	*	*
halves (Hunt's) 1/2 cup	90	*	*	*	*	8	*	*	3	*	2	—	—	*	3	*	2	4	*	*
cling (Del Monte) 1/2 cup	100	*	*	*	*	8	4	*	—	*	2	—	—	6	8	—	—	—	*	*
freestone (Del Monte) 1/2 cup	100	*	*	*	*	8	4	*	—	*	2	—	—	2	2	—	—	—	*	*
melba (Del Monte) 1/2 cup	100	*	*	*	*	8	4	*	—	*	2	—	—	6	8	—	—	—	*	*
slices (Hunt's) 1/2 cup	90	*	*	*	*	8	*	*	3	*	2	—	—	*	3	*	2	4	*	*
cling (Del Monte) 1/2 cup	100	*	*	*	*	8	4	*	—	*	*	—	—	6	8	—	—	—	*	*
freestone (Del Monte) 1/2 cup	100	*	*	*	*	8	4	*	—	*	*	—	—	2	2	—	—	—	*	*
spiced (generic) 1 fruit	66	*	*	*	*	6	4	*	2	*	*	*	2	6	8	*	2	2	*	*
whole cling (Del Monte) 1/2 cup	100	*	*	*	*	8	3	*	—	*	4	—	—	6	8	—	—	—	*	*
in juice (generic) 1/2 cup	55	*	*	*	*	5	4	*	5	*	2	*	2	9	7	*	*	4	*	*
in light syrup (generic) 1/2 cup	68	*	*	*	*	6	4	*	3	*	2	*	2	9	5	*	2	4	*	*
in peach juice (Del Monte Snack Cups) 1 container	60	*	*	*	*	5	4	*	—	*	2	—	—	6	8	—	—	—	*	*
in water (generic) 1/2 cup	29	*	*	*	*	2	4	*	3	*	2	*	2	13	6	*	*	3	*	*
PEACH, DEHYDRATED																				
sulfured 1/2 cup	189	5	*	*	*	16	—	*	22	2	18	3	8	16	10	2	4	14	*	*
cooked 1/2 cup	161	4	*	*	*	14	—	*	19	2	15	3	7	10	14	*	4	12	*	*
PEACH, DRIED (Del Monte Snap-E-Tom) 1/4 cup	51	2	*	*	*	5	12	*	—	*	3	—	—	7	6	—	—	—	*	*
cooked w/ out sugar 1/2 cup halves	99	2	*	*	*	8	12	*	12	*	9	2	4	5	8	*	2	10	*	*
w/ sugar 1/2 cup halves	139	2	*	*	*	12	12	*	11	*	9	2	4	5	8	*	2	9	*	*
sulfured 1/2 cup halves	191	5	*	*	*	16	28	*	23	2	18	3	8	35	6	*	10	18	*	*

	Calories	Protein	Fat	Sat. Fat	Cholesterol	Carbohydrates	Fiber	Sodium	Potassium	Calcium	Iron	Zinc	Magnesium	Vitamin A	Vitamin C	Thiamin	Riboflavin	Niacin	Vitamin B12	Folic acid
PEACH, FROZEN																				
sweetened 1 cup slices	235	3	*	*	*	20	16	*	9	*	5	*	3	14	392	2	5	8	*	*
PEACH BUTTER																				
(Smucker's) 1 tbsp	15	*	*	*	*	*	*	*	*	*	*	*	*	*	*	*	*	*	*	*
PEACH DRINK																				
from concentrate (Mott's Fruit Basket) 8 fl oz	130	*	*	*	*	11	*	*	6	*	2	—	—	6	25	*	*	*	—	—
PEACH GLAZE																				
(Marie's) 2 1/3 oz	90	*	*	*	*	7	*	5	—	*	*	—	—	*	*	*	*	*	—	—
PEACH JUICE																				
(Farmer's Market) 8 fl oz	120	*	*	*	*	10	*	*	2	*	*	—	—	*	4	—	—	—	—	—
(Smucker's) 8 fl oz	120	*	*	*	*	10	*	*	11	*	23	*	*	10	10	2	4	4	*	*
PEACH NECTAR																				
(generic) 8 fl oz	134	*	*	*	*	12	4	*	3	*	3	*	2	13	22	*	2	4	*	*
(Knudsen Exotic Blends) 8 fl oz	120	*	*	*	*	10	*	*	5	2	6	—	—	*	6	—	—	—	—	—
vitamin C added (generic) 8 fl oz	134	*	*	*	*	12	—	*	3	*	3	*	2	13	111	*	2	4	*	*
PEANUT																				
all types raw (generic) 1 oz	161	12	22	10	*	2	10	*	6	3	7	6	12	*	*	12	3	17	*	17
Spanish raw (generic) 1 oz	162	13	22	11	*	2	10	*	6	3	6	4	14	*	*	13	3	23	*	17
Valencia raw (generic) 1 oz	162	12	21	11	*	2	8	*	3	2	4	7	13	*	*	12	5	19	*	18
Virginia raw (generic) 1 oz	160	12	21	9	*	2	8	*	6	3	4	9	12	*	*	13	2	18	*	17
all types dry-roasted salted (generic) 1 oz	166	11	22	10	*	2	10	10	6	2	4	6	13	*	*	9	2	19	*	11
unsalted (generic) 1 oz	166	11	22	10	*	2	10	*	6	2	4	6	13	*	*	9	2	19	*	11
golden roast (Fisher) 1 oz	160	12	18	10	*	3	8	*	—	—	2	—	—	*	*	—	—	—	—	—
in shell salted (Fisher) 1 oz	170	12	22	10	*	2	8	7	—	*	8	—	—	*	*	—	—	—	—	—
oil roasted (Fisher) 1 oz	170	12	23	13	*	2	8	5	—	*	2	—	—	*	*	—	—	—	—	—
w/ salt (generic) 1 oz	165	12	22	10	*	2	8	5	6	2	3	13	13	*	*	5	2	20	*	9
oil-roasted salted (generic) 1 oz	165	13	22	10	*	2	10	5	6	3	3	13	13	*	*	5	2	20	*	9
unsalted (generic) 1 oz	165	13	22	10	*	2	10	*	6	3	3	13	13	*	*	5	2	20	*	9
barbecue (Fisher) 1 oz	160	12	17	10	*	3	8	9	—	*	*	—	—	*	*	—	—	—	—	—
honey roasted (Fisher) 1 oz	160	10	22	13	*	2	4	5	—	*	2	—	—	*	*	—	—	—	—	—
(Weight Watchers) 1 bag (3/4 oz)	160	12	8	5	*	2	8	4	4	*	2	—	—	*	*	—	—	—	—	—
dry roasted (Fisher) 1 oz	170	10	20	13	*	2	4	5	—	*	2	—	—	*	*	—	—	—	—	—
hot (Frito-Lay) 1/4 cup	280	20	32	25	*	2	16	14	—	—	—	—	—	—	—	—	—	—	—	—

	Calories	Protein	Fat	Sat. Fat	Cholesterol	Carbohydrates	Fiber	Sodium	Potassium	Calcium	Iron	Zinc	Magnesium	Vitamin A	Vitamin C	Thiamin	Riboflavin	Niacin	Vitamin B_{12}	Folic acid
PEANUT (continued)																				
salted (Frito-Lay) 1 oz	180	12	23	25	*	*	12	7												
Spanish (Fisher) 1 oz	180	8	25	13	*	2	8	5	—	*	2	—	—	*	*	—	—	—	—	—
oil-roasted salted (generic) 1 oz	164	13	22	11	*	2	8	5	7	3	4	4	12	*	*	6	2	21	*	9
unsalted (generic) 1 oz	164	13	22	11	*	2	8	*	7	3	4	4	12	*	*	6	2	21	*	9
Valencia oil-roasted salted (generic) 1 oz	167	13	23	12	*	2	8	9	5	2	3	6	12	*	*	2	3	21	*	9
unsalted (generic) 1 oz	167	13	23	12	*	2	8	*	5	2	3	6	12	*	*	2	3	21	*	9
Virginia oil-roasted salted (generic) 1 oz	164	12	21	9	*	2	8	5	6	3	3	13	14	*	*	5	2	21	*	9
unsalted (generic) 1 oz	164	12	21	9	*	2	8	*	6	3	3	13	14	*	*	5	2	21	*	9
PEANUT BUTTER																				
crunchy (Jif) 2 tbsp	190	13	25	15	*	2	8	6	—	*	4	—	—	*	*	—	2	20	—	—
(Peter Pan) 2 tbsp	190	15	25	10	*	2	8	5	7	—	4	—	—	*	*	—	*	20	—	—
(Skippy) 2 tbsp	190	15	26	10	*	*	*	5	—	*	2	—	—	*	*	*	*	20	*	*
(Smucker's) 2 tbsp	200	13	25	15	*	2	—	5	—	*	4	*	*	*	*	*	*	25	*	*
all natural no salt added (Smucker's) 2 tbsp	200	13	25	15	*	2	—	*	—	*	4	*	*	*	*	—	*	25	*	*
honey nut (Skippy) 2 tbsp	190	13	26	10	*	2	*	4	—	*	2	—	—	*	*	*	*	20	*	*
reduced sugar/sodium (Jif) 2 tbsp	190	13	25	15	*	2	8	2	—	*	4	—	—	*	*	—	2	20	—	—
salt free (Peter Pan) 2 tbsp	190	15	26	10	*	2	8	*	7	2	4	—	—	*	*	*	*	20	—	—
salted (generic) 2 tbsp	188	13	25	16	*	2	8	6	7	*	3	6	13	*	*	3	2	22	*	7
unsalted (generic) 2 tbsp	188	13	25	16	*	2	8	*	7	*	3	6	13	*	*	3	2	22	*	7
smooth (Hollywood) 2 tbsp	140	12	20	--	*	16	*	*	*	—	--	--	*	*	*	*	8	20	--	—
(Jif) 2 tbsp	190	13	25	15	*	2	8	6	—	*	4	—	—	*	*	—	2	20	—	—
(Peter Pan) 2 tbsp	190	15	25	10	*	2	8	6	7	*	6	—	—	*	*	—	*	20	—	—
(Skippy) 2 tbsp	190	15	26	10	*	*	*	6	—	*	2	*	*	*	*	*	*	20	*	*
(Smucker's) 2 tbsp	200	13	25	15	*	2	—	5	—	*	4	*	*	*	*	*	*	25	*	*
all natural no salt added (Smucker's) 2 tbsp	200	13	25	15	*	2	—	*	—	*	4	*	*	*	*	—	*	25	*	*
blend w/ grape jelly (Smucker's Goober Grape) 2 tbsp	180	8	15	10	*	6	—	5	—	*	2	*	*	*	*	*	—	15	*	*
blend w/ strawberry jelly (Smucker's Goober Strawbwerry) 2 tbsp	180	8	15	10	*	6	—	5	—	*	2	*	*	*	*	—	*	15	*	*
honey nut (Skippy) 2 tbsp	190	13	26	10	*	2	*	4	—	*	2	*	*	*	*	*	*	20	*	*
honey sweetened (Smucker's) 2 tbsp	200	12	25	15	*	2	—	6	—	*	4	*	*	*	*	—	*	25	*	*
reduced sugar/sodium (Jif) 2 tbsp	190	13	25	15	*	2	8	—	—	*	4	—	—	*	*	—	2	20	—	—
salt free (Peter Pan) 2 tbsp	190	15	26	10	*	2	8	*	7	2	4	—	—	*	*	*	*	20	—	—

Food	Calories	Protein	Fat	Sat. Fat	Cholesterol	Carbohydrates	Fiber	Sodium	Potassium	Calcium	Iron	Zinc	Magnesium	Vitamin A	Vitamin C	Thiamin	Riboflavin	Niacin	Vitamin B12	Folic acid
PEANUT BUTTER (continued)																				
salted *(generic)* 2 tbsp	190	13	25	17	*	2	8	6	6	*	3	6	13	*	*	2	2	21	*	6
unsalted *(generic)* 2 tbsp	190	13	25	17	*	2	8	*	6	*	3	6	13	*	*	2	2	21	*	6
PEANUT BUTTER CHIPS																				
(Reese's) 1/4 cup	230	15	20	—	2	6	—	4	6	*	22	11	12	*	*	*	6	20	—	—
PEANUT FLOUR																				
defatted																				
(generic) 1 cup	196	52	*	*	*	7	—	4	22	8	7	20	56	*	*	28	17	81	*	37
w/ salt *(generic)* 1 tbsp	13	3	*	*	*		—	*	*	*	*	*	4	*	*	2	*	5	*	*
low fat																				
(generic) 1 cup	257	34	20	9	*	6	—	*	23	8	16	24	7	*	*	18	6	34	*	20
PEANUT OIL																				
(generic) 1 tbsp	119	*	22	12	*	*	*	*	*	*	*	*	*	*	*	*	*	*	*	*
w/ added vitamin E *(Hollywood)* 1 tbsp	120	*	22	10	*	*	*	*	*	*	*	*	*	*	*	*	*	*	*	*
PEAR																				
Asian 1 fruit	51	*	*	*	*	4	16	*	4	*	*	*	2	*	8	*	*	*	—	2
European 1 fruit	98	*	*	*	*	8	16	x	6	2	2	x	2	*	11	2	4	*	—	3
1/2 cup slices	50	*	*	*	*	4	8	*	3	*	*	*	*	*	6	*	2	*	—	2
PEAR, CANNED																				
in extra heavy syrup *(generic)* 1/2 cup	127	*	*	*	*	11	—	*	2	*	2	*	*	*	2	*	2	2	—	*
in extra light syrup *(Del Monte Snack Cups)* 1 container	60	*	*	*	*	5	4	*	—	*	*	*	*	4	—	—	—	—	—	
(generic) 1/2 cup	58	*	*	*	*	5	—	*	2	*	*	*	2	*	4	*	*	2	—	*
halves *(Del Monte)* 1/2 cup	60	*	*	*	*	5	4	*	—	*	*	—	*	4	—	—	—	—		
slices *(Del Monte)* 1/2 cup	60	*	*	*	*	5	4	*	—	*	*	*	4	—	—	—	—			
in fruit juice halves *(Del Monte)* 1/2 cup	60	*	*	*	*	5	4	*	—	*	*	—	*	4	—	—	—	—		
in heavy syrup *(Del Monte Snack Cups)* 1 container	90	*	*	*	*	8	4	*	—	*	*	*	4	—	—	—	—			
(generic) 1/2 cup	95	*	*	*	*	8	12	*	2	*	2	*	*	*	2	*	2	2	—	*
halves *(Del Monte)* 1/2 cup	100	*	*	*	*	8	4	*	—	*	*	*	4	—	—	—	—			
(Hunt's) 1/2 cup	90	*	*	*	*	7	*	*	2	*	2	—	—	*	1	*	*	15	—	
slices *(Del Monte)* 1/2 cup	100	*	*	*	*	8	4	*	—	*	*	*	4	—	—	—	—			
in juice *(generic)* 1/2 cup	62	*	*	*	*	5	8	*	3	*	2	*	2	*	3	*	*	*	—	*
in light syrup *(generic)* 1/2 cup	72	*	*	*	*	6	12	*	2	*	2	*	*	*	*	*	*	*	—	*
in water *(generic)* 1/2 cup	35	*	*	*	*	3	8	*	2	*	*	*	*	*	2	*	*	*	—	*
PEAR, DRIED																				
cooked w/ out sugar 1/2 cup halves	163	2	*	*	*	14	32	*	9	2	7	2	5	*	9	*	2	2	—	—
w/ sugar 1/2 cup halves	196	2	*	*	*	17	32	*	10	2	8	2	5	*	9	*	2	2	—	—

	Calories	Protein	Fat	Sat. Fat	Cholesterol	Carbohydrates	Fiber	Sodium	Potassium	Calcium	Iron	Zinc	Magnesium	Vitamin A	Vitamin C	Thiamin	Riboflavin	Niacin	Vitamin B₁₂	Folic acid
PEAR, DRIED (continued)																				
sulfured																				
1/2 cup halves	236	3	*	*	*	21	28	*	14	3	10	2	7	*	10	*	8	6	—	—
PEAR DRINK																				
pear cruz, organic																				
(Santa Cruz Natural) 8 fl oz	125	*	*	*	*	10	*	*	4	4	2	—	—	*	40	—	—	—	—	—
PEAR JUICE																				
organic																				
(Heinke's) 8 fl oz	120	*	*	*	*	10	*	*	8	*	4	—	—	*	4	—	—	—	—	—
(Knudsen) 8 fl oz	120	*	*	*	*	10	*	*	8	*	4	—	—	*	4	—	—	—	—	—
vitamin C added																				
(generic) 8 fl oz	150	*	*	*	*	13	—	*	*	*	4	*	2	*	112	*	2	2	*	*
PECAN																				
dried																				
1 oz	189	4	30	8	*	2	8	*	3	*	3	10	9	*	*	16	2	*	*	3
dry roasted																				
1 oz	187	4	28	8	*	2	—	*	3	*	3	11	9	*	*	6	2	*	*	3
w/ salt																				
1 oz	187	4	28	8	*	2	8	9	3	*	3	11	9	*	*	6	2	*	*	3
oil roasted																				
1 oz	195	3	31	8	*	2	—	*	3	*	3	10	9	*	*	6	2	*	*	3
w/ salt																				
1 oz	195	3	31	8	*	2	8	9	3	*	3	10	9	*	*	6	2	*	*	3
PECAN FLOUR																				
1 oz	93	15	*	*	*	5	—	*	3	*	3	10	9	*	*	15	2	*	*	3
PECAN-CARAMEL SWIRL PASTRY																				
(Hostess) 1 pastry	240	5	23	35	3	8	7	7	2	6	8	*	*	*	*	8	8	4	—	—
PECAN SPINNER PASTRY																				
(Hostess) 1 pastry	220	5	15	10	2	10	6	6	2	4	8	*	*	*	*	8	8	4	—	—
PECAN TOPPING																				
in syrup																				
(Smucker's) 2 tbsp	130	3	2	—	*	9	*	*	—	*	2	*	*	*	*	6	2	*	*	*
PECTIN DESSERT																				
from mix, all flavors																				
(generic) 1/4 package	39	*	*	*	*	4	—	*	*	*	2	*	*	*	*	*	*	*	*	*
PEPPER, BANANA																				
hot																				
chunks																				
(Vlasic) 1 oz	4	*	*	*	*	*	*	20	—	*	*	—	—	*	*	*	*	*	—	—
rings																				
(Vlasic) 1 oz	4	*	*	*	*	*	*	20	—	*	*	—	—	*	15	*	*	*	—	—
mild																				
chunks																				
(Vlasic) 1 oz	4	*	*	*	*	*	*	20	—	*	*	—	—	*	*	*	*	*	—	—
rings																				
(Vlasic) 1 oz	4	*	*	*	*	*	*	20	—	*	*	—	—	*	*	*	*	*	—	—
sweet																				
rings																				
(Vlasic) 1 oz	8	*	*	*	*	*	*	20	—	*	*	—	—	*	*	*	*	*	—	—
PEPPER, BELL																				
all types																				
raw																				
1/2 cup chopped	14	*	*	*	*	*	4	*	3	*	*	*	*	6	74	2	*	*	*	3
1 pepper	20	*	*	*	*	2	4	*	4	*	2	*	2	9	110	3	*	2	*	4
red																				
raw																				
1/2 cup chopped	14	*	*	*	*	*	4	*	3	*	*	*	*	57	158	2	*	*	*	3
yellow																				
raw																				
1 large pepper	50	3	*	*	*	4	—	*	11	2	5	2	6	9	569	3	3	8	*	12

	Calories	Protein	Fat	Sat. Fat	Cholesterol	Carbohydrates	Fiber	Sodium	Potassium	Calcium	Iron	Zinc	Magnesium	Vitamin A	Vitamin C	Thiamin	Riboflavin	Niacin	Vitamin B₁₂	Folic acid
PEPPER, BELL (continued)																				
all types																				
boiled 1/2 cup chopped	19	*	*	*	*	2	4	*	3	*	2	*	2	8	84	3	*	2	*	3
cooked w/ salt 1/2 cup chopped	19	*	*	*	*	2	—	7	3	*	2	*	2	51	194	3	*	2	*	3
green																				
boiled w/ salt 3 oz	15	*	*	*	*	*	—	8	2	*	2	*	*	5	58	3	2	5	*	2
cooked w/ salt 1/2 cup chopped	19	*	*	*	*	2	—	7	3	*	2	*	2	8	84	3	*	2	*	3
red																				
cooked 1/2 cup chopped	19	*	*	*	*	2	4	*	3	*	2	*	2	51	194	3	*	2	*	3
PEPPER, BELL, CANNED																				
all types																				
solid & liquid (generic) 1/2 cup halves	13	*	*	*	*	*	4	40	3	3	3	*	2	2	54	*	*	2	*	3
fried																				
(Progresso) 1/2 jar	37	*	5	*	*	*	4	*	3	*	4	—	—	8	160	2	2	*	—	—
red																				
solid & liquid (generic) 1/2 cup halves	13	*	*	*	*	*	—	40	3	3	3	*	2	7	54	*	—	—	—	—
roasted																				
(Progresso) 1 piece	20	*	*	*	*	*	*	5	—	—	—	—	—	—	—	—	—	—	—	—
PEPPER, BELL, FREEZE-DRIED																				
green																				
diced 1 tbsp	1	*	*	*	*	*	*	*	*	*	*	*	*		13	*	*	*	*	*
red																				
diced 1 tbsp	1	*	*	*	*	*	—	*	*	*	*	*	*	6	13	*	*	*	*	*
PEPPER, BELL, FROZEN																				
green																				
boiled 3 oz	15	*	*	*	*	*	—	*	2	*	2	*	*	5	58	3	2	5	*	2
chopped 3 oz	17	2	*	*	*	*	4	*	2	*	3	*	2	6	83	4	2	6	*	3
red																				
boiled 3 oz	15	*	*	*	*	*	—	*	2	*	2	*	*	57	58	3	2	5	*	2
boiled w/ salt 3 oz	15	*	*	*	*	*	—	8	2	*	2	*	*	57	58	3	2	5	*	2
PEPPER, BLACK																				
1 tbsp	16	*	*	*	*	*	8	*	2	3	10	*	3	*	—	*	*	*	*	—
PEPPER, CHERRY																				
hot																				
(Progresso) 1/4 cup	95	*	15	*	*	*	2	3	*	*	2	—	—	14	100	1	1	*	—	—
(Vlasic) 1 oz	8	*	*	*	*	*	*	20	—	*	*	—	—	2	10	*	*	*	—	—
hot pickled																				
(Progresso) 1/4 cup	65	*	9	*	*	*	2	2	*	*	2	—	—	4	95	1	1	*	—	—
mild																				
(Vlasic) 1 oz	8	*	*	*	*	*	*	20	—	*	*	—	—	2	10	*	*	*	—	—
PEPPER, CHILI																				
fresh																				
green																				
(generic) 1 pepper	18	*	*	*	*	*	4	*	4	*	3	*	3	7	182	3	2	2	*	3
raw																				
(generic) 2 tbsp chopped	8	*	*	*	*	*	*	*	2	*	*	*	*	3	76	*	*	*	*	*
red raw																				
(generic) 2 tbsp chopped	8	4	*	*	*	*	*	*	2	*	*	*	*	41	76	*	*	*	*	*

	Calories	Protein	Fat	Sat. Fat	Cholesterol	Carbohydrates	Fiber	Sodium	Potassium	Calcium	Iron	Zinc	Magnesium	Vitamin A	Vitamin C	Thiamin	Riboflavin	Niacin	Vitamin B₁₂	Folic acid
PEPPER, CHILI (continued)																				
(Del Monte) 1 oz	10	*	*	*	*	*	2	25	—	*	2	—	—	*	45	—	—	—	—	—
canned																				
(Vlasic) 2 tbsp	8	*	*	*	*	*	*	20	—	*	*	—	—	*	*	*	*	*	—	—
green chopped																				
(Old El Paso) 2 tbsp	8	*	*	*	*	*	*	3	—	4	2	—	—	*	20	*	*	*	—	—
whole																				
(Old El Paso) 2 tbsp	8	*	*	*	*	*	*	4	—	6	2	—	—	*	20	*	*	*	—	—
solid & liquid																				
(generic) 2 tbsp chopped	4	*	*	*	*	*	*	8	*	*	*	*	*	4	19	*	*	2	*	*
(generic) 1 pepper	18	*	*	*	*	*	4	36	4	*	2	*	3	9	83	*	2	3	*	2
sun-dried																				
(generic) 10 peppers	17	*	*	*	*	*	8	*	3	*	2	*	*	29	3	*	4	2	*	*
PEPPER, HOT																				
canned																				
solid & liquid																				
(generic) 2 tbsp chopped	4	*	*	*	*	*	*	8	*	*	*	*	*	41	17	*	*	*	*	*
PEPPER, JALAPEÑO																				
canned																				
solid & liquid																				
(generic) 2 tbsp chopped	4	*	*	*	*	*	—	10	*	*	3	*	*	6	8	*	*	*	*	*
whole																				
(Del Monte) 2 med whole	5	*	*	*	*	*	2	23	—	*	*	—	—	2	10	—	—	—	—	—
(Del Monte) 1 large	3	*	*	*	*	*	2	9	—	*	*	—	—	*	6	—	—	—	—	—
pickled																				
chipotle in spice sauce																				
(Del Monte) 2 tbsp	20	*	*	*	*	*	4	18	—	*	*	—	—	20	6	—	—	—	—	—
sliced																				
(Del Monte) 2 tbsp	5	*	*	*	*	*	3	22	—	*	*	—	—	2	10	—	—	—	—	—
sliced nacho chiles																				
(Del Monte) 2 tbsp	5	*	*	*	*	*	3	14	—	*	*	—	—	2	10	—	—	—	—	—
PEPPER, PEPPERONICI																				
canned																				
(Vlasic) 1 oz	4	*	*	*	*	*	*	18	—	*	*	—	—	*	*	*	*	*	—	—
PEPPER, PICCALILLI																				
canned																				
(Progresso) 2 tbsp	48	*	8	*	*	*	*	3	*	*	2	*	*	10	60	*	*	*	—	—
PEPPER, RED CAYENNE																				
1 tbsp	17	*	*	*	*	*	4	*	3	*	2	*	2	44	7	*	3	2	*	—
PEPPER SAUCE																				
bottled																				
(General Mills Recipe Sauce)																				
1/6 jar (4 oz)	45	2	2	3	*	3	—	22	2	*	*	*	*	*	*	*	*	*	*	*
from mix																				
(Knorr) 1/4 cup	20	*	2	—	*	*	—	16	—	*	*	*	*	4	*	2	*	*	*	*
PEPPER, TUSCAN																				
canned																				
(Progresso) 1/4 cup	10	*	*	*	*	*	2	*	2	*	2	—	—	9	65	1	*	*	—	—
PEPPER, WHITE																				
1 tbsp	21	*	*	20	*	2	—	*	*	2	6	*	2	*	—	*	*	*	*	—
PEPPERED LOAF																				
pork & beef																				
1 1 oz slice	42	8	3	3	4	*	*	18	3	2	2	6	*	*	12	7	5	4	9	*
PEPPERONI																				
(generic) 1 1 oz slice	141	10	19	23	7	*	*	24	3	*	2	5	*	*	*	6	4	7	12	*
(Hormel) 1 oz	138	10	20	25	10	*	—	19	3	1	3	6	1	2	*	7	5	7	—	—
(Oscar Mayer) 1 slice	10	*	*	2	*	*	—	2	*	*	*	*	*	*	*	—	—	—	—	—
sliced																				
(Hormel) 1 oz	140	8	20	30	10	*	—	19	3	1	3	5	1	3	*	7	5	7	—	—
(Rosa Grande) 1 oz	138	10	20	25	10	*	—	19	3	1	3	6	1	2	*	7	5	7	—	—

	Calories	Protein	Fat	Sat. Fat	Cholesterol	Carbohydrates	Fiber	Sodium	Potassium	Calcium	Iron	Zinc	Magnesium	Vitamin A	Vitamin C	Thiamin	Riboflavin	Niacin	Vitamin B$_{12}$	Folic acid
PERCH																				
fresh																				
baked/broiled 1 fillet	61	20	2	*	9	*	*	2	5	7	3	2	5	*	*	4	4	6	10	*
raw 1 fillet	60	20	2	*	9	*	*	2	5	7	3	2	5	*	*	5	4	6	11	*
frozen																				
battered (Van de Kamp's) 1 fillet	155	10	16	10	5	3	*	11	4	*	3	—	—	*	*	5	5	5	—	*
crispy batter (Gorton's) 1 fillet	150	10	16	18	4	3	*	12	—	*	*	—	—	*	*	*	4	*	—	*
PERSIMMON																				
Japanese																				
dried 1 fruit	93	*	*	*	*	8	20	*	8	*	*	*	3	4	*	—	*	—	—	—
fresh 1 fruit	118	2	*	*	*	10	24	*	8	*	*	*	4	73	21	3	2	*	—	3
native																				
fresh 1 fruit	32	*	*	*	*	3	—	*	2	*	3	—	—	—	*	—	—	—	—	—
PESTO see PASTA SAUCE																				
PESTO DIP																				
from mix (Knorr) 1 tbsp	30	*	5	—	2	*	—	3	—	*	*	*	*	*	*	*	*	*	*	*
PHEASANT																				
breast w/out skin																				
raw 3 oz	113	35	4	5	16	*	*	*	6	*	4	4	4	2	8	5	6	36	12	*
leg																				
raw 1 leg	143	40	7	8	29	*	*	2	9	3	11	11	5	4	11	5	13	20	15	3
meat w/out skin																				
raw 3 oz	113	33	5	6	19	*	*	*	6	*	5	5	4	3	8	4	8	29	12	*
meat w/skin																				
raw 3 oz	154	32	12	12	20	*	*	*	6	*	5	5	4	3	8	4	7	27	11	*
PICANTE SAUCE																				
hot																				
(Chi-Chi's) 1 oz	10	2	2	3	*	*	—	11	3	14	1	*	1	1	2	1	1	1	—	—
(Tostitos) 2 tbsp	15	*	*	*	*	*	4	11		—	—	—	—	—	—	—	—	—	—	—
chunky (Rosarita) 3 tbsp	18	*	*	*	*	*	*	21	3	*	3	—	—	*	10	3	6	3		
medium																				
(Chi-Chi's) 1 oz	8	2	2	3	*	*	—	8	2	1	1	*	*	*	2	*	*	*	—	—
(Tostitos) 2 tbsp	15	*	*	*	*	*	4	10		—	—	—	—	—	—	—	—	—	—	—
chunky (Old El Paso) 3 tbsp	9	*	*	*	*	*	*	18	2	*	*	*	*	9	*	*	*	*	—	—
(Rosarita) 3 tbsp	16	*	*	*	*	*	*	27	4	*	*	—	—	*	10	3	6	3		
mild																				
(Chi-Chi's) 1 oz	9	2	2	3	*	*	—	8	3	1	*	*	*	*	3	*	*	*	—	—
(Tostitos) 2 tbsp	15	*	*	*	*	*	4	6		—	—	—	—	—	—	—	—	—	—	—
chunky (Rosarita) 3 tbsp	25	2	*	*	*	2	*	26	4	*	*	—	—	*	33	3	6	3	—	—
PICKLE																				
bread & butter																				
chips (Vlasic) 1 oz	25	*	*	*	*	2	*	7	*	*	*	*	*	*	*	*	*	*	*	*
old-fashioned (Vlasic) 1 oz	45	*	*	*	*	4	*	9	*	*	*	*	*	*	*	*	*	*	*	*

PICKLE (continued)

	Calories	Protein	Fat	Sat. Fat	Cholesterol	Carbohydrates	Fiber	Sodium	Potassium	Calcium	Iron	Zinc	Magnesium	Vitamin A	Vitamin C	Thiamin	Riboflavin	Niacin	Vitamin B₁₂	Folic acid
chunks old fashioned *(Vlasic)* 1 oz	24	*	*	*	*	2	*	6	*	*	*	*	*	*	*	*	*	*	*	*
sticks *(Vlasic)* 1 oz	20	*	*	*	*	2	*	5	*	*	*	*	*	*	*	*	*	*	*	*
whole old fashioned *(Vlasic)* 1 oz	25	*	*	*	*	2	*	7	*	*	*	*	*	*	*	*	*	*	*	*
butter chips sweet low salt *(Vlasic)* 1 oz	30	*	*	*	*	2	*	4	*	*	*	*	*	*	*	*	*	*	*	*
dill *(generic)* 1 slice	1	*	*	*	*	*	*	3	*	*	*	*	*	*	*	*	*	*	*	*
baby zesty *(Vlasic)* 1 oz	4	*	*	*	*	*	*	12	*	*	*	*	*	*	*	*	*	*	*	*
chips, hamburger *(Del Monte)* 1 oz	5	*	*	*	*	*	*	13	*	6	*	*	*	*	*	*	*	*	*	*
(Vlasic) 1 oz	4	*	*	*	*	*	*	16	*	*	*	*	*	*	*	*	*	*	*	*
crunchy zesty *(Vlasic)* 1 oz	4	*	*	*	*	*	*	12	*	—	*	*	*	*	*	*	*	*	*	*
halves *(Del Monte)* 1 oz	5	*	*	*	*	*	2	15	*	4	*	*	*	*	*	*	*	*	*	*
hamburger low salt *(Vlasic)* 1 oz	4	*	*	*	*	*	*	7	*	*	*	*	*	*	*	*	*	*	*	*
kosher halves *(Vlasic Hearty)* 1 oz	4	*	*	*	*	*	*	13	*	*	*	*	*	*	*	*	*	*	*	*
miniatures *(Vlasic Hearty)* 1 oz	4	*	*	*	*	*	*	13	*	*	*	*	*	*	*	*	*	*	*	*
tiny *(Del Monte)* 1 oz	5	*	*	*	*	*	3	10	*	2	*	*	*	*	*	*	*	*	*	*
wholes *(Vlasic Hearty)* 1 oz	4	*	*	*	*	*	*	13	*	*	*	*	*	*	*	*	*	*	*	*
low salt *(generic)* 1 slice	1	*	*	*	*	*	—	*	*	*	*	*	*	*	*	*	*	*	*	*
original *(Vlasic)* 1 oz	4	*	*	*	*	*	*	16	*	*	*	*	*	*	*	*	*	*	*	*
Polish *(Vlasic)* 1 oz	4	*	*	*	*	*	*	12	*	*	*	*	*	*	*	*	*	*	*	*
snack chunks *(Vlasic)* 1 oz	4	*	*	*	*	*	*	12	*	*	*	*	*	*	*	*	*	*	*	*
zesty *(Vlasic)* 1 oz	4	*	*	*	*	*	*	12	*	*	*	*	*	*	*	*	*	*	*	*
spears zesty *(Vlasic)* 1 oz	4	*	*	*	*	*	*	12	*	*	*	*	*	*	*	*	*	*	*	*
whole *(Del Monte)* 1 oz	5	*	*	*	*	*	2	15	*	4	*	*	*	*	*	*	*	*	*	*
garlic halves *(Vlasic Hearty)* 1 oz	4	*	*	*	*	*	*	12	*	*	*	*	*	*	*	*	*	*	*	*
wholes *(Vlasic Hearty)* 1 oz	4	*	*	*	*	*	*	13	*	*	*	*	*	*	*	*	*	*	*	*
kosher baby dills *(Vlasic)* 1 oz	4	*	*	*	*	*	*	9	*	*	*	*	*	*	*	*	*	*	*	*

PERCENTAGE DAILY VALUE

	Calories	Protein	Fat	Sat. Fat	Cholesterol	Carbohydrates	Fiber	Sodium	Potassium	Calcium	Iron	Zinc	Magnesium	Vitamin A	Vitamin C	Thiamin	Riboflavin	Niacin	Vitamin B12	Folic acid
PICKLE (continued)																				
crunchy low salt *(Vlasic)* 1 oz	4	*	*	*	*	*	*	5	*	*	*	*	*	*	*	*	*	*	*	*
crunchy dills *(Vlasic)* 1 oz	4	*	*	*	*	*	*	16	*	*	*	*	*	*	*	*	*	*	*	*
dill gherkins *(Vlasic)* 1 oz	4	*	*	*	*	*	*	9	*	*	*	*	*	*	*	*	*	*	*	*
dill spears *(Vlasic)* 1 oz	4	*	*	*	*	*	*	9	*	*	*	*	*	*	*	*	*	*	*	*
low salt *(Vlasic)* 1 oz	4	*	*	*	*	*	*	5	*	*	*	*	*	*	*	*	*	*	*	*
hamburger dill chips *(Vlasic)* 1 oz	4	*	*	*	*	*	*	7	*	*	*	*	*	*	*	*	*	*	*	*
snack chunks *(Vlasic)* 1 oz	4	*	*	*	*	*	*	9	*	*	*	*	*	*	*	*	*	*	*	*
no garlic																				
crunchy dills *(Vlasic)* 1 oz	4	*	*	*	*	*	*	9	*	*	*	*	*	*	*	*	*	*	*	*
dill spears *(Vlasic)* 1 oz	4	*	*	*	*	*	*	9	*	*	*	*	*	*	*	*	*	*	*	*
sour *(generic)* 1 slice	1	*	*	*	*	*	*	4	*	*	*	*	*	*	*	*	*	*	*	*
low salt *(generic)* 1 slice	1	*	*	*	*	*	*	*	*	*	*	*	*	*	*	*	*	*	*	*
sweet *(generic)* 1 slice	7	*	*	*	*	*	*	2	*	*	*	*	*	*	*	*	*	*	*	*
chips *(Del Monte)* 1 oz	40	*	*	*	*	3	3	9	*	*	*	*	*	*	*	*	*	*	*	*
(Vlasic) 1 oz	45	*	*	*	*	3	*	7	*	*	2	*	*	*	*	*	*	*	*	*
gherkins *(Del Monte)* 1 oz	40	*	*	*	*	3	3	9	*	*	*	*	*	*	*	*	*	*	*	*
(Vlasic) 1 oz	45	*	*	*	*	3	*	7	*	*	2	*	*	*	*	*	*	*	*	*
low salt *(generic)* 1 slice	7	*	*	*	*	*	*	*	*	*	*	*	*	*	*	*	*	*	*	*
midget *(Del Monte)* 1 oz	40	*	*	*	*	3	3	9	*	*	*	*	*	*	*	*	*	*	*	*
(Vlasic) 1 oz	45	*	*	*	*	4	*	9	*	*	2	*	*	*	*	*	*	*	*	*
whole *(Del Monte)* 1 oz	40	*	*	*	*	3	3	9	*	*	*	*	*	*	*	*	*	*	*	*
PICKLE LOAF																				
(Bryan) 1 oz slice	50	5	6	—	7	*	*	14	—	—	—	—	—	—	—	—	—	—	—	—
PICKLE & PIMIENTO LOAF																				
(generic) 1 1 oz slice	74	5	9	11	3	*	*	16	3	3	2	3	*	*	7	6	4	3	6	*
(Oscar Mayer) 1 slice	62	5	6	7	4	*	*	15	2	5	2	2	2	*	*	—	—	—	—	—
PICNIC LOAF																				
pork & beef *(generic)* 1 1 oz slice	66	7	7	9	4	*	*	14	2	*	2	4	*	*	9	7	4	3	7	*
PIE CRUST																				
(Oronoque) 1/8 crust	90	12	9	7	*	2	*	3	—	—	—	—	—	—	—	—	—	—	—	—
frozen																				
all vegetable shortening *(Pet-Ritz)* 1/6 of 9" shell	120	3	12	10	*	4	*	3	*	*	*	—	*	*	*	*	*	*	—	—
deep dish *(Pet-Ritz)* 1/6 of 9" shell	140	3	14	15	*	4	*	4	*	*	*	—	*	*	*	*	*	*	—	—
deep dish *(Oronque)* 1/6 of 9" shell	130	4	14	10	*	4	—	5	*	*	4	—	*	*	8	2	6	—	—	
(Pet-Ritz) 1/6 of 9" shell	130	3	14	10	*	4	*	5	*	*	4	—	—	*	*	8	2	6	—	—

	Calories	Protein	Fat	Sat. Fat	Cholesterol	Carbohydrates	Fiber	Sodium	Potassium	Calcium	Iron	Zinc	Magnesium	Vitamin A	Vitamin C	Thiamin	Riboflavin	Niacin	Vitamin B₁₂	Folic acid
PIE CRUST (continued)																				
graham cracker																				
(Pet-Ritz) 1/6 of 9″ shell	110	2	9	—	2	3	*	3	*	*	2	—	—	*	*	*	2	*	—	—
regular																				
(Oronque) 1/6 of 9″ shell	120	2	12	10	*	3	—	5	*	*	4	—	—	*	*	8	2	6	—	—
(Pet-Ritz) 1/6 of 9″ shell	120	3	12	10	*	3	*	5	*	*	4	—	—	*	—	8	2	6	—	—
graham																				
(Honey Maid) 3/4 oz	110	2	9	5	*	5	—	4	*	*	4	—	—	*	*	4	4	4	—	—
from mix																				
(Betty Crocker) 1/8 mix	120	3	12	10	*	3	—	6	*	*	2	—	—	*	*	4	2	2	—	—
(Pillsbury) 1/8 crust	200	5	20	15	*	7	—	12	*	*	4	—	—	*	*	10	6	6	—	—
from refrigerated dough																				
(Pillsbury) 1/8 crust	240	3	23	30	—	8	—	*	*	*	*	—	—	*	*	*	*	*	—	—
(Nilla) 3/4 oz	110	2	9	5	2	5	—	2	*	*	4	—	—	*	*	2	2	4	—	—
(Oreo) 3/4 oz	110	2	9	5	*	5	—	6	*	*	6	—	—	*	*	2	2	4	—	—
PIE FILLING																				
canned																				
apple																				
(generic) 1/8 can	75	*	*	*	*	6	4	*	*	*	*	*	*	*	*	*	*	*	*	*
cherry																				
(generic) 1/8 can	85	*	*	*	*	7	*	*	2	*	*	*	*	3	4	*	*	*	*	*
pumpkin																				
(generic) 1/2 cup	140	2	*	*	*	12	—	12	5	5	8	2	5	224	8	*	9	3	*	12
(Libby's) 1/2 cup	100	*	*	*	23	8	8	6	—	2	4	—	—	160	2	—	—	—	—	—
from mix																				
banana cream prep w/ whole milk																				
(Jell-O) amount for 1/6 pie	100	6	5	—	3	6	*	7	4	10				2	*	2	8	*	—	
coconut cream prep w/ whole milk																				
(Jell-O) amount for 1/6 pie	110	6	6	—	3	5	*	6	4	10				2	*	2	8	*	—	
lemon prep w/ whole milk																				
(Jell-O) amount for 1/6 pie	170	4	3	—	30	13	*	4	*	*				*	*	*	2	*	—	
PIE, FROM MIX																				
Boston cream																				
(Betty Crocker Classic) 1/8 pie	270	7	9	10	10	17	—	16	3	15	4			2	*	6	8	2	—	—
PIE, FROZEN																				
apple																				
(Banquet) 3 1/3 oz (1/6 pie)	250	3	17	—	—	12	—	12	—	*	4			*	4	*	*	*	—	
(Mrs. Smith's) 1/6 of 8″ pie	270	3	17	10	*	14	4	12		2	—	—	—	—	—	—	—	—	—	—
apple cranberry																				
(Mrs. Smith's) 1/6 of 8″ pie	280	3	17	10	*	14	4	12		2	—	—	—	—	—	—	—	—	—	—
banana cream																				
(Banquet) 2 1/3 oz	180	3	15	—	—	7	—	6	—	2	4			*	*	*	2	*	—	
(Mrs. Smith's) 1/5 of 8″ pie	250	3	14	13	*	13	4	7		3	—	—	—	—	—	—	—	—	—	—
(Pet-Ritz) 1/6 pie	170	3	14	—	—	7	—	6	2	2	5			*	*	4	2	3	—	
berry																				
(Mrs. Smith's) 1/6 of 8″ pie	280	3	17	10	*	15	*	14		2	—	—	—	—	—	—	—	—	—	—
blackberry																				
(Banquet) 3 1/3 oz (1/6 pie)	270	5	17	—	—	13	—	15	—	2	4			*	8	*	*	*	—	
(Mrs. Smith's) 1/6 of 8″ pie	280	3	17	10	*	14	4	13		2	—	—	—	—	—	—	—	—	—	—
blueberry																				
(Banquet) 3 1/3 oz (1/6 pie)	270	5	17	—	—	13	—	15	—	*	4			*	4	2	*	*	—	
(Mrs. Smith's) 1/6 of 8″ pie	260	3	17	10	*	13	4	13		*	—	—	—	—	—	—	—	—	—	—
Boston cream																				
(Mrs. Smith's) 1/5 of 8″ pie	170	3	8	8	8	10	*	6		*	—	—	—	—	—	—	—	—	—	—
cheese yogurt dessert																				
blueberry																				
(Mrs. Smith's SmartStyle) 1/4 of 7″ pie	270	5	12	15	3	16	4	11		2	—	—	—	—	—	—	—	—	—	—

PIE, FROZEN (continued)

	Calories	Protein	Fat	Sat. Fat	Cholesterol	Carbohydrates	Fiber	Sodium	Potassium	Calcium	Iron	Zinc	Magnesium	Vitamin A	Vitamin C	Thiamin	Riboflavin	Niacin	Vitamin B12	Folic acid
peach (Mrs. Smith's SmartStyle) 1/4 of 7" pie	270	5	12	15	3	15	4	10	4	—	—	—	—	—	—	—	—	—	—	—
yogurt (Mrs. Smith's SmartStyle) 1/4 of 7" pie	240	5	8	5	*	16	4	8	4	—	—	—	—	—	—	—	—	—	—	—
cherry (Banquet) 3 1/3 oz (1/6 pie)	250	5	17	—	—	12	—	11	—	*	4	—	—	2	2	2	2	*	—	—
(Mrs. Smith's) 1/6 of 8" pie	270	3	17	10	*	14	4	13	3	—	—	—	—	—	—	—	—	—	—	—
chocolate cream (Banquet) 2 1/3 oz	190	3	15	—	—	8	—	5	—	2	4	—	—	*	*	*	2	*	—	—
(Mrs. Smith's) 1/5 of 8" pie	290	3	22	20	*	12	4	7	4	—	—	—	—	—	—	—	—	—	—	—
(Pet-Ritz) 1/6 pie	190	2	12	—	—	9	—	6	2	2	5	—	—	*	*	5	2	3	—	—
chocolate mocha (Weight Watchers) 2 3/4 oz	160	10	6	5	2	10	8	6	6	8	4	—	—	*	*	—	—	—	—	—
coconut cream (Banquet) 2 1/3 oz	190	3	17	—	—	7	—	5	—	2	4	—	—	*	*	*	2	*	—	—
(Mrs. Smith's) 1/5 of 8" pie	280	3	22	20	*	*	*	6	2	—	—	—	—	—	—	—	—	—	—	—
(Pet-Ritz) 1/6 pie	190	2	12	—	—	9	—	6	*	2	5	—	—	*	*	5	2	3	—	—
coconut custard (Mrs. Smith's) 1/5 of 8" pie	280	12	18	25	25	12	*	15	7	—	—	—	—	—	—	—	—	—	—	—
Dutch apple (Mrs. Smith's) 1/6 of 8" pie	310	5	20	13	*	16	4	11	2	—	—	—	—	—	—	—	—	—	—	—
French silk cream (Mrs. Smith's) 1/5 of 8" pie	410	5	32	30	2	18	4	10	*	—	—	—	—	—	—	—	—	—	—	—
lemon cream (Banquet) 2 1/3 oz	170	3	14	—	—	8	—	5	—	2	4	—	—	*	2	*	2	*	—	—
(Mrs. Smith's) 1/6 of 8" pie	320	5	20	13	*	*	4	14	4	—	—	—	—	—	—	—	—	—	—	—
(Pet-Ritz) 1/6 pie	190	3	14	—	—	9	—	6	*	2	5	—	—	*	*	4	2	3	—	—
lemon meringue (Mrs. Smith's) 1/5 of 8" pie	300	5	12	10	22	18	*	9	*	—	—	—	—	—	—	—	—	—	—	—
mince (Banquet) 3 1/3 oz (1/6 pie)	260	5	17	—	—	13	—	15	—	*	4	—	—	*	*	2	*	*	—	—
(Mrs. Smith's) 1/6 of 8" pie	300	3	17	10	*	16	8	17	4	—	—	—	—	—	—	—	—	—	—	—
Mississippi mud (Weight Watchers) 3 1/2 oz	180	7	8	8	2	10	8	5	4	6	4	—	—	*	*	—	—	—	—	—
Neapolitan cream (Pet-Ritz) 1/6 pie	180	2	15	—	—	6	—	8	2	*	4	—	—	*	*	*	*	2	—	—
peach (Banquet) 3 1/3 oz (1/6 pie)	245	5	17	—	—	12	—	12	—	*	4	—	—	4	20	*	*	2	—	—
(Mrs. Smith's) 1/6 of 8" pie	260	3	17	10	*	13	4	13	3	—	—	—	—	—	—	—	—	—	—	—
pecan (Mrs. Smith's) 1/6 of 8" pie	520	8	35	20	*	24	4	19	3	—	—	—	—	—	—	—	—	—	—	—
pumpkin (Banquet) 3 1/3 oz (1/6 pie)	200	5	12	—	—	10	—	15	—	4	4	—	—	35	2	2	4	2	—	—
hearty (Mrs. Smith's) 1/5 of 8" pie	280	8	15	15	20	15	8	15	9	—	—	—	—	—	—	—	—	—	—	—
regular (Mrs. Smith's) 1/5 of 8" pie	270	8	12	10	15	15	4	15	7	—	—	—	—	—	—	—	—	—	—	—
raspberry (Mrs. Smith's) 1/6 of 8" pie	280	3	17	10	*	14	*	13	2	—	—	—	—	—	—	—	—	—	—	—
strawberry cream (Banquet) 2 1/3 oz	170	3	14	—	—	7	—	5	—	2	4	—	—	*	10	*	2	*	—	—
(Pet-Ritz) 1/6 pie	170	3	14	—	—	7	—	6	2	2	5	—	—	*	*	4	2	3	—	—
strawberry rhubarb (Mrs. Smith's) 1/6 of 8" pie	280	3	17	10	*	15	*	16	4	—	—	—	—	—	—	—	—	—	—	—

PIG'S FEET see PORK

	Calories	Protein	Fat	Sat. Fat	Cholesterol	Carbohydrates	Fiber	Sodium	Potassium	Calcium	Iron	Zinc	Magnesium	Vitamin A	Vitamin C	Thiamin	Riboflavin	Niacin	Vitamin B12	Folic acid
PIGEON PEA																				
boiled 1/2 cup	85	8	2	*	*	5	—	*		3	7	4	—	2	36	18	8	8	*	19
boiled w/ salt 1/2 cup	85	8	2	*	*	5	—	8		3	7	4	—	2	36	18	8	8	—	
PIGEON see SQUAB																				
PIKE, NORTHERN																				
raw 1/2 fillet	174	64	2	*	26	*	*	3	15	11	6	9	15	3	13	8	7	23	66	*
baked/broiled 1/2 fillet	175	64	2	*	26	*	*	3	15	11	6	9	16	3	10	7	7	22	59	*
PIKE, WALLEYE																				
raw 1 fillet	148	51	3	2	46	*	*	3	18	17	11	7	12	2	*	29	15	18	53	*
broiled/baked 1 fillet	148	51	3	2	45	*	*	3	18	17	11	7	12	2	*	26	14	17	48	*
PILAF see RICE DISH																				
PIMIENTO																				
canned 1 tbsp	3	*	*	*	*	*	—	*	*	*	*	*	*	6	17	*	*	*	*	*
PINA COLADA																				
homemade 1 cocktail (4 1/2 oz)	262	*	4	6	*	13	—	*	3	*	2	*	3	*	*	3	*	*	*	4
PINA COLADA, CANNED																				
canned 6 3/4 fl oz	526	2	26	73	*	20	*	7	5	*	3	3	*	*	3	*	*	*	*	3
PINE NUT																				
pignolia (generic) 1 oz	146	11	22	11	*	*	4	*	5	*	15	8	17	*	*	15	3	5	*	4
(Progresso) 1 tbsp	60	5	8	5	*	*	—	*	2	*	4	*	*	*	*	4	*	*	—	—
pinyon (generic) 1 oz	161	5	27	14	*	2	12	*	5	*	5	8	17	*	*	24	4	6	*	4
PINEAPPLE																				
1/2 cup cubes	37	*	*	*	*	3	4	*	2	*	2	*	3	*	19	5	2	2	—	2
1 slice	41	*	*	*	*	3	4	*	3	*	2	*	3	*	22	5	2	2	—	2
PINEAPPLE, CANNED																				
in extra heavy syrup (generic) 1/2 cup	108	*	*	*	*	9	*	*	4	2	3	*	5	*	16	8	2	2	—	*
in heavy syrup (generic) 1/2 cup	96	*	*	*	*	8	4	*	4	2	3	*	5	*	15	7	2	2	—	*
chunks (Del Monte) 1/2 cup	90	*	*	*	*	8	4	*	—	*	2	—	—	*	20	—	—	—	—	—
crushed (Del Monte) 1/2 cup	90	*	*	*	*	8	4	*	—	*	2	—	—	*	20	—	—	—	—	—
sliced (Del Monte) 1/2 cup	90	*	*	*	*	8	4	*	—	*	2	—	—	*	20	—	—	—	—	—
in juice (generic) 1/2 cup	75	*	*	*	*	7	4	*	4	2	2	*	4	*	20	8	*	2	—	*
in light syrup (generic) 1/2 cup	66	*	*	*	*	6	4	*	4	2	3	*	5	*	16	8	2	2	—	*
in own juice (Del Monte Snack Cups) 1 container	60	*	*	*	*	6	4	*	—	*	2	—	—	4	20	—	—	—	—	—
chunks (Del Monte) 1/2 cup	70	*	*	*	*	6	4	*	—	*	2	—	—	*	20	—	—	—	—	—
crushed (Del Monte) 1/2 cup	70	*	*	*	*	6	4	*	—	*	2	—	—	*	20	—	—	—	—	—
sliced (Del Monte) 1/2 cup	60	*	*	*	*	5	4	*	—	*	2	—	—	*	20	—	—	—	—	—

	Calories	Protein	Fat	Sat. Fat	Cholesterol	Carbohydrates	Fiber	Sodium	Potassium	Calcium	Iron	Zinc	Magnesium	Vitamin A	Vitamin C	Thiamin	Riboflavin	Niacin	Vitamin B₁₂	Folic acid
PINEAPPLE, CANNED (continued)																				
tidbits (Del Monte) 1/2 cup	70	*	*	*	*	6	4	*	—	*	2	—	—	*	20	—	—	—	—	—
in water (generic) 1/2 cup	39	*	*	*	*	3	4	*	4	2	3	*	6	*	16	8	2	2	—	*
PINEAPPLE, FROZEN																				
sweetened (generic) 1/2 cup chunks	104	*	*	*	*	9	4	*	3	*	3	*	3	*	16	8	2	2	—	3
PINEAPPLE DRINK																				
(Sunny Delight) 8 fl oz	120	*	*	*	*	10	*	5	—	*	*	*	*	20	100	20	*	*	*	*
pineapple float (Knudsen) 8 fl oz	140	2	*	*	*	11	*	2	3	4	4			*	15	—	—	—	—	—
PINEAPPLE JUICE																				
(Del Monte) 8 fl oz	110	*	*	*	*	9	*	*	—	*	2	4	—	—	*	100	—	—	—	—
(generic) 8 fl oz	140	*	*	*	*	11	*	*	10	4	4	2	8	*	45	9	3	3	*	14
from concentrate (generic) 8 fl oz	130	2	*	*	*	11	*	*	10	3	4	2	6	*	50	12	3	3	*	7
vitamin C added (generic) 8 fl oz	140	*	*	*	*	11	—	*	10	4	4	2	8	*	160	9	3	3	*	14
PINEAPPLE-APRICOT JUICE																				
organic (Santa Cruz Natural) 8 fl oz	110	*	*	*	*	9	*	*	3	10	4			*	4	—	—	—	—	—
PINEAPPLE-BANANA DRINK																				
(Welch's Orchard) 8 1/2 oz (1 box)	140	*	*	*	*	11	*	*	5	*	*	*	*	*	*	*	*	*	*	*
aseptic pack (Welch's) 8 1/2 oz (1 box)	140	*	*	*	*	12	*	*	5	*	*	*	*	*	*	*	*	*	*	*
from concentrate (Welch's) 6 fl oz	100	*	*	*	*	8	*	*	4	*	*	*	*	*	*	*	*	*	*	*
PINEAPPLE-COCONUT JUICE																				
(Farmer's Market) 8 fl oz	120	*	*	*	*	10	*	*	3	*	*			*	—	—	—	—	—	—
(Knudsen Tropical Blend) 8 fl oz	130	*	*	*	*	11	*	2	6	4	2			8	6	—	—	—	—	—
PINEAPPLE-GRAPEFRUIT DRINK																				
(generic) 8 fl oz	118	*	*	*	*	10	*	*	4	2	4	*	4	2	192	5	2	3	*	7
PINEAPPLE-GRAPEFRUIT JUICE																				
(Tropicana) 6 fl oz	100	*	*	*	*	8	*	—	2	2	*			*	2	10	4	*	—	—
PINEAPPLE-ORANGE DRINK																				
(generic) 8 fl oz	125	5	*	*	*	10	*	*	3	*	4	*	4	27	94	5	3	3	*	7
(Mott's) 10 fl oz	170	*	*	*	*	14	*	*	*	2	*	*	*	*	*	*	*	*	—	—
PINEAPPLE TOPPING																				
(generic) 2 tbsp	106	*	*	*	*	9	*	*	4	*	*	*	*	*	41	*	*	*	*	*
(Kraft) 2 tbsp	100	*	*	*	*	8	*	*	6	*	*	*	*	—	*	—	—	—	—	—
(Smucker's) 2 tbsp	130	*	*	*	*	11	*	*	—	*	*	*	*	*	*	*	*	*	—	—
PINK BEAN																				
cooked 1/2 cup	125	13	*	*	*	8	16	*	12	4	11	5	14	*	*	14	3	2	*	35
salted 1/2 cup	125	13	*	*	*	8	16	8	12	4	11	5	14	*	*	14	3	2	*	35
PINTO BEAN																				
boiled 1/2 cup	116	12	*	*	*	7	28	*	11	4	12	6	12	*	3	11	5	2	*	37
boiled, salted 1/2 cup	116	12	*	*	*	7	—	8	11	4	12	6	12	*	3	11	5	2	*	37
PINTO BEAN, CANNED																				
(Bush Bros) 1/2 cup	110	10	*	*	*	6	24	18	—	4	10	—	—	*	*	—	—	—	—	—
(Gebhardt) 1/2 cup	100	10	*	*	*	6	20	25	11	4	10	—	—	*	2	11	4	2	—	—
(generic) 1/2 cup	94	9	*	*	*	6	16	21	10	4	11	6	8	*	*	8	4	2	*	18
(Hain) 1/2 cup	70	12	2	*	*	5	24	9	9	4	10	—	—	*	*	6	2	2	—	—

	Calories	Protein	Fat	Sat. Fat	Cholesterol	Carbohydrates	Fiber	Sodium	Potassium	Calcium	Iron	Zinc	Magnesium	Vitamin A	Vitamin C	Thiamin	Riboflavin	Niacin	Vitamin B₁₂	Folic acid
PINTO BEAN, CANNED (continued)																				
(Old El Paso) 1/2 cup	100	10	*	*	*	6	32	13	10	6	15	—	—	*	4	10	4	*	—	—
(Progresso) 1/2 cup	110	13	*	*	*	7	26	17	6	4	8	—	—	*	*	4	2	*	—	—
w/ bacon (Bush Bros) 1/2 cup	110	10	2	3	*	6	24	22	—	4	8	—	—	*	*	—	—	—	—	—
w/ bacon & jalapeño (Bush Bros) 1/2 cup	110	12	2	3	*	6	24	23	—	4	10	—	—	*	*	—	—	—	—	—
cowboy (Bush Bros) 1/2 cup	120	10	2	3	*	7	24	15	—	4	8	—	—	*	*	—	—	—	—	—
dry, canned in brine (Green Giant/Joan of Arc) 1/2 cup	45	10	*	*	*	4	10	6	4	3	4	—	—	*	*	—	—	—	—	—
w/ pork (Bush Bros) 1/2 cup	120	10	4	5	*	6	24	22	—	4	8	—	—	*	*	—	—	—	—	—
PISTACHIO NUT																				
dried (generic) 1 oz (47 kernels)	164	10	21	9	*	2	12	*	9	4	11	3	11	*	3	16	3	2	*	4
dry-roasted (generic) 1 oz	172	7	23	10	*	3	12	*	8	2	5	3	9	*	3	8	4	2	*	4
w/ salt (generic) 1 oz	172	7	23	10	*	3	12	9	8	2	5	3	9	*	3	8	4	2	*	4
natural (Blue Diamond) 1 oz	140	10	18	10	*	*	12	9	8	2	8	6	10	*	*	*	4	*	*	—
red (Blue Diamond) 1 oz	140	10	18	10	*	*	12	5	7	2	8	4	10	*	*	*	4	*	*	—
PITA BREAD see BREAD																				
PITANGA																				
raw 1 fruit	2	*	*	*	*	*	—	*	*	*	*	—	*	2	3	*	*	*	*	—
1/2 cup slices	28	*	*	*	*	2	—	*	3	*	*	—	3	26	37	2	2	*	*	—
PIZZA																				
bacon cheddar (Stouffer's) 11 3/8 oz	440	—	34	35	10	15	16	39	9	25	20	—	—	6	10	—	—	—	—	—
Bianca (Weight Watchers) 5 3/4 oz	330	33	14	25	7	14	20	20	7	40	10	—	—	15	4	—	—	—	—	—
Canadian bacon (Jeno's) 1/2 pizza (4 oz)	240	17	15	10	2	9	4	28	5	15	10	—	—	8	4	20	15	10	—	—
(Totino's Party) 1/2 pizza (5 1/3 oz)	330	25	20	10	3	14	12	36	7	20	8	—	—	2	*	10	20	10	—	—
cheese (Jeno's) 1/2 pizza (3 3/4 oz)	240	18	15	15	3	9	4	21	3	20	10	—	—	6	4	15	10	10	—	—
(Jeno's Pizza Rolls) 3 oz	200	15	8	10	7	10	6	15	4	15	4	—	—	2	*	6	4	4	—	—
(Kid Cuisine) 6 3/4 oz	380	18	18	—	8	19	—	16	9	15	15	—	—	25	6	30	15	10	—	—
(Mrs. Paterson's) 1 pie (5 1/2 oz)	470	20	42	50	25	15	—	37	8	15	11	11	6	17	*	21	19	15	—	—
(Pepperidge Farm Croissant) 4 1/3 oz	430	30	35	—		14	—	27	—	35	10	—	—	6	4	4	10	10	—	—
(Stouffer's) 10 3/8 oz	350	27	22	25	5	14	12	27	7	25	15	—	—	8	10	30	20	15	—	—
(Stouffer's Lean Cuisine) 5 1/8 oz	300	28	14	15	5	13	—	13	9	25	15	—	—	6	10	25	20	20	—	—
(Swanson Kids') 8 oz	350	25	15	—	—	16	—	16	—	30	8	—	—	8	*	10	15	10	—	—
(Totino's Party) 1/2 pizza (5 oz)	290	22	15	15	5	13	8	22	7	25	4	—	—	2	*	6	10	6	—	—
(Totino's Party, Family Size) 1/4 pizza (4 oz)	320	18	17	15	5	14	8	24	7	25	6	—	—	2	*	6	10	8	—	—
French bread (Healthy Choice) 5 2/3 oz	300	35	5	—	7	16	—	21	9	30	20	—	—	2	*	30	15	15	—	—
microwave (Pillsbury Oven Lovin') 1 piece (5 3/4 oz)	350	28	22	25	5	14	—	29	6	35	6	—	—	10	8	20	15	10	—	—

PIZZA (continued)

	Calories	Protein	Fat	Sat. Fat	Cholesterol	Carbohydrates	Fiber	Sodium	Potassium	Calcium	Iron	Zinc	Magnesium	Vitamin A	Vitamin C	Thiamin	Riboflavin	Niacin	Vitamin B₁₂	Folic acid
(Pillsbury Oven Lovin') 1/2 pizza (3 1/3 oz)	250	18	18	20	3	8	—	18	4	25	10	—	—	8	6	10	10	10	—	—
(Totino's) 1 pizza (4 oz)	250	18	15	20	5	10	—	23	4	20	10	—	—	8	6	10	15	10	—	—
pan style (Totino's) 1/6 pizza (4 oz)	290	25	15	20	7	12	—	18	5	30	6	—	—	10	6	8	10	8	—	—
cheeseburger (Stouffer's) 11 7/8 oz	440	—	40	45	18	20	—	46	8	25	15	—	—	15	20	—	—	—	—	—
combination (Jeno's) 1/2 pizza (4 oz)	280	17	23	20	5	9	4	28	5	15	10	—	—	8	4	20	15	15	—	—
(Jeno's Pizza Rolls) 3 oz	220	17	14	15	5	9	8	10	6	6	4	—	—	*	*	2	6	8	—	—
(Totino's Party) 1/2 pizza (5 1/3 oz)	370	25	26	20	7	14	12	38	9	20	6	—	—	2	*	10	20	10	—	—
(Totino's Party, Family Size) 1/4 pizza (4 1/3 oz)	400	21	28	20	7	16	12	41	9	25	8	—	—	2	*	10	20	10	—	—
(Weight Watchers) 7 oz	330	40	12	20	8	14	24	16	17	40	15	—	—	10	4	—	—	—	—	—
French bread microwave (Pillsbury Oven Lovin') 1 piece (6 1/2 oz)	420	30	32	50	10	14	—	38	8	30	10	—	—	10	10	30	20	20	—	—
microwave (Pillsbury Oven Lovin') 1/2 pizza (4 oz)	310	22	28	35	7	9	—	24	5	25	10	—	—	8	6	20	15	15	—	—
(Totino's) 1 pizza (4 1/4 oz)	290	15	20	15	5	11	—	32	5	15	10	—	—	10	8	20	15	10	—	—
deluxe (Pepperidge Farm Croissant) 5 oz	440	30	35	—	—	14	—	33	—	30	15			4	2	15	10	15	—	—
(Stouffer's) 12 3/8 oz	440	35	34	35	12	14	20	41	9	20	15	—	—	10	30	30	25	20	—	—
(Stouffer's Lean Cuisine) 6 1/8 oz	350	37	17	20	10	13	—	24	13	20	20	—	—	8	10	30	25	20	—	—
(Stouffer's Lunch Express) 6 5/8 oz	220	—	38	40	15	13	16	42	10	25	15	—	—	6	20	—	—	—	—	—
French bread (Healthy Choice) 6 1/4 oz	330	38	12	—	12	14	—	20	10	25	25	—	—	8	*	30	20	20	—	—
double cheese (Stouffer's) 11 3/4 oz	420	37	29	35	10	15	20	33	7	35	15	—	—	6	15	30	30	20	—	—
(Stouffer's Lunch Express) 5 7/8 oz	170	—	29	35	12	14	12	30	7	40	15	—	—	6	10	—	—	—	—	—
garden vegetable (Stouffer's) 12 5/8 oz	340	—	18	20	5	15	16	22	7	20	15	—	—	6	50	—	—	—	—	—
hamburger (Jeno's) 1/2 pizza (4 oz)	280	18	22	20	5	9	4	14	5	15	10	—	—	6	4	50	15	10	—	—
(Jeno's Pizza Rolls) 3 oz	220	17	12	15	7	9	8	13	6	8	4	—	—	*	*	2	6	6	—	—
(Kid Cuisine) 6 3/4 oz	330	18	15	—	5	17	—	29	8	15	10	—	—	4	6	15	15	20	—	—
(Totino's Party) 1/2 pizza (5 1/2 oz)	350	27	26	20	5	12	12	32	8	20	8	—	—	4	*	8	20	20	—	—
Italian turkey sausage French bread (Healthy Choice) 6 1/2 oz	320	38	11	—	10	14	—	18	10	25	25	—	—	6	*	30	20	20	—	—
pepperoni (Jeno's) 1/2 pizza (3 3/4 oz)	280	17	23	20	5	9	4	30	4	15	10	—	—	8	4	15	15	15	—	—
(Jeno's Pizza Pockets) 1 (4 1/2 oz)	370	20	31	30	8	12	—	33	6	15	10	—	—	8	10	20	10	15	—	—
(Jeno's Pizza Rolls) 3 oz	220	15	14	15	7	9	7	15	6	6	4	—	—	*	*	6	8	6	—	—
(Pepperidge Farm Croissant) 4 1/2 oz	420	25	34	—	—	14	—	29	—	25	10			6	6	20	15	15	—	—
(Stouffer's) 11 1/4 oz	420	32	31	30	12	14	12	39	9	25	20	—	—	10	10	35	25	20	—	—
(Stouffer's Lean Cuisine) 5 1/4 oz	340	32	17	25	8	14	—	24	11	20	20	—	—	10	10	30	25	25	—	—

	Calories	Protein	Fat	Sat. Fat	Cholesterol	Carbohydrates	Fiber	Sodium	Potassium	Calcium	Iron	Zinc	Magnesium	Vitamin A	Vitamin C	Thiamin	Riboflavin	Niacin	Vitamin B12	Folic acid
PIZZA (continued)																				
(Stouffer's Lunch Express) 5 3/4 oz	200	—	35	40	13	13	16	40	9	25	20	—	—	10	20	—	—	—	—	—
(Totino's Party) 1/2 pizza (5 1/4 oz)	380	23	29	20	5	14	12	41	7	20	6	—	—	2	*	10	15	15	—	—
(Totino's Party, Family Size) 1/4 pizza (4 1/4 oz)	410	20	31	20	7	15	12	44	7	25	6	—	—	2	*	10	20	15	—	—
(Weight Watchers) 6 oz	350	45	14	25	10	13	24	22	13	35	10	—	—	15	15	—	—	—	—	—
French bread (Healthy Choice) 6 1/4 oz	320	37	12	—	10	14	—	20	11	20	25	—	—	15	*	35	20	20	—	—
microwave (Pillsbury Oven Lovin') 1 piece (6 oz)	410	30	32	40	12	13	—	41	8	30	10	—	—	10	8	25	20	20	—	—
(Pillsbury Oven Lovin') 1/2 pizza (3 3/4 oz)	300	22	26	30	8	8	—	26	5	25	10	—	—	8	6	15	15	10	—	—
(Totino's) 1 pizza (4 oz)	270	17	20	15	5	10	—	28	4	15	10	—	—	8	8	15	15	10	—	—
pan style (Pappalo's) 1/4 pizza (6 1/2 oz)	350	46	17	30	17	13	12	30	9	30	30	—	—	15	6	45	35	25	—	—
(Totino's) 1/6 pizza (4 1/3 oz)	330	27	23	30	10	12	—	26	6	25	8	—	—	10	6	10	10	10	—	—
traditional crust (Pappalo's) 1/4 of 12" pizza (5 1/4 oz)	350	37	17	25	15	13	16	29	9	30	25	—	—	15	8	40	35	25	—	—
(Pappalo's) 1/3 of 9" pizza (4 oz)	390	26	22	30	15	16	16	36	11	50	25	—	—	10	2	45	25	30	—	—
pepperoni & mushroom (Stouffer's) 12 1/4 oz	430	32	32	30	10	14	12	42	10	25	15	—	—	8	15	50	25	25	—	—
sandwich (Weight Watchers Entree) 5 oz	300	28	5	13	16	16	—	20	7	15	8	—	—	10	6	—	—	—	—	—
sausage (Jeno's) 1/2 pizza (4 oz)	280	17	23	15	3	9	4	27	5	15	10	—	—	8	4	20	15	10	—	—
(Jeno's Pizza Pockets) 1 (4 1/2 oz)	360	18	29	35	5	12	—	27	5	15	10	—	—	8	8	25	15	15	—	—
(Jeno's Pizza Rolls) 3 oz	210	15	11	10	5	9	6	14	6	6	4	—	—	*	*	6	8	6	—	—
(Stouffer's) 12 oz	420	33	31	25	12	14	16	37	10	25	15	—	—	8	10	40	25	20	—	—
(Stouffer's Lean Cuisine) 6 oz	350	37	15	20	12	14	—	25	13	25	20	—	—	6	10	25	30	25	—	—
(Stouffer's Lunch Express) 6 1/2 oz	220	—	38	40	13	13	12	45	11	20	20	—	—	8	15	—	—	—	—	—
(Totino's Party) 1/2 pizza (5 1/2 oz)	370	25	26	20	3	15	12	33	8	20	6	—	—	2	*	10	15	10	—	—
(Totino's Party, Family Size) 1/4 pizza (4 1/2 oz)	410	20	28	20	5	16	16	36	9	20	6	—	—	2	*	10	20	10	—	—
French bread microwave (Pillsbury Oven Lovin') 1 piece (6 1/3 oz)	400	30	31	50	8	14	—	35	8	30	10	—	—	10	8	30	20	20	—	—
(Pillsbury Oven Lovin') 1/2 pizza (4 oz)	290	20	25	35	5	9	—	21	8	20	10	—	—	8	6	20	15	10	—	—
(Totino's) 1 pizza (4 1/4 oz)	280	17	20	15	3	10	—	28	6	15	10	—	—	8	8	20	15	15	—	—
pan style (Pappalo's) 1/4 pizza (6 1/2 oz)	350	46	17	25	13	13	12	22	7	30	25	—	—	10	6	45	30	30	—	—
(Totino's) 1/6 pizza (4 1/3 oz)	320	27	20	35	7	12	—	21	6	25	6	—	—	10	6	15	10	10	—	—
traditional crust (Pappalo's) 1/4 of 12" pizza (5 1/4 oz)	350	37	18	30	13	13	16	25	8	30	25	—	—	15	8	40	30	30	—	—
(Pappalo's) 1/3 of 9" pizza (4 oz)	380	24	20	30	13	16	16	28	11	50	20	—	—	8	2	40	25	30	—	—
sausage and pepperoni (Jeno's Pizza Pockets) 1 (4 1/2 oz)	360	20	31	35	7	12	—	30	6	15	10	—	—	8	8	25	10	15	—	—
(Stouffer's) 12 1/2 oz	460	38	38	35	13	15	16	47	10	20	20	—	—	8	10	50	25	25	—	—

	Calories	Protein	Fat	Sat. Fat	Cholesterol	Carbohydrates	Fiber	Sodium	Potassium	Calcium	Iron	Zinc	Magnesium	Vitamin A	Vitamin C	Thiamin	Riboflavin	Niacin	Vitamin B12	Folic acid
PIZZA (continued)																				
(Stouffer's Lunch Express) 6 3/8 oz	240	—	42	45	20	14	16	47	10	25	20	—	—	15	20	—	—	—	—	—
pan style (Pappalo's) 1/4 pizza (6 2/3 oz)	360	46	18	30	15	13	12	26	8	30	25	—	—	10	6	45	35	30	—	—
(Totino's) 1/6 pizza (4 1/2 oz)	330	27	23	35	8	12	—	23	6	25	8	—	—	10	6	15	10	10	—	—
traditional crust (Pappalo's) 1/4 of 12" pizza (5 1/2 oz)	360	38	18	30	15	13	16	30	9	30	25	—	—	15	8	40	30	30	—	—
(Pappalo's) 1/3 of 9" pizza (4 oz)	390	26	23	35	15	15	16	27	10	40	20	—	—	8	2	45	25	30	—	—
supreme (Jeno's Pizza Pockets) 1 (4 1/2 oz)	370	20	29	35	7	12	—	30	9	15	15	—	—	10	120	25	15	15	—	—
microwave (Pillsbury Oven Lovin') 1/2 pizza (4 1/3 oz)	310	22	28	35	7	9	—	24	8	25	10	—	—	10	100	20	15	15	—	—
pan style (Pappalo's) 1/4 pizza (6 3/4 oz)	340	46	18	30	15	12	12	25	11	30	25	—	—	15	80	45	30	30	—	—
traditional crust (Pappalo's) 1/4 of 12" pizza (5 2/3 oz)	350	37	18	30	15	13	16	27	11	25	25	—	—	15	110	35	30	25	—	—
(Pappalo's) 1/3 of 9" pizza (4 1/3 oz)	400	28	25	35	15	15	16	29	11	45	20	—	—	8	2	45	30	30	—	—
three cheese (Weight Watchers) 6 oz	320	38	9	15	7	14	20	15	13	40	8	—	—	20	6	—	—	—	—	—
pan style (Pappalo's) 1/4 pizza (6 oz)	310	42	12	25	10	13	12	20	7	30	6	—	—	4	2	25	15	6	—	—
traditional crust (Pappalo's) 1/4 of 12" pizza (5 oz)	310	33	11	20	10	14	16	18	7	35	6	—	—	4	2	25	10	4	—	—
(Pappalo's) 1/3 of 9" pizza (3 2/3 oz)	350	23	17	30	10	16	16	27	9	60	20	—	—	15	2	30	25	25	—	—
three-cheese (Stouffer's Lean Cuisine) 5 1/2 oz	330	38	15	15	7	13	—	15	10	40	15	—	—	6	10	25	30	15	—	—
vegetable deluxe (Stouffer's) 12 3/4 oz	380	30	26	30	8	14	20	35	6	30	15	—	—	25	4	30	25	20	—	—
white (Stouffer's) 10 1/8 oz	460	—	43	40	8	14	20	32	3	35	15	—	—	5	*	—	—	—	—	—
PIZZA SAUCE																				
original (Contadina) 1/4 cup	35	4	2	*	*	2	4	15	—	2	4	—	—	8	8	—	—	—	—	—
pizza squeeze (Contadina) 1/4 cup	35	4	2	*	*	2	4	15	—	2	4	—	—	8	8	—	—	—	—	—
w/ Italian cheeses (Contadina) 1/4 cup	40	4	2	*	*	2	4	17	—	2	4	—	—	8	8	—	—	—	—	—
w/ pepperoni (Contadina) 1/4 cup	40	4	3	3	*	2	4	17	—	2	4	—	—	8	8	—	—	—	—	—
PLANTAIN																				
raw 1 fruit	218	4	*	*	*	19	16	*	25	*	6	2	17	40	55	6	6	6	—	—
1/2 cup slices	90	2	*	*	*	8	8	*	11	*	2	*	7	17	23	3	2	3	—	—
cooked 1/2 cup slices	89	*	*	*	*	8	8	*	10	*	2	*	6	14	14	2	2	3	—	5
PLUM																				
1 fruit	36	*	*	*	*	3	4	*	3	*	*	*	*	4	10	2	4	2	—	*
1/2 cup slices	46	*	*	*	*	4	4	*	4	*	*	*	*	5	13	2	5	2	—	*

	Calories	Protein	Fat	Sat. Fat	Cholesterol	Carbohydrates	Fiber	Sodium	Potassium	Calcium	Iron	Zinc	Magnesium	Vitamin A	Vitamin C	Thiamin	Riboflavin	Niacin	Vitamin B$_{12}$	Folic acid
PLUM, CANNED																				
in extra heavy syrup 1/2 cup	133	*	*	*	*	12	—	*	3	*	6	*	2	7	*	*	3	2	—	*
in heavy syrup 1/2 cup	115	*	*	*	*	10	4	*	3	*	6	*	2	7	*	*	3	2	—	*
in juice 1/2 cup	73	*	*	*	*	6	4	*	6	*	2	*	3	25	6	2	4	3	—	*
in light syrup 1/2 cup	79	*	*	*	*	7	4	*	3	*	6	*	2	7	*	*	3	2	—	*
in water 1/2 cup	51	*	*	*	*	5	4	*	5	*	*	*	2	23	6	2	3	2	—	*
PLUM SAUCE																				
from mix, spicy (Knorr) 1 3/4 oz	220	60	8	—	—	5	—	34	—	2	6	*	*	*	*	*	4	6	50	*	*
POI 1/2 cup	134	*	*	*	*	11	*	*	6	2	6	2	7	*	8	10	3	7	*	6
POKEBERRY SHOOT																				
raw 1/2 cup	18	3	*	*	*	*	4	*	6	4	8	*	4	139	181	4	16	5	*	3
boiled 1/2 cup	16	3	*	*	*	*	4	*	4	4	5	*	3	143	112	4	12	5	*	2
boiled w/ salt 1/2 cup	16	3	*	*	*	*	—	9	4	4	5	*	3	143	112	4	12	5	*	2
POLISH SAUSAGE see KIELBASA																				
POLLOCK, ATLANTIC																				
raw 1/2 fillet	178	63	3	*	46	*	*	7	20	12	5	6	32	*	*	6	21	32	102	*
broiled/baked 1/2 fillet	178	63	3	*	46	*	*	7	20	12	5	6	32	*	*	5	20	30	92	*
POLLOCK, WALLEYE																				
raw 1 fillet	62	22	*	*	18	*	*	3	7	*	*	2	11	*	*	3	3	5	40	*
baked/broiled 1 fillet	68	24	*	*	19	*	*	3	7	*	*	2	11	*	*	3	3	5	42	*
POMEGRANATE																				
raw 1 fruit	105	2	*	*	*	9	4	*	11	*	3	—	*	*	16	3	3	2	*	*
POMEGRANATE JUICE *(Knudsen)* 8 fl oz	150	*	*	*	*	12	*	*	12	*	6	—	—	*	45	—	—	—	—	—
POMPANO																				
raw 1 fillet	184	34	16	20	19	*	*	3	12	2	4	5	8	2	*	42	8	17	24	*
baked/broiled 1 fillet	186	35	16	20	19	*	*	3	16	4	3	4	7	2	*	40	8	17	18	*
POPCORN																				
air popped (Orville Redenbacher's) 3 cups	40	2	*	*	*	3	12	*	2	*	2	*	*	*	*	*	*	*	—	—
white (generic) 1 cup	31	2	*	*	*	2	—	*	*	*	*	2	3	*	*	*	*	*	*	*
yellow (generic) 1 cup	31	2	*	*	*	2	4	*	*	*	*	2	3	*	*	*	*	*	*	*
butter (Chester's) 3 cups	160	3	18	8	*	5	12	14						—	—	*	*	*	—	—
(Smartfood) 3 cups	150	3	14	10	2	5	4	10						—	—	—	—	—	—	—
(Weight Watchers) 1 bag (2/3 oz)	90	3	4	*	*	5	12	4	*	*	2	—	—	*	*	—	—	—	—	—
butter toffee (Weight Watchers) 1 bag (1 oz)	110	2	4	5	*	7	4	4	*	*	4	—	—	*	*	—	—	—	—	—
caramel (generic) 1 cup	152	2	7	7	*	9	8	3	*	2	3	*	3	*	*	2	4	*	4	*

POPCORN (continued)

	Calories	Protein	Fat	Sat. Fat	Cholesterol	Carbohydrates	Fiber	Sodium	Potassium	Calcium	Iron	Zinc	Magnesium	Vitamin A	Vitamin C	Thiamin	Riboflavin	Niacin	Vitamin B12	Folic acid
(Health Valley) 1 oz	100	2	*	*	*	7	—	2	2	*	2	—	—	2	*	2	*	*	—	—
(Slim-Fast) 1 oz	110	10	3	—	*	8	12	*	*	10	2	4	*	10	10	10	10	10	10	10
(Weight Watchers) 1 bag (1 oz)	100	2	2	*	*	7	4	2	2	*	4	—	—	*	*	—	—	—	—	—
caramel apple cinnamon (Health Valley) 1 oz	100	2	*	*	*	7	—	2	*	*	2	—	—	2	*	2	*	*	—	—
caramel peanut (Health Valley) 1 oz	100	2	*	*	*	7	—	3	*	*	2	—	—	2	*	2	*	*	—	—
cheddar (Smartfood) 3 cups	285	7	28	19	2	8	12	19			—									
cheddar, white (Weight Watchers) 1 bag (2/3 oz)	90	3	6	5	*	4	8	5	2	*	2	—	—	*	*	—	—	—	—	—
cheese (Chester's) 3 cups	190	5	20	13	*	6	12	12			—									
cheese flavor (generic) 3 cups	174	6	18	12	*	6	12	12	*	*	*	*	9	*	*	*	6	*	*	*
flamin' hot (Chester's) 3 cups	170	5	14	8	*	6	4	14			—									
maple & walnut (Crunch & Munch) 2/3 cup	140	2	6	3	1	8	3	7	—	*	2	—	—	2	*	—	—	—	—	—
microwave (Chester's) 3 cups	120	3	18	8	*	7	16	12			—									
(Weight Watchers) 1 bag (1 oz)	90	5	2	*	*	7	28	*	2	*	4	—	—	*	*	—	—	—	—	—
butter flavor (Orville Redenbacher's) 3 cups	100	3	9	7	*	4	12	10	2	*	2	—	—	*	*	*	*	*	—	—
(Pop Secret) 3 cups	120	3	12	10	*	4	—	7	2	*	2	—	—	*	*	*	*	*	—	—
(Pop Secret Light) 3 cups	70	3	5	3	*	4	—	5	—	*	2	—	—	*	*	*	*	*	—	—
(Pop Secret Pop Quiz) 2 3/4 cups	80	2	8	5	*	3	—	5	*	*	2	—	—	*	*	*	*	*	—	—
frozen (Orville Redenbacher's) 3 cups	100	3	9	7	*	4	12	10	2	*	2	—	—	*	*	*	*	*	—	—
light (Orville Redenbacher's) 3 cups	70	3	5	3	*	3	12	5	2	*	2	—	—	*	*	*	*	*	—	—
salt free (Pop Secret) 3 cups	120	3	12	10	*	4	—	*	2	*	2	—	—	*	*	*	*	*	—	—
butter toffee (Orville Redenbacher's) 3 cups	210	4	18	15	*	9	8	4	3	*	4	—	—	*	*	*	*	*	—	—
cheddar cheese (Orville Redenbacher's) 3 cups	130	3	12	9	*	5	12	12	2	*	2	—	—	*	*	*	3	*	—	—
(Cape Cod) 1 oz	170	7	18	13	3	4	8	11	—	6	2	—	—	2	*	—	—	—	—	—
light (Orville Redenbacher's) 3 cups	70	3	5	3	*	3	12	5	2	*	2	—	—	*	*	*	*	*	—	—
natural flavor (Orville Redenbacher's) 3 cups	100	3	9	7	*	4	12	8	2	*	2	—	—	*	*	*	*	*	—	—
(Pop Secret) 3 cups	120	3	12	10	*	4	—	7	2	*	2	—	—	*	*	*	*	*	—	—
(Pop Secret Light) 3 cups	70	3	5	3	*	4	—	7	—	*	2	—	—	*	*	*	*	*	—	—
frozen (Orville Redenbacher's) 3 cups	100	3	9	7	*	4	12	8	2	*	2	—	—	*	*	*	*	*	—	—
salt free (Orville Redenbacher's) 3 cups	100	3	9	7	*	4	12	*	2	*	2	—	—	*	*	*	*	*	—	—
salt free butter flavor (Orville Redenbacher's) 3 cups	100	3	9	7	*	4	12	*	2	*	2	—	—	*	*	*	*	*	—	—
sour cream 'n' onion (Orville Redenbacher's) 3 cups	160	3	18	14	*	4	12	11	3	2	2	—	—	*	2	*	4	2	—	—
oil-popped (generic) 1 cup	55	2	5	3	*	2	4	4	*	*	2	2	3	*	*	*	*	*	—	*
white (generic) 1 cup	55	2	5	3	*	2	—	4	*	*	2	2	3	*	*	*	*	*	*	*
w/ peanuts (generic) 2 oz	227	6	7	3	*	15	8	7	6	4	12	5	11	*	*	2	4	6	*	2

PERCENTAGE DAILY VALUE

	Calories	Protein	Fat	Sat. Fat	Cholesterol	Carbohydrates	Fiber	Sodium	Potassium	Calcium	Iron	Zinc	Magnesium	Vitamin A	Vitamin C	Thiamin	Riboflavin	Niacin	Vitamin B₁₂	Folic acid

POPCORN (continued)

plain

	Calories	Protein	Fat	Sat. Fat	Cholesterol	Carbohydrates	Fiber	Sodium	Potassium	Calcium	Iron	Zinc	Magnesium	Vitamin A	Vitamin C	Thiamin	Riboflavin	Niacin	Vitamin B12	Folic acid
(Slim-Fast) 1 oz	60	10	3	—	*	3	8	*	*	10	2	4	*	10	10	10	10	10	10	10
(Smartfood) 3 cups	150	2	17	8	*	4	4	6		—	—	—	—	—	—	—	—	—	—	—
toffee																				
(Crunch & Munch) 2/3 cup	140	3	6	4	1	8	4	7	—	*	*	—	—	2	*	—	—	—	—	—
triple mix																				
(Chester's) 3 cups	280	3	22	10	*	13	8	21												
white																				
(Orville Redenbacher's) 3 cups	80	2	6	—	*	3	12	*	2	*	2	—	*	*	*	*	*	*	—	—
(Orville Redenbacher's) 3 cups	80	2	6	—	*	3	12	*	2	*	2	—	*	*	*	*	*	*	—	—
POPCORN CAKES																				
(generic) 2 cakes	77	3	*	*	*	5	4	2	2	*	2	5	8	*	*	*	2	6	*	*
POPCORN OIL																				
(Orville Redenbacher's) 1 tbsp	120	*	22	10	*	*	*	*	*	*	*	*	*	*	*	*	*	*	*	*
POPPY SEED																				
1 tbsp	47	3	6	2	*	*	12	*	2	13	5	6	7	*	—	5	*	*	*	—
CHITTERLINGS see PORK																				
PORK																				
backrib																				
raw																				
3 oz	240	23	31	37	23	*	*	3	6	3	4	13	4	*	*	33	13	19	12	*
salt pork																				
raw																				
1 oz	212	2	35	42	8	*	*	17	*	*	*	2	*	*	*	4	*	2	*	*
blade																				
lean & fat																				
braised																				
3 oz	275	31	33	41	24	*	*	2	7	3	5	19	5	*	*	27	12	15	9	*
broiled																				
3 oz	272	32	32	40	24	*	*	2	8	2	4	19	4	*	*	37	15	17	12	*
roasted																				
3 oz	275	34	32	39	26	*	*	*	8	3	5	19	5	*	*	30	15	18	10	*
lean only																				
braised																				
3 oz	191	35	17	20	24	*	*	2	8	2	6	22	6	*	*	30	14	17	10	*
broiled																				
3 oz	199	36	18	22	24	*	*	3	9	2	5	22	5	*	*	42	17	19	13	*
fried																				
3 oz	291	30	36	43	24	*	*	2	8	3	4	18	4	*	*	35	15	17	12	*
roasted																				
3 oz	210	38	19	23	26	*	*	*	8	2	6	22	6	*	*	33	17	20	11	*
Boston blade																				
lean & fat																				
braised																				
3 oz	271	41	28	34	32	*	*	2	9	3	9	28	9	*	*	38	18	17	13	*
broiled																				
3 oz	220	36	22	26	27	*	*	2	8	2	7	26	9	*	*	39	20	17	15	*
roasted																				
3 oz	229	33	25	30	24	*	*	2	8	2	7	22	7	*	*	36	18	17	12	*
lean only																				
braised																				
3 oz	232	44	20	24	33	*	*	3	10	2	10	32	10	*	*	41	20	18	14	*
broiled																				
3 oz	193	38	16	19	27	*	*	3	8	3	7	28	7	*	*	42	22	18	16	*
roasted																				
3 oz	197	34	19	22	24	*	*	3	10	2	7	24	7	*	*	63	20	21	16	2
brains																				
braised																				
3 oz	117	17	12	9	723	*	*	3	5	*	9	8	9	*	20	4	11	14	20	*

	Calories	Protein	Fat	Sat. Fat	Cholesterol	Carbohydrates	Fiber	Sodium	Potassium	Calcium	Iron	Zinc	Magnesium	Vitamin A	Vitamin C	Thiamin	Riboflavin	Niacin	Vitamin B₁₂	Folic acid

PORK (continued)

center loin
fried

	Calories	Protein	Fat	Sat. Fat	Cholesterol	Carbohydrates	Fiber	Sodium	Potassium	Calcium	Iron	Zinc	Magnesium	Vitamin A	Vitamin C	Thiamin	Riboflavin	Niacin	Vitamin B₁₂	Folic acid
1 chop	160	37	11	13	21	*	*	2	9	2	4	11	4	*	*	57	13	21	9	*
3 oz	236	42	22	26	26	*	*	3	10	2	4	13	4	*	*	64	15	24	10	*
center rib fried																				
1 chop	193	32	19	23	18	*	*	2	9	2	3	10	3	*	*	39	13	20	9	*
lean & fat braised																				
1 chop	188	33	17	22	18	*	*	*	8	2	4	10	4	*	*	30	10	19	7	*
broiled																				
1 chop	195	35	18	21	20	*	*	2	8	2	3	11	3	*	*	51	13	21	9	*
roasted																				
1 chop	189	34	17	22	18	*	*	*	9	2	4	10	4	*	*	36	13	23	8	*
lean only braised																				
1 chop	138	32	10	13	16	*	*	*	8	*	4	9	4	*	*	28	10	17	6	*
broiled																				
1 chop	147	34	10	12	18	*	*	2	8	2	3	11	3	*	*	50	13	21	8	*
roasted																				
1 chop	154	33	12	15	16	*	*	*	9	2	4	10	4	*	*	35	13	22	8	*
chitterlings cooked																				
3 oz	258	15	38	43	40	*	*	*	*	2	17	29	17	*	*	*	4	*	15	*
cut loin lean & fat braised																				
1 chop	205	39	18	22	24	*	*	2	8	2	5	12	5	*	*	43	10	19	7	*
broiled																				
1 chop	197	39	16	20	22	*	*	2	8	3	4	12	4	*	*	58	14	21	10	*
roasted																				
1 chop	197	37	17	22	22	*	*	2	8	2	5	11	5	*	*	48	12	22	8	*
lean only braised																				
1 chop	149	37	9	12	21	*	*	2	8	2	5	11	5	*	*	41	10	18	6	*
broiled																				
1 chop	149	37	9	11	20	*	*	2	8	2	3	12	3	*	*	57	13	21	9	*
roasted																				
1 chop	153	35	11	13	20	*	*	2	8	2	4	11	4	*	*	47	12	21	7	*
ears simmered																				
1 ear	184	29	18	22	33	*	*	8	*	2	9	*	9	*	*	*	5	3	*	*
feet pickled																				
3 oz	173	19	21	*	2	*	*	33	6	3	3	7	3	*	*	2	18	*	*	*
simmered																				
3 oz	165	27	16	18	28	*	*	*	4	4	2	6	2	*	*	*	3	2	3	*
ground cooked																				
3 oz	253	36	27	33	27	*	*	3	9	2	6	18	6	*	*	40	11	18	8	*
heart braised																				
1 cup	215	57	11	10	107	*	*	2	9	*	47	30	47	*	5	54	145	44	91	2
kidneys braised																				
1 cup	211	59	10	11	224	*	*	5	6	2	41	39	41	7	25	37	131	40	181	14
lard																				
1 tbsp	115	*	20	*	*	*	*	*	*	*	*	*	*	*	*	*	*	*	*	*
leaf fat																				
3 oz	729	2	123	193	31	*	*	*	*	*	*	*	*	*	*	6	3	5	3	*

	Calories	Protein	Fat	Sat. Fat	Cholesterol	Carbohydrates	Fiber	Sodium	Potassium	Calcium	Iron	Zinc	Magnesium	Vitamin A	Vitamin C	Thiamin	Riboflavin	Niacin	Vitamin B12	Folic acid
PORK (continued)																				
lings																				
braised 3 oz	84	24	4	5	110	*	*	3	4	*	77	14	77	*	11	4	16	6	29	*
liver																				
braised 3 oz	140	37	6	6	101	*	*	2	4	*	85	38	85	306	33	15	110	36	264	35
loin																				
lean & fat braised 1 chop	213	40	19	23	24	*	*	2	9	2	5	14	5	*	*	37	13	20	8	*
broiled 1 chop	211	40	19	23	23	*	*	2	10	2	4	14	4	*	*	51	16	22	10	*
roasted 1 chop	221	40	20	24	24	*	*	2	10	2	5	14	5	*	*	59	16	25	10	*
lean only braised 1 chop	167	39	12	14	22	*	*	2	9	*	5	14	5	*	*	36	13	19	7	*
broiled 1 chop	166	38	12	15	21	*	*	2	10	*	4	13	4	*	*	49	16	21	9	*
roasted 1 chop	169	39	12	14	22	*	*	2	10	*	5	14	5	*	*	55	16	24	10	*
picnic																				
lean & fat braised 3 oz	280	40	30	36	31	*	*	3	9	2	8	24	8	*	*	31	15	22	9	*
roasted 3 oz	270	33	31	38	27	*	*	2	8	2	6	20	6	*	*	30	15	17	10	*
lean only braised 3 oz	211	46	16	18	32	*	*	4	10	*	9	28	9	*	*	34	18	25	11	*
roasted 3 oz	194	38	16	19	27	*	*	3	9	*	7	23	7	*	*	33	18	18	11	*
rib																				
lean & fat braised 3 oz	252	34	28	34	25	*	*	2	8	2	6	20	6	*	*	29	13	16	10	*
lean only braised 3 oz	199	37	18	21	24	*	*	2	8	2	7	23	7	*	*	31	14	17	10	*
roasted 3 oz	210	38	19	23	26	*	*	*	8	2	6	22	6	*	*	33	17	20	11	*
shoulder																				
lean & fat roasted 3 oz	248	33	28	34	25	*	*	2	8	2	6	21	6	*	*	33	16	17	11	*
lean only roasted 3 oz	196	36	18	21	25	*	*	3	8	2	7	24	7	*	*	36	19	18	12	*
sirloin																				
lean & fat braised 1 chop	196	34	19	22	22	*	*	2	7	*	5	13	5	*	*	35	12	15	7	*
braised 3 oz	161	38	11	13	23	*	*	2	9	*	5	13	5	*	*	39	14	17	8	*
broiled 1 chop	154	38	10	11	22	*	*	2	8	*	5	13	5	*	*	50	17	17	10	*
roasted 1 chop	201	35	19	22	22	*	*	2	8	2	4	12	4	*	*	38	14	20	10	*
roasted 3 oz	176	40	12	15	24	*	*	2	10	*	6	14	6	*	*	50	19	22	11	*

	Calories	Protein	Fat	Sat. Fat	Cholesterol	Carbohydrates	Fiber	Sodium	Potassium	Calcium	Iron	Zinc	Magnesium	Vitamin A	Vitamin C	Thiamin	Riboflavin	Niacin	Vitamin B$_{12}$	Folic acid
PORK (continued)																				
lean only																				
braised																				
3 oz	149	38	9	10	23	*	*	2	9	*	5	13	5	*	*	39	14	17	8	*
broiled																				
1 chop	137	37	7	8	22	*	*	2	8	*	5	13	5	*	*	49	17	17	10	*
roasted																				
3 oz	184	41	14	16	24	*	*	2	9	2	5	15	5	*	*	45	17	24	11	*
sparerib																				
cooked																				
3 oz	338	41	40	*	3	*	*	3	8	4	9	26	9	*	*	22	274	3	5	*
sweetbreads																				
pancreas braised																				
3 oz	186	40	14	16	89	*	*	*	4	*	13	24	13	*	8	5	33	14	241	*
spleen braised																				
3 oz	127	40	4	5	143	*	*	4	6	*	105	20	105	*	16	8	13	25	39	*
tail																				
simmered																				
3 oz	337	24	47	53	37	*	*	*	4	*	4	9	4	*	*	4	4	5	8	*
tenderloin																				
lean & fat																				
broiled																				
1 chop	153	38	10	11	24	*	*	2	10	*	6	15	6	*	*	49	17	19	12	*
roasted																				
3 oz	147	39	8	9	22	*	*	2	10	*	7	15	7	*	*	53	19	20	8	*
lean only																				
broiled																				
1 chop	137	37	7	8	23	*	*	2	9	*	6	14	6	*	*	48	17	19	12	*
roasted																				
3 oz	139	40	6	7	22	*	*	2	11	*	7	15	7	*	*	53	20	20	8	*
tongue																				
braised																				
3 oz	230	34	24	8	*	*	*	4	6	2	24	26	24	*	2	18	26	23	34	*
top loin																				
lean & fat																				
1 chop	189	35	17	19	20	*	*	2	11	2	4	11	4	*	*	54	15	24	9	2
3 oz	162	29	15	17	17	*	*	2	9	2	3	9	3	*	*	45	13	20	7	*
braised																				
3 oz	198	39	17	20	21	*	*	*	10	2	5	12	5	*	*	31	13	19	6	*
broiled																				
1 chop	163	35	12	14	19	*	*	2	8	2	3	11	3	*	*	40	13	18	8	*
roasted																				
3 oz	192	41	15	18	22	*	*	2	8	*	4	13	4	*	*	35	15	22	8	2
lean only																				
braised																				
3 oz	172	41	11	14	21	*	*	*	10	2	5	12	5	*	*	32	13	20	6	*
broiled																				
1 chop	134	34	8	9	18	*	*	2	8	2	3	10	3	*	*	39	13	17	8	2
fried																				
1 chop	142	32	10	12	16	*	*	*	9	*	3	10	3	*	*	35	14	18	7	*
roasted																				
3 oz	165	43	9	11	22	*	*	2	9	*	5	13	5	*	*	36	16	23	8	2
PORK, CANNED																				
loin																				
Cajun style																				
(Bryan) 3 oz	160	28	15	—	17	*	*	47	—	—	—	—	—	—	—	—	—	—	—	—
lemon pepper																				
(Bryan) 3 oz	160	28	15	—	17	*	*	49	—	—	—	—	—	—	—	—	—	—	—	—
regular																				
(Bryan) 3 oz	160	28	15	—	17	*	*	2	—	—	—	—	—	—	—	—	—	—	—	—

	Calories	Protein	Fat	Sat. Fat	Cholesterol	Carbohydrates	Fiber	Sodium	Potassium	Calcium	Iron	Zinc	Magnesium	Vitamin A	Vitamin C	Thiamin	Riboflavin	Niacin	Vitamin B_{12}	Folic acid
PORK, CANNED (continued)																				
southern style (Bryan) 3 oz	160	28	15	—	17	*	*	49	—	—	—	—	—	—	—	—	—	—	—	—
tenderloin (Bryan) 3 oz	110	28	6	—	17	*	*	2	—	—	—	—	—	—	—	—	—	—	—	—
PORK, CURED																				
picnic 3 oz	238	29	28	33	16	*	*	38	6	*	4	14	4	*	*	35	10	18	13	*
shoulder lean & fat roasted 3 oz	229	23	29	34	15	*	*	44	7	*	4	13	4	*	*	31	11	12	18	*
PORK DINNER, FROZEN																				
loin (Swanson) 10 3/4 oz	270	40	15	—	—	9		34	—	4	8	—	—	80	10	30	8	25	—	—
PORK ENTREE, FROZEN																				
barbecue sandwich (Hormel Quickmeal) 4 1/4 oz	350	27	22	25	22	13	—	23	9	4	15	14	8	*	*	30	15	20		
sweet & sour (Chun King) 13 oz	400	18	8	—	8	26	—	61	9	2	10	—	—	30	20	30	10	10	—	—
PORK GRAVY																				
canned (Franco-American) 2 oz	40	*	5	—	*	*	*	14	—	*	*	—	—	*	*	*	*	*	*	*
from mix (generic) 1 cup	26	*	*	—	—	*	—	17	*	*	*	*	*	—	—	*	*	*	*	*
PORK SKINS																				
barbecue flavor (generic) 1/2 oz	76	14	7	8	5	*	—	16	*	*	*	*	*	4	*	*	4	2	*	*
plain (generic) 1/2 oz	77	14	7	8	4	*	—	11	*	*	*	*	*	*	*	*	2	*	2	*
POTATO																				
flesh only raw 1/2 cup diced	59	3	*	*	*	4	4	*	12	*	3	2	4	*	25	4	2	6	*	2
1 medium	88	4	*	*	*	7	8	*	17	*	5	3	6	*	37	7	2	8	*	4
baked 1/2 cup	57	2	*	*	*	4	4	*	7	*	*	*	4	*	13	4	*	4	*	*
1 medium	145	5	*	*	*	11	8	*	17	*	3	3	10	*	33	11	2	11	*	4
baked w/ salt 1/2 cup	57	2	*	*	*	4	—	6	7	*	*	*	4	*	13	4	*	4	*	*
boiled 1/2 cup	67	2	*	*	*	5	4	*	7	*	*	*	4	*	10	5	*	5	*	2
1 medium	116	4	*	*	*	9	8	*	13	*	2	2	7	*	17	9	2	9	*	3
boiled w/ salt 1 medium	118	4	*	*	*	9	8	*	15	*	2	3	7	*	29	10	2	10	*	3
1/2 cup	67	2	*	*	*	5	8	8	7	*	*	*	4	*	10	5	*	5	*	2
microwaved, salted 1 medium	156	5	*	*	*	12	—	*	18	*	4	3	10	*	39	13	2	13	*	5
flesh & skin baked 1 medium	220	8	*	*	*	17	20	*	24	2	15	4	14	*	43	14	4	17	*	6
baked, salted 1/2 cup mashed	103	3	*	*	*	8	—	10	10	3	2	2	5	*	41	5	7	3	*	6
boiled, salted 1/2 cup	68	2	*	*	*	5	8	8	8	*	*	2	4	*	17	6	*	6	*	2
microwave 1 medium	212	8	*	*	*	16	—	*	26	2	14	5	14	*	51	16	4	17	*	6
microwave, salted 1 medium	212	8	*	*	*	16	—	21	26	2	14	5	14	*	51	16	4	17	*	6

	Calories	Protein	Fat	Sat. Fat	Cholesterol	Carbohydrates	Fiber	Sodium	Potassium	Calcium	Iron	Zinc	Magnesium	Vitamin A	Vitamin C	Thiamin	Riboflavin	Niacin	Vitamin B$_{12}$	Folic acid
POTATO (continued)																				
skin																				
raw																				
skin from 1 potato	22	2	*	*	*	2	—	*	4	*	7	*	2	*	7	*	*	2	*	2
baked																				
skin from 1 potato	115	4	*	*	*	9	8	*	9	2	23	2	6	*	13	5	4	9	*	3
baked w/ salt																				
skin from 1 potato	115	4	*	*	*	9	—	6	9	2	23	2	6	*	13	5	4	9	*	3
boiled																				
skin from 1 potato	27	2	*	*	*	2	—	*	4	2	11	*	3	*	3	*	*	2	*	*
boiled w/ salt																				
skin from 1 potato	27	2	*	*	*	2	—	4	4	2	11	*	3	*	3	*	*	2	*	*
microwaved																				
skin from 1 potato	77	4	*	*	*	6	—	*	11	3	19	2	5	*	15	3	3	6	*	2
microwaved w/ salt																				
skin from 1 potato	77	4	*	*	*	6	—	6	11	3	19	2	5	*	15	3	3	6	*	2
POTATO, CANNED																				
new																				
(Hunt's) 1/2 cup	70	3	*	*	*	5	*	10	6	*	8	—	—	*	5	4	*	5	—	—
sliced																				
(Del Monte) 2/3 cup	60	2	*	*	*	4	8	15	—	2	2	—	—	*	20	—	—	—	—	—
whole																				
(Del Monte) 2 whole	60	2	*	*	*	4	8	15	—	2	2	—	—	*	20	—	—	—	—	—
white																				
(Bush Bros) 1/2 cup	50	3	*	*	*	3	4	17	—	6	6	—	—	*	4	—	—	—	—	—
drained																				
(generic) 1/2 cup	54	2	*	*	*	4	—	10	6	*	6	2	3	*	8	4	*	4	*	*
solid & liquid																				
(generic) 1/2 cup	60	3	*	*	*	4	8	19	10	5	8	4	5	*	31	3	2	7	*	2
POTATO, FROZEN																				
French-fried																				
10 strips	107	3	6	10	*	5	8	*	6	*	4	*	3	*	11	5	*	6	*	2
cooked in vegetable & animal fat																				
10 strips	158	3	13	17	2	7	8	4	10	*	2	*	4	*	9	6	*	8	*	4
cooked in vegetable oil																				
10 strips	158	3	13	13	*	7	8	4	10	*	2	*	4	*	9	6	*	8	*	4
crinkle-cut																				
10 strips	99	3	6	9	*	5	—	*	6	*	4	*	3	*	9	4	*	6	*	2
salted																				
10 strips	100	3	6	3	*	5	8	6	6	*	3	*	3	*	8	4	*	5	*	2
unsalted																				
10 strips	100	3	6	3	*	5	8	*	6	*	3	*	3	*	8	4	*	5	*	2
hash browns																				
cooked																				
1/2 cup	170	4	14	18	—	7	8	*	10	*	7	2	3	*	8	6	*	9	*	*
whole																				
boiled																				
1 medium	131	7	*	*	*	10	—	2	17	*	9	3	6	*	32	14	3	13	*	4
boiled, salted																				
1 medium	131	7	*	*	*	10	—	22	17	*	9	3	6	*	32	14	3	13	*	4
POTATO CHIPS & CRISPS																				
barbecue																				
(generic) 2 oz	278	7	28	23	—	10	9	18	20	3	6	4	11	2	32	8	7	13	—	12
(Lay's) 2 oz	300	4	30	20	*	10	8	18		—	—	—	—	—	—	—	—	—	—	—
(Pringle's Right Crisp) 2 oz	280	6	22	20	*	12	8	14	—	2	2	—	—	2	12	—	—	—	—	—
(Ruffles) 2 oz	300	4	28	30	*	10	8	10		—	—	—	—	—	—	—	—	—	—	—
K.C. Masterpiece (Lay's) 2 oz	300	6	28	26	*	10	8	22		—	—	—	—	—	—	—	—	—	—	—

PERCENTAGE DAILY VALUE

	Calories	Protein	Fat	Sat. Fat	Cholesterol	Carbohydrates	Fiber	Sodium	Potassium	Calcium	Iron	Zinc	Magnesium	Vitamin A	Vitamin C	Thiamin	Riboflavin	Niacin	Vitamin B₁₂	Folic acid
POTATO CHIPS & CRISPS (continued)																				
cheddar & sour cream (Ruffles) 2 oz	320	4	30	26	*	10	8	20	—	—	—	—	—	—	—	—	—	—	—	—
cheese flavor (generic) 2 oz	281	8	24	24	*	11	—	19	25	4	6	3	11	—	51	6	5	14	—	—
from dried potatoes (generic) 2 oz	351	7	36	31	*	11	—	20	7	7	6	3	8	—	9	8	4	8	—	3
choice (Ruffles) 2 oz	260	6	18	10	*	12	8	10	—	—	—	—	—	—	—	—	—	—	—	—
double crunch (Lay's) 2 oz	300	6	28	26	*	10	4	8	—	—	—	—	—	—	—	—	—	—	—	—
flamin' hot (Lay's) 2 oz	300	4	30	26	*	10	8	14	—	—	—	—	—	—	—	—	—	—	—	—
light (generic) 2 oz	267	7	18	12	*	13	—	12	28	*	4	—	13	—	24	8	9	20	—	4
from dried potatoes (generic) 2 oz	284	5	22	15	*	12	8	10	16	2	5	2	9	—	11	7	2	12	—	3
onion & garlic (Lay's) 2 oz	300	6	28	26	*	10	8	18	—	—	—	—	—	—	—	—	—	—	—	—
plain (Lay's) 2 oz	300	6	30	26	*	10	8	10	—	—	—	—	—	—	—	—	—	—	—	—
(Ruffles) 2 oz	300	6	30	30	*	10	8	10	—	—	—	—	—	—	—	—	—	—	—	—
from dried potatoes (generic) 2 oz	355	6	38	30	—	11	9	17	18	2	5	3	9	—	9	9	4	10	—	*
(Pringle's) 2 oz	320	6	34	26	*	10	8	14	—	*	*	—	—	*	12	—	—	—	—	—
(Pringle's Right Crisp) 2 oz	280	4	22	20	*	12	8	12	—	*	*	—	—	*	12	—	—	—	—	—
ranch (Lay's) 2 oz	300	6	28	26	*	10	8	18	—	—	—	—	—	—	—	—	—	—	—	—
(Ruffles) 2 oz	300	6	28	26	*	10	8	24	—	—	—	—	—	—	—	—	—	—	—	—
ranch flavor from dried potatoes (Pringle's) 2 oz	300	6	30	26	*	10	8	10	—	*	2	—	—	*	12	—	—	—	—	—
rippled from dried potatoes (Pringle's) 2 oz	320	6	34	30	*	10	8	12	—	*	2	—	—	*	12	—	—	—	—	—
salted (generic) 2 oz	304	7	30	31	*	10	11	14	21	*	5	4	9	—	29	6	7	11	—	6
salt & vinegar (Lay's) 2 oz	300	6	30	26	*	10	8	28	—	—	—	—	—	—	—	—	—	—	—	—
Saratoga style (Bachman) 2 oz	300	6	24	10	*	10	10	12	—	20	4	—	—	*	*	—	—	—	—	—
sour cream & onion (Lay's) 2 oz	300	6	28	26	*	10	8	14	—	—	—	—	—	—	—	—	—	—	—	—
(Ruffles) 2 oz	300	6	30	30	*	10	8	14	—	—	—	—	—	—	—	—	—	—	—	—
from dried potatoes (generic) 2 oz	348	7	36	30	*	11	—	19	9	4	5	3	9	10	10	8	4	8	—	4
(Pringle's) 2 oz	320	6	30	26	*	10	8	12	—	*	*	—	—	*	12	—	—	—	—	—
(Pringle's Right Crisp) 2 oz	280	6	22	20	*	12	8	10	—	*	*	—	—	*	12	—	—	—	—	—
sour cream & onion flavored (generic) 2 oz	301	8	30	25	*	10	12	15	21	4	5	4	10	2	35	7	7	11	9	9
unsalted (generic) 2 oz	304	7	30	31	*	10	—	—	21	*	5	4	9	—	29	6	7	11	—	6
(Lay's) 2 oz	300	6	30	26	*	10	8	*	—	—	—	—	—	—	—	—	—	—	—	—
wavy au gratin (Lay's) 2 oz	300	6	30	26	*	10	8	16	—	—	—	—	—	—	—	—	—	—	—	—
wavy original (Lay's) 2 oz	320	6	30	26	*	10	8	10	—	—	—	—	—	—	—	—	—	—	—	—
POTATO FLOUR 1 cup	628	24	2	2	*	48	44	3	81	6	171	19	39	*	57	50	15	30	*	23

	Calories	Protein	Fat	Sat. Fat	Cholesterol	Carbohydrates	Fiber	Sodium	Potassium	Calcium	Iron	Zinc	Magnesium	Vitamin A	Vitamin C	Thiamin	Riboflavin	Niacin	Vitamin B$_{12}$	Folic acid
POTATO SALAD																				
1/2 cup	179	6	16	9	28	5	—	27	9	2	5	3	5	5	21	6	4	6	*	2
POTATO SIDE DISH																				
au gratin (homemade) 1/2 cup	161	10	14	29	9	5	8	22	14	15	4	6	6	6	20	5	8	6	*	2
prep. w/ margarine (homemade) 1/2 cup	161	10	14	22	6	5	—	22	14	15	4	6	6	6	20	5	8	6	*	2
hash browns (homemade) 1/2 cup	119	3	17	21	—	2	8	*	7	*	4	2	4	*	7	4	*	8	*	2
prep. w/ butter (homemade) 3 oz	151	3	12	15	7	7	—	4	8	3	5	2	3	2	5	3	2	6	*	3
prep w/ milk (homemade) 1/2 cup	81	3	*	*	*	6	8	13	9	3	2	2	5	*	12	6	2	6	*	2
mashed prep w/ milk & butter (homemade) 1/2 cup	111	3	7	15	4	6	—	13	9	3	2	2	5	4	11	6	2	6	*	2
o'brien (homemade) 1/2 cup	79	4	2	4	*	5	—	9	7	3	3	2	4	9	27	5	3	5	*	2
pancake (homemade) 2 pancakes	413	16	36	23	49	14	12	32	34	4	13	8	13	4	56	14	15	16	5	9
scalloped (homemade) 1/2 cup	105	6	7	14	5	4	8	17	13	7	4	3	6	3	22	6	7	6	*	3
prep. w/ margarine (homemade) 1/2 cup	105	6	7	9	2	4	—	17	13	7	4	3	6	3	22	6	7	6	*	3
POTATO SIDE DISH, FROM MIX																				
American cheese (General Mills Homestyle) 1/2 cup	150	5	9	—	—	7	—	26	9	6	2	—	—	4	*	2	6	4	—	—
au gratin (General Mills) 1/2 cup	150	5	9	—	—	7	—	24	8	8	2	—	—	4	*	*	6	4	—	—
(Kraft) 1/2 cup	130	6	8	10	13	6	—	24	8	10	*	—	—	2	*	8	6	2	—	—
w/ broccoli (General Mills Homestyle) 1/2 cup	140	5	9	—	—	6	—	23	9	4	2	—	—	4	*	*	4	4	—	—
(Kraft) 1/2 cup	150	8	8	10	13	7	—	22	8	10	2	—	—	2	*	8	6	4	—	—
tangy (Pillsbury) 1/2 cup	140	5	9	15	5	7	4	22	6	6	2	—	—	4	2	*	4	4	—	—
bacon & cheddar (Twice Baked Potatoes) 1/2 cup	200	10	15	—	—	7	—	24	12	6	4	—	—	6	*	15	10	4	—	—
cheddar & bacon (General Mills) 1/2 cup	150	5	9	270	97	7	—	—	—	4	*	—	—	4	*	*	6	4	—	—
(Pillsbury) 1/2 cup	140	5	9	15	5	6	4	20	6	6	*	—	—	2	2	2	2	6	—	—
cheddar cheese (General Mills Homestyle) 1/2 cup	150	5	9	—	—	7	—	22	9	6	2	—	—	4	*	2	4	4	—	—
hash browns (General Mills) 1/2 cup	160	3	9	—	—	8	—	19	13	*	2	—	—	4	*	*	*	8	—	—
no salt added (General Mills) 1/2 cup	160	3	9	—	—	8	—	4	13	*	2	—	—	4	*	*	*	8	—	—
julienne (General Mills) 1/2 cup	130	5	8	—	—	6	—	24	7	8	2	—	—	4	*	*	6	4	—	—
mashed flakes (generic) 1/2 cup	119	3	9	18	5	5	8	15	7	5	*	*	5	4	17	8	3	4	*	2
(Hungry Jack) 1/2 cup	120	3	8	*	*	5	4	8	6	4	*	—	—	4	*	2	2	6	—	—
(Idaho Spuds) 1/2 cup	130	5	9	3	*	5	4	15	6	4	*	—	—	6	*	2	2	6	—	—
no salt added (Hungry Jack) 1/2 cup	120	3	8	*	*	5	4	4	6	4	*	—	—	4	*	2	2	6	—	—
no salt added (Idaho Spuds) 1/2 cup	130	5	9	3	*	5	4	4	6	4	*	—	—	6	*	2	2	6	—	—

	Calories	Protein	Fat	Sat. Fat	Cholesterol	Carbohydrates	Fiber	Sodium	Potassium	Calcium	Iron	Zinc	Magnesium	Vitamin A	Vitamin C	Thiamin	Riboflavin	Niacin	Vitamin B$_{12}$	Folic acid
POTATO SIDE DISH, FROM MIX																				
prep w/ milk & margarine (generic) 1/2 cup	119	3	9	8	*	5	—	15	7	5	*	*	5	4	17	8	3	4	*	2
granules (generic) 1/2 cup	83	3	4	4	*	5	—	10	10	3	3	2	4	2	5	2	3	4	*	2
prep w/milk & butter (generic) 1/2 cup	113	4	8	16	5	5	—	11	4	4	*	2	5	4	10	6	5	4	*	2
prep w/milk & margarine (generic) 1/2 cup	111	3	7	6	*	6	—	13	9	3	2	2	5	4	11	6	2	6	*	2
mild cheddar w/ onion (Twice Baked Potatoes) 1/2 cup	200	8	17	—	—	7	—	27	11	6	4	—	—	6	*	2	10	4	—	—
pancakes (Pillsbury) 3 3" pancakes	90	5	3	*	18	5	4	17	4	10	4	—	—	*	*	*	2	4	—	—
potato stroganoff (Hamburger Helper) 1 cup	330	33	25	—	—	9	—	41	17	6	15	—	—	*	*	4	10	25	—	—
potatoes & cheese 2 cheese (Kraft) 1/2 cup	130	6	6	10	3	6	—	22	9	10	*	—	—	2	*	8	6	2	—	—
scalloped (General Mills) 1/2 cup	140	5	8	—	—	7	—	24	8	4	2	—	—	4	*	*	2	6	—	—
(generic) 1/6 of 5.5 oz pkg., prep.	127	5	9	18	—	6	8	19	8	5	3	2	5	4	8	2	5	7	*	3
(Kraft) 1/2 cup	140	6	8	10	8	7	—	21	9	10	*	—	—	2	*	8	6	4	—	—
cheesy (General Mills Homestyle) 1/2 cup	150	5	9	—	—	7	—	23	9	6	2	—	—	4	*	2	6	4	—	—
(Pillsbury) 1/2 cup	150	5	9	15	5	7	4	20	6	4	2	—	—	2	2	*	4	6	—	—
w/ ham (General Mills) 1/2 cup	170	7	11	—	—	7	—	26	8	4	2	—	—	4	*	*	6	6	—	—
(Kraft) 1/2 cup	150	8	8	10	5	7	—	21	9	10	*	—	—	2	*	8	6	2	—	—
w/ white sauce (Pillsbury) 1/2 cup	150	5	9	20	5	7	4	21	6	6	2	—	—	4	2	*	4	4	—	—
smokey cheddar (General Mills) 1/2 cup	140	5	8	—	—	7	—	24	8	8	2	—	—	4	*	*	6	4	—	—
sour cream & chives (General Mills) 1/2 cup	150	5	9	—	—	7	—	22	8	2	2	—	—	4	*	*	2	4	—	—
(Kraft) 1/2 cup	150	6	8	10	3	7	—	25	9	10	*	—	—	2	*	8	6	4	—	—
(Twice Baked Potatoes) 1/2 cup	200	8	17	—	—	6	—	24	10	4	2	—	—	6	*	2	8	6	—	—
POTATO SIDE DISH, FROZEN																				
au gratin (Green Giant) 1/2 cup	120	5	8	10	2	6	6	18	6	4	2	—	—	6	*	*	*	10	—	—
(Stouffer's Side Dishes) 11 1/2 oz	130	8	9	13	5	5	4	25	6	10	*	—	—	*	6	*	6	4	—	—
baked broccoli & cheddar (Stouffer's Lean Cuisine) 10 3/8 oz	290	23	14	20	7	12	—	25	25	40	8	—	—	8	80	15	25	10	—	—
(Stouffer's Lean Cuisine) 10 1/4 oz	280	—	14	20	8	9	24	20	22	30	6	—	—	8	60	—	—	—	—	—
broccoli & cheese (Budget Gourmet Light & Healthy) 10 1/2 oz	300	20	15	20	10	13	—	31	25	30	10	—	—	20	30	20	25	15	—	—
(Green Giant One Serving) 1 pkg (5 1/2 oz)	130	7	6	10	2	6	8	24	13	8	4	—	—	35	15	4	6	6	—	—
(Healthy Choice) 9 1/2 oz	240	13	8	10	5	14	—	21	29	10	15	—	—	*	25	15	10	6	—	—
(Stouffer's) 10 1/8 oz	320	—	23	30	8	10	16	32	26	40	8	—	—	4	50	—	—	—	—	—
(Weight Watchers) 10 oz	230	20	11	10	3	11	24	21	24	25	8	—	—	20	15	—	—	—	—	—
cheddar cheese & bacon (Stouffer's) 9 3/8 oz	380	—	34	40	13	10	20	37	24	30	6	—	—	2	10	—	—	—	—	—
sour cream (Stouffer's Lean Cuisine) 10 3/8 oz	220	15	9	10	5	11	—	24	26	15	6	—	—	50	40	10	20	8	—	—

	Calories	Protein	Fat	Sat. Fat	Cholesterol	Carbohydrates	Fiber	Sodium	Potassium	Calcium	Iron	Zinc	Magnesium	Vitamin A	Vitamin C	Thiamin	Riboflavin	Niacin	Vitamin B₁₂	Folic acid
POTATO SIDE DISH, FROZEN (continued)																				
vegetable primavera (Weight Watchers) 10 oz	220	17	11	15	2	11	24	19	21	25	10	—	—	15	20	—	—	—	—	—
casserole (Healthy Choice Quick Meals) 9 1/4 oz	180	20	6	10	7	8	—	15	17	25	6	—	—	20	25	15	20	*	—	—
cheddared (Budget Gourmet Side Dish) 5 1/2 oz	260	10	25	—	12	7	—	25	9	15	4	—	—	6	10	10	10	10	—	—
w/ broccoli (Budget Gourmet Side Dish) 5 oz	150	8	11	—	7	5	—	17	7	15	2	—	—	10	25	6	8	6	—	—
o'brien (generic) 3 oz	173	3	17	14	—	6	—	2	11	2	5	3	7	3	15	3	7	6	*	3
puff (generic) 1/2 cup	138	3	10	16	*	6	8	19	7	2	5	*	3	*	7	8	3	7	*	3
scalloped (Stouffer's Side Dishes) 11 1/2 oz	130	7	9	5	2	6	8	19	6	10	*	—	—	*	8	2	8	4	—	—
w/ ham (Swanson) 9 oz	300	40	22	—	—	8	—	43	—	25	6	—	—	4	15	20	15	15	—	—
(Hormel Micro Cup) 7 1/2 oz	260	13	25	30	11	7	—	32	12	4	4	6	6	*	19	6	6	11	—	—
three cheese (Budget Gourmet Side Dish) 5 3/4 oz	220	11	17	—	10	8	—	20	11	15	2	—	—	6	10	10	10	8	—	—
POTATO STICKS																				
(generic) 1/2 cup	94	2	10	8	*	3	4	2	6	*	2	*	3	*	14	*	*	4	*	2
POTATO, SWEET see SWEET POTATO																				
POULTRY, see specific listings																				
POULTRY SALAD SPREAD																				
1 oz	56	5	6	5	3	*	*	4	*	*	*	2	*	*	*	*	*	*	2	2
POULTRY SEASONING																				
1 tbsp	11	*	*	18	*	*	*	*	*	4	7	*	2	2	*	*	*	*	*	*
POUT, OCEAN																				
raw 1/2 fillet	139	49	2	3	30	*	*	4	20	2	3	12	6	*	*	9	6	18	26	*
broiled/baked 1/2 fillet	140	49	2	3	31	*	*	4	20	2	3	12	6	*	*	8	6	18	24	*
PRESERVES see JAM, JELLY & PRESERVES																				
PRETZEL																				
(Bachman) 1 oz	120	3	1	1	*	7	3	61	—	*	8	—	—	*	*	—	—	—	—	—
Bavarian (Rold Gold) 1 oz	110	5	3	3	*	7	4	18		—	—	—	—	—	—	—	—	—	—	—
bits garlic (Rold Gold) 1 oz	140	3	12	5	*	5	4	12		—	—	—	—	—	—	—	—	—	—	—
honey mustard (Rold Gold) 1 oz	140	3	12	5	*	6	4	10		—	—	—	—	—	—	—	—	—	—	—
chips cheese (Rold Gold) 1 oz	120	3	4	3	*	7	4	16		—	—	—	—	—	—	—	—	—	—	—
plain (Rold Gold) 1 oz	110	3	2	*	*	8	4	15		—	—	—	—	—	—	—	—	—	—	—
Dutch style (Mr. Salty) 1 oz (1/2 oz)	110	5	2	3	*	7	—	18	*	*	6	—	—	*	*	8	8	8	—	—

	Calories	Protein	Fat	Sat. Fat	Cholesterol	Carbohydrates	Fiber	Sodium	Potassium	Calcium	Iron	Zinc	Magnesium	Vitamin A	Vitamin C	Thiamin	Riboflavin	Niacin	Vitamin B₁₂	Folic acid
PRETZEL (continued)																				
fat free																				
low sodium (Rold Gold) 1 oz	110	5	*	*	*	8	4	14	—	—	—	—	—	—	—	—	—	—	—	—
hard																				
chocolate-covered (generic) 1 pretzel	50	*	3	4	*	3	—	3	*	*	*	*	*	*	*	*	*	*	*	*
salted (generic) 10 twists	229	9	3	3	*	16	8	43	3	2	14	3	5	*	*	18	22	16	*	13
unenriched, plain (generic) 10 twists	229	9	3	3	*	16	—	7	3	2	6	3	5	*	*	7	4	6	*	13
unenriched, salted (generic) 10 twists	229	9	3	3	*	16	—	43	3	2	6	3	5	*	*	7	4	6	*	13
unsalted (generic) 10 twists	229	9	3	3	*	16	8	7	3	2	14	3	5	*	*	18	22	16	*	13
whole wheat (generic) 1 oz	103	5	*	*	*	8	—	3	4	*	4	*	*	*	*	9	5	10	*	4
mini																				
(Mr. Salty) 1 oz (1/2 oz)	110	5	2	3	*	7	—	19	*	*	6	—	—	*	*	8	8	8	—	—
nuggets																				
oat bran (Weight Watchers) 1 bag (1/2 oz)	170	7	4	*	*	11	12	10	2	*	4	—	—	*	*	—	—	—	—	—
rods																				
(Rold Gold) 1 oz	110	5	2	3	*	7	4	15	—	—	—	—	—	—	—	—	—	—	—	—
snack mix																				
(Rold Gold) 1 oz	140	5	9	5	*	6	4	13	—	—	—	—	—	—	—	—	—	—	—	—
sourdough																				
(Rold Gold) 1 oz	90	3	2	*	*	6	4	8	—	—	—	—	—	—	—	—	—	—	—	—
sticks																				
(Rold Gold) 1 oz	110	5	2	*	*	8	4	18	—	—	—	—	—	—	—	—	—	—	—	—
fat free (Mr. Salty) 1 oz (1/2 oz)	110	5	*	*	*	8	—	16	*	*	8	—	—	*	*	8	8	8	—	—
(Rold Gold) 1 oz	110	5	*	*	*	8	4	22	—	—	—	—	—	—	—	—	—	—	—	—
thin																				
(Mr. Salty) 1 oz (1/2 oz)	110	5	2	3	*	7	—	25	*	*	8	—	—	*	*	8	8	8	—	—
thin & light																				
(Bachman) 1 oz	120	5	2	1	*	8	5	27	—	*	8	—	—	*	*	—	—	—	—	—
twists																				
(Mr. Salty) 1 oz (1/2 oz)	110	5	3	3	*	7	—	24	*	*	8	—	—	*	*	8	8	8	—	—
fat free (Mr. Salty) 1 oz (1/2 oz)	110	5	*	*	*	8	—	16	*	*	8	—	—	*	*	8	8	8	—	—
(Rold Gold) 1 oz	100	5	*	*	*	8	4	17	—	—	—	—	—	—	—	—	—	—	—	—
thin (Rold Gold) 1 oz	110	5	2	*	*	7	4	21	—	—	—	—	—	—	—	—	—	—	—	—
tiny																				
(Rold Gold) 1 oz	110	5	2	*	*	7	4	17	—	—	—	—	—	—	—	—	—	—	—	—
wheat																				
(Bachman) 1 oz	110	5	1	*	*	8	4	35	—	*	6	—	—	*	*	—	—	—	—	—
PRETZEL CHIP																				
fat free																				
(Mr. Phipps) 1 oz	60	3	*	*	*	3	—	13	*	2	4	—	—	*	*	4	4	4	—	—
lightly salted																				
(Mr. Phipps) 1 oz	60	3	2	3	*	3	—	8	*	2	4	—	—	*	*	2	4	4	—	—
original																				
(Mr. Phipps) 1 oz	60	3	2	3	*	3	—	13	*	2	4	—	—	*	*	2	4	4	—	—
(Slim-Fast) 1 oz	100	10	2	—	*	7	16	4	*	10	10	10	*	10	10	10	10	10	10	10
sesame																				
(Mr. Phipps) 1 oz	60	3	3	3	*	3	—	10	*	2	4	—	—	*	*	2	4	4	—	—

	Calories	Protein	Fat	Sat. Fat	Cholesterol	Carbohydrates	Fiber	Sodium	Potassium	Calcium	Iron	Zinc	Magnesium	Vitamin A	Vitamin C	Thiamin	Riboflavin	Niacin	Vitamin B₁₂	Folic acid
PRICKLY PEAR																				
1 fruit	42	*	*	*	*	3	16	*	6	6	2	—	22	*	24	*	4	2	*	—
PROVENÇALE SAUCE																				
from mix																				
(Knorr) 3 3/4 oz	200	60	8	—	23	3	—	25	—	2	6	*	*	*	*	4	6	50	*	*
PRUNE																				
canned																				
in heavy syrup																				
1/2 cup	123	2	*	*	*	11	16	*	8	2	3	*	4	19	5	3	8	5	*	*
dehydrated																				
1/2 cup	224	4	*	*	*	20	—	*	20	5	13	3	11	23	*	5	6	10	*	*
cooked																				
1/2 cup	158	3	*	*	*	14	—	*	14	3	9	2	7	15	*	4	2	7	*	*
dried																				
1/2 cup	194	4	*	*	*	17	24	*	17	4	11	3	9	32	4	4	8	8	*	*
cooked																				
w/ out sugar																				
1/2 cup	113	2	*	*	*	10	28	*	10	2	7	2	5	6	5	2	6	4	*	*
w/ sugar																				
1/2 cup	148	2	*	*	*	13	20	*	11	2	7	2	6	7	5	2	7	4	*	*
pitted																				
(Del Monte Snap-E-Tom) 1/4 cup	120	2	*	*	*	10	11	*	—	*	2	—	—	10	4	—	—	—	*	*
unpitted																				
(Del Monte Snap-E-Tom) 1/4 cup	62	2	*	*	*	5	6	*	—	*	2	—	—	6	2	—	—	—	*	*
PRUNE JUICE																				
(Del Monte) 8 fl oz	170	2	*	*	*	14	4	*	—	2	6	—	—	*	30	—	—	—	*	*
(generic) 8 fl oz	182	3	*	*	*	15	12	*	20	3	17	4	9	*	17	3	11	10	*	*
organic																				
(Knudsen) 8 fl oz	170	2	*	*	*	15	*	*	*	4	6	—	—	*	4	—	—	—	*	*
PUDDING																				
bread																				
(homemade) 1/2 cup	212	11	11	15	28	10	—	12	8	14	8	4	6	6	2	8	17	4	—	4
caramel custard																				
(homemade) 1/2 cup	220	11	10	15	47	12	—	4	5	13	3	5	4	6	*	3	18	*	7	3
egg custard																				
(homemade) 1/2 cup	148	12	10	17	41	5	—	5	6	16	2	5	5	6	*	3	19	*	7	3
flan																				
(homemade) 1/2 cup	220	11	10	15	47	12	—	4	5	13	3	5	4	6	*	3	18	*	7	3
rice																				
(homemade) 1/2 cup	217	9	7	13	6	13	—	4	8	16	6	5	6	3	2	8	13	4	4	2
tapioca																				
(homemade) 1/2 cup	190	12	10	17	41	9	—	12	6	16	3	5	5	6	2	4	19	*	9	3
vanilla																				
(homemade) 1/2 cup	130	7	6	13	5	7	—	5	5	15	*	3	4	3	*	2	12	*	4	*
PUDDING, FROM MIX																				
banana																				
prep w/ low-fat milk																				
(generic) 1/2 cup	143	7	4	8	3	8	—	10	5	15	*	3	5	5	2	3	12	*	6	*
prep w/ whole milk																				
(generic) 1/2 cup	157	7	6	13	6	8	—	10	5	15	*	3	5	3	2	3	12	*	6	*
butterscotch																				
prep w/ skim milk																				
(D-Zerta) 1/2 cup	70	10	*	*	*	4	*	3	7	15	*	—	—	4	2	2	10	*	—	*
prep w/ whole milk																				
(Jell-O) 1/2 cup	170	8	6	—	5	10	*	8	5	15	*	—	—	2	*	2	10	*	—	*
caramel custard																				
prep w/ low-fat milk																				
(generic) 1/2 cup	136	7	4	8	3	6	—	3	6	15	*	3	5	5	2	3	12	*	6	*
prep w/ whole milk																				
(generic) 1/2 cup	150	7	6	13	5	8	—	3	5	15	*	3	4	3	2	3	12	*	6	*

PUDDING, FROM MIX (continued)

	Calories	Protein	Fat	Sat. Fat	Cholesterol	Carbohydrates	Fiber	Sodium	Potassium	Calcium	Iron	Zinc	Magnesium	Vitamin A	Vitamin C	Thiamin	Riboflavin	Niacin	Vitamin B₁₂	Folic acid
chocolate																				
(Maizena) 1/2 cup	170	6	6	—	7	10	—	4	—	15	*	*	*	2	*	2	10	*	*	*
prep w/ low-fat milk (generic) 1/2 cup	206	8	6	10	3	13	—	6	7	16	4	5	10	6	2	3	13	*	6	2
prep w/ low-fat milk sugar-free (Jell-O) 1/2 cup	90	10	5	—	3	4	*	7	9	15	2	—	—	4	*	4	10	*	—	—
prep w/ skim milk (D-Zerta) 1/2 cup	60	10	*	*	*	4	—	3	9	15	—	—	—	4	2	4	10	*	—	—
prep w/ whole milk (generic) 1/2 cup	221	8	9	16	6	13	—	6	7	15	4	5	9	4	2	3	13	*	6	2
(Jell-O) 1/2 cup	160	10	6	—	5	9	*	7	9	15	*	—	—	2	*	4	10	*	—	—
chocolate fudge																				
prep w/ whole milk (Jell-O) 1/2 cup	160	10	6	—	5	9	*	7	10	15	*	—	—	2	*	4	10	*	—	—
coconut																				
prep w/ whole milk (generic) 1/2 cup	160	7	8	18	6	8	—	9	6	16	2	3	6	3	2	3	12	*	6	*
(Maizena) 1/2 cup	170	6	6	—	*	10	—	5	—	15	*	*	*	2	*	2	10	*	*	*
coconut cream																				
prep w/ low-fat milk (generic) 1/2 cup	146	7	5	13	3	8	—	9	6	16	2	3	6	5	2	3	12	*	6	*
egg custard																				
prep w/ low-fat milk (generic) 1/2 cup	162	9	8	15	27	8	—	8	8	19	2	5	6	4	2	5	17	*	10	3
prep w/ whole milk (generic) 1/2 cup	149	9	6	10	25	8	—	8	8	20	2	5	7	6	2	5	17	*	10	3
prep w/ whole milk (Jell-O Americana) 1/2 cup	150	10	6	—	5	8	*	8	8	20	—	—	—	2	*	4	15	*	—	—
flan																				
prep w/ low-fat milk (generic) 1/2 cup	136	7	4	8	3	8	—	3	6	15	*	3	4	5	2	3	12	*	6	*
prep w/ whole milk (generic) 1/2 cup	150	7	6	13	5	8	—	3	5	15	*	3	4	3	2	3	12	*	6	*
(Jell-O) 1/2 cup	150	8	6	—	5	9	*	3	5	15	*	—	—	2	*	2	10	*	—	—
w/ sauce (Knorr) 1/2 cup	190	8	6	—	7	11	—	3	—	15	*	*	*	2	*	2	10	*	*	*
French vanilla																				
prep w/ whole milk (Jell-O) 1/2 cup	170	8	6	—	5	10	*	8	5	15	*	—	—	2	*	2	10	*	—	—
lemon																				
prep w/ whole milk (generic) 1/2 cup	164	2	3	3	26	12	—	4	*	*	*	2	*	2	*	*	3	*	3	2
1/2 cup	170	6	6	—	7	10	—	4	—	15	*	*	*	2	*	2	10	*	*	*
prep w/ low-fat milk (generic) 1/2 cup	154	7	4	8	3	8	*	16	5	15	*	3	4	5	2	3	12	*	7	*
milk chocolate																				
prep w/ whole milk (Jell-O) 1/2 cup	160	10	6	—	5	9	*	7	*	15	—	—	—	2	*	2	10	*	—	—
pineapple																				
prep w/ whole milk (Maizena) 1/2 cup	170	6	6	—	7	10	—	6	—	15	*	*	*	2	*	2	10	*	*	*
rice																				
prep w/ low-fat milk (generic) 1/2 cup	161	8	4	8	3	10	—	5	5	15	3	4	5	3	2	7	12	3	6	2
prep w/ whole milk (generic) 1/2 cup	176	8	6	13	5	10	—	7	5	15	3	4	5	3	2	7	12	3	6	2
rice pudding																				
prep w/ whole milk (Jell-O Americana) 1/2 cup	170	10	6	—	5	10	*	7	5	15	2	—	—	2	*	6	10	2	—	—

	Calories	Protein	Fat	Sat. Fat	Cholesterol	Carbohydrates	Fiber	Sodium	Potassium	Calcium	Iron	Zinc	Magnesium	Vitamin A	Vitamin C	Thiamin	Riboflavin	Niacin	Vitamin B$_{12}$	Folic acid
PUDDING, FROM MIX (continued)																				
tapioca																				
prep w/ low-fat milk (generic) 1/2 cup	147	7	4	8	3	9	—	7	5	15	*	3	4	5	2	3	12	*	6	*
prep w/ whole milk (generic) 1/2 cup	161	7	6	13	6	9	—	7	5	15	*	3	4	3	2	3	12	*	6	*
vanilla																				
prep w/ low-fat milk (generic) 1/2 cup	141	7	4	8	3	9	—	9	6	15	*	3	5	5	2	3	12	*	6	*
sugar-free (Jell-O) 1/2 cup	80	10	3	—	3	4	*	8	5	15	*	—	—	4	*	2	10	*	—	—
prep w/ skim milk (D-Zerta) 1/2 cup	70	10	*	*	*	4	*	3	6	15	*	—	—	4	2	2	10	*	—	—
prep w/ whole milk (generic) 1/2 cup	155	7	6	13	6	9	*	9	5	15	*	3	5	3	2	3	12	*	6	*
(Jell-O) 1/2 cup	160	8	6	—	5	9	*	8	5	15	*	—	—	2	*	2	10	*	—	—
(Maizena) 1/2 cup	170	6	6	—	7	10	—	6	—	15	*	—	—	2	*	2	10	*	*	*
vanilla tapioca																				
prep w/ whole milk (Jell-O Americana) 1/2 cup	150	8	6	—	5	9	*	7	5	15	*	—	—	2	*	2	10	*	—	—
PUDDING, INSTANT																				
banana																				
prep w/ low-fat milk (generic) 1/2 cup	153	7	4	8	3	10	—	18	6	15	*	3	4	5	2	3	12	*	7	2
sugar-free (Jell-O) 1/2 cup	90	10	3	—	3	4	*	16	5	15	*	—	—	4	*	2	10	*	—	—
prep w/ whole milk (generic) 1/2 cup	166	7	7	13	5	10	—	18	5	15	*	3	4	3	2	3	12	*	7	2
banana cream																				
prep w/ whole milk (Jell-O) 1/2 cup	160	8	6	—	5	9	*	17	5	15	*	—	—	2	*	2	10	*	—	—
butter pecan																				
prep w/ whole milk (Jell-O) 1/2 cup	170	10	8	—	5	9	*	17	5	15	*	—	—	2	*	4	10	*	—	—
butterscotch																				
prep w/ low-fat milk sugar-free (Jell-O) 1/2 cup	90	10	3	—	3	4	*	16	5	15	*	—	—	4	*	2	10	*	—	—
prep w/ whole milk (Jell-O) 1/2 cup	160	8	6	—	5	9	*	19	5	15	*	—	—	2	*	2	10	*	—	—
chocolate																				
prep w/ low-fat milk (generic) 1/2 cup	150	8	4	8	3	9	—	17	7	15	2	4	7	5	2	3	12	*	8	2
sugar-free (Jell-O) 1/2 cup	100	10	5	—	3	5	*	16	7	15	*	—	—	4	*	4	10	*	—	—
prep w/ skim milk (Weight Watchers) 1/2 cup	90	13	2	*	2	6	4	17	4	25	*	—	—	6	*	—	—	—	—	—
prep w/ whole milk (generic) 1/2 cup	163	8	7	14	5	9	4	17	7	15	2	4	7	3	2	3	12	*	7	2
(Jell-O) 1/2 cup	180	10	6	—	5	10	*	20	8	15	2	—	—	2	*	4	10	*	—	—
chocolate fudge																				
prep w/ low-fat milk sugar-free (Jell-O) 1/2 cup	100	10	5	—	3	5	*	15	9	15	*	—	—	4	*	4	15	*	—	—
prep w/ whole milk (Jell-O) 1/2 cup	180	10	8	—	5	10	*	18	9	15	2	—	—	2	*	4	10	*	—	—
chocolate mousse																				
prep w/ skim milk (Weight Watchers) 1/2 cup	60	5	5	10	2	2	8	2	9	15	*	—	—	*	*	—	—	—	—	—
coconut																				
prep w/ whole milk (generic) 1/2 cup	172	7	8	16	5	9	—	15	5	15	*	3	5	3	2	3	12	*	7	2

	Calories	Protein	Fat	Sat. Fat	Cholesterol	Carbohydrates	Fiber	Sodium	Potassium	Calcium	Iron	Zinc	Magnesium	Vitamin A	Vitamin C	Thiamin	Riboflavin	Niacin	Vitamin B₁₂	Folic acid

PUDDING, INSTANT (continued)

coconut cream

	Calories	Protein	Fat	Sat. Fat	Cholesterol	Carbohydrates	Fiber	Sodium	Potassium	Calcium	Iron	Zinc	Magnesium	Vitamin A	Vitamin C	Thiamin	Riboflavin	Niacin	Vitamin B$_{12}$	Folic acid
prep w/ low-fat milk (generic) 1/2 cup	157	7	5	10	3	9	—	15	6	15	*	3	5	5	2	3	12	*	7	2
prep w/ whole milk (Jell-O) 1/2 cup	180	10	9	—	5	9	*	13	6	15	*	—	—	2	*	4	10	*	—	—
French vanilla prep w/ whole milk (Jell-O) 1/2 cup	160	8	6	—	5	9	*	17	5	15	*	—	—	2	*	2	10	*	—	—
lemon prep w/ whole milk (generic) 1/2 cup	169	7	7	13	5	10	—	16	5	15	*	3	4	3	2	3	12	*	7	2
(Jell-O) 1/2 cup	170	8	6	—	5	10	*	15	5	15	*	—	—	2	*	2	10	*	—	—
milk chocolate prep w/ whole milk (Jell-O) 1/2 cup	180	10	8	—	5	10	*	20	8	15	2	—	—	2	*	4	10	*	—	—
pistachio prep w/ low-fat milk sugar-free (Jell-O) 1/2 cup	90	10	5	—	3	4	*	16	6	15	*	—	—	4	*	4	10	*	—	—
prep w/ whole milk (Jell-O) 1/2 cup	170	10	8	—	5	9	*	17	5	15	*	—	—	2	*	2	10	*	—	—
vanilla prep w/ low-fat milk (generic) 1/2 cup	148	7	4	7	3	9	—	17	5	15	*	3	4	5	2	3	12	*	7	*
sugar-free (Jell-O) 1/2 cup	90	10	3	—	3	4	*	16	5	15	*	—	—	4	*	2	10	*	—	—
prep w/ skim milk (Weight Watchers) 1/2 cup	90	10	*	*	2	6	4	21	2	25	*	—	—	6	*	—	—	—	—	—
prep w/ whole milk (generic) 1/2 cup	162	6	6	13	5	9	*	17	5	14	*	3	4	3	2	3	11	*	7	*
(Jell-O) 1/2 cup	170	8	6	—	5	10	*	17	5	15	*	—	—	2	*	2	10	*	—	—
white chocolate almond mousse prep w/ skim milk (Weight Watchers) 1/2 cup	70	—	5	5	—	2	4	4	*	15	—	—	—	*	*	—	—	—	—	—

PUDDING, READY-TO-EAT

banana

	Calories	Protein	Fat	Sat. Fat	Cholesterol	Carbohydrates	Fiber	Sodium	Potassium	Calcium	Iron	Zinc	Magnesium	Vitamin A	Vitamin C	Thiamin	Riboflavin	Niacin	Vitamin B$_{12}$	Folic acid
(Del Monte Snack Cups) 1 container	140	2	6	5	*	8	*	8	—	6	*	—	—	*	*	—	—	—	—	—
(generic) 1 can	180	6	8	4	*	10	—	12	4	12	*	3	3	3	*	2	12	*	4	—
(SnackPack) 4 1/4 oz	145	3	9	7	*	7	*	7	2	6	*	—	—	*	*	*	4	*	—	—
butterscotch (Del Monte Snack Cups) 1 container	140	2	6	5	*	8	*	7	—	6	*	—	—	*	*	—	—	—	—	—
(Rich's) 3 oz	130	3	9	—	*	6	*	5	3	3	*	*	*	*	*	7	*	*	—	—
(SnackPack) 4 1/4 oz	170	3	9	7	*	9	*	9	3	7	*	*	*	*	*	*	5	*	—	—
(Swiss Miss) 1/2 cup	180	3	9	6	2	10	*	6	4	6	*	—	—	*	*	2	6	*	—	—
(Ultra Slim-Fast Plus) 4 oz	100	10	—	—	*	7	8	10	*	10	10	10	10	10	10	10	10	10	10	10
butterscotch/chocolate/vanilla swirl (Jello-O Pudding Snacks) 4 oz cup	180	6	9	—	*	9	*	8	5	10	*	—	—	2	*	*	6	*	—	—
caramello (Hershey's) 4 oz	156	5	8	—	*	8	—	7	—	8	4	—	—	*	*	*	6	*	—	—
chocolate (Del Monte Snack Cups) 1 container	160	3	6	5	*	9	*	5	—	6	2	—	—	*	*	—	—	—	—	—
(Hershey's) 4 oz	160	6	8	—	*	8	—	9	—	9	5	—	—	*	—	*	7	*	—	—
(Jell-O Free) 4 oz cup	100	6	*	*	*	8	*	8	6	10	2	—	—	2	*	*	6	*	—	—
(Jell-O Pudding Snacks) 4 oz cup	160	6	8	—	*	9	*	8	8	10	4	—	—	2	*	*	6	*	—	—
(Rich's) 3 oz	140	3	11	35	*	6	*	5	3	5	2	*	*	*	*	5	6	*	—	—

PUDDING, READY-TO-EAT (continued)

	Calories	Protein	Fat	Sat. Fat	Cholesterol	Carbohydrates	Fiber	Sodium	Potassium	Calcium	Iron	Zinc	Magnesium	Vitamin A	Vitamin C	Thiamin	Riboflavin	Niacin	Vitamin B₁₂	Folic acid
(SnackPack) 4 1/4 oz	170	3	9	7	*	9	*	5	4	6	*	—		*	*	*	4	*	—	
(Swiss Miss) 1/2 cup	180	3	9	7	2	10	*	7	7	10	6	—	—	*	*	2	6	*	—	—
(Ultra Slim-Fast) 4 oz	100	10	—	—	*	7	8	10	*	10	10	10	10	10	10	10	10	10	10	10
light (Del Monte Snack Cups) 1 container	100	3	2	*	*	6	*	6	—	6	*	—		*	*		—	—	—	—
(SnackPack) 4 oz	100	5	3	*	*	7	*	5	6	10	3	—	—	*	*	2	5	*	—	—
(Swiss Miss) 1/2 cup	100	5	2	*	*	7	*	5	6	8	3	—	—	*	*	2	6	*	—	—
chocolate & almond (Hershey's) 4 oz	160	5	8	—	*	9	—	7	—	8	4	—		*	—	*	6	*	—	
chocolate fudge (Del Monte Snack Cups) 1 container	150	3	6	5	*	8	*	8	—	6	2	—		*	*	—	—	—	—	
(Jell-O Pudding Snacks) 4 oz cup	160	6	8	—	*	9	*	8	7	10	4	—	—	2	*	*	6	*	—	—
(SnackPack) 4 1/4 oz	165	3	9	6	*	9	*	5	4	6	*			*	*	*	4	*	—	
(Swiss Miss) 1/2 cup	220	5	9	8	2	13	*	7	7	10	6	—	—	*	*	2	6	*	—	—
light (Swiss Miss) 1/2 cup	100	5	2	*	*	7	*	5	5	8	*	—	—	*	*	*	6	*	—	—
Chocolate Kisses (Hershey's) 4 oz	162	5	8	—	*	8	—	6	—	9	5	—		*	—	*	7	*	—	
chocolate marshmallow (SnackPack) 4 1/4 oz	165	3	9	7	*	9	*	5	3	6	*	—		*	*	*	4	*	—	
chocolate parfait (Swiss Miss) 1/2 cup	170	5	9	7	*	9	*	8	8	10	4	—	—	*	*	2	7	*	—	—
chocolate peanut butter (Del Monte Snack Cups) 1 container	160	3	6	5	*	9	*	11	—	6	2	—	—	*	*		—	—	—	—
chocolate sundae (Swiss Miss) 1/2 cup	220	3	11	9	2	12	*	6	6	8	8	—	—	*	*	*	5	*	—	—
chocolate/vanilla swirl (Jell-O Free) 4 oz cup	100	6	*	*	*	8	*	9	5	10	*	—	—	2	*	*	6	*	—	—
(Jell-O Pudding Snacks) 4 oz cup	170	6	9	—	*	9	*	8	6	10	*	—	—	2	*	*	6	*	—	—
chocolate/caramel swirl (Jell-O Pudding Snacks) 4 oz cup	170	6	9	—	*	9	*	8	6	10	2	—	—	2	*	*	6	*	—	—
chocolate/mint swirl (Jell-O Free) 4 oz cup	100	6	*	*	*	8	*	9	6	10	*	—	—	2	*	*	6	*	—	—
lemon (generic) 1 can	178	*	7	3	*	12	—	8	*	*	*	*	*	*	*	*	*	*	*	*
(SnackPack) 4 1/4 oz	150	*	6	4	*	10	*	3	*	*	*	—	—	*	*	*	*	*	—	—
peppermint patty (Hershey's) 4 oz	162	5	8	—	*	8	—	7	—	8	3	—	—	*	—	*	6	*	—	—
rice (generic) 1 can	231	5	16	9	*	10	—	5	2	7	2	5	3	3	*	2	6	*	5	*
special dark (Hershey's) 4 oz	150	6	6	—	*	9	—	7	—	8	12	—		*	—	*	6	*	—	
tapioca (Del Monte Snack Cups) 1 container	140	2	6	5	*	8	*	5	—	6	*	—	—	*	*	—	—	—	—	—
(generic) 1 can	169	5	8	5	*	9	*	7	4	12	2	3	3	*	2	2	8	2	3	*
(Jell-O Pudding Snacks) 4 oz cup	170	6	6	—	*	10	*	7	4	10	*	—	—	2	*	*	6	*	—	—
(SnackPack) 4 1/4 oz	150	3	8	6	*	8	*	5	4	9	*	—	—	*	*	2	6	*	—	—
(Swiss Miss) 1/2 cup	160	3	8	5	2	9	*	7	4	10	*	—	—	*	*	2	6	*	—	—

	Calories	Protein	Fat	Sat. Fat	Cholesterol	Carbohydrates	Fiber	Sodium	Potassium	Calcium	Iron	Zinc	Magnesium	Vitamin A	Vitamin C	Thiamin	Riboflavin	Niacin	Vitamin B$_{12}$	Folic acid
PUDDING, READY-TO-EAT (continued)																				
light (SnackPack) 4 oz	100	3	3	2	*	6	*	4	2	6	*	—	—	*	*	*	4	*	—	—
vanilla (Del Monte Snack Cups) 1 container	150	2	6	5	*	8	*	6	—	6	*		—	*	*		—	—	*	—
(generic) 1/2 cup	147	4	6	3	3	8	*	6	4	10	*	2	2	*	*	2	9	*	2	*
(Jell-O Free) 4 oz cup	100	6	*	*	*	8	*	10	4	10	*	—	—	2	*	*	6	*	—	—
(Jell-O Pudding Snacks) 4 oz cup	160	6	8	—	*	8	*	7	4	10	*	—	—	2	*	*	6	*	—	—
(Rich's) 3 oz	130	3	9	—	*	6	*	7	3	3	*	—	—	*	*	5	*	*	—	—
(SnackPack) 4 1/4 oz	170	3	9	7	*	9	*	6	2	6	*	—	—	*	*	*	4	*	—	—
light (Del Monte Snack Cups) 1 container	90	2	2	*	*	6	*	8	—	6	*		—	*	*		—	—	*	—
(Swiss Miss) 1/2 cup	100	3	2	*	*	7	*	4	3	6	*	—	—	*	*	*	4	*	—	—
Vanilla Kisses (Hershey's) 4 oz	162	5	8	—	*	8	—	6	—	9	5	—	—	*	*	*	7	*	—	—
vanilla parfait (Swiss Miss) 1/2 cup	180	3	9	7	*	10	*	6	5	10	4	—	—	*	*	*	2	6	*	—
vanilla sundae (Swiss Miss) 1/2 cup	220	3	11	8	2	12	*	7	4	7	4	—	—	*	*	*	*	5	*	—
vanilla/chocolate parfait light (Swiss Miss) 1/2 cup	100	3	2	*	*	7	*	5	4	8	*	—	—	*	*	*	2	6	*	—
vanilla/chocolate swirl (Jell-O Pudding Snacks) 4 oz cup	180	6	9	—	*	9	*	8	5	10	*	—	—	2	*	*	6	*	—	—
PUDDING POP																				
chocolate (generic) 1 pop	72	3	3	—	*	4	*	3	3	7	*	*	2	*	*	*	5	*	4	*
(Jell-O) 1 bar	80	4	3	—	*	4	*	4	3	8	*	*	2	*	*	*	6	*	*	*
chocolate fudge (Jell-O) 1 bar	80	4	3	—	*	4	*	4	2	8	*	*	2	*	*	*	6	*	*	*
chocolate/vanilla swirl (Jell-O) 1 bar	80	4	3	—	*	4	*	29	2	8	*	*	2	*	*	*	6	*	2	*
double chocolate swirl (Jell-O) 1 bar	80	4	3	—	*	4	*	4	2	8	*	*	2	*	*	*	6	*	*	*
milk chocolate (Jell-O) 1 bar	80	4	3	—	*	4	*	2	*	8	*	*	2	*	*	*	6	*	*	*
vanilla (generic) 1 pop	75	3	3	—	*	4	*	2	2	6	*	*	*	*	*	2	2	5	*	3
(Jell-O) 1 bar	80	4	3	—	*	4	*	2	*	8	*	*	*	*	*	*	6	*	4	*
PUFF PASTRY DOUGH SHEET (Pepperidge Farm) 1 shell (1/2 oz)	260	6	26	—	—	7	—	12	—	*	4	—	—	*	*	2	2	2	—	—
PUFF PASTRY SHELL																				
mini (Pepperidge Farm) 1 shell	52	*	6	—	*	*	*	2	*	*	*	*	*	*	*	*	*	*	*	*
regular (Pepperidge Farm) 1 shell	210	4	23	—	—	5	—	7	—	*	2	—	—	*	*	4	2	2	—	—
PUMMELO																				
raw 1 fruit	231	8	*	*	*	20	24	*	37	2	4	3	9	*	619	14	10	7	*	—
1/2 cup sections	32	*	*	*	*	3	4	*	5	*	*	*	*	*	86	2	*	*	*	—
PUMPKIN																				
raw 1/2 cup	15	*	*	*	*	*	4	*	6	*	3	*	2	19	9	2	4	2	*	2

	Calories	Protein	Fat	Sat. Fat	Cholesterol	Carbohydrates	Fiber	Sodium	Potassium	Calcium	Iron	Zinc	Magnesium	Vitamin A	Vitamin C	Thiamin	Riboflavin	Niacin	Vitamin B12	Folic acid
PUMPKIN (continued)																				
boiled 1/2 cup mashed	24	*	*	*	*	2	—	*	8	2	4	2	3	26	10	3	6	3	*	3
boiled w/ salt 1/2 cup mashed	24	*	*	*	*	2	—	12	8	2	4	2	3	26	10	3	6	3	*	3
PUMPKIN, CANNED *(Libby's)* 1/2 cup	60	3	*	*	*	5	16	*	—	2	10	—	—	350	8	—	—	—	—	—
cooked (generic) 1/2 cup	41	2	*	*	*	3	12	*	7	3	9	*	7	538	9	2	4	2	*	4
cooked w/ salt (generic) 1/2 cup	41	2	*	*	*	3	12	12	7	3	9	*	7	538	9	—	—	—	—	—
PUMPKIN FLOWER *raw* 1/2 cup	3	*	*	*	*	*	—	*	*	*	*	—	*	7	8	*	*	*	*	3
boiled 1/2 cup	10	*	*	*	*	*	4	*	2	2	3	—	4	23	6	*	*	*	*	7
boiled w/ salt 1/2 cup	10	*	*	*	*	*	—	7	2	2	3	—	4	23	6	*	*	*	*	7
PUMPKIN KERNEL *dried* 1 oz (142 kernels)	154	12	20	13	*	2	16	*	7	*	24	14	38	2	*	4	5	2	*	4
roasted 1 oz	148	16	18	12	*	*	—	*	7	*	24	14	38	2	*	4	5	2	*	4
roasted w/ salt 1 oz	148	16	18	12	*	*	8	7	7	*	24	14	38	2	*	4	5	2	*	4
PUMPKIN LEAF *raw* 1/2 cup	4	*	*	*	*	*	—	*	2	*	2	*	2	8	4	*	2	*	*	2
boiled 1/2 cup	7	2	*	*	*	*	4	*	4	2	6	*	3	17	*	2	3	*	*	2
boiled w/ salt 1/2 cup	7	2	*	*	*	*	—	4	4	2	6	*	3	17	*	2	3	*	*	2
PUMPKIN SEED *roasted* 1 oz (85 seeds)	127	9	8	5	*	5	—	*	7	2	5	19	19	*	*	*	*	*	*	*
roasted w/ salt 1 oz (85 seeds)	127	9	8	5	*	5	—	7	7	2	5	19	19	*	*	*	*	*	*	*
PUMPKIN BUTTER *(Smucker's Autumn Harvest)* 1 tbsp	12	*	*	*	*	*	*	*	*	*	*	*	*	*	*	*	*	*	*	*
PUMPKIN PIE SPICE 1 tbsp	19	*	*	20	*	*	4	*	*	*	4	6	*	2	*	2	*	*	*	—
PUNCH see FRUIT PUNCH																				
PURSLANE *raw* 1/2 cup	4	*	*	*	*	*	—	*	3	*	2	*	4	6	8	*	*	*	*	*
1 plant	1	*	*	*	*	*	—	*	*	*	*	*	*	*	*	*	*	*	*	*
boiled 1/2 cup	10	*	*	*	*	*	—	*	8	5	2	*	10	21	10	*	3	*	*	*
boiled w/ salt 1/2 cup	10	*	*	*	*	*	—	7	8	5	2	*	10	21	10	*	3	*	*	*
QUAIL *breast* 1 breast	69	21	3	3	11	*	*	*	4	*	7	10	4	*	5	9	8	23	4	*
meat w/ out skin 1 quail	123	33	6	6	21	*	*	2	6	*	23	17	6	*	11	17	15	38	7	2
meat w/ skin 1 quail	209	36	20	19	28	*	*	2	7	*	24	18	6	5	11	18	17	41	8	2
QUINCE 1 fruit	52	*	*	*	*	5	8	*	5	*	4	—	2	*	23	*	2	*	*	—

	Calories	Protein	Fat	Sat. Fat	Cholesterol	Carbohydrates	Fiber	Sodium	Potassium	Calcium	Iron	Zinc	Magnesium	Vitamin A	Vitamin C	Thiamin	Riboflavin	Niacin	Vitamin B₁₂	Folic acid
RABBIT																				
domesticated																				
roasted																				
3 oz	175	41	14	10	23	*	*	*	9	*	11	12	5	*	*	5	11	36	117	*
stewed																				
3 oz	175	43	15	10	24	*	*	*	8	*	12	12	5	*	*	4	9	30	92	*
wild																				
stewed																				
3 oz	149	47	6	5	39	*	*	*	9	*	23	—	7	*	*	*	3	27	—	—
RACCOON																				
roasted																				
3 oz	216	41	25	—	—	*	*	—	—	—	—	—	—	*	*	—	27	—	—	—
RADDICCHIO																				
raw																				
1/2 cup shredded	5	*	*	*	*	*	—	*	2	*	*	*	*	*	3	*	*	*	*	3
4 medium	7	*	*	*	*	*	—	*	3	*	*	*	*	*	4	*	*	*	*	5
RADISH																				
raw																				
10 radishes	8	*	*	*	*	*	4	*	3	*	*	*	*	*	17	*	*	*	*	3
1/2 cup slices	10	*	*	*	*	*	4	*	4	*	*	*	*	*	22	*	2	*	*	4
RADISH, DAIKON																				
raw																				
1/2 cup slices	8	*	*	*	*	*	4	*	3	*	*	*	2	*	16	*	*	*	*	3
1 large	61	3	*	*	*	5	20	3	22	9	8	3	14	*	124	5	4	3	*	24
boiled																				
1/2 cup slices	13	*	*	*	*	*	4	*	6	*	*	*	2	*	19	*	*	*	*	3
boiled w/ salt																				
1/2 cup slices	13	*	*	*	*	*	4	8	6	*	*	*	2	*	19	*	*	*	*	3
dried																				
1/2 cup	157	8	*	*	*	12	—	7	58	36	22	8	25	*	*	10	23	10	*	43
RADISH, WHITE ICICLE																				
raw																				
1/2 cup slices	7	*	*	*	*	*	—	*	4	*	2	*	*	*	24	*	*	*	*	2
4 radishes	10	*	*	*	*	*	—	*	5	2	3	*	2	*	33	*	*	*	*	2
RADISH SPROUT																				
raw																				
1/2 cup	8	*	*	*	*	*	—	*	*	*	*	*	2	*	9	*	*	3	*	5
RAISIN																				
golden																				
(Del Monte Snap-E-Tom) 1/4 cup	130	2	*	*	*	10	9	*	—	*	6	*	*	*	*	*	—	—	—	*	*
(generic) 1/4 cup	125	2	*	*	*	10	12	*	8	2	4	*	3	*	2	*	4	2	*	*
(Sun-Maid) 1/4 cup	130	*	*	*	*	*	9	*	—	2	6	*	*	*	*	—	—	—	*	*
muscat																				
(Sun-Maid) 1/4 cup	135	2	*	*	*	11	—	*	10	2	8	*	3	*	4	2	3	2	*	*
regular																				
(Del Monte Snap-E-Tom) 1/4 cup	130	2	*	*	*	10	9	*	—	*	6	*	—	*	*	*	—	—	—	*
(Sun-Maid) 1/4 cup	130	*	*	*	*	*	9	*	—	2	6	*	*	*	*	*	—	—	*	*
yogurt covered																				
strawberry																				
(Del Monte Snap-E-Tom)																				
1 oz bag	110	3	4	14	*	7	3	*	—	4	*	*	—	*	*	—	—	—	*	*
vanilla																				
(Del Monte Snap-E-Tom)																				
1 oz bag	110	3	4	14	*	7	3	*	—	4	*	*	—	*	*	—	—	—	*	*
RANCH DIP																				
cracked pepper																				
from mix																				
(Knorr) 1 tbsp	50	*	—	—	3	*	—	3	—	*	*	*	*	*	*	*	*	*	*	*

	Calories	Protein	Fat	Sat. Fat	Cholesterol	Carbohydrates	Fiber	Sodium	Potassium	Calcium	Iron	Zinc	Magnesium	Vitamin A	Vitamin C	Thiamin	Riboflavin	Niacin	Vitamin B12	Folic acid
RASPBERRY DRINK																				
from concentrate raspberry nectar (Knudsen) 8 fl oz	120	*	*	*	*	10	*	*	3	*	2	—	—	*	10	—	—	—	*	*
float (Knudsen) 8 fl oz	140	2	*	*	*	11	*	2	3	4	4	—	—	*	15	—	—	—	*	*
from mix (Kool-Aid) 8 fl oz	70	*	*	*	*	6	*	*	*	*	*	*	*	*	10	*	*	*	*	*
unsweetened (Kool-Aid) 8 fl oz prep w/ out sugar	2	*	*	*	*	*	*	*	*	*	*	*	*	*	10	*	*	*	*	*
sugar added (Kool-Aid) 8 fl oz prep w/ sugar	100	*	*	*	*	8	*	*	*	*	*	*	*	*	10	*	*	*	*	*
organic (Santa Cruz Natural) 8 fl oz	100	*	*	*	*	9	*	*	6	4	4	—	—	*	*	—	—	—	*	*
RASPBERRY JUICE																				
(Farmer's Market) 8 fl oz	120	*	*	*	*	10	*	*	2	*	*	—	—	*	4	—	—	—	*	*
(Heinke's) 8 fl oz	120	*	*	*	*	10	*	*	5	*	2	—	—	*	6	—	—	—	*	*
(Smucker's) 8 fl oz	120	*	*	*	*	10	*	*	9	2	4	*	*	2	20	2	4	2	*	*
RASPBERRY NECTAR																				
(Knudsen Exotic Blends) 8 fl oz	120	*	*	*	*	10	*	*	3	*	2	—	—	*	10	—	—	—	*	*
RASPBERRY-CRANBERRY DRINK																				
(Ocean Spray) 8 fl oz	140	*	*	*	*	12	*	*	—	*	*	—	—	*	100	—	—	—	*	*
low calorie (Lightstyle) 8 fl oz	40	*	*	*	*	3	*	*	—	*	*	—	—	*	100	—	—	—	*	*
reduced calorie (Ocean Spray) 8 fl oz	50	*	*	*	*	4	*	*	3	*	*	—	—	*	100	—	—	—	*	*
RASPBERRY-GUAVA DRINK																				
organic (Santa Cruz Natural) 8 fl oz	100	*	*	*	*	8	*	*	3	4	4	—	—	*	2	—	—	—	*	*
RASPBERRY-LEMON JUICE																				
organic (Santa Cruz Natural) 8 fl oz	120	*	*	*	*	10	*	*	2	*	*	—	—	*	8	—	—	—	*	*
RASPBERRY-PEACH JUICE																				
(Knudsen Exotic Blends) 8 fl oz	120	*	*	*	*	10	*	*	5	2	*	—	—	*	*	—	—	—	*	*
RAVIOLI see PASTA																				
RED BEAN																				
canned (Bush Bros) 1/2 cup	110	10	*	*	*	6	24	19	—	4	8	—	—	*	*	—	—	—	—	—
(Hunt's) 1/2 cup	90	10	*	*	*	6	24	17	10	2	9	—	—	*	*	9	2	3	—	—
dry, canned in brine (Green Giant/Joan of Arc) 1/2 cup	45	10	*	*	*	3	10	7	3	2	4	—	—	*	*	2	*	*	—	—
REFRIED BEAN see BEAN, REFRIED																				
RELISH																				
corn (Nance's) 1 tbsp	13	*	*	*	*	*	*	5	*	*	*	*	*	*	*	*	*	*	*	*
cranberry-orange (generic) 1 oz	31	*	*	*	*	3	—	*	*	*	*	*	*	*	5	*	*	*	*	*
dill (Vlasic) 1 oz	2	*	*	*	*	—	*	19	—	*	*	*	*	*	*	*	*	*	—	—
hamburger (Del Monte) 1 tbsp	20	*	*	*	*	2	2	9	—	*	*	—	—	4	*	—	—	—	—	—
(generic) 1 tbsp	20	*	*	*	*	*	2	7	*	*	*	*	*	*	*	*	*	*	*	*
(Vlasic) 1 oz	35	*	*	*	*	3	*	11	—	*	*	—	—	*	2	*	*	*	—	—
hot dog (Del Monte) 1 tbsp	15	*	*	*	*	*	2	6	—	*	*	—	—	*	*	—	—	—	—	—
(generic) 1 tbsp	14	*	*	*	*	*	—	7	*	*	*	*	*	*	*	*	*	*	*	*
(Vlasic) 1 oz	40	*	*	*	*	3	*	11	—	*	*	—	—	*	2	*	*	*	—	—

	Calories	Protein	Fat	Sat. Fat	Cholesterol	Carbohydrates	Fiber	Sodium	Potassium	Calcium	Iron	Zinc	Magnesium	Vitamin A	Vitamin C	Thiamin	Riboflavin	Niacin	Vitamin B₁₂	Folic acid
RELISH (continued)																				
India																				
(Vlasic) 1 oz	30	*	*	*	*	3	*	11	—	*	*	—	—	*	*	*	*	*	—	—
jalapeño																				
(Old El Paso) 1tbsp	8	*	*	*	*	2	2	2	*	*	*	—	—	2	5	*	*	*	—	—
picalilli																				
hot																				
(Vlasic) 1 oz	35	*	*	*	*	3	*	7	—	*	*	—	—	2	*	*	*	*	—	—
mild																				
(Vlasic) 1 oz	35	*	*	*	*	3	*	7	—	*	*	—	—	2	*	*	*	*	—	—
sweet																				
(America's Choice) 1 tbsp	20	*	*	*	*	2	*	6	*	*	*	*	*	*	*	*	*	*	*	*
(Del Monte) 1 tbsp	20	*	*	*	*	2	*	5	—	*	*	—	*	*	*	*	—	*	*	*
(generic) 1 tbsp	20	*	*	*	*	*	—	5	*	*	*	*	*	*	*	*	*	*	*	*
(Heinz) 1 tbsp	15	*	*	*	*	*	*	5	*	*	*	*	*	*	*	*	*	*	*	*
(Vlasic) 1 oz	35	*	*	*	*	3	*	11	—	*	*	—	—	*	*	*	*	*	—	—
RENNIN DESSERT																				
chocolate																				
from mix																				
made w/ low-fat milk																				
(generic) 1/2 cup	110	7	4	9	3	6	—	3	7	17	2	5	7	5	2	3	12	*	7	2
made w/whole milk																				
(generic) 1/2 cup	125	7	7	14	5	6	—	3	7	17	2	5	7	3	2	3	12	*	7	2
vanilla																				
(homemade) 1/2 cup	112	7	6	13	5	5	—	4	5	15	*	3	4	3	2	3	12	*	7	*
from mix																				
made w/ low-fat milk																				
(generic) 1/2 cup	101	7	4	8	3	5	—	3	5	16	*	3	4	5	2	3	12	*	7	2
made w/whole milk																				
(generic) 1/2 cup	116	7	6	13	6	5	—	3	5	16	*	3	4	3	2	3	12	*	7	2
RENNIN TABLET																				
unsweetened																				
(generic) 1 tablet	1	*	*	*	*	*	—	10	*	3	*	*	*	*	*	*	*	*	*	*
RICE																				
basmati																				
(President's Choice) 1/2 cup	100	3	*	*	*	7	—	*	—	*	4	—	*	*	*	6	2	6	—	—
brown																				
(Uncle Ben's) 1/2 cup	157	7	2	*	*	11	5	*	3	*	3	—	14	*	*	12	*	14	—	—
boil-in-bag																				
(Success) 1/2 cup	103	4	*	*	*	7	—	*	—	*	4	—	—	*	*	2	*	2	—	—
fast cooking																				
(Uncle Ben's) 1/2 cup	157	6	2	*	*	12	6	*	*	*	2	—	*	*	*	3	*	6	—	—
instant																				
(Minute) 1/2 cup	120	4	2	—	*	9	*	*	*	*	2	—	—	*	*	2	*	6	—	—
long grain																				
(Carolina) 1/2 cup	110	4	*	*	*	8	—	*	—	*	2	—	—	—	*	6	*	8	—	—
(Mahatma) 1/2 cup	110	4	*	*	*	8	—	—	—	*	2	—	—	*	*	6	*	8	—	—
medium grain																				
(River) 1/2 cup	110	4	*	*	*	8	—	*	—	*	2	—	—	*	*	6	*	8	—	—
long grain & wild																				
(Minute) 1/2 cup	150	4	6	—	3	8	—	24	*	*	6	—	—	2	*	10	*	10	—	—
white																				
boil-in-bag																				
(Minute) 1/2 cup	90	4	*	*	*	7	—	*	*	*	4	—	*	*	*	8	*	4	—	—
boil-in-bag																				
(Uncle Ben's) 1/2 cup	94.2	3	*	*	*	7	2	*	*	*	4	—	*	*	*	8	*	5	—	—
converted																				
(Uncle Ben's) 1/2 cup	122	5	*	*	*	9	*	*	2	*	6	—	2	*	*	10	*	6	—	—

	Calories	Protein	Fat	Sat. Fat	Cholesterol	Carbohydrates	Fiber	Sodium	Potassium	Calcium	Iron	Zinc	Magnesium	Vitamin A	Vitamin C	Thiamin	Riboflavin	Niacin	Vitamin B$_{12}$	Folic acid
RICE (continued)																				
fast cooking (Uncle Ben's Rice in an Instant) 1/2 cup	111	4	*	*	*	8	2	*	*	*	5	—	*	*	*	*	9	*	6	—	—
instant (Carolina) 1/2 cup	110	2	*	*	*	8	—	—	—	*	4	—	—	*	*	8	*	6	—	—
(Mahatma) 1/2 cup	110	2	*	*	*	8	—	—	—	*	4	—	—	*	*	8	*	6	—	—
(Minute) 1/2 cup	120	4	*	*	*	9	—	*	*	*	6	—	—	*	*	10	*	6	—	—
long grain (Carolina) 1/2 cup	100	2	*	*	*	7	—	—	—	*	4	—	—	*	*	8	*	6	—	—
(Mahatma) 1/2 cup	100	2	*	*	*	7	—	—	—	*	4	—	—	*	*	8	*	6	—	—
(Minute) 1/2 cup	120	4	*	*	*	9	—	*	*	*	6	—	—	*	*	10	*	6	—	—
(Success) 1/2 cup	90	2	*	*	*	7	—	*	—	*	4	—	—	*	*	8	*	4	—	—
medium grain (River) 1/2 cup	100	2	*	*	*	7	—	—	—	*	4	—	—	*	*	8	*	6	—	—
(Water Maid) 1/2 cup	100	2	*	*	*	7	—	—	—	*	4	—	—	*	*	8	*	6	—	—
RICE DISH, CANNED																				
Spanish rice (Bush Bros) 1 cup	85	4	3	3	*	5	8	25	—	*	5	—	—	25	*	—	—	—	—	—
RICE DISH, FROM MIX																				
almond beef (Mahatma) 1/2 cup	100	4	*	*	—	7	—	14	—	*	4	—	—	*	*	10	4	8	—	—
basmati w/ tomato & fine herbs (Knorr Pilaf) 1/2 cup	230	6	8	—	*	11	—	19	—	*	*	—	*	20	*	4	4	4	*	*
beef (Lipton Rice & Sauce) 1/2 cup	150	5	5	—	—	9	—	25	—	*	8	2	—	6	*	10	4	10	—	—
beef & broccoli (Lipton Rice & Sauce) 1/2 cup	140	5	5	—	—	8	—	23	—	*	4	2	—	2	8	10	4	8	—	—
beef oriental (Success) 1/2 cup	100	2	*	*	—	6	—	15	—	*	6	—	—	10	*	10	*	8	—	—
broccoli almondine (Uncle Ben's Country Inn) 1/2 cup	124	6	2	—	*	8	3	14	*	2	6	—	*	*	4	9	9	6	—	—
broccoli au gratin (Uncle Ben's Country Inn) 1/2 cup	116	6	3	—	*	7	4	14	*	4	6	—	*	*	5	8	7	5	—	—
broccoli & cheese (Success) 1/2 cup	120	4	—	—	—	8	—	13	—	50	25	—	—	*	*	4	4	25	—	—
broccoli & white cheddar (Uncle Ben's Country Inn) 1/2 cup	131	7	4	—	*	8	3	12	*	4	5	—	*	*	2	9	5	5	—	—
brown & wild (Success) 1/2 cup	120	4	*	*	—	8	—	21	—	*	2	—	—	*	*	4	4	6	—	—
(Uncle Ben's Country Inn) 1/2 cup	120	6	*	*	*	9	6	16	5	*	4	—	28	*	3	7	6	12	—	—
Cajun style (Lipton Rice & Sauce) 1/2 cup	160	14	5	3	*	9	15	12	—	3	8	—	—	3	*	—	—	—	—	—
chicken (Lipton Rice & Sauce) 1/2 cup	150	5	6	—	—	8	—	20	—	*	6	2	—	6	*	15	4	10	—	—
(Success) 1/2 cup	100	4	*	*	—	6	—	17	—	*	2	—	—	2	*	4	2	4	—	—
chicken & broccoli (Lipton Rice & Sauce) 1/2 cup	150	7	6	—	—	8	—	21	—	2	8	2	—	10	6	20	6	15	—	—
chicken stock rice (Uncle Ben's Country Inn) 1/2 cup	123	7	2	—	*	8	2	11	2	2	6	—	2	*	2	13	5	10	—	—
chicken w/ wild rice (Uncle Ben's Country Inn) 1/2 cup	108	5	*	*	*	8	2	15	*	*	5	—	*	*	*	9	4	7	—	—
couscous (Knorr Pilaf) 1/2 cup	160	8	2	—	*	10	—	15	—	4	6	*	*	*	*	25	15	10	*	*

RICE DISH, FROM MIX (continued)

	Calories	Protein	Fat	Sat. Fat	Cholesterol	Carbohydrates	Fiber	Sodium	Potassium	Calcium	Iron	Zinc	Magnesium	Vitamin A	Vitamin C	Thiamin	Riboflavin	Niacin	Vitamin B₁₂	Folic acid
(Near East) 1/2 cup	100	6	*	*	*	7	4	*	—	*	3	—	—	*	*	—	—	—	—	—
creamy chicken & mushrooms (Uncle Ben's Country Inn) 1/2 cup	138	6	5	—	*	8	4	16	*	3	6	—	—	*	*	10	7	8		
creamy chicken & wild rice (Uncle Ben's Country Inn) 1/2 cup	135	7	2	—	*	9	2	14	*	5	5	—	—	*	*	10	11	8		
drumstick mix (Minute) 1/2 cup	150	4	6	—	*	8	—	29	*	*	6	—	—	*	2	*	8	*	6	
florentine (Uncle Ben's Country Inn) 1/2 cup	121	6	2	—	*	8	4	15	4	3	6	—	6	*	*	10	8	8		
fried (Minute) 1/2 cup	160	4	8	—	*	8	—	24	*	*	6	—	—	*	*	*	8	*	6	
Chinese style (La Choy) 1/2 cup	125	4	*	*	*	9	*	11	*	*	10	—	—	*	*	7	*	14		
w/ chicken (Chun King) 1/2 cup	130	12	3	—	13	7	—	31	3	*	10	—	—	5	5	25	5	3		
w/ pork (Chun King) 1/2 cup	135	9	5	—	*	9	—	25	3	*	8	—	—	*	3	10	5	3		
green bean almondine (Uncle Ben's Country Inn) 1/2 cup	128	6	3	—	*	8	3	12	*	3	6	—	—	*	2	13	6	7		
harvest medley (Knorr Pilaf) 1/2 cup	110	4	2	—	*	8	—	17	—	*	6	*	*	20	*	10	4	8	*	*
herbed rice au gratin (Uncle Ben's Country Inn) 1/2 cup	119	6	2	—	*	8	3	15	*	4	5	—	—	*	*	11	7	6		
homestyle chicken & vegetable (Uncle Ben's Country Inn) 1/2 cup	139	7	5	—	2	8	4	12	2	2	6	—	2	*	*	9	7	8		
lemon herb jasmine (Knorr Pilaf) 1/2 cup	140	4	2	—	*	10	—	16	*	*	*	*	*	*	*	6	2	2	*	*
long grain & wild chicken stock sauce (Uncle Ben's Country Inn) 1/2 cup	132	7	3	—	2	8	4	25	2	2	6	—	2	*	9	7	5	8	—	—
fast cooking (Uncle Ben's Country Inn) 1/2 cup	101	5	*	*	*	7	3	19	*	*	5	—	2	*	*	11	2	6	—	—
garden vegetable blend (Uncle Ben's Country Inn) 1/2 cup	128	6	2	—	*	9	4	25	4	2	5	—	3	*	*	8	6	8	—	—
original (Uncle Ben's Country Inn) 1/2 cup	96	5	*	*	*	7	2	15	3	2	5	—	4	*	4	7	2	6	—	—
Mexican (Old El Paso) 1/2 cup	140	3	3	—	—	9	—	15	—	6	4	—	—	*	8	15	6	6	—	
milanese risotto (Knorr) 1/2 cup	180	4	6	—	*	11	—	22	—	*	*	*	*	2	*	2	2	4	*	*
mushroom risotto (Knorr) 1/2 cup	180	4	6	—	*	11	—	26	—	*	*	*	*	2	*	2	4	4	*	*
onion herb risotto (Knorr) 1/2 cup	200	6	8	—	*	11	—	34	4	*	*	*	*	2	*	4	4	4	*	*
pilaf (Mahatma) 1/2 cup	100	4	*	*	—	7	—	20	—	*	2	—	—	*	*	4	*	*	—	—
(Success) 1/2 cup	120	4	*	*	—	8	—	17	—	*	6	—	—	6	*	10	2	10	—	—
primavera risotto (Knorr) 1/2 cup	180	4	6	—	*	11	—	22	—	*	*	*	*	2	*	*	*	*	*	*

	Calories	Protein	Fat	Sat. Fat	Cholesterol	Carbohydrates	Fiber	Sodium	Potassium	Calcium	Iron	Zinc	Magnesium	Vitamin A	Vitamin C	Thiamin	Riboflavin	Niacin	Vitamin B$_{12}$	Folic acid
RICE DISH, FROM MIX (continued)																				
red beans & rice (Mahatma) 1/2 cup	200	2	*	*	—	15	—	38	—	14	25	—	—	*	*	40	4	8	—	—
rice, buttery (Tuna Helper) 1/2 cup	178	12	12	—	—	8	—	27	5	4	3	—	—	10	*	6	4	7	—	—
saffron yellow (Mahatma) 1/2 cup	100	2	*	*	—	7	—	20	—	*	6	—	—	2	*	10	2	6	—	—
sesame chicken (Mahatma) 1/2 cup	100	2	*	*	—	7	—	26	—	2	8	—	—	*	*	10	4	6	—	—
Spanish (Lipton Rice & Sauce) 1/2 cup	140	5	5	—	—	8	—	23	—	4	4	2	—	4	6	4	8	*	—	—
(Mahatma) 1/2 cup	100	2	*	*	—	7	—	8	—	*	2	—	—	4	*	10	*	6	—	—
(Success) 1/2 cup	110	4	*	*	—	8	—	19	—	4	3	—	—	*	*	12	2	12	—	—
tomato risotto (Knorr) 1/2 cup	190	4	8	—	*	11	—	26	—	*	*	*	*	2	*	2	4	4	*	*
vegetable pilaf (Uncle Ben's Country Inn) 1/2 cup	115	5	*	*	*	8	3	15	*	*	5	—	*	*	3	10	4	7	—	*
wild (Mahatma) 1/2 cup	100	4	*	*	—	7	—	20	—	*	10	—	—	*	*	15	2	6	—	—
RICE DISH, FROZEN																				
w/ broccoli (Green Giant Rice Originals) 1/2 cup	120	5	6	5	2	6	—	21	2	4	8	—	—	20	10	15	2	8	—	—
w/ broccoli in cheese flavored sauce (Green Giant One Serving) 1 pkg (5 1/2 oz)	160	8	8	10	2	9	8	20	4	6	10	—	—	50	6	10	2	15	—	—
pilaf (Green Giant Rice Originals) 1/2 cup	110	3	2	3	*	7	—	22	2	*	4	—	—	*	*	15	*	10	—	—
w/ green beans (Budget Gourmet Side Dish) 5 1/2 oz	230	6	17	—	3	10	—	21	2	4	2	—	—	8	15	8	4	8	—	—
rice florentine (Green Giant Rice Originals) 1/2 cup	140	7	6	10	3	7	—	17	3	8	4	—	—	10	*	10	*	8	—	—
rice medley (Green Giant Rice Originals) 1/2 cup	100	5	2	3	2	6	—	13	2	*	4	—	—	*	*	15	*	10	—	—
vegetables and rice (Stouffer's Lunch Express) 9 7/8 oz	90	—	17	13	10	15	8	31	8	10	4	—	—	40	6	—	—	—	—	—
white 'n' wild (Green Giant Rice Originals) 1/2 cup	130	5	3	3	*	8	—	22	2	*	4	—	—	*	*	10	*	15	—	—
RICE BRAN OIL																				
(generic) 1 tbsp	120	*	22	14	*	*	*	*	*	*	*	*	*	*	*	*	*	*	*	*
(Hollywood) 1 tbsp	120	*	22	15	*	*	*	*	*	*	*	*	*	*	*	*	*	*	*	*
RICE CAKE																				
apple cinnamon (Hain) 5 mini cakes	60	2	*	*	*	4	—	*	*	*	*	*	*	*	*	*	*	4	*	*
barbeque (Hain) 5 mini cakes	70	2	5	—	*	3	—	2	*	*	*	*	*	*	*	*	*	*	*	*
brown rice buckwheat (generic) 2 cakes	68	3	*	*	*	5	4	*	2	*	*	3	7	*	*	*	*	7	*	*
unsalted (generic) 2 cakes	68	3	*	*	*	5	—	*	2	*	*	3	7	*	*	*	*	7	*	*
corn (generic) 2 cakes	69	3	*	*	*	5	4	2	*	*	*	3	5	*	*	*	*	6	*	*

	Calories	Protein	Fat	Sat. Fat	Cholesterol	Carbohydrates	Fiber	Sodium	Potassium	Calcium	Iron	Zinc	Magnesium	Vitamin A	Vitamin C	Thiamin	Riboflavin	Niacin	Vitamin B12	Folic acid
RICE CAKE (continued)																				
mixed-grain (generic) 2 cakes	70	3	*	*	*	5	4	2	2	*	2	3	6	*	*	*	2	6	*	*
unsalted (generic) 2 cakes	70	3	*	*	*	5	—	*	2	*	2	3	6	*	*	*	2	6	*	*
plain (generic) 2 cakes	70	2	*	*	*	5	4	2	*	*	*	4	6	*	*	*	2	7	*	*
unsalted (generic) 2 cakes	70	2	*	*	*	5	4	*	*	*	*	4	6	*	*	*	2	7	*	*
rye (generic) 2 cakes	69	2	*	*	*	5	4	2	*	*	2	4	6	*	*	*	*	6	*	*
sesame seed (generic) 2 cakes	71	2	*	*	*	5	4	2	*	*	2	4	6	*	*	*	*	6	*	*
unsalted (generic) 2 cakes	71	2	*	*	*	5	—	*	*	*	2	4	6	*	*	*	*	6	*	*
butter flavored (Hain) 1 cake	45	2	2	*	*	3	—	2	*	*	*	*	*	*	*	*	*	4	*	*
caramel (Hain) 5 mini cakes	60	2	*	*	*	4	—	5	*	*	*	*	*	*	*	*	2	*	*	*
cheese (Hain) 5 mini cakes	60	2	5	—	*	3	—	4	*	*	*	*	*	*	*	*	*	*	*	*
honey nut (Hain) 5 mini cakes	60	2	3	—	*	3	—	2	*	*	*	*	*	*	*	*	*	4	*	*
nacho cheese (Hain) 5 mini cakes	70	2	3	—	*	3	—	2	*	*	*	*	*	*	*	*	*	*	*	*
plain																				
salted (Hain) 1 cake	35	2	*	*	*	3	—	2	*	*	*	*	*	*	*	*	*	4	*	*
(Hain) 5 mini cakes	50	2	*	*	*	4	—	*	*	*	*	*	*	*	*	*	*	*	*	*
unsalted (Hain) 5 mini cakes	50	2	*	*	*	4	—	*	*	*	*	*	*	*	*	*	*	*	*	*
popcorn																				
butter flavor (Hain) 5 mini cakes	60	2	3	—	*	3	—	2	*	*	*	*	*	*	*	*	*	2	*	*
mild cheddar flavor (Hain) 5 mini cakes	60	2	3	—	*	3	—	3	*	*	*	2	*	*	*	*	*	4	*	*
plain (Hain) 5 mini cakes	60	2	2	—	*	4	—	*	*	*	*	*	*	*	*	*	*	2	*	*
white cheddar flavor (Hain) 5 mini cakes	60	2	3	—	*	3	—	3	*	*	*	2	*	*	*	*	*	4	*	*
ranch (Hain) 5 mini cakes	70	2	5	—	*	3	—	4	*	*	*	*	*	*	*	*	*	*	*	*
teriyaki (Hain) 5 mini cakes	50	2	*	*	*	4	—	5	*	*	*	*	*	*	*	*	4	*	*	*
white cheddar (Hain) 1 cake	45	2	2	*	*	3	—	6	*	*	*	*	*	*	*	*	*	4	*	*
ROCKFISH																				
raw 1 fillet	180	60	5	4	22	*	*	5	22	2	4	5	12	7	*	5	8	31	32	*
baked/broiled 1 fillet	180	60	5	4	22	*	*	5	22	2	4	5	13	7	*	4	7	29	30	*
ROE																				
raw 1 oz	39	10	3	2	35	*	*	*	2	*	*	2	*	*	7	4	12	3	46	*
broiled/baked 1 oz	58	14	4	3	45	*	*	*	2	*	*	2	2	*	8	5	16	3	54	*
ROLL, DINNER																				
bakery style																				
original (Wonder) 1 roll	140	8	3	3	*	8	—	12	—	6	10	—	—	*	*	15	6	10	—	—

ROLL, DINNER (continued)

	Calories	Protein	Fat	Sat. Fat	Cholesterol	Carbohydrates	Fiber	Sodium	Potassium	Calcium	Iron	Zinc	Magnesium	Vitamin A	Vitamin C	Thiamin	Riboflavin	Niacin	Vitamin B12	Folic acid
sourdough (Wonder) 1 roll	150	10	3	3	*	8	—	12	—	6	10	—	—	*	*	30	10	15	—	—
Bavarian wheat (Bread du Jour) 1 roll	80	5	2	3	*	5	6	7	2	4	8	—	—	*	*	10	6	8	—	—
Bran'nola buns (Arnold) 1 bun	100	8	3	*	*	6	12	6	—	2	10	—	—	*	*	10	8	8	—	—
brown & serve buttermilk (Wonder) 1 roll	70	2	2	3	*	5	2	6	*	6	4	—	—	*	*	8	6	6	—	—
plain (Wonder) 1 roll	70	2	2	3	*	5	2	6	*	6	4	—	—	*	*	8	6	6	—	—
bun enriched (Wonder) 1 roll	70	5	2	3	*	4	3	7	*	6	6	—	—	*	*	8	6	6	—	—
hamburger light (Wonder) 1 roll	80	7	2	3	*	5	18	9	*	8	10	—	—	*	*	15	15	8	—	—
honey wheat (Wonder) 1 roll	130	8	3	3	*	7	8	10	2	10	8	—	—	*	*	10	8	10	—	—
butter flavored butterflake (Pillsbury) 1 roll	140	5	8	5	*	7	—	22	*	*	6	—	—	*	*	10	6	6	—	—
club brown & serve (Pepperidge Farm) 1 roll	100	6	2	*	*	6	2	8	—	4	6	—	—	*	*	15	8	8	—	—
crescent (Pillsbury) 1 roll	100	3	9	5	*	4	—	10	2	2	2	—	—	*	*	4	2	4	—	—
heat & serve (Pepperidge Farm) 1 roll	110	4	9	15	5	4	*	6	—	2	4	—	—	2	*	10	6	6	—	—
crusty Italian (Bread du Jour) 1 roll	80	7	2	3	*	5	3	8	*	6	8	—	—	*	*	12	8	8	—	—
Dutch egg (Arnold) 1 bun	130	6	5	5	*	7	8	7	—	4	6	—	—	*	*	8	6	6	—	—
French (Arnold Francisco) 1 roll	130	6	3	—	—	8	—	6	—	2	4	—	—	*	*	10	6	6	—	—
(DiCarlo's) 1 roll	180	10	3	3	*	12	7	16	2	10	12	—	—	*	*	15	12	15	—	—
brown & serve (Pepperidge Farm) 1 roll	360	20	6	*	*	24	4	32	—	12	20	—	—	*	*	50	30	30	—	—
seven grain (Pepperidge Farm) 1 roll	100	8	3	5	*	6	4	7	—	4	*	—	—	*	*	10	6	8	—	—
sourdough style (Pepperidge Farm) 1 roll	100	6	2	*	*	6	2	10	—	2	6	—	—	*	*	15	8	8	—	—
French style fully baked (Pepperidge Farm) 1 oz	80	4	2	*	*	5	*	6	—	2	4	—	—	*	*	10	6	6	—	—
garlic bread (Pepperidge Farm) 3/4 oz	100	4	9	10	5	4	8	6	—	*	6	—	—	2	*	10	4	6	—	—
garlic & cheese (Pepperidge Farm) 1 1/2 oz	130	6	9	10	2	6	12	10	—	6	8	—	—	6	*	20	10	10	—	—
garlic parmesan (Pepperidge Farm) 1 oz	100	4	8	10	7	4	8	6	—	*	6	—	—	2	*	10	6	6	—	—
golden twist heat & serve (Pepperidge Farm) 1 roll	110	4	8	10	2	5	*	6	—	2	4	—	—	*	*	8	4	6	—	—
hearth (Pepperidge Farm) 1 roll	50	2	2	*	*	3	*	4	—	2	4	—	—	*	*	6	4	4	—	—
homestyle from dough (Rich's) 1 roll	70	3	2	*	*	4	2	6	*	*	3	*	*	*	*	7	47	*	—	—
Italian (Arnold) 1 roll	210	10	5	5	*	13	12	—	—	4	10	—	—	*	*	15	15	10	—	—

	Calories	Protein	Fat	Sat. Fat	Cholesterol	Carbohydrates	Fiber	Sodium	Potassium	Calcium	Iron	Zinc	Magnesium	Vitamin A	Vitamin C	Thiamin	Riboflavin	Niacin	Vitamin B₁₂	Folic acid
ROLL, DINNER (continued)																				
light																				
(Arnold Bakery) 1 roll	80	6	3	*	*	7	16	8	—	2	10	—	—	*	*	10	8	8	—	—
onion																				
(Arnold) 1 roll	170	8	3	—	—	11	—	—	—	4	8	—	—	*	*	15	8	10	—	—
pan																				
(Wonder) 1 roll	80	3	2	3	*	5	2	6	—	4	4	—	—	*	*	8	6	6	—	—
petite party																				
(Arnold) 2 rolls	60	4	3	5	*	3	4	3	—	*	4	—	—	*	*	4	4	4	—	—
plain																				
(Arnold) 1 roll	50	2	2	*	*	3	4	3	—	*	4	—	—	*	*	4	4	4	—	—
(Arnold August Bros.) 1 roll	90	4	2	—	—	6	—	7	—	2	2	—	—	*	*	6	4	4	—	—
potato																				
(Arnold) 1 roll	60	2	2	—	*	3	4	3	—	2	2	—	—	*	*	6	8	2	—	—
(Pepperidge Farm) 1 roll	160	6	6	5	*	9	16	11	—	*	6	—	—	*	*	30	8	25	—	—
potato classic																				
(Pepperidge Farm) 1 roll	80	2	3	*	*	4	—	5	—	*	2	—	—	*	*	10	4	10	—	—
sesame																				
(Arnold) 1 roll	50	2	2	*	*	3	4	3	—	*	4	—	—	*	*	4	4	4	—	—
(Arnold August Bros.) 1 roll	170	10	2	—	*	12	8	13	—	4	15	—	—	*	*	15	10	10	—	—
soft onion																				
(Arnold) 1 roll	140	8	5	—	*	8	8	8	—	4	8	—	—	*	*	10	6	6	—	—
sourdough																				
(Arnold Francisco) 1 roll	90	6	2	—	*	6	4	5	—	4	4	—	—	*	*	8	6	6	—	—
(DiCarlo's) 1 roll	200	13	3	3	*	12	9	13	2	10	15	—	—	*	*	20	15	15	—	—
brown 'n' serve																				
(Arnold Francisco) 1 roll	90	6	2	—	*	5	4	5	—	4	4	—	—	*	*	8	6	6	—	—
brown 'n' serve																				
(Arnold Francisco) 1 oz	70	4	2	*	*	5	4	10	—	4	4	—	—	*	*	8	4	4	—	—
wheat																				
(Home Pride) 1 roll	70	3	3	5	*	3	3	5	*	4	4	—	—	*	*	6	4	4	—	—
bakery style																				
(Wonder) 1 roll	150	10	3	3	*	8	—	12	—	6	10	—	—	*	*	30	10	15	—	—
old fashioned																				
(Arnold) 2 rolls	80	2	5	—	*	4	—	4	—	2	4	—	—	*	*	8	*	4	—	—
white																				
(Home Pride) 1 roll	70	3	3	5	*	3	3	5	*	4	4	—	—	*	*	6	4	4	—	—
from mix																				
(Pillsbury) 1 roll	120	7	3	*	5	7	—	9	*	*	6	—	—	*	*	10	10	8	—	—
old fashioned																				
(Arnold) 2 rolls	80	2	5	—	*	4	—	4	—	2	4	—	—	*	*	8	*	4	—	—
ROLL, HAMBURGER see ROLL, SANDWICH																				
ROLL, HOT DOG																				
(Arnold) 1 bun	110	6	3	5	*	7	4	7	—	2	8	—	—	*	*	10	8	8	—	—
Bran'nola																				
(Arnold) 1 roll	100	8	3	5	*	6	12	6	—	2	10	—	—	*	*	10	8	8	—	—
dijon																				
(Pepperidge Farm) 1 roll	160	8	8	5	*	8	8	10	—	6	10	—	—	*	*	10	10	10	—	—
light																				
(Wonder) 1 roll	80	7	2	3	*	5	18	9	*	8	10	—	—	*	*	15	10	8	—	—
New England style																				
(Arnold) 1 bun	110	6	3	—	*	7	4	7	—	2	8	—	—	*	*	10	8	8	—	—
side sliced																				
(Pepperidge Farm) 1 roll	140	8	5	5	*	8	2	11	—	4	6	—	—	*	*	15	10	10	—	—
sliced																				
(Brownberry) 1 bun	110	6	3	—	*	7	4	9	—	2	6	—	—	*	*	8	6	6	—	—
top sliced																				
(Pepperidge Farm) 1 roll	140	8	5	5	*	8	2	11	—	4	6	—	—	*	*	15	10	10	—	—

	Calories	Protein	Fat	Sat. Fat	Cholesterol	Carbohydrates	Fiber	Sodium	Potassium	Calcium	Iron	Zinc	Magnesium	Vitamin A	Vitamin C	Thiamin	Riboflavin	Niacin	Vitamin B12	Folic acid
ROLL, KAISER																				
(Arnold) 1 roll	170	8	3	—	—	11	—	—	—	4	8	—	—	*	*	15	8	10	—	—
(Arnold August Bros.) 1 roll	170	10	2	—	*	12	8	13	—	4	15	—	—	*	*	15	10	10	—	—
(Arnold Francisco) 1 roll	90	10	5	—	*	11	8	9	—	4	10	—	—	*	*	15	10	10	—	—
hearth (Brownberry) 1 roll	150	8	5	5	3	9	8	13	—	6	8	—	—	*	*	15	8	10	—	—
ROLL, ONION																				
(Arnold August Bros.) 1 roll	160	10	2	—	*	—	8	13	—	4	15	—	—	*	*	15	10	10	—	—
premium (Arnold) 1 roll	180	10	2	—	*	13	8	14	—	2	10	—	—	*	*	15	10	10	—	—
w/ poppy seeds (Pepperidge Farm) 1 roll	150	8	5	5	*	9	2	11	—	4	8	—	—	*	*	15	8	10	—	—
ROLL, SANDWICH																				
fat free (Pepperidge Farm) 1 roll	130	8	*	*	*	9	2	10	—	8	10	—	—	*	*	15	8	8	—	—
hamburger bun (Arnold) 1 bun	120	6	3	—	*	7	8	8	—	2	8	—	—	*	*	10	6	8	—	—
hearty (Pepperidge Farm) 1 roll	230	15	3	10	*	13	16	16	—	6	15	—	—	*	*	30	15	15	—	—
sesame (Arnold) 1 roll	130	6	5	—	*	8	8	9	—	4	8	—	—	*	*	8	8	6	—	—
sliced (Pepperidge Farm) 1 roll	130	8	5	5	*	7	—	9	—	2	8	—	—	*	*	20	8	8	—	—
soft (Arnold) 1 roll	110	6	5	—	*	6	8	7	—	2	8	—	—	x	x	8	6	8	—	—
soft hoagie (Pepperidge Farm) 1 roll	210	15	8	5	*	11	4	13	—	6	8	—	—	*	2	10	10	15	—	—
sub roll (Levy) 1 roll	180	8	3	—	—	11	—	10	—	4	10	—	—	*	*	15	10	10	—	—
super sub loaf (Arnold Francisco) 1 slice	70	4	2	—	*	4	4	6	—	2	6	—	—	*	*	6	4	4	—	—
w/ sesame seeds (Pepperidge Farm) 1 roll	140	8	5	5	*	8	2	10	—	4	8	—	—	*	*	20	10	8	—	—
wheat (Brownberry) 1 bun	130	6	5	—	*	8	8	10	—	2	6	—	—	*	*	10	6	6	—	—
white (Brownberry) 1 bun	130	6	5	—	*	8	8	9	—	4	6	—	—	*	*	10	6	6	—	—
ROSEMARY, DRIED 1 tbsp	11	*	*	*	*	*	*	*	*	4	5	*	2	2	3	*	2	*	—	—
ROUGHY																				
raw 3 oz	107	21	9	*	6	*	*	2	7	3	*	4	6	*	*	6	7	13	28	*
broiled/baked 3 1/2 oz	89	31	*	*	9	*	*	3	11	4	*	6	10	2	*	8	11	18	38	*
RUM 1 1/2 fl oz	97	*	*	*	*	*	*	*	*	*	*	*	*	*	*	*	*	*	*	*
RUTABAGA																				
raw 1/2 cup cubes	25	*	*	*	*	2	8	*	7	3	2	2	4	8	29	4	2	2	*	4
boiled 1/2 cup cubes	33	2	*	*	*	2	8	*	8	4	3	2	5	10	27	5	2	3	*	3
boiled w/ salt 1/2 cup cubes	33	2	*	*	*	2	8	9	8	4	3	2	5	10	27	5	2	3	*	3
RYE BREAD see BREAD																				
RYE FLOUR																				
medium (Pillsbury Best) 1 cup	367	17	3	2	*	26	34	*	8	2	7	—	—	*	*	21	6	6	—	—
RYE-WHEAT FLOUR																				
Bohemian style (Pillsbury Best) 1 cup	357	21	2	*	*	25	—	*	4	2	20	—	—	*	*	31	15	20	—	—

	Calories	Protein	Fat	Sat. Fat	Cholesterol	Carbohydrates	Fiber	Sodium	Potassium	Calcium	Iron	Zinc	Magnesium	Vitamin A	Vitamin C	Thiamin	Riboflavin	Niacin	Vitamin B₁₂	Folic acid
SABLEFISH																				
raw																				
1/2 fillet	376	43	45	31	32	*	*	4	20	7	14	4	27	12	*	13	10	39	48	*
broiled/baked																				
1/2 fillet	378	43	46	31	32	*	*	5	20	7	14	4	27	10	*	12	10	39	36	*
smoked																				
3 oz	218	25	26	18	18	*	*	26	11	4	8	2	16	7	*	7	6	23	28	*
SAFFLOWER KERNEL																				
dried																				
(generic) 1 oz	147	8	17	5	*	3	—	*	6	2	8	10	25	*	*	22	7	3	*	11
SAFFLOWER MEAL																				
partially defatted																				
(generic) 1 oz	97	17	*	*	*	5	—	*	*	2	8	9	25	*	*	22	7	3	*	11
SAFFLOWER OIL																				
w/ added vitamin E																				
(Hollywood) 1 tbsp	120	*	22	5	*	*	*	*	*	*	*	*	*	*	*	*	*	*	*	*
SAGE, GROUND																				
1 tbsp	6	*	*	*	*	*	*	*	*	3	3	*	2	2	*	*	*	*	*	*
SALAD DRESSING																				
cooked																				
(homemade) 1 tbsp	25	*	2	3	3	*	*	5	*	*	*	*	*	*	*	*	*	*	*	*
w/ stick margarine																				
(homemade) 1 tbsp	25	*	2	*	*	*	*	5	*	*	*	—	*	5	*	*	*	*	—	—
w/ tub margarine																				
(homemade) 1 tbsp	25	*	2	*	*	*	*	5	*	*	*	—	*	5	*	*	*	*	*	*
French																				
(homemade) 1 tbsp	88	*	15	9	*	*	*	4	*	*	*	*	*	*	*	*	*	*	*	*
oil & vinegar																				
(homemade) 1 tbsp	70	*	12	7	*	*	*	*	*	*	*	*	*	*	*	*	*	*	*	*
SALAD DRESSING, BOTTLED																				
bacon, creamy																				
reduced calorie																				
(Kraft) 1 tbsp	30	*	3	*	*	*	*	6	*	*	*	*	*	*	*	*	*	*	—	—
bacon & tomato																				
(Kraft) 1 tbsp	70	*	11	5	*	*	*	5	*	*	*	*	*	*	*	*	*	*	*	*
reduced calorie																				
(Kraft) 1 tbsp	30	*	3	*	*	*	*	6	*	*	*	—	*	*	*	*	*	*	*	*
blue cheese																				
(generic) 1 tbsp	77	*	12	8	*	*	*	7	*	*	*	*	*	*	*	*	*	*	*	*
(Kraft) 1 tbsp	60	*	9	5	—	*	*	10	*	*	*	—	*	*	*	*	*	*	*	*
(Roka) 1 tbsp	60	*	9	5	3	*	*	7	*	2	*	—	*	*	*	*	*	*	*	*
reduced calorie																				
(Marie's) 1/2 oz	100	*	15	10	3	*	*	4	—	*	*	*	*	*	*	*	*	*	*	*
(Marie's Lite & Luscious) 1/2 oz	50	*	6	*	*	*	—	5	—	*	*	*	*	*	*	*	*	*	*	*
(Roka) 1 tbsp	16	*	2	5	2	*	*	12	*	*	*	*	*	*	*	*	*	*	*	*
unsalted																				
(generic) 1 tbsp	77	*	12	8	*	*	*	*	*	*	*	*	*	*	*	*	*	*	*	*
blue cheese, creamy																				
reduced calorie																				
(Kraft) 1 tbsp	30	*	3	5	—	*	*	10	*	*	*	*	*	*	*	*	*	*	*	*
buttermilk																				
(Kraft) 1 tbsp	80	*	12	5	*	*	*	5	*	*	*	*	*	*	*	*	*	*	*	*
(Seven Seas) 1 tbsp	80	*	12	5	2	*	*	5	*	*	*	*	*	*	*	*	*	*	*	*
buttermilk, creamy																				
reduced calorie																				
(Kraft) 1 tbsp	30	*	5	*	—	*	*	5	*	*	*	*	*	*	*	*	*	*	*	*
buttermilk ranch																				
reduced calorie																				
(Seven Seas Light) 1 tbsp	50	*	8	5	*	*	*	6	*	*	*	—	—	*	*	*	*	*	—	—

SALAD DRESSING, BOTTLED (continued)

	Calories	Protein	Fat	Sat. Fat	Cholesterol	Carbohydrates	Fiber	Sodium	Potassium	Calcium	Iron	Zinc	Magnesium	Vitamin A	Vitamin C	Thiamin	Riboflavin	Niacin	Vitamin B₁₂	Folic acid
buttermilk spice, ranch style (Marie's) 1/2 oz	90	*	14	10	3	*	*	5	—	*	*	—	—	*	*	*	*	*	—	—
Caesar (Kraft) 1 tbsp	70	*	11	5	*	*	*	7	*	*	*	*	*	*	*	*	*	*	—	—
reduced calorie (Weight Watchers) 1 tbsp	5	*	*	*	*	*	8	8	*	*	*	*	*	*	*	—	—	—	—	—
Caesar, creamy (Marie's) 1/2 oz	100	*	15	10	3	*	*	4	—	*	*	—	—	*	*	*	*	*	—	—
catalina fat free (Kraft Free) 1 tbsp	16	*	*	*	*	*	*	5	*	*	*	—	—	6	*	*	*	*	—	—
cole slaw (Kraft) 1 tbsp	70	*	9	5	3	*	*	8	*	*	*	*	*	*	*	*	*	*	—	—
(Marie's) 1/2 oz	70	*	10	—	—	*	*	5	—	*	*	—	*	*	*	*	*	*	—	—
creamy (Rancher's Choice) 1 tbsp	90	*	15	5	2	*	*	6	*	*	*	*	*	*	*	*	*	*	—	—
creamy Italian (Seven Seas) 1 tbsp	70	*	11	5	*	*	*	10	*	*	*	*	*	*	*	*	*	*	—	—
reduced calorie (Weight Watchers) 1 tbsp	15	*	*	*	*	*	10	8	*	*	*	*	*	*	*	—	—	—	—	—
creamy peppercorn reduced calorie (Weight Watchers) 1 tbsp	4	*	*	*	*	*	8	2	*	*	*	*	*	*	*	—	—	—	—	—
cucumber (Kraft) 1 tbsp	70	*	12	5	*	*	*	8	*	*	*	*	*	*	*	*	*	*	—	—
cucumber, creamy reduced calorie (Kraft) 1 tbsp	25	*	3	*	*	*	*	9	*	*	*	—	—	*	*	*	*	*	—	—
(Weight Watchers) 1 tbsp	9	*	*	*	*	*	10	2	—	*	*	—	—	*	*	—	—	—	—	—
dijon vinaigrette (Hain) 1 tbsp	50	*	8	—	*	*	*	7	*	*	*	*	*	*	*	*	*	*	*	*
French (Catalina) 1 tbsp	60	*	8	5	*	*	*	7	*	*	*	*	*	—	*	*	*	*	—	—
(generic) 1 tbsp	67	*	10	8	3	*	*	9	*	*	*	*	*	*	*	*	*	*	*	*
(Kraft) 1 tbsp	60	*	9	5	*	*	*	5	*	*	*	—	—	6	*	*	*	*	—	—
(Kraft Miracle) 1 tbsp	70	*	9	5	*	*	*	10	*	*	*	—	—	*	*	*	*	*	—	—
low calorie (generic) 1 tbsp	22	*	*	*	*	*	*	5	*	*	*	*	*	*	*	*	*	*	*	*
low calorie no salt (generic) 1 tbsp	22	*	*	*	*	*	—	*		*	*	—		3	*	*	*	*	—	—
no salt (generic) 1 tbsp	67	*	10	8	*	*	*		*	*	*	*	—	*	*	*	*	*	—	—
reduced calorie (Kraft) 1 tbsp	20	*	2	*	*	*	*	5	*	*	*	—	—	8	*	*	*	*	—	—
(Kraft Free) 1 tbsp	20	*	*	*	*	*	*	5	*	*	*	—	—	6	*	*	*	*	—	—
(Seven Seas Light) 1 tbsp	35	*	5	*	*	*	*	9	*	*	*	—	—	*	*	*	*	*	—	—
(Weight Watchers) 1 tbsp	20	*	*	*	*	*	18	4	*	*	*	—	—	*	*	—	—	—	—	—
French, creamy (Marie's) 1/2 oz	70	*	9	5	*	*	—	5	—	*	*	—	*	2	*	*	*	*	—	—
(Seven Seas) 1 tbsp	60	*	9	5	*	*	*	10	*	*	*	*	*	*	*	*	*	*	—	—
garlic (Kraft) 1 tbsp	50	*	8	5	*	*	*	7	*	*	*	—	*	*	*	*	*	*	—	—
herb & spice (Seven Seas) 1 tbsp	60	*	9	5	*	*	*	7	*	*	*	—	—	*	*	*	*	*	—	—
reduced calorie (Seven Seas Light) 1 tbsp	30	*	5	*	*	*	*	8	*	*	*	—	—	*	*	*	*	*	—	—

SALAD DRESSING, BOTTLED (continued)

	Calories	Protein	Fat	Sat. Fat	Cholesterol	Carbohydrates	Fiber	Sodium	Potassium	Calcium	Iron	Zinc	Magnesium	Vitamin A	Vitamin C	Thiamin	Riboflavin	Niacin	Vitamin B12	Folic acid
herb vinaigrette reduced calorie (Marie's Zesty) 1/2 oz	16	*	*	*	*	*	*	5	—	*	*	*	*	*	*	*	*	*	—	—
honey dijon reduced calorie (Weight Watchers) 1 tbsp	23	*	*	*	*	2	10	3	*	*	*	—	*	*	*	*	—	—	—	—
honey mustard (Marie's) 1/2 oz	80	*	11	—	*	*	—	3	—	*	*	*	*	*	*	*	*	*	—	—
Italian (generic) 1 tbsp	69	*	11	5	*	*	*	5	*	*	*	*	*	*	*	*	*	*	*	*
(Kraft) 1 tbsp	60	*	9	5	*	*	*	5	*	*	*	—	*	*	*	*	*	*	—	—
(Kraft Presto) 1 tbsp	70	*	11	5	*	*	*	6	*	*	*	—	*	*	*	*	*	*	—	—
(Marie's) 1/2 oz	100	*	15	10	3	*	—	5	—	*	*	*	—	*	*	*	*	*	—	—
(Seven Seas) 1 tbsp	50	*	8	5	*	*	*	10	*	*	*	—	*	*	*	*	*	*	—	—
no salt (generic) 1 tbsp	69	*	11	5	3	*	*	*	*	*	*	—	*	*	*	*	*	*	—	—
oil-free (Kraft) 1 tbsp	4	*	*	*	*	*	*	9	*	*	*	—	*	*	*	*	*	*	—	—
reduced calorie (generic) 1 tbsp	16	*	2	*	*	*	*	5	*	*	*	*	*	*	*	*	*	*	*	*
(Kraft) 1 tbsp	30	*	3	*	*	*	*	5	*	*	*	—	*	*	*	*	*	*	—	—
(Kraft Free) 1 tbsp	6	*	*	*	*	*	*	9	*	*	*	—	*	*	*	*	*	*	—	—
(Seven Seas Free) 1 tbsp	4	*	*	*	*	*	*	9	*	*	*	—	*	*	*	*	*	*	—	—
(Seven Seas Light) 1 tbsp	30	*	5	*	*	*	*	10	*	*	*	—	*	*	*	*	*	*	—	—
(Weight Watchers) 1 tbsp	5	*	*	*	*	*	2	8	*	*	*	—	*	*	*	—	—	—	—	—
no salt (generic) 1 tbsp	16	*	2	*	*	*	—	*	*	*	*	—	*	*	*	*	*	*	—	—
w/ sour cream (Kraft) 1 tbsp	50	*	8	5	*	*	*	5	*	*	*	—	*	*	*	*	*	*	—	—
reduced calorie and zesty (Kraft) 1 tbsp	20	*	3	*	*	*	*	10	*	*	*	—	*	*	*	*	*	*	—	—
zesty (Kraft) 1 tbsp	50	*	8	5	*	*	*	11	*	*	*	—	*	*	*	*	*	*	—	—
Italian, creamy (Hain) 1 tbsp	80	*	12	—	*	*	*	4	*	*	*	*	*	*	*	*	*	*	*	*
(Hollywood) 1 tbsp	90	*	14	5	*	*	*	6	*	*	*	*	*	*	*	*	*	*	*	*
reduced calorie (Kraft) 1 tbsp	25	*	3	*	*	*	*	5	*	*	*	—	*	*	*	*	*	*	—	—
(Seven Seas Light) 1 tbsp	45	*	6	5	*	*	*	10	*	*	*	—	*	*	*	*	*	*	—	—
Italian garlic (Marie's) 1/2 oz	100	*	15	10	3	*	—	4	—	*	*	*	—	*	*	*	*	*	—	—
reduced calorie (Marie's Lite & Luscious) 1/2 oz	40	*	5	*	*	*	—	5	—	*	*	*	—	*	*	*	*	*	—	—
Italian herb & romano (Marie's) 1/2 oz	100	*	15	10	3	*	—	4	—	*	*	*	—	*	*	*	*	*	—	—
Italian vinaigrette reduced calorie (Marie's Zesty) 1/2 oz	16	*	*	*	*	*	*	6	—	*	*	*	—	*	*	*	*	*	—	—
mayonnaise type (generic) 1 tbsp	57	*	8	4	*	*	*	4	*	*	*	—	*	*	*	*	*	*	*	*
oil & vinegar (Kraft) 1 tbsp	70	*	12	5	*	*	*	9	*	*	*	—	*	*	*	*	*	*	—	—
old fashioned buttermilk (Hain) 1 tbsp	70	*	11	—	*	*	*	4	*	*	*	*	*	*	*	*	*	*	*	*
poppy seed (Marie's) 1/2 oz	70	*	9	—	*	*	*	4	*	*	*	*	*	*	*	*	*	*	—	—
poppyseed rancher's (Hain) 1 tbsp	60	*	11	—	*	*	*	4	*	*	*	*	*	*	*	*	*	*	*	*

	Calories	Protein	Fat	Sat. Fat	Cholesterol	Carbohydrates	Fiber	Sodium	Potassium	Calcium	Iron	Zinc	Magnesium	Vitamin A	Vitamin C	Thiamin	Riboflavin	Niacin	Vitamin B$_{12}$	Folic acid
SALAD DRESSING, BOTTLED (continued)																				
ranch																				
(Marie's) 1/2 oz	100	*	15	10	3	*	—	4	—	*	*	*	*	*	*	*	*	*	—	—
(Seven Seas) 1 tbsp	80	*	12	5	2	*	*	6	*	*	*	*	*	*	*	*	*	*	—	—
reduced calorie																				
(Kraft Free) 1 tbsp	16	*	*	*	*	*	*	6	*	*	*	*	*	*	*	10	*	*	—	—
(Marie's Lite & Luscious) 1/2 oz	45	*	5	*	*	*	—	5	—	*	*	*	*	*	*	*	*	*	—	—
(Rancher's Choice) 1 tbsp	30	*	5	*	2	*	*	6	*	*	*	*	*	*	*	*	*	*	—	—
(Seven Seas Free) 1 tbsp	16	*	*	*	*	*	*	5	*	*	*	*	*	*	*	10	*	*	—	—
(Seven Seas Light) 1 tbsp	50	*	8	5	2	*	*	5	*	*	*	*	*	*	*	*	*	*	—	—
(Weight Watchers) 1 tbsp	18	*	*	*	*	*	6	6	*	*	*	*	—	*	*	—	—	—	—	—
red wine vinaigrette																				
(Kraft) 1 tbsp	60	*	6	5	*	*	*	8	*	*	*	*	—	*	*	*	*	*	—	—
(Seven Seas) 1 tbsp	70	*	11	5	*	*	*	12	*	*	*	*	—	*	*	*	*	*	—	—
reduced calorie																				
(Marie's Zesty) 1/2 oz	20	*	*	*	*	2	*	6	—	*	*	*	*	*	*	*	*	*	—	—
(Seven Seas Free) 1 tbsp	6	*	*	*	*	*	*	8	*	*	*	*	—	*	*	*	*	*	—	—
(Seven Seas Light) 1 tbsp	45	*	6	5	*	*	*	8	*	*	*	*	—	*	*	*	*	*	—	—
Russian																				
(generic) 1 tbsp	76	*	12	6	*	*	*	6	*	*	*	*	*	2	2	*	*	*	*	*
(Kraft) 1 tbsp	60	*	8	5	2	*	*	6	*	*	*	*	—	*	*	*	*	*	—	—
reduced calorie																				
(generic) 1 tbsp	23	*	*	*	*	*	*	6	*	*	*	*	*	*	2	*	*	*	*	*
(Kraft) 1 tbsp	30	*	2	*	*	*	*	5	*	*	*	*	—	*	*	*	*	*	—	—
(Weight Watchers) 1 tbsp	45	*	2	*	3	3	*	8	*	*	*	*	—	—	4	*	—	—	—	—
w/ honey																				
(Kraft) 1 tbsp	60	*	8	5	*	*	*	5	*	*	*	*	—	2	*	*	*	*	—	—
sesame seed																				
(generic) 1 tbsp	68	*	10	5	*	*	—	6	*	*	*	*	*	2	*	*	*	*	*	*
sour cream & dill																				
(Marie's) 1/2 oz	50	*	6	*	*	*	*	5	—	*	*	*	*	*	*	*	*	*	—	—
sour, filled																				
(generic) 1 tbsp	21	*	3	8	*	*	*	*	*	*	*	*	*	*	*	*	*	*	*	*
thousand island																				
(Hain) 1 tbsp	50	*	8	—	*	*	*	4	*	*	*	*	*	*	*	*	*	*	*	*
(Kraft) 1 tbsp	60	*	8	5	2	*	*	6	*	*	*	*	—	—	*	*	*	*	*	
(Marie's) 1/2 oz	80	*	12	5	3	*	—	5	—	*	*	*	—	*	*	*	*	*	—	—
reduced calorie																				
(generic) 1 tbsp	24	*	2	*	*	*	*	6	*	*	*	*	*	*	*	*	*	*	*	*
(Kraft) 1 tbsp	20	*	2	*	*	*	*	6	*	*	*	*	—	*	*	*	*	*	—	—
(Kraft Free) 1 tbsp	20	*	*	*	*	2	*	6	*	*	*	*	—	*	*	10	*	*	—	—
(Seven Seas Light) 1 tbsp	30	*	3	*	2	*	*	7	*	*	*	*	—	*	*	*	*	*	—	—
(Weight Watchers) 1 tbsp	45	*	2	*	3	3	*	8	*	*	*	*	—	—	4	*	—	—	—	—
regular																				
(generic) 1 tbsp	59	*	9	5	*	*	*	5	*	*	*	*	*	*	*	*	*	*	*	*
w/ bacon																				
(Kraft) 1 tbsp	60	*	9	5	*	*	*	4	*	*	*	*	—	*	*	*	*	*	—	—
thousand island, creamy																				
(Seven Seas) 1 tbsp	50	*	8	5	2	*	*	6	*	*	*	*	—	*	*	*	*	*	—	—
three cheese Caesar																				
reduced calorie																				
(Weight Watchers) 1 tbsp	40	2	3	*	3	2	*	8	*	2	*	*	—	*	*	*	—	—	—	—
white wine vinaigrette																				
reduced calorie																				
(Marie's Zesty) 1/2 oz	20	*	*	*	*	2	*	6	—	*	*	*	*	*	*	*	*	*	—	—
SALAD DRESSING MIX																				
bleu cheese & herbs																				
(Good Seasons) 1 tbsp	70	*	12	—	*	*	*	6	*	*	*	*	*	*	*	*	*	*	*	*

Encyclopedia of Daily Values

SALAD DRESSING MIX (continued)

	Calories	Protein	Fat	Sat. Fat	Cholesterol	Carbohydrates	Fiber	Sodium	Potassium	Calcium	Iron	Zinc	Magnesium	Vitamin A	Vitamin C	Thiamin	Riboflavin	Niacin	Vitamin B12	Folic acid
blue cheese																				
reduced calorie (Weight Watchers) 1 tbsp	8	*	*	*	—	*	—	5	—	*	*	—	—	*	*	—	—	—	—	—
buttermilk farm style (Good Seasons) 1 tbsp	60	*	9	—	2	*	*	6	*	*	*	*	*	*	*	*	*	*	*	*
cheese garlic (Good Seasons) 1 tbsp	70	*	12	—	*	*	*	7	*	*	*	*	*	*	*	*	*	*	*	*
cheese Italian (Good Seasons) 1 tbsp	70	*	12	—	*	*	*	5	2	*	*	*	*	*	*	*	*	*	*	*
reduced calorie (Good Seasons) 1 tbsp	25	*	5	—	*	*	*	5	2	*	*	*	*	*	*	*	*	*	*	*
classic dill (Good Seasons) 1 tbsp	70	*	12	—	*	*	*	6	*	*	*	*	*	*	*	*	*	*	*	*
creamy Italian																				
fat free (Good Seasons) 1 tbsp (prep w/ out oil)	8	*	*	*	*	*	*	6	2	*	*	*	*	*	*	*	*	*	*	*
reduced calorie (Weight Watchers) 1 tbsp	3	*	*	*	—	*	—	7	—	*	*	—	—	*	*	*	—	—	—	—
French																				
reduced calorie (Weight Watchers) 1 tbsp	3	*	*	*	—	*	—	6	—	*	*	—	—	*	*	*	—	—	—	—
garlic & herbs (Good Seasons) 1 tbsp	70	*	12	—	*	*	*	8	*	*	*	*	*	*	*	*	*	*	*	*
honey mustard (Good Seasons) 1 tbsp	80	*	12	—	*	*	*	5	*	*	*	*	*	*	*	*	*	*	*	*
fat free (Good Seasons) 1 tbsp (prep w/ out oil)	10	*	*	*	*	*	*	5	*	*	*	*	*	*	*	*	*	*	*	*
Italian (Good Seasons) 1 tbsp	70	*	12	—	*	*	*	7	*	*	*	*	*	*	*	*	*	*	*	*
fat free (Good Seasons) 1 tbsp (prep w/ out oil)	6	*	*	*	*	*	*	7	*	*	*	*	*	*	*	*	*	*	*	*
reduced calorie (Good Seasons) 1 tbsp	25	*	5	—	*	*	*	7	*	*	*	*	*	*	*	*	*	*	*	*
(Weight Watchers) 1 tbsp	2	*	*	*	—	*	—	6	—	*	*	—	—	*	*	*	—	—	—	—
Italian, mild (Good Seasons) 1 tbsp	70	*	12	—	*	*	*	8	*	*	*	*	*	*	*	*	*	*	*	*
Italian, zesty (Good Seasons) 1 tbsp	70	*	12	—	*	*	*	5	*	*	*	*	*	*	*	*	*	*	*	*
reduced calorie (Good Seasons) 1 tbsp	25	*	5	—	*	*	*	5	*	*	*	*	*	*	*	*	*	*	*	*
lemon & herbs (Good Seasons) 1 tbsp	70	*	12	—	*	*	*	6	*	*	*	*	*	*	*	*	*	*	*	*
ranch (Good Seasons) 1 tbsp	60	*	9	—	*	*	*	5	*	*	*	*	*	*	*	*	*	*	*	*
reduced calorie (Good Seasons) 1 tbsp	30	*	3	—	*	*	*	5	*	*	*	*	*	*	*	*	*	*	*	*
Russian																				
reduced calorie (Weight Watchers) 1 tbsp	4	*	*	*	—	*	—	5	—	*	*	—	—	*	*	*	—	—	—	—
thousand island																				
reduced calorie (Weight Watchers) 1 tbsp	4	*	*	*	—	*	—	6	—	*	*	—	—	*	*	*	—	—	—	—
zesty herb																				
fat free (Good Seasons) 1 tbsp (prep w/ out oil)	6	*	*	*	*	*	*	6	*	*	*	*	*	*	*	*	*	*	*	*

	Calories	Protein	Fat	Sat. Fat	Cholesterol	Carbohydrates	Fiber	Sodium	Potassium	Calcium	Iron	Zinc	Magnesium	Vitamin A	Vitamin C	Thiamin	Riboflavin	Niacin	Vitamin B₁₂	Folic acid
SALAMI																				
beef																				
(Bryan) 1 oz	70	7	8	—	7	*	*	13	—	—	—	—	—	—	—	—	—	—	—	—
(Machiaeh) 1 slice	60	5	8	12	5	*	*	11	*	*	3	3	*	*	*	—	—	—	—	—
beef & pork																				
(Bryan) 1 oz	60	7	6	—	7	*	*	14	—	—	—	—	—	—	—	—	—	—	—	—
cooked																				
beef (generic) 1 1 oz slice	74	7	9	13	6	*	*	14	2	*	3	4	*	*	8	2	3	5	14	*
beef & pork (generic) 1 1 oz slice	71	7	9	12	6	*	*	13	2	*	4	4	*	*	6	5	6	5	17	*
cotto																				
(Oscar Mayer) 1 slice	55	5	7	9	6	*	*	12	*	*	3	3	*	*	*	—	—	—	—	—
beef (Oscar Mayer) 1 slice	46	5	5	8	6	*	*	12	*	*	3	3	*	*	*	—	—	—	—	—
dry																				
pork (generic) 1 1 oz slice	115	11	15	17	7	*	*	27	3	*	2	8	2	*	*	18	6	8	13	*
pork & beef (generic) 1 1 oz slice	119	11	15	18	7	*	*	22	3	*	2	6	*	*	12	11	5	7	9	*
for beer																				
(Oscar Mayer) 1 slice	53	5	7	8	5	*	*	12	*	*	*	3	*	*	*	—	—	—	—	—
genoa																				
(Di Lusso) 1 oz	88	10	11	15	9	*	—	21	5	*	3	7	2	*	*	14	6	10	—	—
(Oscar Mayer) 1 slice	35	3	5	5	3	*	*	7	*	*	*	2	*	*	*	4	2	2	2	—
hard																				
(Homeland) 1 oz	117	10	15	20	10	*	—	19	4	1	4	6	1	*	13	7	5	7	—	—
(Oscar Mayer) 1 slice	34	3	4	5	3	*	*	7	*	*	*	2	*	*	*	3	*	2	3	*
SALAMI, TURKEY see TURKEY																				
SALMON																				
chinook raw 1/2 fillet	356	66	32	25	44	*	*	4	22	4	8	6	47	18	13	5	14	78	98	*
chum raw 1/2 fillet	238	66	12	9	49	*	*	4	24	2	6	6	11	4	*	11	21	69	99	*
pink raw 1/2 fillet	184	53	8	5	28	*	*	4	15	2	7	6	10	4	*	18	6	56	79	*
sockeye raw 1/2 fillet	333	70	26	15	41	*	*	4	22	*	5	7	12	8	*	27	17	57	164	*
Atlantic farmed broiled/baked 1/2 fillet	367	66	34	23	37	*	*	5	19	*	—	5	13	2	11	40	14	72	83	*
raw 1/2 fillet	362	66	33	22	39	*	*	5	20	*	—	5	14	2	13	45	14	74	92	*
wild broiled/baked 1/2 fillet	280	65	19	10	36	*	*	4	28	2	9	8	14	*	*	28	44	78	78	*
raw 1/2 fillet	281	65	19	10	36	*	*	4	28	2	9	8	14	2	*	30	44	78	105	*
chinook broiled/baked 1/2 fillet	356	66	32	25	44	*	*	4	22	4	8	6	47	15	11	5	14	77	73	*
smoked (lox) 3 oz	99	26	6	4	7	*	*	71	4	*	4	2	4	*	*	*	5	20	15	*
chum broiled/baked 1/2 fillet	237	66	11	9	49	*	*	4	24	2	6	6	11	4	*	9	20	66	88	*

Encyclopedia of Daily Values 495

PERCENTAGE DAILY VALUE

	Calories	Protein	Fat	Sat. Fat	Cholesterol	Carbohydrates	Fiber	Sodium	Potassium	Calcium	Iron	Zinc	Magnesium	Vitamin A	Vitamin C	Thiamin	Riboflavin	Niacin	Vitamin B₁₂	Folic acid
SALMON (continued)																				
coho																				
farmed																				
broiled/baked																				
1 fillet	255	58	18	14	30	*	*	3	19	2	3	4	12	6	4	10	10	53	75	*
raw																				
1 fillet	254	56	19	15	27	*	*	3	20	2	3	5	12	6	3	10	10	54	70	*
wild																				
broiled/baked																				
1/2 fillet	247	70	12	10	33	*	*	4	22	*	—	7	15	5	4	9	15	71	148	*
poached/steamed																				
1/2 fillet	285	71	18	13	29	*	*	3	20	7	6	5	14	3	3	12	14	60	115	*
raw																				
1/2 fillet	289	71	18	13	30	*	*	4	24	7	6	5	15	4	3	15	16	72	137	*
pink																				
broiled/baked																				
1/2 fillet	185	53	8	5	28	*	*	4	15	2	7	6	10	3	*	16	5	53	71	*
sockeye																				
baked/broiled																				
1/2 fillet	335	71	26	15	45	*	*	4	17	2	5	5	12	6	*	22	16	52	149	*
SALMON, CANNED																				
chum																				
salted																				
(generic) 1/2 can	261	33	8	7	12	*	*	19	8	23	4	6	7	*	*	*	9	32	135	*
unsalted																				
(generic) 1/2 can	261	33	8	7	12	*	*	3	8	23	4	6	7	*	*	*	9	32	135	*
keta																				
(Libby's) 3 3/4 oz	130	45	9	10	13	*	*	19	10	20	2	4	8	*	*	*	8	30	80	—
pink																				
(Libby's) 3 3/4 oz	150	45	11	10	13	*	*	17	10	20	4	4	8	*	*	*	10	30	60	—
salted																				
(generic) 1/2 can	314	37	11	9	21	*	*	26	11	24	5	7	10	*	*	2	12	37	165	*
unsalted																				
(generic) 1/2 can	314	37	11	9	21	*	*	4	11	24	5	7	10	*	*	2	12	37	166	*
skinless & boneless																				
(Libby's) 3 1/4 oz	110	35	6	5	17	*	*	17	9	*	4	2	6	*	*	*	10	30	60	—
sockeye																				
(Libby's) 3 3/4 oz	150	45	11	10	13	*	*	16	10	25	6	6	8	2	*	*	10	30	75	—
in water																				
(generic) 1/2 can	283	31	10	8	14	*	*	21	10	22	5	6	7	3	*	*	10	25	9	*
unsalted																				
(generic) 1/2 can	283	31	10	8	14	*	*	3	10	22	5	6	7	3	*	*	10	25	9	*
SALMON OIL																				
1 tbsp	123	*	22	14	22	*	*	*	*	*	*	*	*	*	*	*	*	*	*	*
SALSA																				
(generic) 2 tbsp	6	*	*	*	*	*	*	2	*	*	*	*	*	2	5	*	*	*	*	*
chili caliente																				
from mix																				
(Knorr) 2 tbsp	100	*	16	—	6	*	—	6	—	*	*	*	*	*	*	*	*	*	*	*
green chili																				
chunky																				
(Old El Paso) 2 tbsp	3	*	*	*	*	*	*	11	*	*	*	*	*	*	*	*	*	*	*	*
hot																				
(Chi-Chi's) 1 oz	8	2	2	3	*	*	—	6	3	1	1	1	1	1	4	1	1	1	—	—
(Tostitos) 2 tbsp	15	*	*	*	*	*	2	11		—	—	—	—							—
chunky																				
(Hain) 2 tbsp	6	*	*	*	*	*	*	5	2	*	*	*	*	4	4	*	*	*	*	*
(Old El Paso) 2 tbsp	6	*	*	*	*	*	*	7	—	*	*	—	—	4	2	*	8	*	—	—
(Rosarita) 2 tbsp	16	*	*	*	*	*	*	8	*	*	2	—	—	*	11	2	8	3	—	—

	Calories	Protein	Fat	Sat. Fat	Cholesterol	Carbohydrates	Fiber	Sodium	Potassium	Calcium	Iron	Zinc	Magnesium	Vitamin A	Vitamin C	Thiamin	Riboflavin	Niacin	Vitamin B$_{12}$	Folic acid
SALSA (continued)																				
medium																				
(Chi-Chi's) 1 oz	7	2	2	3	*	*	—	6	3	2	1	*	1	1	6	1	1	1	—	—
(Tostitos) 2 tbsp	15	*	*	*	*	*	2	11			—									
chunky																				
(Hain) 2 tbsp	6	*	*	*	*	*	*	4	2	*	*	*	*	6	4	*	*	*	*	*
(Old El Paso) 2 tbsp	6	*	*	*	*	*	*	7	—	*	*	—	—	4	2	*	8	*	—	—
chunky for tacos																				
(Rosarita) 2 tbsp	16	*	*	*	*	*	*	8	*	*	2	—	—	*	10	2	8	3	—	—
mexicana																				
(Del Monte) 2 tbsp	5	*	*	*	*	*	4	8	—	*	—	—	—	6	2	—	—	—	—	—
mild																				
(Tostitos) 2 tbsp	15	*	*	*	*	*	4	10			—									—
chunky																				
(Hain) 2 tbsp	6	2	*	*	*	*	*	4	2	*	*	*	*	4	6	*	*	*	*	*
(Old El Paso) 2 tbsp	6	*	*	*	*	*	*	7	—	*	*	—	—	4	2	*	8	*	—	—
(Rosarita) 2 tbsp	16	*	*	*	*	*	*	9	*	2	*	—	—	*	11	2	12	3	—	—
chunky for tacos																				
(Rosarita) 2 tbsp	16	*	*	*	*	*	*	8	*	*	2	—	—	*	10	2	8	3	—	—
picante																				
hot																				
(Old El Paso) 2 tbsp	10	*	*	*	*	*	*	7	—	*	*	—	—	10	2	*	4	*	—	—
medium																				
(Old El Paso) 2 tbsp	10	*	*	*	*	*	*	7	—	*	*	—	—	10	2	*	4	*	—	—
mild																				
(Old El Paso) 2 tbsp	10	*	*	*	*	*	*	7	—	*	*	—	—	10	2	*	4	*	—	—
salsa																				
mild																				
(Chi-Chi's) 1 oz	7	2	2	3	*	*	—	5	3	2	1	*	1	1	4	1	*	1	—	—
taquera																				
(Del Monte) 2 tbsp	5	*	*	*	*	*	4	9	—	*	*	—	—	8	2	—	—	—	—	—
verde																				
(Del Monte) 2 tbsp	10	*	*	*	*	*	2	12	—	*	4	—	—	*	4	—	—	—	—	—
chunky																				
(Old El Paso) 2 tbsp	10	*	*	*	*	*	4	6	3	*	*	*	*	2	10	*	*	2	*	*
SALSIFY																				
raw																				
1/2 cup slices	55	4	*	*	*	4	8	*	7	4	3	2	4	*	9	4	9	2	*	4
boiled																				
1/2 cup slices	46	3	*	*	*	3	8	*	5	3	2	*	3	*	5	3	7	*	*	3
boiled w/ salt																				
1/2 cup slices	46	3	*	*	*	3	—	7	5	3	2	*	3	*	5	3	7	*	*	3
SALT, TABLE																				
1 tsp	0	*	*	*	*	*	*	97	*	*	*	*	*	*	*	*	*	*	*	*
Kosher																				
(Morton) 1 tsp	0	*	*	*	*	*	—	78	—	*	*	*	*	*	*	*	*	*	*	*
lite																				
(Morton) 1 tsp	0	*	*	*	*	*	—	46	—	*	*	*	*	*	*	*	*	*	*	*
non-iodized																				
(Morton) 1 tsp	0	*	*	*	*	*	—	96	—	*	*	*	*	*	*	*	*	*	*	*
sea																				
(Hain) 1 tsp	0	*	*	*	*	*	—	94	—	*	*	*	*	*	*	*	*	*	*	*
SANDWICH SPREAD																				
(generic) 1 oz	67	4	8	9	4	*	*	12	*	*	*	*	2	*	*	*	3	2	2	5	*
(Oscar Mayer) 1 oz	67	3	7	9	3	*	*	11	*	*	*	*	2	*	*	*	3	2	2	5	*
SARDINE																				
in mustard sauce																				
(Underwood) 3 3/4 oz	220	27	25	—	—	*	*	27	7	25	10	—	—	6	*	*	8	20	—	—

	Calories	Protein	Fat	Sat. Fat	Cholesterol	Carbohydrates	Fiber	Sodium	Potassium	Calcium	Iron	Zinc	Magnesium	Vitamin A	Vitamin C	Thiamin	Riboflavin	Niacin	Vitamin B12	Folic acid
SARDINE (continued)																				
in oil																				
(generic) 1/2 can	96	9	4	2	11	*	*	5	3	20	4	2	2	*	*	*	3	6	68	*
(Underwood) 3 3/4 oz	230	27	28	—	—	*	*	17	6	25	10	—	—	4	*	*	8	20	—	—
in tomato sauce																				
(Del Monte) 1 fish	50	8	4	5	8	*	3	5	—	8	10	—	—	*	15	—	—	—	—	—
(generic) 1/2 can	329	25	17	15	19	*	4	16	9	22	12	9	8	7	2	3	13	19	276	*
(Underwood) 3 3/4 oz	220	27	25	—	—	*	*	21	8	25	10	—	—	6	*	*	8	20	—	—
SARDINE OIL																				
1 tbsp	123	*	22	21	32	*	*	*	*	*	*	*	*	*	*	*	*	*	*	*
SAUERKRAUT																				
(Bush Bros) 1/2 cup	30	2	*	*	*	2	8	32	—	4	6	—	—	4	15	—	—	—	—	—
(Del Monte) 1/2 cup	15	2	*	*	*	2	8	30	—	*	2	—	—	*	30	—	—	—	—	—
Bavarian																				
(Bush Bros) 1/2 cup	60	2	*	*	*	5	12	20	—	4	4	—	—	*	15	—	—	—	—	—
old fashioned																				
(Vlasic) 1 oz	4	*	*	*	*	*	*	12	—	2	2	—	—	*	4	*	*	*	—	—
solid & liquid																				
1/2 cup	22	2	*	*	*	2	12	32	6	4	10	*	4	*	29	2	2	*	*	7
SAUERKRAUT JUICE																				
(Bush Bros) 8 fl oz	14	3	*	*	*	*	*	69	—	6	15	—	—	*	*	—	—	—	—	—
SAUSAGE																				
raw																				
pork																				
(generic) 2 4" links	108	5	16	19	6	*	*	7	2	*	3	*	*	*	*	9	3	4	5	*
beef smokie links																				
(Oscar Mayer) 1 slice	123	9	17	23		*	*	18	2	*	4	9	2	*	*	—	—	—	—	
cheese smokies																				
(Oscar Mayer) 1 slice	129	9	18	22	10	*	*	19	2	2	3	6	2	*	*	—	—	—	—	
chicken																				
smoked																				
(Bryan) 1 oz	90	5	12	—	7	*	*	12								—	—	—	—	
cocktail																				
beef																				
(Bryan) 1 oz	90	7	12	—	7	*	*	12								—	—	—	—	
regular																				
(Bryan) 1 oz	90	7	12	—	7	*	*	12								—	—	—	—	
cooked																				
pork																				
(generic) 2 4" links	96	9	12	14	7	*	*	14	3	*	2	4	*	*	*	13	4	6	7	*
pork & beef																				
(generic) 2 4" links	103	6	14	17	6	*	*	9	*	*	2	3	*	*	*	6	2	4	2	*
smoked																				
(generic) 3 oz	265	20	35	49	19	*	*	40	4	*	8	16	3	*	17	3	7	14	26	*
links																				
(Jimmy Dean) 2 links	180	12	26	—	—	*	*	16	—	*	4	—	—	*	*	10	6	10	—	—
little smokies																				
(Oscar Mayer) 1 slice	27	2	4	5	2	*	*	4	*	*	*	*	*	*	*	—	—	—	—	
New England																				
(generic) 1 1 oz slice	46	8	3	4	5	*	*	14	3	*	*	5	*	*	10	12	4	5	6	*
(Oscar Mayer) 1 slice	28	6	2	3	4	*	*	12	2	*	*	4	*	*	*	—	—	—	—	
patty																				
extra mild																				
(Jimmy Dean) 1 oz slice	140	8	20	—	—	*	*	12	—	*	2	—	—	*	*	8	4	8	—	—
pork																				
(Jimmy Dean) 1 oz slice	120	7	17	—	—	*	*	10	—	*	2	—	—	*	*	6	4	6	—	—
hot																				
(Jimmy Dean) 1 oz slice	120	7	17	—	—	*	*	10	—	*	2	—	—	*	*	6	4	6	—	—

	Calories	Protein	Fat	Sat. Fat	Cholesterol	Carbohydrates	Fiber	Sodium	Potassium	Calcium	Iron	Zinc	Magnesium	Vitamin A	Vitamin C	Thiamin	Riboflavin	Niacin	Vitamin B$_{12}$	Folic acid
SAUSAGE (continued)																				
w/ sage (Jimmy Dean) 1 oz slice	120	7	17	—		*	*	10	—	*	2			*	*	6	4	6	—	—
patty, ready made (Jimmy Dean) 1 patty	140	8	20	—		*	*	12	—	*	2			*	*	8	4	8	—	—
Polish pork (generic) 1 oz	92	7	12	15	7	*	*	10	2	*	4			*	*	9	2	5	5	*
pork (Hormel Little Sizzlers) 1 oz	130	5	20	25	6	*	*	8	2	*	1	2	1	*	*	6	2	4	—	—
links (Oscar Mayer) 1 slice	85	7	11	13	7	*	*	9	2	*	2	4	*	*	*	—	—	—	—	—
patties (Oscar Mayer) 1 slice	143	9	21	24	9	*	*	12	2	*	3	5	*	*	*	—	—	—	—	—
precooked (Oscar Mayer) 1 slice	84	6	12	14	5	*	*	7	*	*	2	3	*	*	*	—	—	—	—	—
smoked (generic) 1 link	265	25	33	39	15	*	*	42	6	2	4	13	3	*	2	32	10	15	18	*
pork & beef smoked (generic) 1 link	228	15	32	36	16	*	*	27	4	*	5	10	2	*	22	12	7	11	17	*
smoked (Bryan) 1 oz	90	5	12	—	7	*	*	12	—	—	—	—	—	—	—	—	—	—	—	—
(Oscar Mayer) 1 slice	82	6	11	14	6	*	*	12	*	*	3	4	*	*	*	—	—	—	—	—
beef (Bryan) 1 oz	80	7	11	—	7	*	*	12	—	—	—	—	—	—	—	—	—	—	—	—
bun size beef (Bryan) 2 oz	180	12	25	—	13	*	*	25	—	—	—	—	—	—	—	—	—	—	—	—
regular (Bryan) 2 oz	180	12	25	—	13	*	*	25	—	—	—	—	—	—	—	—	—	—	—	—
traditional (Bryan) 1 oz	80	7	11	—	7	*	*	12	—	—	—	—	—	—	—	—	—	—	—	—
smokies (Oscar Mayer) 1 slice	129	9	18	20	9	*	*	18	2	*	3	6	2	*	*	—	—	—	—	—
smoky hollow (Bryan) 1 oz	90	5	12	—	7	*	*	12	—	—	—	—	—	—	—	—	—	—	—	—
sweet morsel smoked (Oscar Mayer) 1 slice	70	6	9	12	6	*	*	11	*	*	3	5	*	*	*	5	4	3	5	—
SAUSAGE, MEATLESS (generic) 1 link	64	8	7	4	*	*	4	9	2	2	5	2	2	3	*	39	6	14	*	2
(generic) 1 patty	97	12	11	6	*	*	4	14	3	2	8	4	3	5	*	59	9	21	*	2
SAVORY, GROUND 1 tbsp	12	*	*	*	*	*	—	*	*	9	9	*	4	5	—	*	11	*	—	—
SCALLION (see ONION, SPRING)																				
SCALLOP *raw* 1 large or 5 small	26	8	*	*	3	*	*	2	3	*	*	2	4	*	*	*	*	2	8	*
breaded & fried 2 large scallops	67	9	5	4	6	*	—	6	3	*	*	2	5	*	*	*	2	2	7	*
frozen fried (Mrs. Paul's) 3 1/2 oz	160	20	11	15	3	6	*	13	—	2	*	—	—	*	*	*	4	4	—	—
SCALLOP, IMITATION see SURIMI																				
SCALLOPED SQUASH see SQUASH																				
SCREWDRIVER 1 cocktail (7 fl oz)	175	2	*	*	*	6	—	*	9	*	*	*	4	3	*	9	2	2	*	19
SCUP *raw* 1 fillet	67	20	3	2	11	*	*	*	5	3	2	2	4	*	*	5	4	13	15	*

	Calories	Protein	Fat	Sat. Fat	Cholesterol	Carbohydrates	Fiber	Sodium	Potassium	Calcium	Iron	Zinc	Magnesium	Vitamin A	Vitamin C	Thiamin	Riboflavin	Niacin	Vitamin B12	Folic acid
SCUP (continued)																				
broiled/baked 1 fillet	68	20	3	—	11	*	*	*	5	3	2	2	4	*	*	4	4	12	13	*
SEAFOOD see specific listings																				
SEAWEED																				
agar raw 3 oz	22	*	*	*	*	2	*	*	5	5	9	3	14	*	*	*	*	*	*	18
Irish moss raw 3 oz	42	2	*	*	*	3	4	2	2	6	42	11	31	2	—	*	23	3	*	39
kelp raw 3 oz	37	2	*	*	*	3	4	8	2	14	13	7	26	2	—	3	7	2	*	38
laver raw 3 oz	30	8	*	*	*	*	*	2	9	6	8	6	*	88	55	6	22	6	*	31
spirulina raw 3 oz	22	8	*	*	*	*	—	3	3	*	13	*	4	*	*	13	17	5	*	2
wakame raw 3 oz	38	4	*	*	*	3	*	31	*	13	10	2	23	6	4	3	11	7	*	42
agar dried 3 oz	260	9	*	*	*	23	28	4	27	53	101	33	164	*	*	*	11	*	*	124
spirulina dried 3 oz	247	81	10	12	*	7	12	37	33	10	134	11	41	10	14	135	183	54	*	20
SESAME BUTTER PASTE 1 oz	169	9	22	10	*	2	8	*	5	27	30	14	26	*	*	5	3	10	*	7
SESAME CRUNCH 20 pieces	181	7	18	8	*	6	12	*	4	25	8	9	22	*	*	13	4	6	*	6
SESAME FLOUR *high-fat* 1 oz	149	15	16	8	*	3	—	*	3	5	24	20	26	*	*	51	5	19	*	2
low-fat 1 oz	95	24	*	*	*	3	—	*	3	4	22	19	24	*	*	48	4	18	*	2
partially defatted 1 oz	108	19	5	3	*	3	—	*	3	4	23	20	26	*	*	48	5	18	*	2
SESAME KERNEL *toasted* 1 oz	161	8	21	10	*	2	20	*	3	4	12	19	25	*	*	23	8	8	*	7
toasted, salted 1 oz	161	8	21	10	*	2	20	7	3	4	12	19	25	*	*	23	8	8	*	7
SESAME MEAL *partially defatted* 1 oz	161	8	21	10	*	2	—	*	3	4	23	19	25	*	*	49	5	18	*	2
SESAME OIL 1 tbsp	120	*	22	10	*	*	*	*	*	*	*	*	*	*	*	*	*	*	*	*
SESAME SEED *dried* 1 tbsp	52	3	7	3	*	*	4	*	*	9	7	5	8	*	*	5	*	2	*	2
roasted 1 oz	160	8	21	10	*	2	16	*	4	28	23	14	25	*	*	15	4	7	*	7
SESAME STICK *salted* 2 oz	307	10	32	19	*	9	8	35	3	10	2	4	6	*	*	5	2	4	*	3
unsalted 2 oz	307	10	32	19	*	9	—	*	3	10	2	4	6	*	*	5	2	4	*	3

	Calories	Protein	Fat	Sat. Fat	Cholesterol	Carbohydrates	Fiber	Sodium	Potassium	Calcium	Iron	Zinc	Magnesium	Vitamin A	Vitamin C	Thiamin	Riboflavin	Niacin	Vitamin B₁₂	Folic acid
SESBANIA FLOWER																				
raw 1/2 cup	3	*	*	*	*	*	—	*	*	*	—	*	*	*	12	*	*	*	*	3
steamed 1/2 cup	11	*	*	*	*	*	—	*	2	*	2	—	2	*	32	2	*	*	*	7
w/ salt 1/2 cup	11	*	*	*	*	*	—	5	2	*	2	—	2	*	32	2	*	*	*	7
SHAD, AMERICAN																				
raw 1 fillet	362	52	39	41	46	*	*	4	20	9	10	5	14	4	*	18	26	77	5	*
broiled/baked 1 fillet	363	52	39	—	46	*	*	4	20	9	10	5	14	3	*	18	26	78	3	*
SHALLOT																				
raw 3 oz	61	4	*	*	*	5	—	*	8	3	6	2	4	212	11	3	*	*	*	7
freeze-dried 1 tbsp	3	*	*	*	*	*	—	*	*	*	*	*	*	*	11	*	*	*	*	*
SHARK																				
raw 3 oz	111	30	6	4	14	*	*	3	4	3	4	2	10	4	*	2	3	12	21	*
battered & fried 3 oz	194	26	18	14	17	2	*	4	4	4	5	3	9	3	*	4	5	12	17	*
SHEEPSHEAD																				
raw 1 fillet	257	80	9	7	40	*	*	7	27	5	6	6	19	5	*	2	6	18	79	*
baked/broiled 1 fillet	234	81	5	4	40	*	*	6	27	7	7	8	16	4	*	*	5	17	71	*
SHERBET BAR																				
orange (generic) 1 bar	91	*	2	4	*	7	—	*	2	4	*	2	*	*	5	*	3	*	*	*
SHERBET (see also SORBET)																				
orange (generic) 1/2 cup	132	2	3	6	2	10	—	2	3	5	*	3	2	*	7	2	4	*	2	*
SHORTENING																				
all-purpose (Crisco) 1 tbsp	110	*	18	15	*	*	*	*	*	*	*	*	*	*	*	*	*	*	*	*
(generic) 1 tbsp	113	*	22	20	*	*	*	*	*	*	*	*	*	*	*	*	*	*	*	*
(Wesson) 1 tbsp	100	*	18	20	*	*	*	*	*	*	*	*	*	*	*	*	*	*	*	*
lard & vegetable oil (generic) 1 tbsp	115	*	22	26	2	*	*	*	*	*	*	*	*	*	*	*	*	*	*	*
soy & cottonseed (generic) 1 tbsp	113	*	20	20	*	*	*	*	*	*	*	*	*	*	*	*	*	*	*	*
baking (generic) 1 tbsp	113	*	22	19	*	*	*	*	*	*	*	*	*	*	*	*	*	*	*	*
butter flavor (Crisco) 1 tbsp	110	*	18	15	*	*	*	*	*	*	*	*	*	4	*	*	*	*	*	*
cake soybean (generic) 1 tbsp	113	*	22	18	*	*	*	*	*	*	*	*	*	*	*	*	*	*	*	*
cake & icing (generic) 1 tbsp	113	*	22	13	*	*	*	*	*	*	*	*	*	*	*	*	*	*	*	*
confectionery coconut & palm oil (generic) 1 tbsp	113	*	20	59	*	*	*	*	*	*	*	*	*	*	*	*	*	*	*	*
frying heavy beef tallow & cottonseed oil (generic) 1 tbsp	115	*	315	29	4	*	*	*	*	*	*	*	*	*	*	*	*	*	*	*
palm oil (generic) 1 tbsp	113	*	20	31	*	*	*	*	*	*	*	*	*	*	*	*	*	*	*	*

	Calories	Protein	Fat	Sat. Fat	Cholesterol	Carbohydrates	Fiber	Sodium	Potassium	Calcium	Iron	Zinc	Magnesium	Vitamin A	Vitamin C	Thiamin	Riboflavin	Niacin	Vitamin B₁₂	Folic acid
SHORTENING (continued)																				
regular																				
soy & cottonseed oil																				
(generic) 1 tbsp	113	*	20	10	*	*	*	*	*	*	*	*	*	*	*	*	*	*	*	*
SHRIMP																				
raw																				
4 large shrimp	30	9	*	*	14	*	*	2	*	*	4	2	3	*	*	*	*	4	5	*
breaded & fried																				
4 large shrimp	73	11	6	3	18	*	*	4	2	2	2	3	3	*	*	3	2	5	9	*
steamed/poached																				
4 large shrimp	22	8	*	*	14	*	*	2	*	*	4	2	2	*	*	*	*	3	5	*
SHRIMP, CANNED																				
1/2 cup	77	12	*	*	18	*	*	2	2	2	5	3	3	*	*	*	*	4	12	*
SHRIMP, FROZEN																				
breaded																				
butter flavored																				
(Mrs. Paul's) 5 1/2 oz	320	45	23	10	42	9	*	33	—	8	6	—	—	*	*	15	10	15	—	—
Cajun popcorn style																				
(Gorton's) 1/3 package	220	10	20	6	20	6	*	24	—	6	8	—	—	*	*	4	6	2	—	—
garlic & herb																				
(Mrs. Paul's) 5 1/2 oz	250	40	22	10	43	4	*	40	—	10	8	—	—	*	*	15	10	15	—	—
microwave																				
(Gorton's) 1/2 package	150	10	12	5	8	5	*	15	—	2	2	—	—	*	*	2	2	*	—	—
Oriental seasoning																				
(Gorton's) 5 shrimp	170	10	14	10	18	5	*	17	—	10	2	—	—	*	*	2	4	2	—	—
original seasoning																				
(Gorton's) 5 shrimp	210	10	20	10	22	6	*	16	—	10	2	—	—	*	*	4	4	4	—	—
scampi seasoning																				
(Gorton's) 5 shrimp	240	10	23	15	22	6	*	17	—	10	2	—	—	*	*	2	4	2	—	—
special recipe																				
(Mrs. Paul's) 5 1/2 oz	300	45	15	10	40	11	*	35	—	10	8	—	—	*	*	15	10	15	—	—
SHRIMP, IMITATION see SURIMI																				
SHRIMP DINNER, FROZEN																				
Creole																				
(Armour Classics Lite) 11 1/4 oz	260	10	3	—	15	18	—	37	12	4	15	—	—	6	190	10	8	6	—	—
marinara																				
(Healthy Choice) 10 1/2 oz	260	17	2	3	20	17	—	13	11	6	15	—	—	15	190	15	8	6	—	—
SHRIMP ENTREE, FROZEN																				
marinara																				
(Weight Watchers) 8 oz	150	13	2	*	8	9	12	17	11	8	10	—	—	8	10	—	—	—	—	—
SISYMBRIUM SEED																				
dried																				
(generic) 1 oz	90	6	2	*	*	5	—	*	17	46	*	*	22	*	15	4	7	24	*	7
SLOPPY JOE, CANNED																				
(Hormel Not-so-Sloppy Joe)																				
2 1/4 oz	70	2	2	*	2	5	—	30	—	2	2	—	—	4	2	2	2	2	—	—
(Manwich)																				
1 sandwich prepared	310	28	20	24	17	10	4	26	15	4	20	—	—	*	3	10	15	20	—	—
extra thick & chunky																				
(Manwich)																				
1 sandwich prepared	330	28	20	24	17	12	12	36	17	4	20	—	—	*	4	25	20	25	—	—
Mexican																				
(Manwich)																				
1 sandwich prepared	310	28	20	24	17	10	8	29	15	6	20	—	—	*	3	10	10	20	—	—
SLOPPY JOE, FROM MIX																				
(Manwich)																				
1 sandwich prepared	320	28	20	24	17	10	8	25	17	4	20	—	—	*	3	15	10	25	—	—
bake																				
(Hamburger Helper) 1 cup	340	30	23	—		11	—	46	11	10	15	—	—	2	*	20	15	20	—	—

	Calories	Protein	Fat	Sat. Fat	Cholesterol	Carbohydrates	Fiber	Sodium	Potassium	Calcium	Iron	Zinc	Magnesium	Vitamin A	Vitamin C	Thiamin	Riboflavin	Niacin	Vitamin B12	Folic acid
SLOPPY JOE, FROZEN																				
sandwich (Swanson Kids') 7 2/3 oz	260	15	12	—	—	—	—	22	—	4	10	—	—	6	20	6	8	8	—	—
SLOPPY JOE SAUCE																				
(Del Monte) 1/4 cup	70	2	*	*	*	5	*	29	—	2	6	—	—	35	20	—	—	—	—	—
(Libby's) 1/4 cup	45	2	*	*	*	3	4	18	—	2	2	—	—	6	10	—	—	—	—	—
SMELT, RAINBOW																				
raw 3 oz	82	25	3	2	20	*	*	2	7	5	4	9	6	*	*	*	6	6	49	*
baked/broiled 3 oz	105	32	4	3	25	*	*	3	9	7	5	12	8	*	*	*	7	8	56	*
SNACKS (see also specific snack)																				
barbecue curls (Weight Watchers) 1 bag (1/2 oz)	60	2	2	*	*	4	4	5	*	*	*	—	—	*	*	*	—	—	—	—
cheese & crackers (Handi-Snacks) 1 package	120	8	12	25	7	3	*	15	2	8	*	—	—	4	*	*	6	*	—	—
w/ bacon (Handi-Snacks) 1 package	130	10	14	20	7	3	*	17	*	10	*	—	—	6	*	*	4	*	—	—
w/ peanut butter (Handi-Snacks) 1 package	190	15	22	20	*	4	*	7	4	*	*	—	—	*	*	*	2	*	—	—
Chex mix																				
barbecue (Ralston) 1 oz	130	4	8	—	*	6	—	16	—	*	20	2	2	*	10	20	4	20	15	15
cheddar (Ralston) 1 oz	130	4	8	—	*	6	—	12	—	*	20	2	2	*	10	20	4	20	15	15
sour cream & onion (Ralston) 1 oz	130	4	8	—	*	6	—	12	—	*	20	2	2	*	10	20	4	20	15	15
traditional (Ralston) 1 oz	120	4	8	—	*	6	—	13	—	*	25	2	4	*	10	20	4	20	15	15
Combos																				
cheddar & pretzel (Combos) 10 nuggets	143	5	9	—	*	6	—	14	*	6	5	*	2	*	*	2	10	5	*	*
other varieties (Combos) 1 bag	240	8	15	—	*	11	—	26	—	10	6	—	—	*	*	2	15	6	—	—
corn cones																				
nacho flavor (generic) 2 oz	303	6	27	76	*	10	—	22	2	*	4	4	4	*	4	4	8	4	4	*
cheese flavored corn puffs																				
(generic) 6 oz bag	314	7	30	19	*	10	—	25	3	3	3	1	3	3	—	10	7	3	1	17
cracker sandwich																				
cheese peanut butter (Nab) 4 (1 oz)	130	5	11	5	*	5	—	13	2	*	4	—	—	*	*	*	6	6	—	—
peanut butter toast (Nab) 4 (1 oz)	130	5	11	5	*	5	—	12	2	*	4	—	—	*	*	*	4	6	—	—
cracker snacks																				
hot (Frito-Lay) 1 pkg	200	7	14	10	*	9	4	20	—	—	—	—	—	—	—	—	—	—	—	—
original (Frito-Lay) 1 pkg	220	7	18	13	*	8	2	21	—	—	—	—	—	—	—	—	—	—	—	—
crisps																				
cinnamon raisin swirl (Pepperidge Farm) 1 oz	140	4	6	*	*	6	*	7	*	*	*	—	—	*	*	8	4	4	—	—
Crunch Taters																				
jalapeño (Frito-Lay) 1 oz	140	2	12	10	*	5	4	6	—	—	—	—	—							—
mesquite (Frito-Lay) 1 oz	140	3	12	10	*	5	4	5												
Flutters																				
butter (Pepperidge Farm) 1 oz	133	3	8	5	2	6	—	8	*	*	*	—	—	*	*	3	*	*	—	—

	Calories	Protein	Fat	Sat. Fat	Cholesterol	Carbohydrates	Fiber	Sodium	Potassium	Calcium	Iron	Zinc	Magnesium	Vitamin A	Vitamin C	Thiamin	Riboflavin	Niacin	Vitamin B_{12}	Folic acid
SNACKS (continued)																				
garden herb (Pepperidge Farm) 1 oz	133	3	8	5	*	6	—	10	*	*	*	—	—	*	*	3	3	*	—	—
sesame (Pepperidge Farm) 1 oz	146	5	11	5	*	6	—	8	*	*	*	—	—	*	*	*	*	*	—	—
toasted wheat (Pepperidge Farm) 1 oz	146	3	11	5	*	6	—	9	*	*	*	—	—	*	*	*	*	*	—	—
Funyuns (Frito-Lay) 1 oz	140	3	11	8	*	6	2	10	—	—	—	—	—	—	—	—	—	—	—	—
mixed grain cheddar (Sunchips) 1 oz	140	3	11	5	*	6	8	7	—	—	—	—	—	—	—	—	—	—	—	—
French onion (Sunchips) 1 oz	140	3	11	5	*	6	8	5	—	—	—	—	—	—	—	—	—	—	—	—
plain (Sunchips) 1 oz	140	3	11	5	*	6	8	7	—	—	—	—	—	—	—	—	—	—	—	—
Munchos (Frito-Lay) 1 oz	150	2	15	13	*	5	4	11	—	—	—	—	—	—	—	—	—	—	—	—
Oriental mix (generic) 2 oz	309	19	36	51	*	6	28	20	8	4	9	17	20	*	*	11	5	30	*	12
pizza curls (Weight Watchers) 1 bag (1/2 oz)	60	2	3	*	*	4	4	5	*	*	*	—	—	*	*	*	*	*	—	—
ranch curls (Weight Watchers) 1 bag (1/2 oz)	60	2	3	*	*	3	4	7	*	*	*	—	—	*	*	*	*	*	—	—
snack mix (Frito-Lay) 1 oz	140	3	12	8	*	6	4	10	—	—	—	—	—	—	—	—	—	—	—	—
cheese (Ritz) 1 oz	130	3	9	5	*	6	—	15	2	4	10	—	—	*	*	6	6	8	—	—
nutty (Pepperidge Farm) 1 oz	150	*	12	10	*	5	8	7	—	6	6	—	—	*	*	8	4	6	—	—
original (Doo Dads) 1 oz	130	5	9	*	*	6	—	15	2	2	6	—	—	*	*	6	4	8	—	—
spicy (Pepperidge Farm) 1 oz	140	*	12	10	*	5	4	14	—	4	*	—	—	*	*	4	4	4	—	—
traditional (Ritz) 1 oz	130	3	9	5	*	6	—	12	2	2	10	—	—	*	*	6	6	8	—	—
zesty herb (Pepperidge Farm) 1 oz	150	*	14	5	*	5	4	10	—	8	6	—	—	*	*	10	4	8	—	—
trail mix chocolate chip (generic) 1/4 cup	177	9	18	11	*	6	—	2	7	4	7	8	15	*	*	10	5	8	*	6
regular (generic) 1/4 cup	174	8	17	11	*	6	—	4	8	3	6	8	15	*	*	11	4	9	*	6
Sierra (Del Monte Snap-E-Tom) 1/4 cup	150	7	12	12	*	5	9	3	—	4	4			*	6	—	—	—	—	—
tropical (generic) 1/4 cup	143	4	9	15	*	8	—	*	7	2	5	3	9	*	5	11	2	3	*	4
unsalted (generic) 1/4 cup	173	17	17	10	*	6	—	8	3	6	8	15		*	*	12	4	9	*	7
SNAP BEAN see GREEN BEAN																				
SNAPPER																				
raw 1 fillet	218	74	4	3	27	*	*	6	26	7	2	5	17	4	6	7	*	3	109	*
baked/broiled 1 fillet	218	74	4	3	27	*	*	4	25	7	2	5	16	4	5	6	*	3	99	*
SOFT DRINK																				
7Up diet 12 fl oz	2	*	*	*	*	*	*	*	*	*	*	*	*	*	*	*	*	*	*	*

SOFT DRINK (continued)

	Calories	Protein	Fat	Sat. Fat	Cholesterol	Carbohydrates	Fiber	Sodium	Potassium	Calcium	Iron	Zinc	Magnesium	Vitamin A	Vitamin C	Thiamin	Riboflavin	Niacin	Vitamin B$_{12}$	Folic acid
regular 12 fl oz	156	*	*	*	*	12	*	*	*	*	*	*	*	*	*	*	*	*	*	*
cherry diet 12 fl oz	2	*	*	*	*	*	*	*	*	*	*	*	*	*	*	*	*	*	*	*
regular 12 fl oz	156	*	*	*	*	13	*	*	*	*	*	*	*	*	*	*	*	*	*	*
apple (Welch's) 12 fl oz	200	*	*	*	*	19	*	*	*	*	*	*	*	*	*	*	*	*	*	*
birch beer (Canada Dry) 8 fl oz	110	*	*	*	*	9	*	2	*	*	*	*	*	*	*	*	*	*	*	*
bitter lemon (Schweppes) 8 fl oz	110	*	*	*	*	9	*	2	*	*	*	*	*	*	*	*	*	*	*	*
black cherry wishniak (Canada Dry) 8 fl oz	130	*	*	*	*	11	*	2	*	*	*	*	*	*	*	*	*	*	*	*
cactus cooler (Sunkist) 8 fl oz	110	*	*	*	*	9	*	2	*	*	*	*	*	*	*	*	*	*	*	*
cherry (Sunkist) 8 fl oz	140	*	*	*	*	12	*	*	*	*	*	*	*	*	*	*	*	*	*	*
citrus diet (Sunkist) 8 fl oz	0	*	*	*	*	*	*	4	*	*	*	*	*	*	*	*	*	*	*	*
club soda (generic) 5 1/2 fl oz can	0	*	*	*	*	*	*	*	*	*	*	*	*	*	*	*	*	*	*	*
regular (Schweppes) 8 fl oz	0	*	*	*	*	*	*	3	*	*	*	*	*	*	*	*	*	*	*	*
sodium free (seltzer) (Schweppes) 8 fl oz	0	*	*	*	*	*	*	*	*	*	*	*	*	*	*	*	*	*	*	*
Coca-cola 12 fl oz	140	*	*	*	*	13	*	2	*	*	*	*	*	*	*	*	*	*	*	*
diet 12 fl oz	*	*	*	*	*	*	*	2	*	*	*	*	*	*	*	*	*	*	*	*
cola (generic) 12 fl oz can	146	*	*	*	*	12	*	*	*	*	*	*	*	*	*	*	*	*	*	*
diet (Tab) 12 fl oz	*	*	*	*	*	*	*	2	*	*	*	*	*	*	*	*	*	*	*	*
low-calorie sweetened w/ aspartame (generic) 12 fl oz can	4	*	*	*	*	*	*	*	*	*	*	2	*	*	*	*	*	5	*	*
sweetened w/ saccharine (generic) 12 fl oz can	0	*	*	*	*	*	*	2	*	*	*	*	*	*	*	*	*	*	*	*
collins mixer (Schweppes) 8 fl oz	100	*	*	*	*	8	*	2	*	*	*	*	*	*	*	*	*	*	*	*
cream soda (Canada Dry) 8 fl oz	120	*	*	*	*	10	*	2	*	*	*	*	*	*	*	*	*	*	*	*
(generic) 12 fl oz can	181	*	*	*	*	16	*	2	*	2	*	2	*	*	*	*	*	*	*	*
(Hires) 8 fl oz	0	*	*	*	*	11	*	*	*	*	*	*	*	*	*	*	*	*	*	*
(IBC) 12 fl oz	180	*	*	*	*	14	*	*	*	*	*	*	*	*	*	*	*	*	*	*
diet (Hires) 8 fl oz	0	*	*	*	*	*	*	*	*	*	*	*	*	*	*	*	*	*	*	*
Dr. Pepper diet 12 fl oz	2	*	*	*	*	*	*	*	*	*	*	*	*	*	*	*	*	*	*	*
regular 12 fl oz	156	*	*	*	*	13	*	*	*	*	*	*	*	*	*	*	*	*	*	*
caffeine-free diet 12 fl oz	2	*	*	*	*	*	*	*	*	*	*	*	*	*	*	*	*	*	*	*
regular 12 fl oz	156	*	*	*	*	13	*	*	*	*	*	*	*	*	*	*	*	*	*	*

	Calories	Protein	Fat	Sat. Fat	Cholesterol	Carbohydrates	Fiber	Sodium	Potassium	Calcium	Iron	Zinc	Magnesium	Vitamin A	Vitamin C	Thiamin	Riboflavin	Niacin	Vitamin B12	Folic acid
SOFT DRINK (continued)																				
ginger ale																				
(generic) 12 fl oz can	126	*	*	*	*	11	*	*	*	4		*	*	*	*	*	*	*	*	*
ginger ale																				
diet																				
(Canada Dry) 8 fl oz	0	*	*	*	*	*	*	2	*	*	*	*	*	*	*	*	*	*	*	*
(Schweppes) 8 fl oz	0	*	*	*	*	*	*	3	*	*	*	*	*	*	*	*	*	*	*	*
regular																				
(Canada Dry) 8 fl oz	100	*	*	*	*	8	*	*	*	*	*	*	*	*	*	*	*	*	*	*
(Schweppes) 8 fl oz	90	*	*	*	*	7	*	2	*	*	*	*	*	*	*	*	*	*	*	*
ginger beer																				
(Schweppes) 8 fl oz	100	*	*	*	*	8	*	4	*	*	*	*	*	*	*	*	*	*	*	*
grape																				
(generic) 12 fl oz can	157	*	*	*	*	14	*	2	*	*	2	2	*	*	*	*	*	*	*	*
(Schweppes) 8 fl oz	130	*	*	*	*	11	*	2	*	*	*	*	*	*	*	*	*	*	*	*
(Welch's) 12 fl oz	200	*	*	*	*	17	*	2	*	*	*	*	*	*	*	*	*	*	*	*
grapefruit																				
(Schweppes) 8 fl oz	110	*	*	*	*	9	*	3	*	*	*	*	*	*	*	*	*	*	*	*
lemon sour																				
(Schweppes) 8 fl oz	110	*	*	*	*	9	*	*	*	*	*	*	*	*	*	*	*	*	*	*
lemon-lime																				
(Fresca) 12 fl oz	*	*	*	*	*	*	*	*	*	*	*	*	*	*	*	*	*	*	*	*
(generic) 12 fl oz can	149	*	*	*	*	13	*	2	*	*	*	*	*	*	*	*	*	*	*	*
(Schweppes) 8 fl oz	100	*	*	*	*	8	*	3	*	*	*	*	*	*	*	*	*	*	*	*
malt drink																				
(generic) 8 fl oz	22	*	*	*	*	*	*	*	*	2	*	*	6	*	*	*	4	6	*	4
(Malta India) 12 fl oz	250	2	*	*	*	12	*	1	*	*	*	*	*	*	*	*	*	*	*	*
mocha																				
diet																				
(Hires) 8 fl oz	5	*	*	*	*	*	*	2	*	*	*	*	*	*	*	*	*	*	*	*
regular																				
(Hires) 8 fl oz	100	*	*	*	*	8	*	2	*	*	*	*	*	*	*	*	*	*	*	*
orange																				
(generic) 12 fl oz can	177	*	*	*	*	15	*	2	*	2	*	2	*	*	*	*	*	*	*	*
(Welch's) 12 fl oz	200	*	*	*	*	17	*	*	*	*	*	*	*	*	*	*	*	*	*	*
diet																				
(Sunkist) 8 fl oz	5	*	*	*	*	*	*	3	*	*	*	*	*	*	*	*	*	*	*	*
regular																				
(Sunkist) 8 fl oz	140	*	*	*	*	12	*	2	*	*	*	*	*	*	*	*	*	*	*	*
peach																				
(Sunkist) 8 fl oz	120	*	*	*	*	10	*	2	*	*	*	*	*	*	*	*	*	*	*	*
(Welch's) 12 fl oz	220	*	*	*	*	17	*	*	*	*	*	*	*	*	*	*	*	*	*	*
pepper type																				
(generic) 12 fl oz can	153	*	*	*	*	13	*	2	*	*	*	*	*	*	*	*	*	*	*	*
Pepsi-cola																				
diet																				
8 fl oz	0	*	*	*	*	12	*	*	*	*	*	*	*	*	*	*	*	*	*	*
regular																				
8 fl oz	150	*	*	*	*	12	*	*	*	*	*	*	*	*	*	*	*	*	*	*
pineapple																				
(Sunkist) 8 fl oz	140	*	*	*	*	12	*	*	*	*	*	*	*	*	*	*	*	*	*	*
(Welch's) 12 fl oz	210	*	*	*	*	18	*	2	*	*	*	*	*	*	*	*	*	*	*	*
raspberry ginger ale																				
diet																				
(Schweppes) 8 fl oz	0	*	*	*	*	*	*	3	*	*	*	*	*	*	*	*	*	*	*	*
regular																				
(Schweppes) 8 fl oz	100	*	*	*	*	9	*	2	*	*	*	*	*	*	*	*	*	*	*	*
root beer																				
(Barrelhead) 8 fl oz	110	*	*	*	*	9	*	*	*	*	*	*	*	*	*	*	*	*	*	*

	Calories	Protein	Fat	Sat. Fat	Cholesterol	Carbohydrates	Fiber	Sodium	Potassium	Calcium	Iron	Zinc	Magnesium	Vitamin A	Vitamin C	Thiamin	Riboflavin	Niacin	Vitamin B₁₂	Folic acid
SOFT DRINK (continued)																				
(generic) 12 fl oz can	150	*	*	*	*	13	*	2	*	2	*	2	*	*	*	*	*	*	*	*
(IBC) 12 fl oz	168	*	*	*	*	14	*	*	*	*	*	*	*	*	*	*	*	*	*	*
diet																				
(Hires) 8 fl oz	0	*	*	*	*	*	*	3	*	*	*	*	*	*	*	*	*	*	*	*
(IBC) 12 fl oz	2	*	*	*	*	*	*	3	*	*	*	*	*	*	*	*	*	*	*	*
regular																				
(Hires) 8 fl oz	130	*	*	*	*	10	*	2	*	*	*	*	*	*	*	*	*	*	*	*
seltzer																				
fruit flavors																				
(Canada Dry) 8 fl oz	0	*	*	*	*	*	*	*	*	*	*	*	*	*	*	*	*	*	*	*
(Schweppes) 8 fl oz	0	*	*	*	*	*	*	*	*	*	*	*	*	*	*	*	*	*	*	*
plain																				
(Canada Dry) 8 fl oz	0	*	*	*	*	*	*	*	*	*	*	*	*	*	*	*	*	*	*	*
Sprite																				
12 fl oz	*	*	*	*	*	9	*	2	*	*	*	*	*	*	*	*	*	*	*	*
diet																				
12 fl oz	*	*	*	*	*	*	*	*	*	*	*	*	*	*	*	*	*	*	*	*
strawberry																				
(Canada Dry) 8 fl oz	110	*	*	*	*	9	*	2	*	*	*	*	*	*	*	*	*	*	*	*
(Sunkist) 8 fl oz	140	*	*	*	*	11	*	*	*	*	*	*	*	*	*	*	*	*	*	*
(Welch's) 12 fl oz	200	*	*	*	*	17	*	*	*	*	*	*	*	*	*	*	*	*	*	*
tonic																				
citrus																				
(Schweppes) 8 fl oz	90	*	*	*	*	7	*	*	*	*	*	*	*	*	*	*	*	*	*	*
cranberry																				
(Schweppes) 8 fl oz	90	*	*	*	*	7	*	*	*	*	*	*	*	*	*	*	*	*	*	*
tonic water																				
(generic) 12 fl oz	125	*	*	*	*	11	*	*	*	*	*	2	*	*	*	*	*	*	*	*
diet																				
(Canada Dry) 8 fl oz	0	*	*	*	*	*	*	*	*	*	*	*	*	*	*	*	*	*	*	*
regular																				
(Canada Dry) 8 fl oz	100	*	*	*	*	8	*	*	*	*	*	*	*	*	*	*	*	*	*	*
wild cherry																				
(Canada Dry) 8 fl oz	110	*	*	*	*	9	*	2	*	*	*	*	*	*	*	*	*	*	*	*
Wink																				
diet																				
(Hires) 8 fl oz	5	*	*	*	*	*	*	4	*	*	*	*	*	*	*	*	*	*	*	*
regular																				
(Hires) 8 fl oz	130	*	*	*	*	10	*	*	*	*	*	*	*	*	*	*	*	*	*	*
SOLE																				
frozen																				
(Mrs. Paul's Light) 4 1/4 oz	240	35	15	10	17	7	*	—	—	4	4	—	—	2	*	6	8	8	—	—
(Van de Kamp's) 4 oz	100	37	3	5	12	*	*	4	7	*	*	—	—	*	*	4	8	8	—	—
country herb																				
(Gorton's Select) 2 fillets	110	35	5	5	25	*	*	14	—	2	2	—	—	*	*	2	4	8	—	—
light																				
(Van de Kamp's) 1	250	28	18	10	15	6	*	20	6	2	8	—	—	*	*	10	15	10	—	—
seafood stuffed																				
(Gorton's Select) 1 fillet	170	30	5	—	18	6	*	30	—	10	8	—	—	*	*	10	10	10	—	—
SORBET (see also SHERBET)																				
orange																				
(Haagen-Dazs Sorbet & Cream) 1 bar	200	4	12	20	20	10	*	*	3	6	*	—	—	8	10	2	6	4	—	—
raspberry																				
(Haagen-Dazs Sorbet & Cream) 1 bar	180	4	11	20	20	9	*	*	3	6	*	—	—	8	*	*	8	2	—	—
SORGHUM SYRUP																				
1 tbsp	61	*	*	*	*	5	*	*	6	3	4	*	5	*	*	*	2	*	*	*

	Calories	Protein	Fat	Sat. Fat	Cholesterol	Carbohydrates	Fiber	Sodium	Potassium	Calcium	Iron	Zinc	Magnesium	Vitamin A	Vitamin C	Thiamin	Riboflavin	Niacin	Vitamin B₁₂	Folic acid
SOUFFLÉ, FROM MIX																				
chocolate																				
(Knorr) 1 ramekin	100	*	2	—	*	6	*	8	—	*	*	*	*	*	*	*	*	*	*	*
lemon																				
(Knorr) 1 ramekin	80	*	—	—	*	*	*	7	—	*	*	*	*	*	*	*	*	*	*	*
SOUP, CONDENSED																				
asparagus																				
prep w/ water																				
(generic) 1 cup	163	11	13	—	—	6	4	44	10	18	5	6	5	12	7	7	16	4	8	8
asparagus, cream of																				
(Campbell's) 1 cup	120	3	12	—	2	3	—	34	—	2	2	—	—	2	2	*	2	2	—	—
prep w/ low-fat milk																				
(Campbell's) 1 cup	170	8	15	—	3	5	—	36	—	15	4	—	—	6	4	4	10	2	—	—
prep w/ milk																				
(generic) 1 cup	85	4	6	—	—	4	*	41	5	3	4	6	*	9	4	4	5	4	*	5
prep w/ water																				
(generic) 1 cup	58	4	3	—	—	3	—	33	4	2	3	5	*	5	*	3	3	3	*	2
bean																				
homestyle																				
(Campbell's) 1 cup	130	8	2	—	2	8	24	29	—	6	8	—	—	15	4	6	6	4	—	—
bean & bacon																				
(Campbell's) 1 cup	130	12	6	—	2	7	24	32	—	6	10	—	—	10	*	2	2	2	—	—
(generic) 1 cup	171	13	9	—	—	8	36	39	11	8	11	7	11	18	3	6	2	3	*	8
beans & franks																				
(generic) 1 cup	183	16	10	—	—	7	—	44	13	9	13	8	12	17	2	7	4	5	*	7
beef																				
(Campbell's) 1 cup	80	8	3	—	3	3	—	35	—	*	4	—	—	20	2	2	2	4	—	—
beef boullion																				
(generic) 1 cup	20	2	*	—	*	*	*	57	*	*	*	*	2	*	*	*	*	2	*	*
beef broth																				
(Campbell's) 1 cup	14	3	*	*	2	*	—	34	—	*	*	—	—	*	*	2	2	4	—	—
beef mushroom																				
(Campbell's) 1 cup	60	7	5	—	2	2	—	39	—	*	2	—	—	*	*	2	2	4	—	—
(generic) 1 cup	153	19	9	—	—	4	—	81	9	*	10	18	4	*	*	3	9	11	7	4
beef noodle																				
(Campbell's) 1 cup	60	7	3	—	5	2	—	35	—	*	4	—	—	4	*	6	4	4	—	—
(generic) 1 cup	82	8	5	—	—	3	4	39	3	—	6	10	*	12	*	4	3	5	3	*
homestyle																				
(Campbell's) 1 cup	90	10	6	—	7	3	—	34	—	*	4	—	—	*	2	4	4	8	—	—
black bean																				
(generic) 1 cup	118	10	2	—	—	7	20	51	8	5	12	10	11	10	*	5	3	3	*	6
broccoli, cream of																				
(Campbell's) 1 cup	80	2	8	—	2	3	—	28	—	2	2	—	—	6	10	*	2	*	—	—
prep w/ low-fat milk																				
(Campbell's) 1 cup	140	8	11	—	3	5	—	31	—	15	2	—	—	10	10	2	10	*	—	—
broccoli cheese																				
(Campbell's) 1 cup	110	3	11	—	—	3	—	33	—	6	4	—	—	25	*	*	*	*	—	—
celery, cream of																				
(Campbell's) 1 cup	100	3	11	15	2	3	—	34	—	2	*	—	—	6	*	*	*	*	—	—
prep w/ milk																				
(generic) 1 cup	164	9	15	—	—	5	4	42	9	19	4	*	6	9	2	5	15	2	8	2
prep w/ water																				
(generic) 1 cup	90	3	9	—	—	3	4	39	3	4	4	*	2	6	*	2	3	2	4	*
cheddar cheese																				
(Campbell's) 1 cup	130	5	12	15	5	3	—	31	—	8	4	—	—	15	*	*	6	*	—	—
cheese																				
prep w/ milk																				
(generic) 1 cup	228	16	22	—	—	3	4	42	10	29	4	5	5	25	2	4	19	2	7	2
prep w/ water																				
(generic) 1 cup	156	9	16	—	—	3	—	40	4	14	4	4	*	22	*	*	8	2	*	*

PERCENTAGE DAILY VALUE

	Calories	Protein	Fat	Sat. Fat	Cholesterol	Carbohydrates	Fiber	Sodium	Potassium	Calcium	Iron	Zinc	Magnesium	Vitamin A	Vitamin C	Thiamin	Riboflavin	Niacin	Vitamin B₁₂	Folic acid

SOUP, CONDENSED (continued)

	Calories	Protein	Fat	Sat. Fat	Cholesterol	Carbohydrates	Fiber	Sodium	Potassium	Calcium	Iron	Zinc	Magnesium	Vitamin A	Vitamin C	Thiamin	Riboflavin	Niacin	Vitamin B₁₂	Folic acid
chicken alphabet (Campbell's) 1 cup	70	5	3	—	3	3	—	33	—	*	4	—	—	15	*	4	4	6	—	—
chicken broth (Campbell's) 1 cup	30	2	3	—	2	*	—	30	—	*	*	—	—	*	*	*	2	6	—	—
(generic) 1 cup	40	8	2	—	—	*	*	33	6	*	3	2	*	*	*	*	4	17	4	*
chicken, cream of (Campbell's) 1 cup	110	3	11	10	5	3	—	34	—	2	2	—	—	10	*	*	2	2	—	—
prep w/ milk (generic) 1 cup	193	13	18	—	—	5	*	44	8	18	4	5	4	14	2	5	15	5	9	2
prep w/ water (generic) 1 cup	116	6	11	—	—	3	*	41	2	3	3	4	*	11	*	2	4	4	2	*
chicken dumpling (generic) 1 cup	94	9	8	—	—	2	4	35	3	*	3	2	*	10	*	*	4	9	3	*
chicken 'n' dumplings (Campbell's) 1 cup	80	7	5	—	8	3	—	40	—	*	2	—	—	8	*	*	2	6	—	—
chicken gumbo (Campbell's) 1 cup	50	3	2	—	2	3	—	37	—	2	2	—	—	2	*	*	*	2	—	—
(generic) 1 cup	55	4	2	—	—	3	8	39	2	2	5	2	*	3	8	2	3	3	*	*
chicken mushroom (generic) 1 cup	274	15	28	—	—	6	4	81	9	6	10	13	4	45	*	3	13	16	2	*
chicken mushroom, creamy (Campbell's) 1 cup	120	5	12	10	5	3	—	38	—	2	2	—	—	15	*	*	4	4	—	—
chicken 'n' stars (Campbell's) 1 cup	60	5	3	—	2	3	—	35	—	*	2	—	—	15	*	4	4	6	—	—
chicken noodle (Campbell's) 1 cup	60	3	3	—	3	3	—	36	—	*	4	—	—	6	*	6	4	4	—	—
(generic) 1 cup	76	7	4	—	—	3	4	47	2	2	4	3	*	15	*	4	4	7	2	*
homestyle (Campbell's) 1 cup	60	5	3	—	3	3	—	37	—	*	4	—	—	15	2	4	4	6	—	—
chicken noodleO's (Campbell's) 1 cup	70	5	3	—	3	3	—	36	—	*	4	—	—	25	*	6	4	8	—	—
chicken rice (Campbell's) 1 cup	60	3	3	—	2	3	—	32	—	*	*	—	—	8	*	*	*	2	—	—
(generic) 1 cup	61	6	3	—	—	2	4	34	3	2	4	2	*	13	*	*	*	6	2	*
chicken vegetable (Campbell's) 1 cup	70	5	3	—	3	4	—	34	—	2	2	—	—	50	4	4	4	6	—	—
(generic) 1 cup	75	6	4	—	—	3	4	39	4	2	5	2	2	53	2	3	3	6	2	*
chili beef (Campbell's) 1 cup	450	10	8	—	3	7	—	34	—	2	8	—	—	15	4	2	2	2	—	—
(generic) 1 cup	166	11	10	—	—	7	36	42	15	4	12	9	7	29	7	4	4	5	5	4
clam chowder Manhattan (Campbell's) 1 cup	70	3	3	—	*	4	—	34	—	2	2	—	—	30	8	*	2	4	—	—
(generic) 1 cup	78	4	3	—	—	4	4	24	5	3	9	7	3	19	7	2	2	4	67	2
prep w/low-fat milk (Campbell's) 1 cup	130	12	5	—	3	6	—	39	—	15	4	—	—	4	4	4	10	4	—	—
New England (Campbell's) 1 cup	80	7	3	—	2	4	—	37	—	2	4	—	—	*	2	*	2	2	—	—
prep w/milk (generic) 1 cup	164	16	10	—	—	6	4	41	9	19	8	5	6	3	6	4	14	5	170	2
prep w/water (generic) 1 cup	95	8	4	—	—	4	4	38	4	4	8	5	2	*	3	*	3	5	133	*
prep w/ milk (Gorton's) 1/4 can	140	10	8	—	7	6	—	31	4	15	4	—	—	2	*	2	10	4	—	—
clam chowder Manhattan chunky (generic) 1 cup	134	12							11	7	15	11	5	66	20	4	4	9	131	2

SOUP, CONDENSED (continued)

	Calories	Protein	Fat	Sat. Fat	Cholesterol	Carbohydrates	Fiber	Sodium	Potassium	Calcium	Iron	Zinc	Magnesium	Vitamin A	Vitamin C	Thiamin	Riboflavin	Niacin	Vitamin B$_{12}$	Folic acid
consommé (Campbell's) 1 cup	25	7	*	*	2	*	—	31	—	*	2	—	—	*	*	*	*	4	—	—
(generic) 1 cup	29	9	*	*	—	*	—	26	4	*	3	2	*	*	2	*	2	4	*	*
curly noodle w/ chicken (Campbell's) 1 cup	70	3	3	—	5	4	—	33	—	*	4	—	—	15	35	4	6	6	—	—
dinosaur vegetable (Campbell's) 1 cup	100	7	3	—	2	6	—	28	—	2	4	—	—	30	*	4	4	4	—	—
double noodle in chicken broth (Campbell's) 1 cup	90	7	3	—		4	—	29	—		4	—	—	30	*	8	8	10	—	—
French onion (Campbell's) 1 cup	60	3	3	—	2	3	—	37	—	2	2	—	—	*	4	2	*	2	—	—
golden corn (Campbell's) 1 cup	110	3	5	—	2	6	—	29	—	*	2	—	—	8	*	2	4	6	—	—
prep w/ low-fat milk (Campbell's) 1 cup	160	10	8	—		8	—	32	—	15	2	—	—	10	*	4	10	6	—	—
golden mushroom (Campbell's) 1 cup	70	3	5	—	2	3	—	35	—	*	2	—	—	15	*	2	4	6	—	—
green pea (Campbell's) 1 cup	150	13	5	—	2	8	16	33	—	2	8	—	—	*	*	8	2	4	—	—
prep w/ milk (generic) 1 cup	233	21	11	—		10	12	43	10	17	11	11	14	7	5	10	15	7	7	2
prep w/ water (generic) 1 cup	159	14	4	—	—	8	12	40	5	3	10	11	10	4	3	7	4	6	*	*
hearty vegetable w/ pasta (Campbell's) 1 cup	70	5	*	*	*	5	—	33	—	2	4	—	—	50	*	4	6	10	—	—
Italian tomato w/ basil & oregano (Campbell's) 1 cup	90	2	*	*	*	7	—	31	—	4	4	—	—	20	15	2	4	4	—	—
minestrone (Campbell's) 1 cup	80	5	3	—	2	4	—	37	—	2	6	—	—	40	*	4	2	4	—	—
prep w/ water (generic) 1 cup	82	7	4	—	—	4	4	38	9	5	5	5	2	47	2	4	3	5	*	4
mushroom barley prep w/ water (generic) 1 cup	75	3	4	—	—	4	4	38	3	*	3	3	3	4	*	2	5	5	*	*
mushroom & beef stock prep w/ water (generic) 1 cup	85	5	6	—	—	3	4	40	5	*	5	9	2	25	2	2	6	6	*	2
mushroom, cream of (Campbell's) 1 cup	100	3	11	10	2	3	—	33	—	2	*	—	—	*	*	*	4	2	—	—
prep w/ milk (generic) 1 cup	203	10	21	—		5	*	45	8	18	3	4	5	3	4	5	16	5	8	2
prep w/ water (generic) 1 cup	129	4	14	—	—	5	*	43	3	5	3	4	*	*	2	3	5	4	*	*
nacho cheese (Campbell's) 1 cup	110	7	12	—	5	3	—	31	—	4	*	—	—	25	2	*	4	*	—	—
prep w/ whole milk (Campbell's) 1 cup	160	12	15	—	7	4	—	33	—	20	*	—	—	30	4	2	10	*	—	—
noodles & ground beef (Campbell's) 1 cup	90	7	6	—	7	3	—	34	—	*	4	—	—	20	*	6	6	6	—	—
onion prep w/ water (generic) 1 cup	57	6	3	—	—	3	4	43	2	3	4	4	*	*	2	2	*	3	*	4
onion, cream of (Campbell's) 1 cup	100	3	8	—	5	4	—	35	—	2	*	—	—	6	*	*	2	*	—	—
prep w/ 1/2 low-fat milk & 1/2 water (Campbell's) 1 cup	140	7	11	—	8	5	—	36	—	8	2	—	—	8	*	2	8	*	—	—
prep w/ milk (generic) 1 cup	188	11	15	—		6	4	42	9	18	4	4	6	9	4	7	16	3	8	3

SOUP, CONDENSED (continued)

	Calories	Protein	Fat	Sat. Fat	Cholesterol	Carbohydrates	Fiber	Sodium	Potassium	Calcium	Iron	Zinc	Magnesium	Vitamin A	Vitamin C	Thiamin	Riboflavin	Niacin	Vitamin B₁₂	Folic acid
prep w/ water (generic) 1 cup	111	5	8	—	—	4	—	40	4	4	4	*	*	6	2	4	5	3	*	2
oyster stew (Campbell's) 1 cup	80	3	8	—	5	2	—	35	—	*	8	—	—	*	4	*	2	2	—	—
prep w/ whole milk (Campbell's) 1 cup	130	10	11	—	7	3	—	37	—	15	10	—	—	4	6	2	15	2	—	—
prep w/ milk (generic) 1 cup	135	10	12	—	—	3	*	44	7	17	6	69	5	5	7	4	14	2	44	2
prep w/ water (generic) 1 cup	58	3	6	—	—	*	—	41	*	2	5	69	*	*	5	*	2	*	36	*
pepperpot (Campbell's) 1 cup	90	8	6	—	8	3	—	40	—	2	4	—	—	20	*	2	2	4	—	—
prep w/ water (generic) 1 cup	108	11	7	—	—	3	4	42	5	3	5	8	*	18	2	4	3	6	3	3
potato, cream of (Campbell's) 1 cup	80	2	5	—	3	4	—	35	—	*	*	—	—	*	*	*	*	*	—	—
prep w/ 1/2 low-fat milk & 1/2 water (Campbell's) 1 cup	120	5	6	—	7	5	—	37	—	8	2	—	—	4	*	2	8	2	—	—
prep w/ milk (generic) 1 cup	152	10	10	—	—	6	4	45	9	17	3	5	4	9	2	6	14	3	8	2
prep w/ water (generic) 1 cup	73	3	4	—	—	4	*	42	4	2	3	4	*	6	*	2	2	3	*	*
Scotch broth (Campbell's) 1 cup	80	7	5	—	3	3	—	36	—	*	2	—	—	15	*	*	2	4	—	—
(generic) 1 cup	83	9	4	—	—	3	4	44	5	2	5	11	*	45	2	*	3	6	5	3
shrimp, cream of (Campbell's) 1 cup	90	3	9	10	7	3	—	34	—	*	*	—	—	*	*	*	*	*	—	—
prep w/ low-fat milk (Campbell's) 1 cup	140	8	15	15	7	4	—	36	—	15	2	—	—	6	*	2	10	*	—	—
prep w/ milk (generic) 1 cup	397	28	35	—	—	11	4	105	17	40	8	13	14	15	5	10	32	6	42	6
prep w/ water (generic) 1 cup	100	5	9	—	—	3	*	45	2	2	3	6	3	3	*	*	2	2	11	*
souper stars w/ chicken (Campbell's) 1 cup	70	3	3	—	2	4	—	35	—	*	4	—	—	20	35	4	4	4	—	—
split pea w/ ham (generic) 1 cup	190	17	7	—	—	9	—	42	11	2	13	9	12	9	3	10	4	7	4	*
split pea w/ ham & bacon (Campbell's) 1 cup	160	15	5	—	2	8	16	32	—	2	10	—	—	10	*	6	2	4	—	—
stockpot (generic) 1 cup	96	8	6	—	—	4	—	43	7	2	5	8	*	78	3	3	3	6	*	2
teddy bear (Campbell's) 1 cup	60	3	2	—	2	4	—	32	—	*	6	—	—	15	35	6	2	4	—	—
tomato (Campbell's) 1 cup	90	2	3	—	*	6	—	28	—	*	2	—	—	8	35	2	*	2	—	—
prep w/ low-fat milk (Campbell's) 1 cup	140	8	6	—	3	7	—	30	—	15	4	—	—	10	40	4	10	4	—	—
prep. w/ milk (generic) 1 cup	151	10	9	—	—	7	*	36	12	15	9	2	5	16	106	8	14	7	7	5
tomato beef noodle (generic) 1 cup	139	7	7	—	—	7	4	38	6	2	6	5	2	11	*	6	5	9	3	2
tomato bisque (Campbell's) 1 cup	120	2	5	—	*	7	—	34	—	4	4	—	—	10	30	2	2	4	—	—
prep. w/ milk (generic) 1 cup	198	10	10	—	—	10	—	46	17	19	5	4	6	18	12	8	16	6	7	5
tomato, cream of homestyle (Campbell's) 1 cup	110	2	3	—	2	6	—	30	—	*	2	—	—	10	40	2	2	2	—	—

	Calories	Protein	Fat	Sat. Fat	Cholesterol	Carbohydrates	Fiber	Sodium	Potassium	Calcium	Iron	Zinc	Magnesium	Vitamin A	Vitamin C	Thiamin	Riboflavin	Niacin	Vitamin B12	Folic acid
SOUP, CONDENSED (continued)																				
prep w/ whole milk homestyle (Campbell's) 1 cup	180	8	11	—	5	8	—	36	—	10	2	—	—	15	40	4	10	2	—	—
tomato rice (generic) 1 cup	118	3	4	—	—	7	4	34	9	2	4	3	*	15	25	4	3	5	*	3
old fashioned (Campbell's) 1 cup	110	2	3	—	*	7	—	30	—	*	2	—	—	8	15	*	*	2	—	—
turkey noodle (Campbell's) 1 cup	70	5	3	—	5	3	—	37	—	*	2	—	—	10	*	6	4	6	—	—
(generic) 1 cup	67	6	3	—	—	3	4	33	2	*	5	4	*	6	*	5	4	7	2	*
turkey vegetable (Campbell's) 1 cup	70	5	3	—	3	3	—	32	—	2	2	—	—	60	*	*	2	4	—	—
(generic) 1 cup	38	3	2	—	—	*	*	20	3	*	2	2	*	26	*	*	*	3	*	*
vegetable (Campbell's) 1 cup	90	5	3	—	2	5	—	35	—	2	2	—	—	40	6	2	2	2	—	—
homestyle (Campbell's) 1 cup	60	3	3	—	*	3	—	37	—	2	2	—	—	40	2	2	2	4	—	—
old fashioned (Campbell's) 1 cup	60	3	3	—	2	3	—	35	—	2	2	—	—	45	*	2	2	4	—	—
vegetarian (Campbell's) 1 cup	80	3	3	—	*	4	—	33	—	*	4	—	—	40	4	2	2	4	—	—
vegetable beef (Campbell's) 1 cup	70	8	3	—	2	3	—	31	—	2	4	—	—	30	*	*	2	4	—	—
(generic) 1 cup	77	9	3	—	—	3	*	39	5	2	6	10	*	37	4	2	3	5	5	3
vegetable beef broth (generic) 1 cup	0	*	*	*	—	*	*	*	*	*	*	*	*	*	*	*	*	*	*	*
vegetarian vegetable (generic) 1 cup	72	3	3	—	—	4	*	34	6	2	6	3	2	60	2	4	3	5	*	3
SOUP, FROM MIX																				
asparagus (Knorr) 1 cup	80	8	5	—	—	4	—	32	—	10	2	*	—	2	8	4	10	*	*	*
asparagus, cream of (generic) 1 cup	52	3	2	—	*	3	—	29	3	2	2	3	4	5	*	2	3	2	*	2
bean & bacon (generic) 1 cup	98	8	3	—	—	5	32	36	9	5	7	4	7	*	2	3	14	2	*	2
beef cube (Wyler's) 1 cube	10	*	*	*	*	*	—	39	*	*	*	*	*	*	*	*	*	*	*	*
beef boullion (Knorr) 1 cup	15	*	2	—	—	—	—	51	—	*	*	*	*	*	*	*	*	*	*	*
cube (Herb-Ox) 1 cube	10	*	*	—	*	*	*	31	—	*	*	*	*	*	*	*	*	*	*	*
beef broth (generic) 1 cup	7	*	*	*	—	*	*	48	*	*	*	*	*	*	*	*	*	*	*	*
(Weight Watchers) 1 packet	10	2	*	*	*	*	*	34	*	*	*	*	*	*	*	—	—	—	—	—
beef flavor ramen (Samwa) 1 1/4 oz dry	140	6	3	5	—	9	*	18	—	2	6	—	—	*	*	10	10	*	—	—
low fat (Samwa) 1 1/2 oz dry	160	8	2	*	—	11	*	37	—	*	10	—	—	*	*	10	6	6	—	—
beef flavor w/ vegetables ramen (Samwa) 2 1/4 oz dry	270	8	15	—	—	13	—	64	—	2	10	—	—	20	*	10	4	10	—	—
low fat (Samwa) 2 1/4 oz dry	220	10	3	—	—	15	—	67	—	2	10	—	—	40	2	10	8	10	—	—
beef noodle (generic) 1 cup	40	4	*	*	—	2	4	43	2	*	2	*	3	*	*	8	4	3	*	*
microwave (Campbell's Cup) 1 cup	140	10	3	—	—	8	—	55	—	2	10	—	—	20	2	20	15	15	—	—

SOUP, FROM MIX

	Calories	Protein	Fat	Sat. Fat	Cholesterol	Carbohydrates	Fiber	Sodium	Potassium	Calcium	Iron	Zinc	Magnesium	Vitamin A	Vitamin C	Thiamin	Riboflavin	Niacin	Vitamin B12	Folic acid
ramen (Samwa) 1 1/2 oz dry	200	6	14	—	—	9	—	35	—	*	6	—	—	*	*	15	6	8	—	—
cup (Samwa) 2 1/2 oz dry	340	10	25	—	—	14	*	56	—	2	15	—	—	*	*	20	10	15	—	—
black bean (Knorr Latin Taste) 1 cup	140	10	2	—	—	8	—	39	—	4	15	*	*	*	4	10	8	4	*	*
boullion chicken cube (Wyler's) 1 cube	10	*	*	*	*	*	—	37	*	*	*	*	*	*	*	*	*	*	*	*
broccoli (Knorr) 1 cup	160	10	12	—	—	5	—	44	—	20	2	*	*	10	30	6	15	*	*	*
cauliflower (generic) 1 cup	69	5	3	—	—	4	—	35	3	*	3	2	*	*	4	5	5	3	3	*
celery, cream of prep w/ water (generic) 1 cup	64	4	2	—	—	3	—	35	3	4	3	*	*	5	*	2	3	2	*	*
chick 'n' pasta (Knorr) 1 cup	90	4	3	—	—	5	—	35	—	2	4	*	*	25	10	2	*	4	*	*
chicken asopao (Knorr Latin Taste) 1 cup	130	4	2	—	—	9	—	52	—	*	6	*	*	*	2	8	*	4	*	*
chicken boullion (Knorr) 1 cup	16	*	*	*	*	*	—	33	—	*	*	*	*	*	*	*	*	*	*	*
chicken broth (generic) 1 cup	23	2	2	—	—	*	*	63	*	2	*	*	*	*	*	*	2	*	*	*
(Weight Watchers) 1 packet	10	2	*	*	*	*	*	37	*	*	4	—	—	*	*	—	—	—	—	—
from cube (generic) 1 cup	12	2	"	*	—	*	—	33	*	*	*	*	*	*	*	*	*	*	*	*
chicken, cream of prep w/ water (generic) 1 cup	103	3	8	—	—	4	*	47	6	7	*	10	*	8	*	7	12	13	4	*
chicken flavor ramen (Samwa) 1 1/4 oz dry	140	6	3	5	*	9	*	17	—	*	6	—	—	*	*	8	8	*	—	—
low fat (Samwa) 1 1/2 oz dry	160	8	2	*	—	11	*	39	—	*	10	—	—	*	*	10	8	8	—	—
chicken flavor noodle (Knorr) 1 cup	100	8	3	—	—	6	—	30	—	*	2	*	*	*	*	*	*	2	*	*
microwave (Campbell's Cup) 1 cup	140	12	3	—	—	8	—	57	—	*	8	—	—	*	*	20	10	15	—	—
chicken flavor w/ vegetables ramen (Samwa) 2 1/4 oz dry	270	8	15	—	—	13	—	61	—	2	10	—	—	20	2	10	4	10	—	—
low fat (Samwa) 2 1/4 oz dry	220	10	3	—	—	15	—	62	—	2	10	—	—	40	2	10	8	10	—	—
chicken noodle (Campbell's Cup) 1 cup	80	7	3	—	—	4	—	37	—	*	4	—	—	*	*	8	8	6	—	—
microwave (Campbell's Cup) 1 cup	100	8	3	—	—	5	—	29	—	*	4	—	—	*	*	15	10	6	—	—
(generic) 1 cup	38	4	*	*	—	2	*	39	*	2	2	*	*	*	*	3	2	3	*	*
(Lipton Cup-A-Soup) 6 fl oz	50	3	2	—	—	3	—	25	—	*	2	—	—	*	2	6	2	4	—	—
ramen (Samwa) 1 1/2 oz dry	200	6	14	—	—	9	—	34	—	*	6	—	—	*	*	15	6	8	—	—
cup (Samwa) 2 1/2 oz dry	330	10	25	—	—	14	*	54	—	2	15	—	—	*	*	20	10	15	—	—
spicy (Samwa) 1 1/2 oz dry	200	6	14	—	—	9	—	33	—	*	6	—	—	*	*	15	6	8	—	—
chicken rice (generic) 1 cup	59	4	2	—	—	3	4	39	*	*	*	*	*	*	*	*	*	2	*	*

	Calories	Protein	Fat	Sat. Fat	Cholesterol	Carbohydrates	Fiber	Sodium	Potassium	Calcium	Iron	Zinc	Magnesium	Vitamin A	Vitamin C	Thiamin	Riboflavin	Niacin	Vitamin B$_{12}$	Folic acid
SOUP, FROM MIX (continued)																				
chicken supreme (Lipton Cup-A-Soup) 6 fl oz	80	2	5	—	—	4	—	29	—	2	*	—	—	*	*	4	6	2	—	—
chicken vegetable (generic) 1 cup	122	11	3	—	—	6	4	83	5	3	8	3	13	*	5	12	7	9	4	2
(Lipton Cup-A-Soup) 6 fl oz	60	3	2	—	—	3	—	23	—	*	*	—	—	*	*	4	*	2	—	—
chicken vegetable, creamy (Lipton Cup-A-Soup) 6 fl oz	100	3	8	—	—	4	—	29	—	4	*	—	—	*	2	8	8	2	—	—
clam chowder Manhattan (generic) 1 cup	60	3	2	—	—	3	—	51	5	2	9	6	2	19	6	2	2	4	66	2
New England (Knorr) 1 cup	100	4	6	—	*	4	—	40	—	2	8	*	*	10	2	4	2	*	*	*
prep w/water (generic) 1 cup	95	4	4	—	—	4	4	38	4	4	8	5	2	*	3	*	3	5	133	*
consomme w/ gelatin (generic) 1 cup	17	4	*	*	—	*	—	137	2	*	*	*	2	*	*	*	2	3	2	*
country barley (Knorr) 10 fl oz	120	6	3	—	—	8	—	39	—	4	10	*	*	25	15	6	2	4	*	*
creamy chicken (Campbell's Cup) 1 cup	90	5	6	—	—	4	—	40	—	2	*	—	—	*	*	*	6	2	—	—
double noodle (Campbell's Cup) 1 cup	200	13	3	—	—	12	—	32	—	2	10	—	—	*	*	25	10	15	—	—
fine herb (Knorr) 1 cup	130	8	9	—	—	5	—	41	—	8	4	*	*	2	2	6	10	2	*	*
fish boullion (Knorr) 1 cup	10	*	—	—	—	—	—	47	—	*	*	*	*	*	*	*	*	*	*	*
French onion (Knorr) 1 cup	50	2	2	—	—	3	—	40	—	*	2	*	*	*	2	*	*	*	*	*
ramen (Samwa) 1 1/2 oz dry	210	6	14	—	—	9	—	29	—	*	6	—	—	*	*	15	6	8	*	*
green pea (Lipton Cup-A-Soup) 6 fl oz	110	5	6	—	—	6	—	27	—	*	2	—	—	*	*	6	2	2	—	—
hot & sour (Knorr) 1 cup	80	6	5	—	—	3	—	29	—	*	4	*	*	2	*	2	4	*	*	*
leek (Knorr) 1 cup	110	8	6	—	—	5	—	33	—	10	4	*	*	*	2	6	8	*	*	*
prep w/ water (generic) 1 cup	11	*	*	*	—	*	*	6	*	*	*	*	*	*	*	*	*	*	*	*
minestrone (generic) 1 cup	79	7	3	—	—	4	—	43	10	4	6	5	2	6	2	5	3	5	*	5
(Knorr) 10 fl oz	130	6	3	—	—	8	—	39	—	6	8	—	—	15	40	8	2	4	*	*
mushroom (generic) 1 cup	96	4	8	—	—	4	4	42	6	7	3	*	*	*	2	19	7	3	4	*
(Knorr) 1 cup	100	8	6	—	—	4	—	36	—	8	2	*	*	*	4	6	10	4	*	*
mushroom, cream of (Lipton Cup-A-Soup) 6 fl oz	70	2	5	—	—	3	—	28	—	2	*	—	—	*	*	*	6	2	—	—
mushroom noodle ramen (Samwa) 1 1/2 oz dry	200	6	14	—	—	9	—	30	—	*	6	—	—	*	*	15	6	8	*	*
noodle (Campbell's Cup) 1 cup	110	7	3	—	—	7	—	31	—	2	8	—	—	*	*	15	8	8	—	—
(Lipton Soup Secrets) 6 fl oz	70	3	3	—	—	3	—	33	—	*	2	—	—	*	*	6	2	4	—	—
noodle w/ chicken broth (Campbell's Cup) 1 cup	90	7	3	—	—	5	—	40	—	2	4	—	—	*	*	10	8	4	—	—
(Knorr Latin Taste) 1 cup	70	4	2	—	—	4	—	36	—	*	2	*	*	*	2	2	*	*	*	*
microwave (Campbell's Cup) 1 cup	140	10	3	—	—	8	—	58	—	*	8	—	—	20	2	15	10	15	—	—

	Calories	Protein	Fat	Sat. Fat	Cholesterol	Carbohydrates	Fiber	Sodium	Potassium	Calcium	Iron	Zinc	Magnesium	Vitamin A	Vitamin C	Thiamin	Riboflavin	Niacin	Vitamin B$_{12}$	Folic acid
SOUP, FROM MIX (continued)																				
onion																				
(Campbell's Cup) 1 cup	30	2	2	—	—	2	—	27	—	*	*	—	—	*	*	2	*	2	—	—
(generic) 1 cup	27	2	*	*	—	2	4	35	2	*	*	*	*	*	*	2	3	2	*	*
Oriental flavor																				
ramen																				
(Samwa) 1 1/4 oz dry	140	6	3	5	*	2	*	18	—	*	8	—	—	*	*	4	8	*	—	—
low fat																				
(Samwa) 1 1/2 oz dry	150	8	2	*	—	10	*	39	—	*	10	—	—	*	*	10	6	6	—	—
Oriental flavor w/ vegetables																				
ramen																				
(Samwa) 2 1/4 oz dry	270	8	15	—	—	13	—	50	—	2	10	—	—	15	2	10	4	10	—	—
low fat																				
(Samwa) 2 1/4 oz dry	220	10	3	—	—	15	—	58	—	2	10	—	—	40	2	8	6	8	—	—
oxtail																				
(generic) 1 cup	68	5	4	—	—	3	*	49	2	*	*	*	2	*	*	2	*	4	4	*
(Knorr) 1 cup	70	2	3	—	—	3	—	47	—	*	4	*	*	4	20	4	2	*	*	*
pork flavor																				
ramen																				
(Samwa) 1 1/4 oz dry	140	6	3	—	—	2	*	19	—	*	6	—	—	*	*	8	6	*	—	—
low fat																				
(Samwa) 1 1/2 oz dry	140	6	3	5	*	9	—	19	—	*	6	—	—	*	*	8	6	*	—	—
pork noodle																				
ramen																				
(Samwa) 1 1/2 oz dry	200	6	14	—	—	9	—	31	—	*	6	—	—	*	*	15	6	8	—	—
seafood flavored asopao																				
(Knorr Latin Taste) 1 cup	140	6	2	—	—	10	—	48	—	*	6	*	*	*	4	8	*	6	*	*
shrimp bisque																				
(Knorr) 1 cup	70	2	6	—	3	2	—	32	—	*	*	*	*	*	*	*	*	*	*	*
shrimp flavor w/ vegetables																				
ramen																				
(Samwa) 2 1/4 oz dry	280	8	15	—	—	13	—	50	—	2	10	—	—	30	4	15	8	10	—	—
low fat																				
(Samwa) 2 1/4 oz dry	230	10	3	—	—	15	—	54	—	2	15	—	—	25	2	30	10	15	—	—
shrimp noodle																				
ramen																				
(Samwa) 1 1/2 oz dry	200	6	14	—	—	9	—	3	—	*	6	—	—	*	*	15	6	8	—	—
snowpea, cream of																				
prep w/ milk																				
(Knorr) 8 fl oz	80	4	3	—	*	4	—	33	—	*	4	—	*	2	15	6	2	*	*	*
spinach																				
(Knorr) 1 cup	100	8	8	—	2	4	—	37	—	10	4	*	*	8	2	4	8	*	*	*
split pea																				
(generic) 1 cup	100	10	2	—	—	6	12	38	5	2	4	3	9	*	*	11	7	5	5	3
spring vegetable w/ herbs																				
(Knorr) 1 cup	30	*	—	—	—	2	—	30	—	*	*	*	*	*	*	*	*	*	*	*
tomato																				
(generic) 1 cup	98	4	4	—	—	6	4	37	8	5	2	*	3	16	7	4	3	4	*	2
tomato flavored w/ letters & numbers																				
(Knorr Latin Taste) 1 cup	70	2	2	—	—	5	—	36	—	*	4	*	*	2	15	10	2	4	*	*
tomato flavored w/ stars																				
(Knorr Latin Taste) 1 cup	70	2	2	—	—	5	—	36	—	*	4	*	*	2	15	10	2	4	*	*
tomato vegetable																				
(generic) 1 cup	56	3	*	*	—	3	4	48	3	*	4	*	5	4	10	4	3	4	*	3
tortellini in brodo																				
(Knorr) 1 cup	60	*	2	—	—	4	—	34	—	*	*	*	*	*	*	*	*	*	*	*
vegetable																				
(Campbell's) 1/2 oz dry	40	*	*	*	—	3	—	30	—	2	*	—	—	10	4	*	*	2	—	—
(Knorr) 1 cup	35	*	2	—	—	2	—	35	—	4	2	*	*	25	20	2	*	*	*	*

	Calories	Protein	Fat	Sat. Fat	Cholesterol	Carbohydrates	Fiber	Sodium	Potassium	Calcium	Iron	Zinc	Magnesium	Vitamin A	Vitamin C	Thiamin	Riboflavin	Niacin	Vitamin B12	Folic acid
SOUP, FROM MIX (continued)																				
vegetable beef																				
(generic) 1 cup	73	7	2	—	—	4	*	57	3	2	7	2	8	7	3	3	3	3	7	3
ramen cup (Samwa) 2 1/2 oz dry	330	10	23	—	—	14	—	71	—	2	15	—	—	*	*	20	10	15	—	—
vegetable beef noodle ramen (Samwa) 1 1/2 oz dry	210	6	14	—	—	9	—	29	—	*	6	—	—	*	*	15	6	8	—	—
vegetable, cream of (generic) 1 cup	45	*	4	—	—	2	*	21	*	*	*	*	*	*	3	34	3	*	*	*
vegetarian vegetable boullion (Knorr) 1 cup	16	*	2	—	—	*	—	41	—	*	*	*	*	*	*	*	*	*	*	*
wild mushroom, cream of prep w/ milk (Knorr) 1 cup	100	4	5	*	—	5	—	39	—	2	4	*	*	*	2	4	10	10	*	*
SOUP, READY-TO-EAT																				
bean & ham (Campbell's Home Cookin') 9 1/2 oz	180	20	5	—	—	9	—	35	—	8	15	—	—	30	2	8	6	10	—	—
(Healthy Choice) 7 1/2 oz	220	20	6	—	2	12	—	20	18	6	10	—	—	6	4	15	10	6	—	—
(Hormel) 7 1/2 oz	190	15	6	5	8	10	—	27	14	9	1	8	15	14	11	85	7	5	—	—
chunky (generic) 9 1/2 fl oz	259	24	15	19	8	10	52	45	14	9	20	8	13	89	8	11	10	10	*	8
old fashioned chunky (Campbell's) 9 1/2 oz	260	22	12	—	—	11	—	40	—	8	15	—	—	70	4	10	6	8	—	—
bean w/ bacon & ham microwave (Campbell's) 8 oz	200	15	8	—	—	10	—	33	—	8	15	—	—	15	*	6	6	8	—	—
beef (Progresso) 9 1/2 oz	160	22	8	10	12	5	*	32	9	4	15	—	—	30	6	6	8	15	—	—
chunky (Campbell's) 9 1/2 oz	180	22	8	—	—	7	—	42	—	4	10	—	—	100	6	6	8	10	—	—
(generic) 1 cup	170	20	8	—	—	7	4	36	10	3	13	18	*	52	12	4	9	14	10	3
hearty (Healthy Choice) 7 1/2 oz	120	15	3	—	7	6	—	24	8	4	4	—	—	15	15	4	6	10	—	—
(Progresso) 9 1/2 oz	160	25	6	10	12	5	—	34	9	4	15	—	—	50	*	2	8	15	—	—
beef barley (Progresso) 9 1/2 oz	130	20	6	10	10	5	16	36	5	4	15	—	—	35	*	20	6	10	—	—
beef broth (generic) 1 14-oz can	28	8	*	2	*	*	*	54	6	2	4	*	2	*	*	*	5	15	5	2
(Swanson) 7 1/4 oz	16	2	2	—	—	*	—	30	—	*	*	—	—	*	*	*	2	6	—	—
natural (Health Valley) 7 oz	10	2	*	*	*	*	*	12	2	*	*	—	—	*	*	*	*	4	—	—
beef noodle (Progresso) 9 1/2 oz	160	25	6	10	12	6	—	42	3	2	20	—	—	20	2	10	10	15	—	—
chunky (Campbell's) 9 1/2 oz	180	40	9	—	—	3	—	37	—	4	10	—	—	*	*	6	20	10	—	—
beef stroganoff style chunky (Campbell's) 10 3/4 oz	320	27	25	—	—	9	—	50	—	8	15	—	—	50	*	8	15	15	—	—
beef vegetable (Hormel) 7 1/2 oz	90	10	2	3	2	5	—	30	10	4	5	7	6	96	3	*	5	8	—	—
(Progresso) 9 1/2 oz	140	23	5	5	10	5	—	34	10	4	15	—	—	60	4	4	8	15	—	—
chunky (Healthy Choice) 7 1/2 oz	110	17	2	—	7	5	—	20	9	2	8	—	—	20	15	8	6	8	—	—
microwave (Healthy Choice) 7 1/2 oz	110	17	2	—	7	5	—	20	9	2	8	—	—	20	15	8	6	8	—	—
black bean (Hain) 10 1/2 oz	140	18	2	*	*	11	46	28	24	6	20	—	—	6	*	10	6	8	—	—

	Calories	Protein	Fat	Sat. Fat	Cholesterol	Carbohydrates	Fiber	Sodium	Potassium	Calcium	Iron	Zinc	Magnesium	Vitamin A	Vitamin C	Thiamin	Riboflavin	Niacin	Vitamin B_{12}	Folic acid
SOUP, READY-TO-EAT (continued)																				
hearty (Progresso) 9 1/2 oz	140	15	3	3	*	11	44	34	20	8	20	—	—	4	*	20	8	10	—	—
black bean & carrot (Health Valley) 7 1/2 oz	70	12	*	*	*	4	44	12	17	6	25	—	—	100	*	20	6	6	—	30
borscht (Rokeach) 1 cup	27	*	*	*	*	2	*	40	—	*	4	*	*	*	30	*	2	*	*	*
chickarina (Progresso) 9 1/2 oz	130	13	8	10	7	4	—	34	5	4	15	—	—	10	*	4	4	15	—	—
chicken chunky (generic) 1 cup	178	21	10	10	10	6	8	37	5	3	10	7	2	26	2	6	10	22	4	*
hearty (Healthy Choice) 7 1/2 oz	150	15	8	—	12	6	—	22	5	4	4	—	—	20	4	6	10	10	—	—
(Progresso) 9 1/2 oz	130	20	6	5	8	4	—	42	6	2	8	—	—	45	*	6	8	25	—	—
homestyle (Progresso) 9 1/2 oz	110	17	5	3	7	4	—	33	5	2	10	—	—	40	*	4	6	20	—	—
old fashioned (Campbell's) 9 1/2 oz	150	18	6	—	—	6	—	43	—	4	6	—	—	110	6	2	8	15	—	—
chicken barley (Progresso) 9 1/4 oz	110	17	9	3	7	5	16	33	7	2	10	—	—	40	*	2	6	20	—	—
chicken broth (Health Valley) 7 1/2 oz	20	6	*	*	*	*	*	12	3	*	2	—	—	*	*	*	2	10	2	—
(Swanson) 7 1/4 oz	25	2	2	—	—	*	—	37	—	*	*	—	—	*	*	*	2	8	—	—
(Swanson Natural Goodness) 7 1/4 oz	20	2	2	—	—	*	—	22	—	*	*	—	—	*	*	*	2	10	—	—
low sodium (Campbell's) 10 1/2 oz	30	5	2	—	—	*	—	4	—	2	*	—	—	*	*	*	2	6	15	—
no salt added (Hain) 9 oz	45	5	5	—	*	*	—	4	5	*	2	—	—	10	*	*	4	25	—	—
regular (Hain) 9 oz	30	3	5	—	2	*	*	40	4	*	*	—	—	8	*	*	2	15	—	—
chicken corn chowder chunky (Campbell's) 9 1/2 oz	270	18	26	—	—	6	—	42	—	4	8	—	—	80	4	4	8	10	—	—
chicken, cream of (Progresso) 9 1/2 oz	190	17	17	23	12	4	2	40	4	*	10	—	—	6	*	2	8	20	—	—
chicken & meatball (generic) 1 cup	99	14	6	6	3	3	—	43	4	3	10	3	2	—	13	8	7	13	4	*
chicken mushroom, creamy chunky (Campbell's) 9 1/2 oz	250	17	28	—	—	4	—	47	—	2	6	—	—	20	*	4	6	10	—	—
chicken noodle (Campbell's Home Cookin') 9 1/2 oz	110	18	5	—	—	3	—	42	—	2	8	—	—	60	*	2	6	15	—	—
(Hormel) 7 1/2 oz	110	12	5	5	6	5	—	29	3	2	4	4	5	4	*	18	8	9	—	—
(Progresso) 9 1/2 oz	190	18	3	3	8	3	—	36	5	2	8	—	—	60	*	8	8	25	—	—
(Progresso Healthy Classics) 8 oz	80	12	3	15	5	3	—	19	4	*	6	—	—	90	*	6	6	15	—	—
(Weight Watchers) 10 1/2 oz	80	13	2	*	3	4	28	40	4	2	10	—	—	10	*	—	—	—	—	—
chunky (Campbell's) 9 1/2 oz	170	20	9	—	—	5	—	39	—	2	8	—	—	20	*	6	8	10	—	—
(generic) 9 1/2 fl oz	197	24	10	8	7	6	16	40	3	3	9	7	3	27	*	5	11	24	—	—
classic chunky (Campbell's) 9 1/2 oz	140	17	6	—	—	6	—	40	—	2	6	—	—	80	*	4	4	10	—	—
low sodium (Campbell's) 10 3/4 oz	170	22	8	—	—	6	—	4	—	2	10	—	—	35	4	10	20	25	—	—
microwave (Campbell's) 7 3/4 oz	90	8	5	—	—	3	—	45	—	2	4	—	—	10	*	2	6	6	—	—

	Calories	Protein	Fat	Sat. Fat	Cholesterol	Carbohydrates	Fiber	Sodium	Potassium	Calcium	Iron	Zinc	Magnesium	Vitamin A	Vitamin C	Thiamin	Riboflavin	Niacin	Vitamin B₁₂	Folic acid
SOUP, READY-TO-EAT (continued)																				
no salt added (Hain) 8 oz	100	12	6	—	7	3	—	3	3	*	8	—	—	30	*	*	2	15	—	—
old fashioned (Healthy Choice) 7 1/2 oz	90	8	5	—	7	3	—	22	4	2	2	—	—	8	20	2	6	10	—	—
regular (Hain) 8 oz	110	13	6	—	7	4	—	33	4	*	6	—	—	15	*	*	4	20	—	—
tub (Weight Watchers) 7 1/2 oz	80	13	2	*	5	4	*	19	4	—	4	—	—	15	*	—	—	—	—	—
chicken noodle & vegetable																				
(Healthy Choice) 7 1/2 oz	160	20	6	—	15	6	—	21	5	2	6	—	—	35	25	10	8	15	—	—
microwave (Healthy Choice) 7 1/2 oz	160	20	6	—	15	6	—	21	5	2	6	—	—	35	25	10	8	10	—	—
chicken nuggets chunky (Campbell's) 9 1/2 oz	180	15	9	—	—	7	—	38	—	4	8	—	—	50	10	6	6	15	—	—
chicken rice (Campbell's Home Cookin') 9 1/2 oz	150	13	6	—	—	7	—	37	—	2	4	—	—	80	*	*	15	15	—	—
(Healthy Choice) 7 1/2 oz	140	8	6	—	5	6	—	21	4	2	2	—	—	8	10	2	4	10	—	—
(Hormel) 7 1/2 oz	110	8	3	5	2	6	—	37	7	4	3	4	6	52	10	3	8	10	—	—
(Progresso) 9 1/2 oz	120	13	5	5	7	5	—	33	5	2	6	—	—	30	*	*	4	15	—	—
chunky (Campbell's) 9 1/2 oz	140	17	6	—	—	5	—	44	—	4	6	—	—	90	6	2	6	15	—	—
(generic) 9 1/2 fl oz	143	23	6	6	4	5	4	42	3	4	12	7	3	132	7	2	7	23	6	*
microwave (Campbell's) 7 3/4 oz	110	5	6	—	—	5	—	43	—	4	6	—	—	30	*	*	*	4	—	—
chicken rice w/ vegetables (Progresso Healthy Classics) 8 oz	80	12	3	15	3	4	—	18	6	2	6	—	—	30	*	*	2	15	—	—
chicken vegetable (Campbell's Home Cookin') 9 1/2 oz	160	15	6	—	—	7	—	35	—	4	6	—	—	140	*	4	10	15	—	—
(Progresso) 9 1/2 oz	130	15	5	5	—	5	80	34	9	4	10	—	—	45	4	4	6	20	—	—
chunky (Campbell's) 9 1/2 oz	170	17	9	—	—	7	—	43	—	4	6	—	—	110	6	2	6	15	—	—
(generic) 9 1/2 fl oz	186	23	8	8	6	7	—	50	12	3	9	16	3	—	10	3	11	19	4	3
no salt added (Hain) 8 oz	100	12	5	—	3	4	—	4	11	2	8	—	—	60	2	2	6	20	—	—
regular (Hain) 8 oz	110	12	5	—	3	4	—	33	9	2	8	—	—	45	2	2	4	20	—	—
chicken & wild rice (Progresso) 9 1/2 oz	120	10	5	3	7	6	—	35	4	*	4	—	—	35	*	*	6	20	—	—
chili beef chunky (Campbell's) 11 oz	300	35	11	—	—	13	—	45	—	6	25	—	—	25	8	8	8	10	—	—
microwave (Campbell's) 8 oz	190	12	6	—	—	11	—	36	—	4	10	—	—	20	2	8	6	8	—	—
clam chowder Manhattan (Progresso) 9 1/2 oz	120	22	3	3	3	4	*	33	15	4	10	—	—	50	6	2	4	10	—	—
chunky (Campbell's) 9 1/2 oz	150	12	6	—	—	7	—	41	—	6	10	—	—	100	10	*	4	6	—	—
New England (Campbell's Home Cookin') 9 1/2 oz	230	12	25	—	—	4	—	45	—	4	10	—	—	*	*	2	2	6	—	—
(Hormel) 7 1/2 oz	130	8	8	10	10	5	—	33	6	2	4	3	5	*	*	*	2	4	—	—
(Progresso) 9 1/4 oz	190	10	17	15	5	6	*	39	7	4	10	—	—	*	15	*	4	6	—	—
(Weight Watchers) 7 1/2 oz	90	8	*	*	*	5	8	14	5	*	6	—	—	*	*	—	—	—	—	—

SOUP, READY-TO-EAT (continued)

	Calories	Protein	Fat	Sat. Fat	Cholesterol	Carbohydrates	Fiber	Sodium	Potassium	Calcium	Iron	Zinc	Magnesium	Vitamin A	Vitamin C	Thiamin	Riboflavin	Niacin	Vitamin B$_{12}$	Folic acid
chunky (Campbell's) 9 1/2 oz	260	13	23	—	—	8	—	45	—	6	10	—	—	*	6	2	2	6	—	—
microwave (Campbell's) 7 3/4 oz	200	8	20	—	—	5	—	37	—	2	8	—	—	*	*	*	2	*	—	—
corn chowder (Progresso) 9 1/4 oz	200	8	15	23	3	7	—	35	11	*	6	—	—	6	10	*	6	15	—	—
corn & vegetable (Health Valley) 7 1/2 oz	70	6	*	*	*	4	20	9	10	4	4	—	—	100	10	6	4	6	—	8
country vegetable (Campbell's Home Cookin') 9 1/2 oz	130	7	3	—	—	8	—	32	—	6	6	—	—	150	*	4	15	10	—	—
(Healthy Choice) 7 1/2 oz	120	5	2	—	*	8	—	22	11	4	4	—	—	20	10	4	4	8	—	—
(Hormel) 7 1/2 oz	90	7	3	3	*	5	—	30	12	4	6	4	7	20	*	4	8	10	—	—
crab (generic) 13 oz can	114	14	4	3	5	5	4	78	14	10	10	15	6	15	*	20	7	10	5	6
Creole style chunky (Campbell's) 9 1/2 oz	230	18	12	—	—	10	—	32	—	6	10	—	—	10	*	8	8	8	—	—
escarole (generic) 9 1/2 fl oz	30	3	3	3	*	*	—	75	8	4	4	16	*	—	8	5	3	13	9	10
(Progresso) 9 1/4 oz	30	3	2	*	*	*	*	46	4	2	4	—	—	15	*	*	4	8	—	—
five bean vegetable (Health Valley) 7 1/2 oz	100	15	*	*	*	5	40	10	20	4	4	—	—	100	8	8	4	4	—	8
garden vegetable (Health Valley) 7 1/2 oz	50	8	*	*	*	2	20	10	10	4	6	—	—	100	10	15	4	10	—	6
gazpacho (generic) 13 oz	85	22	5	2	*	*	24	74	10	8	8	2	3	6	8	5	2	7	*	4
ham & bean (Progresso) 9 1/2 oz	130	18	5	3	5	9	40	41	15	8	15	—	—	30	*	10	6	10	—	—
chunky (Campbell's) 10 3/4 oz	280	22	15	—	—	11	—	49	—	4	10	—	—	60	8	8	6	10	—	—
lentil (Campbell's Home Cookin') 10 3/4 oz	150	17	2	—	—	9	—	40	—	4	20	—	—	70	4	10	6	8	—	—
(Progresso) 9 1/2 oz	130	17	3	3	*	8	28	35	13	6	25	—	—	15	*	8	6	6	—	—
(Progresso Healthy Classics) 8 oz	120	12	2	15	*	6	—	17	10	4	15	—	—	20	*	4	2	6	—	—
lentil & carrot (Health Valley) 7 1/2 oz	90	13	*	*	*	5	28	11	11	6	25	—	—	100	*	6	8	25	—	6
lentil ham (generic) 9 1/2 fl oz	151	17	5	6	3	7	—	60	11	5	16	5	6	—	8	13	7	7	5	14
lentil w/ sausage (Progresso) 9 1/2 oz	170	13	12	10	7	7	20	35	12	*	20	—	—	30	8	4	6	8	—	—
macaroni & bean (Progresso) 9 1/2 oz	140	13	8	3	*	8	26	45	11	6	15	—	—	4	*	8	4	6	—	—
Mediterranean vegetable chunky (Campbell's) 9 1/2 oz	170	8	9	—	—	8	—	39	—	6	8	—	—	110	6	8	8	8	—	—
minestrone (Campbell's Home Cookin') 9 1/2 oz	120	7	5	—	—	7	—	45	—	6	4	—	—	70	*	4	6	6	—	—
(Health Valley) 7 1/2 oz	80	13	*	*	*	4	24	12	13	4	8	—	—	100	10	8	4	4	—	8
(Healthy Choice) 7 1/2 oz	160	10	3	—	*	10	—	22	4	2	2	—	—	8	20	2	6	10	—	—
(Hormel) 7 1/2 oz	100	8	2	3	2	6	—	19	10	4	4	4	7	15	6	6	8	10	—	—
(Progresso) 9 1/2 oz	120	12	5	3	*	7	28	38	10	4	15	—	—	30	*	6	4	6	—	—
(Progresso Healthy Classics) 8 oz	120	7	3	3	*	6	—	20	7	4	8	—	—	25	*	4	4	6	—	—

PERCENTAGE DAILY VALUE

519

	Calories	Protein	Fat	Sat. Fat	Cholesterol	Carbohydrates	Fiber	Sodium	Potassium	Calcium	Iron	Zinc	Magnesium	Vitamin A	Vitamin C	Thiamin	Riboflavin	Niacin	Vitamin B₁₂	Folic acid
SOUP, READY-TO-EAT(continued)																				
beef (Progresso) 9 1/2 oz	160	22	8	10	10	5	—	38	10	4	15	—	—	45	4	6	6	15	—	—
chicken (Progresso) 9 1/2 oz	130	18	6	5	7	4	—	36	9	4	10	—	—	60	*	4	6	25	—	—
chunky (Campbell's) 9 1/2 oz	160	10	6	—	—	8	—	36	—	8	10	—	—	70	6	2	4	6	—	—
(generic) 9 1/2 fl oz	143	10	5	9	2	8	8	40	20	7	11	11	4	98	9	4	8	7	*	9
hearty (Progresso) 9 1/4 oz	90	12	3	*	*	5	16	32	10	4	15	—	—	40	2	6	6	6	—	—
no salt added (Hain) 9 1/2 oz	160	12	6	—	*	9	—	3	11	4	10	—	—	35	2	10	6	6	—	—
regular (Hain) 9 1/2 oz	160	12	5	—	*	9	—	39	13	6	10	—	—	35	4	8	6	6	—	—
zesty (Progresso) 9 1/2 oz	150	10	11	15	5	7	16	30	10	4	15	—	—	35	2	6	8	15	—	—
low sodium (Campbell's) 10 1/2 oz	210	5	22	—	—	6	* —	2	—	6	6	—	—	*	*	2	15	4	—	—
mushroom barley (Hain) 10 1/2 oz	100	7	3	3	2	5	—	30	6	2	8	—	—	20	*	*	10	15	—	—
mushroom, cream of (Progresso) 9 1/4 oz	160	7	15	23	5	5	—	47	6	2	4	—	—	*	*	4	8	10	—	—
(Weight Watchers) 10 1/2 oz	70	3	*	*	*	5	4	52	7	8	4	—	—	4	*	—	—	—	—	—
pepper steak chunky (Campbell's) 9 1/2 oz	160	22	5	—	—	7	—	39	—	4	10	—	—	50	8	4	8	10	—	—
sirloin burger chunky (Campbell's) 9 1/2 oz	210	18	14	—	—	7	—	44	—	4	10	—	—	90	6	4	8	10	—	—
split pea (Progresso) 9 1/2 oz	160	18	5	5	*	9	20	44	11	2	15	—	—	2	*	10	4	6	—	—
low sodium (Campbell's) 10 3/4 oz	230	20	6	—	—	12	—	*	—	4	10	—	—	30	8	10	10	15	—	—
split pea & carrots (Health Valley) 7 1/2 oz	80	10	*	*	*	4	28	12	8	6	10	—	—	100	*	20	20	30	—	2
split pea & ham (Campbell's Home Cookin') 9 1/2 oz	190	22	3	—	—	10	—	43	—	4	15	—	—	45	6	10	8	10	—	—
(generic) 9 1/2 oz	208	20	7	—	—	10	18	45	10	4	14	24	11	109	13	9	6	14	5	2
(Healthy Choice) 7 1/2 oz	170	17	5	—	3	8	—	19	13	2	6	—	—	10	10	10	8	10	—	—
(Progresso) 9 1/2 oz	140	17	8	10	8	7	—	39	10	4	15	—	—	25	2	10	6	15	—	—
tomato (Progresso) 9 1/2 oz	90	—	3	3	*	6	16	47	11	4	10	—	—	30	4	4	6	10	—	—
garden (Campbell's Home Cookin') 9 1/2 oz	140	5	5	—	—	8	—	33	—	8	10	—	—	50	4	4	6	4	—	—
(Healthy Choice) 7 1/2 oz	130	7	5	—	2	7	—	21	13	4	4	—	—	10	10	4	6	6	—	—
tomato beef w/ rotini (Progresso) 9 1/2 oz	160	20	8	5	8	6	—	38	10	4	15	—	—	6	*	6	10	25	—	—
tomato tortellini (Progresso) 9 1/4 oz	130	8	8	8	3	5	—	43	10	4	15	—	—	30	*	20	15	35	—	—
tomato vegetable (Health Valley) 7 1/2 oz	50	8	*	*	*	3	24	10	15	4	6	—	—	100	15	6	4	10	—	8
tomato w/ tomato pieces low sodium (Campbell's) 10 1/2 oz	190	7	9	—	—	10	—	2	—	4	8	—	—	30	60	10	10	15	—	—
tortellini (Progresso) 9 1/2 oz	80	8	3	5	2	8	8	36	5	4	15	—	—	60	*	25	15	30	—	—
tortellini, creamy (Progresso) 9 1/4 oz	240	8	25	43	12	6	*	38	9	15	8	—	—	25	*	6	10	8	—	—

	Calories	Protein	Fat	Sat. Fat	Cholesterol	Carbohydrates	Fiber	Sodium	Potassium	Calcium	Iron	Zinc	Magnesium	Vitamin A	Vitamin C	Thiamin	Riboflavin	Niacin	Vitamin B12	Folic acid
SOUP, READY-TO-EAT(continued)																				
turkey																				
chunky (generic) 9 1/2 fl oz	150	19	8	—	—	6	—	29	12	6	12	17	7	145	12	3	7	20	40	3
turkey rice																				
no salt added (Hain) 8 oz	100	10	5	—	3	4	—	3	5	*	4	—	—	25	*	*	4	15	—	—
regular (Hain) 8 oz	80	12	5	—	5	3	—	34	5	*	6	—	—	25	*	2	4	15	—	—
vegetable (Progresso) 9 1/2 oz	90	5	2	*	*	6	12	34	13	4	8	—	—	70	2	4	6	8	—	—
(Progresso Healthy Classics) 8 oz	80	7	2	3	2	4	—	19	6	2	8	—	—	60	2	4	4	10	—	—
chunky (generic) 9 1/2 fl oz	138	7	6	—	—	7	4	47	13	6	10	23	2	132	11	5	4	7	*	—
microwave (Campbell's) 7 3/4 oz	100	5	3	—	—	6	—	38	—	4	4	—	—	60	2	*	*	*	—	—
vegetable barley (Health Valley) 7 1/2 oz	60	7	*	*	*	3	24	10	11	4	6	—	—	100	10	6	4	4	—	8
vegetable beef (Campbell's Home Cookin') 9 1/2 oz	120	18	3	—	—	5	—	42	—	4	10	—	—	90	2	4	8	10	—	—
(Healthy Choice) 7 1/2 oz	130	13	2	—	5	7	—	22	10	4	4	—	—	15	25	6	6	10	—	—
(Weight Watchers) 7 1/2 oz	80	13	2	*	3	4	*	19	6	2	6	—	—	6	*	—	—	—	—	—
chunky low sodium (Campbell's) 10 3/4 oz	180	23	8	—	—	6	—	4	—	4	10	—	—	100	15	10	15	15	—	—
microwave (Campbell's) 7 3/4 oz	100	12	3	—	—	5	—	39	—	2	6	—	—	60	6	4	6	6	—	—
old fashioned chunky (Campbell's) 9 1/2 oz	170	18	9	—	—	6	—	40	—	4	10	—	—	100	6	4	8	10	—	—
vegetable broth, clear (Swanson Natural Goodness) 7 1/4 oz	20	*	2	—	—	*	—	38	—	*	2	—	—	6	6	*	4	10	—	—
vegetable w/ pasta, hearty (Progresso) 9 1/2 oz	100	8	2	*	*	7	16	35	6	4	8	—	—	70	2	15	15	10	—	—
vegetarian lentil (Hain) 10 1/2 oz	160	17	3	*	*	9	24	34	14	4	25	—	—	30	*	8	8	8	—	—
no salt added (Hain) 10 1/2 oz	150	20	3	*	*	8	24	3	15	2	20	—	—	30	*	6	6	10	—	—
vegetarian split pea (Hain) 10 1/2 oz	180	23	2	*	*	11	18	37	12	2	15	—	—	40	*	15	6	10	—	—
no salt added (Hain) 10 1/2 oz	170	23	2	*	*	10	18	3	12	4	15	—	—	25	*	10	4	10	—	—
vegetarian vegetable no salt added (Hain) 9 1/2 oz	150	8	8	—	*	8	—	3	11	4	10	—	—	120	2	10	6	10	—	—
regular (Hain) 9 1/2 oz	150	7	6	—	*	7	—	33	11	4	8	—	—	100	6	4	6	10	—	—
vegetarian veggie broth (Hain) 10 1/2 oz	45	3	*	*	*	3	—	32	5	*	8	—	—	35	*	*	*	4	—	—
no salt added (Hain) 10 1/2 oz	50	2	*	*	*	3	—	4	4	*	8	—	—	45	*	*	*	4	—	—
wild rice (Hain) 10 1/2 oz	90	5	3	*	*	6	14	35	2	*	4	—	—	25	*	*	*	4	—	—
SOUR CREAM SAUCE																				
from mix (generic) 1 cup	125	6	12	—	—	4	—	13	4	9	*	3	*	*	*	*	*	6	*	*
SOUR CREAM see CREAM, SOUR																				

	Calories	Protein	Fat	Sat. Fat	Cholesterol	Carbohydrates	Fiber	Sodium	Potassium	Calcium	Iron	Zinc	Magnesium	Vitamin A	Vitamin C	Thiamin	Riboflavin	Niacin	Vitamin B$_{12}$	Folic acid
SOY BEAN																				
green																				
raw																				
1/2 cup	188	28	13	5	*	5	20	*	23	25	25	8	21	5	62	37	13	11	*	53
raw																				
1/2 cup	387	57	28	14	*	9	36	*	48	26	81	30	65	*	9	54	48	8	*	87
cooked																				
1/2 cup	149	24	12	6	*	3	20	*	13	9	25	7	18	*	2	9	14	2	*	12
cooked, salted																				
1/2 cup	149	24	12	6	*	3	20	8	13	9	25	7	18	*	2	9	14	2	*	12
dry-roasted																				
1/2 cup	387	57	29	14	*	9	28	*	33	23	19	27	49	*	7	24	38	5	*	44
green																				
boiled																				
1/2 cup	127	19	9	4	*	3	16	*	14	13	12	5	14	3	25	16	8	6	*	25
boiled, salted																				
1/2 cup	127	19	9	4	*	3	16	9	14	13	12	5	14	3	25	16	8	6	*	25
roasted																				
1/2 cup	405	50	34	16	*	10	—	6	36	12	19	18	31	3	3	6	7	6	*	45
SOY BEAN CURD see TOFU																				
SOY BEAN OIL																				
hydrogenated																				
1 tbsp	120	*	22	10	*	*	*	*	*	*	*	*	*	*	*	*	*	*	*	*
regular																				
1 tbsp	120	*	22	10	*	*	*	*	*	*	*	*	*	*	*	*	*	*	*	*
w/ added vitamin E																				
1 tbsp	120	*	22	15	*	*	*	*	*	*	*	*	*	*	*	*	*	*	*	*
SOY BEAN & COTTONSEED OIL																				
hydrogenated																				
1 tbsp	120	*	23	12	*	*	*	*	*	*	*	*	*	*	*	*	*	*	*	*
SOY BEAN SNACK																				
roasted																				
1 oz	129	18	10	5	*	3	4	*	12	4	7	7	12	*	*	2	2	2	*	16
roasted, salted																				
1 oz	129	18	10	5	*	3	—	2	12	4	7	7	12	*	*	2	2	2	*	16
SOY BEAN SPROUT																				
raw																				
1/2 cup	43	8	4	*	*	*	—	*	5	2	4	3	6	*	9	8	2	2	*	15
steamed																				
1/2 cup	38	7	3	*	*	*	*	*	5	3	3	3	7	*	6	6	*	3	*	9
steamed, salted																				
1/2 cup	38	7	3	*	*	*	*	5	5	3	3	3	7	*	6	6	*	3	*	9
stir-fried																				
3 oz	106	19	9	4	*	3	—	*	14	7	2	12	20	*	17	24	9	5	*	27
stir-fried, salted																				
3 oz	106	19	9	—	*	3	—	9	14	7	2	12	20	*	17	24	9	5	*	27
SOY FLOUR																				
defatted																				
(generic) 1 cup stirred	329	78	2	*	*	13	72	*	68	24	51	16	73	*	*	46	15	13	*	77
(generic) 1/2 cup	207	46	2	*	*	8	—	*	43	15	46	21	47	*	*	28	9	8	*	46
low fat																				
(generic) 1 cup stirred	287	68	9	5	*	11	36	*	64	17	29	7	50	*	*	22	15	10	*	90
SOY LECITHIN																				
1 tbsp	104	*	22	10	*	*	*	*	*	*	*	*	*	*	*	*	*	*	*	*
SOY MILK																				
1/2 cup	40	5	4	*	*	*	8	*	5	*	4	2	6	*	*	13	5	*	*	*
Soy Moo																				
(Health Valley) 1 cup	110	10	*	*	*	6	*	*	*	40	40	—	—	20	*	15	6	15	—	—

PERCENTAGE DAILY VALUE

	Calories	Protein	Fat	Sat. Fat	Cholesterol	Carbohydrates	Fiber	Sodium	Potassium	Calcium	Iron	Zinc	Magnesium	Vitamin A	Vitamin C	Thiamin	Riboflavin	Niacin	Vitamin B₁₂	Folic acid

PERCENTAGE DAILY VALUE

	Calories	Protein	Fat	Sat. Fat	Cholesterol	Carbohydrates	Fiber	Sodium	Potassium	Calcium	Iron	Zinc	Magnesium	Vitamin A	Vitamin C	Thiamin	Riboflavin	Niacin	Vitamin B₁₂	Folic acid
SOY SAUCE																				
lite (La Choy) 1 tbsp	3	*	*	*	*	*	*	15	5	*	*	—	—	*	*	*	*	*	—	—
regular (La Choy) 1 tbsp	6	*	*	*	*	*	*	30	*	*	*	—	—	*	*	*	*	*	—	—
soy & wheat (generic) 1 tbsp	10	2	*	*	*	*	*	43	*	*	2	*	2	*	*	*	*	*	3	*	*
tamari (generic) 1 tbsp	11	3	*	*	*	*	*	42	*	*	2	*	2	*	*	*	*	2	4	*	*
w/ vegetable protein (generic) 1 tbsp	7	*	*	*	*	*	*	43	*	*	*	*	*	*	*	*	*	*	3	*	*
SPAGHETTI see PASTA																				
SPAGHETTI SAUCE see PASTA SAUCE																				
SPAGHETTI SQUASH see SQUASH																				
SPARE RIBS see PORK																				
SPICES see specific listings																				
SPINACH																				
raw 1/2 cup chopped	6	*	*	*	*	*	4	*	4	3	4	*	6	38	13	*	3	*	*	14
boiled 1/2 cup	21	4	*	*	*	*	8	3	12	12	18	5	20	147	15	6	12	2	*	33
boiled w/ salt 1/2 cup	21	4	*	*	*	*	—	11	12	12	18	5	20	147	15	6	12	2	*	33
SPINACH, CANNED																				
(Bush Bros) 1/2 cup	30	5	*	*	*	*	8	16	—	10	6	—	—	75	15	—	—	—	—	—
chopped (Del Monte) 1/2 cup	30	3	*	*	*	*	8	15	—	10	6	—	—	50	40	—	—	—	—	—
drained (generic) 1/2 cup	25	5	*	*	*	*	—	*	11	14	14	3	20	188	25	*	9	2	*	26
low salt solid & liquid (generic) 1/2 cup	22	4	*	*	*	*	12	4	8	10	10	3	16	151	26	*	7	2	*	17
no salt added (Del Monte) 1/2 cup	30	3	*	*	*	*	8	4	—	10	6	—	—	60	40	—	—	—	—	—
reduced salt (Del Monte) 1/2 cup	30	3	*	*	*	*	8	8	—	10	6	—	—	60	40	—	—	—	—	—
solid & liquid (generic) 1/2 cup	22	4	*	*	*	*	12	16	8	10	10	3	16	151	26	*	7	2	*	17
whole leaf (Del Monte) 1/2 cup	30	3	*	*	*	*	8	15	—	10	6	—	—	50	40	—	—	—	—	—
SPINACH, FROZEN																				
(Green Giant) 1/2 cup	25	5	*	*	*	2	20	4	7	10	10	—	—	100	30	4	10	4	—	—
(Green Giant Harvest Fresh) 1/2 cup	25	7	*	*	*	2	12	7	15	10	8	—	—	50	10	4	10	2	—	—
boiled (generic) 1/2 cup	27	5	*	*	*	2	12	3	8	14	8	4	16	148	19	4	9	2	*	26
boiled, salted (generic) 1/2 cup	27	5	*	*	*	2	—	13	8	14	8	4	16	148	19	4	9	2	*	26
creamed (Green Giant) 1/2 cup	70	5	5	5	*	3	8	20	11	10	4	—	—	35	4	4	10	2	—	—
microwave (Bird's Eye Deluxe) 4 3/4 oz	90	5	8	—	—	3	4	13	—	8	2	—	—	30	25	6	10	*	—	—
in butter sauce (Green Giant) 1/2 cup	40	5	3	3	2	2	14	16	19	6	2	—	—	140	40	4	10	4	—	—
whole leaf (Bird's Eye) 3 1/3 oz	20	5	*	*	*	*	12	4	—	10	10	*	2	150	45	6	8	2	15	20
SPLIT PEA																				
cooked 1/2 cup	116	14	*	*	*	7	32	*	10	*	7	7	9	*	*	12	3	4	*	16

	Calories	Protein	Fat	Sat. Fat	Cholesterol	Carbohydrates	Fiber	Sodium	Potassium	Calcium	Iron	Zinc	Magnesium	Vitamin A	Vitamin C	Thiamin	Riboflavin	Niacin	Vitamin B₁₂	Folic acid
SPLIT PEA (continued)																				
cooked, salted																				
1/2 cup	116	14	*	*	*	7	—	10	10	*	7	7	9	*	*	12	3	4	*	16
SPORTS DRINK																				
all flavors																				
(Gatorade) 8 fl oz	50	*	*	*	*	5	*	5	—	*	*	*	*	*	*	*	*	*	*	*
Lemon Recharge (Knudsen Sports Beverages) 8 fl oz	70	*	*	*	*	6	*	*	*	*	*	*	—	—	*	4	—	—	—	—
Lemon Recharge, organic (Knudsen Sports Beverages) 8 fl oz	70	*	*	*	*	6	*	*	*	*	*	*	—	—	*	4	—	—	—	—
Orange Recharge (Knudsen Sports Beverages) 8 fl oz	70	7	*	*	*	6	*	*	*	*	*	*	—	—	60	4	—	—	—	—
thirst quencher (generic) 6 fl oz	45	*	*	*	*	4	*	3	*	*	*	*	*	*	*	*	*	*	—	*
Tropical Recharge (Knudsen Sports Beverages) 8 fl oz	70	*	*	*	*	6	*	*	*	*	*	*	—	—	*	4	—	—	—	—
SPOT																				
raw																				
1 fillet	79	20	5	5	13	*	*	*	9	*	*	2	7	*	*	7	8	22	32	*
broiled/baked																				
1 fillet	79	20	5	5	13	*	*	*	9	*	*	2	7	*	*	6	8	21	29	*
SPROUTS see specific listings																				
SQUAB																				
breast																				
raw																				
1 breast	135	37	7	6	30	*	*	2	7	*	13	18	7	*	9	16	14	37	8	*
meat w/ out skin																				
raw																				
1 squab	239	49	19	17	50	*	*	4	11	2	42	30	11	3	20	32	28	58	13	3
meat w/ skin																				
raw																				
1 squab	585	61	73	84	63	*	*	4	11	2	39	29	11	10	17	28	26	60	13	3
SQUASH, ACORN																				
raw																				
1 cup cubes	56	2	*	*	*	5	—	*	14	5	5	*	11	10	26	13	*	5	*	6
1 medium	172	6	*	*	*	15	—	*	43	14	17	4	34	29	79	40	3	15	*	18
baked																				
1/2 cup cubes	57	2	*	*	*	5	—	*	13	4	5	*	11	9	18	11	*	4	*	5
baked w/ salt																				
1/2 cup cubes	57	2	*	*	*	5	—	10	13	4	5	*	11	9	18	11	*	4	*	5
boiled																				
1/2 cup mashed	41	*	*	*	*	4	—	*	9	3	4	*	8	6	13	8	*	3	*	3
boiled w/ salt																				
1/2 cup mashed	41	*	*	*	*	4	—	12	9	3	4	*	8	6	13	8	*	3	*	3
SQUASH, BUTTERNUT																				
raw																				
1/2 cup cubes	32	*	*	*	*	3	—	*	7	3	3	*	6	109	24	5	*	4	*	5
baked																				
1/2 cup cubes	41	2	*	*	*	4	—	*	8	4	3	*	7	143	26	5	*	5	*	5
baked, salted																				
1/2 cup cubes	41	2	*	*	*	4	—	10	8	4	3	*	7	143	26	5	*	5	—	5
frozen																				
3 oz	48	2	*	*	*	4	4	*	5	2	4	*	3	81	9	5	3	3	*	5
boiled																				
1/2 cup mashed	47	2	*	*	*	4	—	*	5	2	4	*	3	80	7	4	3	3	*	5
w/salt																				
1/2 cup mashed	47	2	*	*	*	4	—	12	5	2	4	*	3	80	7	4	3	3	*	5

	Calories	Protein	Fat	Sat. Fat	Cholesterol	Carbohydrates	Fiber	Sodium	Potassium	Calcium	Iron	Zinc	Magnesium	Vitamin A	Vitamin C	Thiamin	Riboflavin	Niacin	Vitamin B₁₂	Folic acid
SQUASH, CROOKNECK																				
raw 1/2 cup slices	12	*	*	*	*	*	—	*	4	*	2	*	3	4	9	2	2	*	*	4
boiled 1/2 cup slices	18	*	*	*	*	*	4	*	5	2	2	2	5	5	8	3	3	2	*	5
boiled, salted 1/2 cup slices	18	*	*	*	*	*	—	9	5	2	2	2	5	5	8	3	3	2	*	5
canned drained 1/2 cup slices	14	*	*	*	*	*	—	*	3	*	4	2	4	3	5	*	2	2	*	3
frozen 1/2 cup slices	13	*	*	*	*	*	4	*	4	*	2	2	4	4	7	2	2	*	*	2
boiled 1/2 cup slices	24	2	*	*	*	2	—	*	7	2	3	2	6	4	11	2	3	2	*	3
boiled, w/ salt 1/2 cup slices	24	2	*	*	*	2	—	10	7	2	3	2	6	4	11	2	3	2	*	3
SQUASH, HUBBARD																				
raw 1/2 cup cubes	23	2	*	*	*	2	—	*	5	*	*	*	3	63	11	3	*	*	*	2
baked 1/2 cup cubes	51	4	*	*	*	4	—	*	10	2	3	*	6	123	16	5	3	3	*	4
baked w/ salt 1/2 cup cubes	51	4	*	*	*	4	—	10	10	2	3	*	6	123	16	5	3	3	*	4
boiled 1/2 cup mashed	35	3	*	*	*	3	12	*	7	*	2	*	4	95	13	3	2	2	*	3
boiled, salted 1/2 cup mashed	35	3	*	*	*	3	12	12	7	*	2	*	4	95	13	3	2	2	*	3
SQUASH, SCALLOPED																				
raw 1/2 cup slices	12	*	*	*	*	*	—	*	3	*	*	*	4	*	19	3	*	2	*	5
boiled 1/2 cup slices	14	2	*	*	*	*	4	*	4	*	2	*	4	2	16	3	*	2	*	5
1/2 cup mashed	19	2	*	*	*	*	4	*	5	2	2	2	6	2	22	4	2	3	*	6
boiled, salted 1/2 cup slices	14	2	*	*	*	*	—	9	4	*	2	*	4	2	16	3	*	2	*	5
SQUASH, SPAGHETTI																				
raw 1/2 cup cubes	17	*	*	*	*	*	—	*	2	*	*	*	*	*	2	*	*	2	*	2
boiled 1/2 cup	23	*	*	*	*	2	4	*	3	2	*	*	2	2	5	2	*	3	*	2
boiled w/ salt 1/2 cup	23	*	*	*	*	2	4	8	3	2	*	*	2	2	5	2	*	3	*	2
SQUASH, SUMMER																				
raw 1/2 cup slices	13	*	*	*	*	*	4	*	4	*	2	*	4	3	16	3	*	2	*	4
boiled 1/2 cup slices	18	*	*	*	*	*	4	*	5	2	2	2	5	5	8	3	2	2	*	5
boiled w/ salt 1/2 cup slices	18	*	*	*	*	*	—	9	5	2	2	2	5	5	8	3	2	2	*	5
SQUASH, WINTER																				
raw 1/2 cup cubes	21	*	*	*	*	2	4	*	6	2	2	*	3	47	12	4	*	2	*	3
baked 1/2 cup cubes	40	2	*	*	*	3	12	*	13	*	2	2	2	73	16	6	*	4	*	7
baked w/ salt 1/2 cup cubes	40	2	*	*	*	3	—	10	13	*	2	2	2	73	16	6	*	4	*	7
SQUASH, YELLOW																				
canned sliced (Bush Bros) 1/2 cup	20	2	*	*	*	*	4	15	—	*	4	—	—	*	4	—	—	—	—	—

	Calories	Protein	Fat	Sat. Fat	Cholesterol	Carbohydrates	Fiber	Sodium	Potassium	Calcium	Iron	Zinc	Magnesium	Vitamin A	Vitamin C	Thiamin	Riboflavin	Niacin	Vitamin B₁₂	Folic acid
SQUASH KERNEL																				
roasted w/ salt																				
1 oz	148	16	18	12	*	*	8	7	7	*	24	14	38	2	*	4	5	2	*	4
SQUASH SEED																				
roasted w/ salt																				
1 oz (85 seeds)	127	9	8	5	*	5	8	7	7	2	5	19	19	*	*	*	*	*	*	*
SQUID																				
raw																				
3 oz	78	22	2	*	66	*	*	2	6	3	3	9	7	*	7	*	21	9	18	*
fried																				
3 oz	149	25	10	8	74	2	*	11	7	3	5	10	8	*	6	3	23	11	17	*
SQUIRREL																				
roasted																				
braised																				
3 oz	146	44	6	2	35	*	*	5	8	*	32	13	6	*	*	4	15	20	117	2
STRAWBERRY, FROZEN																				
sweetened																				
sliced																				
1/2 cup	245	2	*	*	*	22	20	*	7	3	8	*	4	*	176	3	8	5	—	10
whole																				
1/2 cup	100	*	*	*	*	9	*	*	4	*	3	*	2	*	84	*	6	2	—	*
unsweetened																				
1/2 cup	26	*	*	*	*	3	6	*	3	*	3	*	2	*	51	*	*	*	—	3
STRAWBERRY DRINK																				
from mix																				
(Kool-Aid) 8 fl oz	70	*	*	*	*	6	*	*	*	*	*	*	*	*	10	*	*	*	*	*
unsweetened																				
(Kool-Aid) 8 fl oz prep w/out sugar	2	*	*	*	*	*	*	*	*	*	*	*	*	*	10	*	*	*	*	*
sugar added																				
(Kool-Aid) 8 fl oz prep w/ sugar	100	*	*	*	*	8	*	*	*	*	*	*	*	*	10	*	*	*	*	*
strawberry float																				
(Knudsen) 8 fl oz	140	2	*	*	*	11	*	2	3	4	*	*	*	*	15	—	*	*	—	*
STRAWBERRY GLAZE																				
(Marie's) 2 1/3 oz	90	*	*	*	*	7	*	3	—	*	*	*	*	*	*	*	*	*	—	*
STRAWBERRY JUICE																				
(Farmer's Market) 8 fl oz	120	*	*	*	*	10	*	*	2	*	*	*	*	*	4	—	—	—	—	—
STRAWBERRY MILK DRINK																				
from mix																				
(generic)																				
1 cup milk + 2–3 heaping tsps	234	13	13	*	11	11	*	5	11	29	*	6	8	6	4	6	25	*	15	3
(Quik) 2 tbsp & 1 cup																				
low-fat milk	210	16	7	15	6	11	*	5	13	30	*	7	9	10	*	7	*	*	16	22
STRAWBERRY NECTAR																				
(Knudsen Exotic Blends) 8 fl oz	120	*	*	*	*	10	*	*	3	*	2	—	*	*	10	—	—	—	—	—
STRAWBERRY TOPPING																				
(generic) 2 tbsp	107	*	*	*	*	9	*	*	*	*	2	*	*	*	17	*	*	*	*	*
(Kraft) 2 tbsp	100	*	*	*	*	10	*	*	*	*	*	*	*	*	*	*	*	*	*	*
(Smucker's) 2 tbsp	120	*	*	*	*	10	*	*	—	*	*	*	*	*	*	*	*	*	*	*
STRAWBERRY-BANANA JUICE																				
(Knudsen Exotic Blends) 8 fl oz	120	*	*	*	*	10	*	*	3	*	2	—	*	*	10	—	—	—	—	—
STRAWBERRY-GUAVA JUICE																				
(Knudsen Tropical Blend) 8 fl oz	110	*	*	*	*	9	*	*	2	2	4	—	*	4	40	—	—	—	—	—
organic																				
(Santa Cruz Natural) 8 fl oz	100	*	*	*	*	8	*	*	3	4	*	—	*	*	2	—	—	—	—	—
STRAWBERRY-LEMON JUICE																				
organic																				
(Santa Cruz Natural) 8 fl oz	120	*	*	*	*	10	*	*	2	*	*	—	*	*	8	—	—	—	—	—
STROGANOFF SAUCE																				
(General Mills Recipe Sauce)																				
1/6 jar (4 oz)	60	2	6	10	3	2	—	22	2	2	—	*	*	*	*	*	2	*	—	—
from mix																				
(generic) 1/4 cup	21	*	*	—	—	*	*	10	2	4	*	*	*	*	*	*	8	4	2	*

	Calories	Protein	Fat	Sat. Fat	Cholesterol	Carbohydrates	Fiber	Sodium	Potassium	Calcium	Iron	Zinc	Magnesium	Vitamin A	Vitamin C	Thiamin	Riboflavin	Niacin	Vitamin B₁₂	Folic acid

STRUDEL

	Calories	Protein	Fat	Sat. Fat	Cholesterol	Carb.	Fiber	Sodium	Potassium	Calcium	Iron	Zinc	Magn.	Vit. A	Vit. C	Thiamin	Ribo.	Niacin	Vit. B₁₂	Folic acid
apple toaster (Pillsbury) 1 pastry	200	5	14	10	2	9	—	8	*	*	2	—	—	*	*	8	6	6	—	—
blueberry toaster (Pillsbury) 1 pastry	190	5	14	10	2	9	—	9	*	*	2	—	—	*	*	8	6	6	—	—
cinnamon toaster (Pillsbury) 1 pastry	200	8	15	10	2	8	—	8	*	*	2	—	—	*	*	8	6	6	—	—
strawberry toaster (Pillsbury) 1 pastry	190	5	14	10	2	9	—	8	*	*	2	—	—	*	*	8	6	6	—	—

STUFFED PEPPER see VEGETABLE, FROZEN

STUFFING

	Calories	Protein	Fat	Sat. Fat	Cholesterol	Carb.	Fiber	Sodium	Potassium	Calcium	Iron	Zinc	Magn.	Vit. A	Vit. C	Thiamin	Ribo.	Niacin	Vit. B₁₂	Folic acid
apple & raisin (Pepperidge Farm Distinctive) 1 oz	110	4	6	—		7	—	17	—	2	10			*	2	10	6	6		
beef (Stove Top) 1/2 cup	180	6	14	—	*	7	—	25	3	2	6	—	—	10	*	6	4	4		
broccoli & cheese microwave (Stove Top) 1/2 cup	170	6	12	—	2	7	—	24	2	6	6	—	—	4	*	6	6	4		
chicken (General Mills) 1/2 cup	180	7	14	—	—	7	—	26	2	2	8	—	—	6	*	10	6	8		
chicken flavor (Stove Top) 1/2 cup	180	6	14	—	*	7	—	21	2	2	6	—	—	6	*	6	4	4		
flexible serving (Stove Top) 1/2 cup	170	6	14	—	*	7	—	24	2	2	6	—	—	6	*	6	4	4		
microwave (Stove Top) 1/2 cup	160	6	12	—	*	7	—	20	2	2	6	—	—	4	*	6	4	4		
chicken flavor w/ rice (Stove Top) 1/2 cup	180	6	14	—	*	7	—	23	2	2	6	—	—	6	*	6	4	6		
classic chicken (Pepperidge Farm Distinctive) 1 oz	110	6	2	—	—	7	—	17	—	4	8			6	8	10	6	10	—	—
cornbread (Arnold) 1 oz	100	4	4	*	*	6	8	12	—	*	4	—	—	*	*	8	4	4		
(Brownberry) 1 oz	100	4	4	*	*	6	8	12	—	*	4	—	—	*	*	4	4	4		
(Pepperidge Farm) 1 oz	110	4	2	—	—	7	—	13	—	2	6			*	*	10	6	6		
(Stove Top) 1/2 cup	180	4	14	—	*	7	—	23	2	2	6	—	—	8	*	4	2	4		
flexible serving (Stove Top) 1/2 cup	180	6	14	—	*	7	—	25	2	2	6	—	—	6	*	4	4	4		
homestyle microwave (Stove Top) 1/2 cup	160	4	11	—	*	7	—	19	2	*	4	—	—	4	*	4	2	4		
country garden herb (Pepperidge Farm Distinctive) 1 oz	120	6	5	—		6	—	12	—	4	10	—	—	*	4	10	6	6		
country style (Pepperidge Farm) 1 oz	100	6	2	—		7	—	17	—	4	8	—	—	*	*	10	6	8		
cube (Pepperidge Farm) 1 oz	110	4	2	—		7	—	17	—	4	8	—	—	*	*	10	6	8		
harvest vegetable & almond (Pepperidge Farm Distinctive) 1 oz	110	6	8	—		6	—	10	—	4	15	—	—	*	10	10	6	6		
herb seasoned (Arnold) 1 oz	100	4	4	—	*	*	8	12	—	*	4	—	—	*	*	8	4	4	—	—
(Pepperidge Farm) 1 oz	110	6	2	—	—	7	—	16	—	4	8	—	—	*	*	10	6	8		
restaurant style (Pepperidge Farm) 1 oz	110	6	2	*	*	7	—	16	—	4	8	—	—	*	*	10	6	8		
herb, traditional (General Mills) 1/2 cup	180	7	12	—	—	7	—	27	2	2	6	—	—	6	*	10	6	8	—	—

	Calories	Protein	Fat	Sat. Fat	Cholesterol	Carbohydrates	Fiber	Sodium	Potassium	Calcium	Iron	Zinc	Magnesium	Vitamin A	Vitamin C	Thiamin	Riboflavin	Niacin	Vitamin B12	Folic acid
STUFFING (continued)																				
homestyle herb																				
flexible serving																				
(Stove Top) 1/2 cup	170	6	14	—	*	7	—	21	2	4	8	—	—	6	*	6	4	4	—	—
honey pecan cornbread																				
(Pepperidge Farm																				
Distinctive) 1 oz	120	4	2	5	*	6	—	14	—	*	6	—	—	20	4	10	4	10	—	—
long grain & wild rice																				
(Stove Top) 1/2 cup	180	6	14	—	*	7	—	23	2	2	6	—	—	6	*	6	4	6	—	—
mushroom & onion																				
(Stove Top) 1/2 cup	170	6	11	—	*	7	—	21	2	2	6	—	—	4	*	6	4	4	—	—
pork																				
(Stove Top) 1/2 cup	180	6	14	—	*	7	—	23	3	4	6	—	—	8	*	15	4	6	—	—
flexible serving																				
(Stove Top) 1/2 cup	170	6	14	—	*	7	—	26	2	4	6	—	—	6	*	15	4	4	—	—
sage & onion																				
(Arnold) 1 oz	100	4	4	*	*	6	8	20	—	*	8	—	—	*	*	8	4	4	—	—
(Pepperidge Farm																				
Distinctive) 1 oz	100	6	2	*	*	7	8	22	—	2	8	—	—	*	*	15	10	10	—	—
San Francisco																				
(Stove Top) 1/2 cup	170	6	14	—	*	7	—	27	2	2	6	—	—	8	*	6	4	6	—	—
savory herbs flavor																				
(Stove Top) 1/2 cup	180	6	14	—	*	7	—	24	3	4	6	—	—	8	*	6	4	4	—	—
seasoned																				
(Arnold) 1 oz	100	4	4	*	*	6	8	16	—	*	8	—	—	*	*	8	4	4	—	—
turkey flavor																				
(Stove Top) 1/2 cup	180	6	14	—	*	7	—	26	3	4	6	—	—	6	*	6	4	4	—	—
wild rice & mushroom																				
(Pepperidge Farm																				
Distinctive) 1 oz	130	6	2	—	—	6	—	13	—	2	8	—	—	*	8	10	6	6	—	—
STURGEON																				
raw																				
3 oz	89	23	5	4	17	*	*	2	7	*	3	2	7	12	*	4	3	35	31	*
baked/broiled																				
3 oz	115	29	7	5	22	*	*	2	9	*	4	3	10	14	*	5	4	43	35	*
smoked																				
3 oz	147	44	6	5	23	*	*	26	9	*	4	3	10	16	*	5	4	47	41	*
SUCCOTASH																				
boiled w/ salt																				
1/2 cup	110	8	*	*	*	8	—	10	11	2	8	4	13	6	13	11	5	6	*	8
SUCCOTASH, CANNED																				
boiled																				
1/2 cup	110	8	*	*	*	8	—	*	11	2	8	4	13	6	13	11	5	6	*	8
drained																				
1/2 cup	102	6	*	*	*	8	—	14	7	*	4	4	*	4	14	2	5	4	*	15
solid & liquid																				
1/2 cup	81	6	*	*	*	6	28	12	6	*	4	4	6	4	10	2	4	4	*	10
SUCCOTASH, FROZEN																				
boiled																				
1/2 cup	79	6	*	*	*	6	20	2	6	*	4	3	5	4	8	4	3	6	*	7
boiled w/ salt																				
1/2 cup	79	6	*	*	*	6	—	10	6	*	4	3	5	4	8	4	3	6	*	7
SUCKER, WHITE																				
raw																				
1 fillet	146	44	6	4	22	*	*	3	17	11	11	8	12	5	*	*	7	10	53	*
broiled/baked																				
1 fillet	148	44	6	4	22	*	*	3	17	11	11	8	12	5	*	*	6	9	48	*
SUGAR																				
brown																				
(generic) 1 cup	827	*	*	*	*	71	*	4	22	19	23	3	16	*	*	*	*	*	*	*

	Calories	Protein	Fat	Sat. Fat	Cholesterol	Carbohydrates	Fiber	Sodium	Potassium	Calcium	Iron	Zinc	Magnesium	Vitamin A	Vitamin C	Thiamin	Riboflavin	Niacin	Vitamin B12	Folic acid
SUGAR (continued)																				
granulated (generic) 1 tbsp	15	*	*	*	*	*	*	*	*	*	*	*	*	*	*	*	*	*	*	*
maple (generic) 1 piece	100	*	*	*	*	9	*	*	2	3	3	11	*	*	*	*	*	*	*	*
powdered (generic) 1 tbsp	31	*	*	*	*	3	*	*	*	*	*	*	*	*	*	*	*	*	*	*
turbinado (Hain) 1 tbsp	50	*	*	*	*	4	*	*	*	*	*	*	*	*	*	*	*	*	*	*
SUGAR SUBSTITUTE																				
(Sprinkle Sweet) 1 tsp	0	*	*	*	*	*	*	*	*	*	*	*	*	*	*	*	*	*	*	*
(Sweet*10) 1/8 tsp	0	*	*	*	*	*	*	*	*	*	*	*	*	*	*	*	*	*	*	*
SUGAR-APPLE																				
1 fruit	146	5	*	*	*	12	28	*	11	4	5	—	8	*	94	11	10	7	*	—
1/2 cup pulp	118	4	*	*	*	10	24	*	9	3	4	—	7	*	76	9	8	6	*	—
SUMMER SAUSAGE see THURINGER CERVELAT																				
SUMMER SQUASH see SQUASH																				
SUNFISH																				
raw 1 fillet	43	16	*	*	11	*	*	2	5	4	3	5	4	*	*	3	2	3	16	*
broiled/baked 1 fillet	42	15	*	*	11	*	*	2	5	4	3	5	4	*	*	2	2	3	14	*
SUNFLOWER NUT																				
(Fisher) 1 oz	170	13	23	8	*	2	8	7	—	2	*	—	—	*	*	—	—	—	—	—
SUNFLOWER OIL																				
hydrogenated (generic) 1 tbsp	120	*	20	9	*	*	*	*	*	*	*	*	*	*	*	*	*	*	*	*
regular (Wesson) 1 tbsp	120	*	22	9	*	*	*	*	*	*	*	—	*	*	*	*	*	*	*	—
SUNFLOWER SEED																				
(Frito-Lay) 1/3 cup	140	7	12	5	*	4	48	56		—	—	—	—	—	—	—	—	—	—	—
(generic) 1 oz	164	9	21	7	*	3	—	*	*	3	7	10	26	*	*	6	5	8	*	17
dried (generic) 1 oz	162	11	22	8	*	2	12	*	6	3	11	10	25	*	*	43	4	6	*	16
in shell (Fisher) 1 oz	170	13	23	8	*	2	8	5	—	2	6	—	—	*	*	—	—	—	—	—
dry-roasted (generic) 1 oz	165	9	22	8	*	2	12	*	7	2	6	10	9	*	*	2	4	10	*	17
dry-roasted w/ salt (generic) 1 oz	165	9	22	8	*	2	8	9	7	2	6	10	9	*	*	2	4	10	*	17
oil-roasted (generic) 1 oz	175	10	25	9	*	2	8	*	4	2	11	10	9	*	*	6	5	6	*	17
oil-roasted w/ salt (generic) 1 oz	175	10	25	9	*	2	8	7	4	2	11	10	9	*	*	6	5	6	*	17
partially defatted (generic) 1 tbsp	16	4	*	*	*	*	*	*	*	*	2	2	4	*	*	11	*	2	*	3
toasted (generic) 1 oz	176	8	25	9	*	2	—	*	4	2	11	10	9	*	*	6	5	6	*	17
toasted w/ salt (generic) 1 oz	176	8	25	9	*	2	—	7	4	2	11	10	9	*	*	6	5	6	*	17
SURIMI																				
imitation king crab 3 oz	87	17	2	*	6	3	*	30	2	*	2	2	9	*	*	2	*	*	23	*
imitation scallop 3 oz	84	18	*	*	6	3	*	28	3	*	*	2	9	*	*	*	*	*	23	*
imitation shrimp 3 oz	86	18	2	*	10	3	*	25	2	2	3	2	9	*	*	*	*	2	23	*
plain 3 oz	84	21	*	*	8	2	*	5	3	*	*	2	9	*	*	*	*	*	23	*

	Calories	Protein	Fat	Sat. Fat	Cholesterol	Carbohydrates	Fiber	Sodium	Potassium	Calcium	Iron	Zinc	Magnesium	Vitamin A	Vitamin C	Thiamin	Riboflavin	Niacin	Vitamin B₁₂	Folic acid
SWAMP CABBAGE																				
shoot																				
raw																				
1 cup chopped	11	2	*	*	*	*	4	3	5	4	5	*	10	71	51	*	3	3	*	8
boiled																				
1 cup chopped	20	3	*	*	*	*	8	5	8	5	7	*	7	102	26	3	5	2	*	9
boiled w/ salt																				
1/2 cup chopped	10	2	*	*	*	*	—	7	4	3	4	*	4	51	13	2	2	*	*	4
SWEET POTATO																				
raw																				
1 sweet potato (5")	137	4	*	*	*	11	16	*	8	3	4	2	3	522	49	6	11	4	*	5
1/2 cup cubes	70	2	*	*	*	5	8	*	4	*	2	*	2	269	25	3	6	2	*	2
baked																				
1/2 cup mashed	103	3	*	*	*	8	12	*	10	3	2	2	5	436	41	5	7	3	*	6
1 sweet potato (5")	117	3	*	*	*	9	12	*	11	3	3	2	6	498	47	6	9	3	*	6
boiled																				
w/ out skin																				
1 cup mashed	344	9	2	*	*	27	32	2	17	7	10	6	8	1119	93	12	27	10	*	9
w/salt																				
1/2 cup mashed	172	5	*	*	*	13	—	17	9	3	5	3	4	559	47	6	14	—	*	—
candied																				
1 piece	144	2	5	7	3	10	—	3	6	3	7	*	3	88	12	*	3	2	*	3
SWEET POTATO, CANNED																				
in syrup																				
drained																				
1/2 cup	106	2	*	*	*	8	—	2	5	2	5	*	3	140	18	2	2	2	*	2
solid & liquid																				
1/2 cup	101	2	*	*	*	8	8	2	6	2	5	*	4	130	20	2	3	3	*	2
mashed																				
1/2 cup	128	4	*	*	*	10	—	4	8	4	9	2	8	384	11	2	7	6	*	3
vacuum packed																				
1/2 cup pieces	91	3	*	*	*	7	12	2	9	2	5	*	6	160	44	2	3	4	*	4
SWEET POTATO, FROZEN																				
baked																				
(generic) 1/2 cup cubes	88	3	*	*	*	7	12	*	9	3	3	2	5	289	13	4	3	2	*	5
baked, salted																				
(generic) 1/2 cup cubes	88	3	*	*	*	7	—	9	9	3	3	2	5	289	13	4	3	2	*	5
candied																				
(Mrs. Paul's) 1/2 cup	190	*	2	*	*	15	—	6	—	2	2	—	—	110	4	2	4	2	*	—
w/ apples																				
(Mrs. Paul's) 1/2 cup	160	*	*	*	*	13	—	2	—	8	4	—	—	25	50	2	4	*	*	—
SWEET POTATO LEAF																				
raw																				
1/2 cup chopped	6	*	*	*	*	*	—	*	3	*	*	*	3	4	3	2	4	*	*	4
1 leaf	6	*	*	*	*	*	—	*	2	*	*	*	2	3	3	2	3	*	*	3
steamed																				
1/2 cup	11	*	*	*	*	*	4	*	4	*	*	*	5	6	*	2	5	2	*	4
w/ salt																				
1/2 cup	11	*	*	*	*	*	—	3	4	*	*	*	5	6	*	2	5	2	*	4
SWEET PEPPER see PEPPER, BELL																				
SWEET & SOUR SAUCE																				
(Contadina) 1/2 cup	160	*	8	*	*	12	*	20	—	*	8	—	—	*	*	—	—	—	—	—
(General Mills																				
Recipe Sauce) 1/2 cup	130	*	*	*	*	11	—	15	*	*	*	*	*	*	*	*	*	*	—	—
(La Choy) 1/2 cup	200	*	*	*	*	16	*	16	2	*	*	*	*	*	*	*	*	*	—	—
(Sauceworks) 1/2 cup	200	*	*	*	*	16	*	16	2	*	*	*	*	*	*	*	*	*	—	—
from mix																				
(generic) 1/2 cup	294	*	*	*	—	12	2	16	*	2	5	*	1	*	*	*	3	2	*	*
SWEETBREADS see specific meat																				

	Calories	Protein	Fat	Sat. Fat	Cholesterol	Carbohydrates	Fiber	Sodium	Potassium	Calcium	Iron	Zinc	Magnesium	Vitamin A	Vitamin C	Thiamin	Riboflavin	Niacin	Vitamin B12	Folic acid
SWORDFISH																				
raw 1 piece	165	45	8	8	18	*	*	5	11	*	6	10	9	3	2	3	8	66	40	*
baked/broiled 1 piece	164	45	8	8	18	*	*	5	11	*	6	10	9	3	2	3	7	62	36	*
SYRUP, see specific listings																				
TABASCO SAUCE see HOT SAUCE																				
TABOULE																				
(Near East) 3/4 cup	320	8	27	13	*	12	20	22	—	4	8	—	—	20	15	—	—	—	—	—
TACO SAUCE																				
hot (Chi-Chi's) 1 oz	18	2	2	3	*	*	—	11	5	*	*	*	*	4	*	*	*	*	—	—
(Old El Paso) 2 tbsp	10	*	*	*	*	*	*	5	—	*	*	—	—	*	2	*	*	2	—	—
medium (Old El Paso) 2 tbsp	10	*	*	*	*	*	*	5	—	*	*	—	—	*	2	*	*	2	—	—
mild (Old El Paso) 2 tbsp	10	*	*	*	*	*	*	5	—	*	*	—	—	*	2	*	*	2	—	—
thick & chunky (Chi-Chi's) 1 oz	12	2	2	3	*	*	—	6	4	*	*	*	*	3	2	2	3	*	—	—
TACO SEASONING MIX																				
(Hain) 1/10 pkg	10	2	*	*	*	*	*	8	*	*	*	*	*	4	*	*	*	*	*	*
(Old El Paso) 1/12 pkg	8	*	*	*	*	*	*	10	*	*	*	—	—	*	*	*	*	*	—	—
TACO SHELL																				
(Chi-Chi's) 1 shell	140	3	11	—	*	6	—	*	—	*	2	—	—	*	*	6	6	4	—	—
(Gebhardt) 1 shell	50	2	3	9	*	2	*	*	*	*	3	—	—	*	*	8	10	4	—	—
(Old El Paso) 1 shell	50	*	5	—	*	2	2	2	*	*	*	—	—	*	*	*	*	*	—	—
(Rosarita) 1 shell	50	2	3	9	*	2	*	*	*	*	3	—	—	*	*	8	4	4	—	—
mini (Old El Paso) 3 shells	70	2	6	—	*	2	2	2	*	2	2	—	—	*	*	*	*	*	—	—
super (Old El Paso) 1 shell	100	2	9	—	*	4	6	4	*	2	2	—	—	*	*	*	*	2	—	—
tostaco shell (Old El Paso) 1 shell	100	2	8	—	*	4	4	*	*	2	6	—	—	*	*	4	2	6	—	—
white corn (Old El Paso) 1 shell	60	2	5	—	*	2	*	*	*	*	*	—	—	*	*	*	*	*	—	—
TAHINI KERNEL																				
raw (generic) 1 oz	162	8	21	10	*	2	12	*	3	12	4	9	7	*	*	24	9	8	*	7
roasted (generic) 1 oz	169	8	24	11	*	2	12	*	3	12	14	9	7	*	*	23	8	8	*	7
unroasted (generic) 1 oz	172	8	25	11	*	2	12	*	4	4	10	20	25	*	*	30	2	8	*	7
TAHINI see SESAME BUTTER PASTE																				
TAMALE, CANNED (Old El Paso) 2 tamales	190	8	18	—	7	5	—	16	5	2	18	—	—	*	*	*	6	8	—	—
TAMALE, FROZEN (Patio) 13 oz	470	20	32	—	12	19	—	77	19	10	20	—	—	30	*	15	15	8	—	—
TAMALE, REFRIGERATED																				
(Derby) 2 tamales	160	13	11	15	8	5	4	24	4	*	8	—	—	*	1	5	5	10	—	—
(Gebhardt) 2 tamales	290	8	34	40	18	6	8	30	5	3	11	—	—	*	2	14	8	9	—	—
jumbo (Gebhardt) 2 tamales	400	12	46	57	25	9	12	43	8	5	15	—	—	*	3	20	12	13	—	—
TAMARI (*see also* **SOY SAUCE**) (Season) 1/4 tsp	1	*	*	*	*	*	*	10	—	*	*	*	*	*	*	*	*	*	*	*
TAMARIND																				
1 fruit	5	*	*	*	*	*	*	*	*	*	*	*	—	*	*	*	*	*	*	*
1/2 cup pulp	143	3	*	*	*	12	12	*	11	4	9	—	14	*	3	17	5	6	*	—
TANGERINE 1 fruit	37	*	*	*	*	3	8	*	4	*	*	*	3	15	43	6	*	*	—	4

	Calories	Protein	Fat	Sat. Fat	Cholesterol	Carbohydrates	Fiber	Sodium	Potassium	Calcium	Iron	Zinc	Magnesium	Vitamin A	Vitamin C	Thiamin	Riboflavin	Niacin	Vitamin B12	Folic acid
TANGERINE (continued)																				
1/2 cup sections	43	*	*	*	*	4	8	*	4	*	2	*	3	18	50	7	*	*	—	5
TANGERINE, CANNED																				
in juice																				
1/2 cup	46	*	*	*	*	4	4	*	5	*	2	4	3	21	71	7	2	3	—	*
in light syrup																				
1/2 cup	77	*	*	*	*	7	4	*	3	*	3	*	3	21	42	4	3	3	—	*
TANGERINE JUICE																				
fresh																				
8 fl oz	106	2	*	*	*	8	*	*	13	4	3	*	5	21	128	10	3	*	—	2
canned																				
sweetened																				
8 fl oz	125	2	*	*	*	10	*	*	13	3	3	*	5	21	91	10	3	*	—	3
frozen																				
from concentrate sweetened																				
6 fl oz	79	*	*	*	*	6	*	*	6	*	3	*	3	20	69	6	2	*	—	2
TAPIOCA see PUDDING																				
TARO CHIPS																				
10 chips	115	*	9	8	*	5	8	3	5	*	2	*	5	*	2	3	*	*	*	*
TARO LEAF																				
raw																				
1 cup	12	2	*	*	*	*	4	*	5	3	3	*	3	27	24	4	8	2	*	9
1 leaf	4	*	*	*	*	*	*	*	2	*	*	*	*	10	9	*	3	*	*	3
steamed																				
1/2 cup	18	3	*	*	*	*	—	*	10	6	5	*	4	63	44	7	17	5	*	9
steamed w/ salt																				
1/2 cup	18	3	*	*	*	*	—	7	10	6	5	*	4	63	44	7	17	5	*	9
TARO ROOT																				
raw																				
1/2 cup slices	56	*	*	*	*	5	8	*	9	2	2	*	4	*	4	3	*	2	*	3
cooked																				
1/2 cup slices	94	*	*	*	*	8	12	*	9	*	3	*	5	*	5	5	*	2	*	3
cooked w/ salt																				
1/2 cup slices	94	*	*	*	*	8	—	7	9	*	3	*	5	*	5	5	*	2	*	3
TARO ROOT, TAHITIAN																				
raw																				
1/2 cup slices	25	3	*	*	*	*	—	*	11	8	4	*	7	25	99	3	9	3	*	*
cooked																				
1/2 cup slices	30	5	*	*	*	2	—	2	12	10	6	*	9	24	43	2	8	2	*	*
cooked w/ salt																				
1/2 cup slices	30	5	*	*	*	2	—	8	12	10	6	*	9	24	43	2	8	2	*	*
TARO SHOOT																				
raw																				
1/2 cup slices	5	*	*	*	*	*	—	*	4	*	*	*	*	15	*	*	2	*	*	*
1 shoot	9	*	*	*	*	*	—	*	8	*	3	3	2	*	29	2	2	3	*	*
cooked																				
1/2 cup slices	10	*	*	*	*	*	—	*	7	*	2	3	*	*	22	2	2	3	*	*
cooked w/ salt																				
1/2 cup slices	10	*	*	*	*	*	—	7	7	*	2	3	*	*	22	2	2	3	*	*
TARRAGON, GROUND																				
1 tbsp	14	2	*	20	*	*	*	*	4	5	9	*	4	4	—	*	4	2	*	—
TARTAR SAUCE																				
(Best) 1 tbsp	70	*	12	5	2	*	*	8	*	*	*	*	*	*	*	*	*	*	*	*
(Hellman's) 1 tbsp	70	*	12	5	2	*	*	8	*	*	*	*	*	*	*	*	*	*	*	*
(Sauceworks) 1 tbsp	50	*	8	5	2	*	*	4	*	*	*	*	*	*	*	*	*	*	*	*
lemon & herb																				
(Sauceworks) 1 tbsp	70	*	12	5	2	*	*	4	*	*	*	*	*	*	*	*	*	*	*	*
reduced fat																				
(Best) 1 tbsp	30	*	3	*	*	*	*	6	*	*	*	*	*	*	*	*	*	*	*	*
(Hellman's) 1 tbsp	30	*	3	*	*	*	*	6	*	*	*	*	*	*	*	*	*	*	*	*

Item	Calories	Protein	Fat	Sat. Fat	Cholesterol	Carbohydrates	Fiber	Sodium	Potassium	Calcium	Iron	Zinc	Magnesium	Vitamin A	Vitamin C	Thiamin	Riboflavin	Niacin	Vitamin B12	Folic acid
TEA																				
black (generic) 1 cup	3	*	*	*	*	*	*	*	3	*	*	*	2	*	*	*	2	*	*	3
chamomile (generic) 1 cup	2	*	*	*	*	*	*	*	*	*	*	*	*	*	*	*	*	*	*	*
herbal (generic) 1 cup	2	*	*	*	*	*	*	*	*	*	*	*	*	*	*	*	*	*	*	*
instant (generic) 1 cup	2	*	*	*	*	*	*	*	*	*	*	*	*	*	*	*	*	*	*	*
sugar-free (generic) 1 cup	5	*	*	*	*	*	*	*	*	*	*	*	*	*	*	*	*	*	*	*
w/ lemon (generic) 1 cup	5	*	*	*	*	*	*	*	*	*	*	*	*	*	*	*	*	*	*	*
w/ sugar & lemon (generic) 1 cup	88	*	*	*	*	7	*	*	*	*	*	*	*	*	39	*	3	*	*	2
TEA, ICED (Schweppes) 1 cup	90	*	*	*	*	7	*	2	—	*	*	*	*	*	*	*	*	*	*	*
hibiscus cooler (Knudsen Herbal Tea Coolers) 1 cup	90	*	*	*	*	8	*	2	2	2	*	*	*	*	*	—	—	—	—	—
lemon tea cooler (Knudsen Herbal Tea Coolers) 1 cup	90	*	*	*	*	8	*	2	2	2	*	*	*	*	*	—	—	—	—	—
mango tea cooler (Knudsen Herbal Tea Coolers) 1 cup	90	*	*	*	*	8	*	2	2	2	*	*	*	*	*	—	—	—	—	—
orange tea cooler (Knudsen Herbal Tea Coolers) 1 cup	90	*	*	*	*	8	*	2	2	2	*	*	*	*	*	—	—	—	—	—
raspberry tea cooler (Knudsen Herbal Tea Coolers) 1 cup	90	*	*	*	*	8	*	2	2	2	*	*	*	*	*	—	—	—	—	—
TEA, ICED, FROM MIX (Country Time) 1 cup	70	*	*	*	*	6	*	*	—	*	*	*	*	*	10	*	*	*	*	*
decaffeinated (Crystal Light) 1 cup	4	*	*	*	*	*	*	*	—	*	*	*	*	*	10	*	*	*	*	*
TEMPEH see also TOFU (generic) 1/2 cup	165	26	10	5	*	5	—	*	9	8	10	10	15	11	*	7	5	19	14	11
TEQUILA LIME SAUCE from mix (Knorr) 1 1/2 oz	190	60	8	—	23	3	—	30	—	2	6	*	*	2	4	4	6	50	*	*
TEQUILA SUNRISE canned 6 3/4 fl oz	232	*	*	*	*	8	*	5	*	*	*	8	4	4	*	5	2	2	*	6
homemade 1 cocktail (5 1/2 oz)	189	*	*	*	*	5	—	*	5	*	3	*	3	3	*	4	2	2	*	5
TERIYAKI ENTREE, FROZEN stir-fry (Stouffer's Lean Cuisine) 9 oz	45	—	8	5	10	13	16	23	9	2	8	—	—	20	20	—	—	—	—	—
TERIYAKI SAUCE (General Mills Recipe Sauce) 1/6 jar (4 oz)	60	3	*	*	*	4	—	34	4	*	2	—	—	4	*	*	*	*	—	—
(generic) 1 tsp	5	*	*	*	—	*	*	9	*	*	2	*	*	*	*	*	*	*	*	*
for basting (La Choy) 1 tsp	2	*	*	*	*	*	*	5	*	*	*	—	—	*	*	*	*	*	—	—
lite (La Choy) 1 tsp	5	*	*	*	*	*	*	4	*	*	*	—	—	*	*	*	*	*	—	—
regular (La Choy) 1 tsp	5	*	*	*	*	*	*	12	*	*	*	—	—	*	*	*	*	*	—	—

	Calories	Protein	Fat	Sat. Fat	Cholesterol	Carbohydrates	Fiber	Sodium	Potassium	Calcium	Iron	Zinc	Magnesium	Vitamin A	Vitamin C	Thiamin	Riboflavin	Niacin	Vitamin B₁₂	Folic acid
THURINGER CERVELAT																				
beef																				
(Oscar Mayer) 1 slice	71	6	10	14	6	*	*	13	2	*	3	4	*	*	*	2	5	5	21	*
beef & pork																				
(generic) 1 slice	95	7	13	17	7	*	*	15	2	*	4	5	*	*	9	3	6	6	26	*
(Oscar Mayer) 1 slice	71	6	10	13	6	*	*	14	*	*	*	3	*	*	*	3	4	5	14	*
THYME, FRESH																				
1 tsp	1	*	*	*	*	*	*	*	*	*	*	*	*	*	2	*	*	*	*	*
THYME, GROUND																				
1 tbsp	12	*	*	*	*	*	4	*	*	8	29	2	2	3	*	*	*	*	*	*
TILEFISH																				
raw																				
1/2 fillet	185	56	7	5	32	*	*	4	24	5	3	5	14	2	*	15	18	28	70	*
baked/broiled																				
1/2 fillet	221	61	11	7	32	*	*	4	22	4	3	5	12	2	*	14	17	26	62	*
TOASTER CAKE																				
plain																				
banana nut																				
(Thomas') 1 pastry	110	2	6	5	3	6	4	8	*	*	2	—	—	*	*	4	4	2	—	—
blueberry																				
(Thomas') 1 pastry	100	2	5	5	3	6	4	7	*	*	*	—	—	*	*	6	6	4	—	—
chocolate chip																				
(Thomas') 1 pastry	100	2	6	—	—	5	8	6	*	*	2	—	—	*	*	8	4	4	—	—
corn																				
(Thomas') 1 pastry	120	2	6	5	3	7	4	8	*	*	*	—	—	*	*	6	6	4	—	—
TOASTER PASTRY																				
plain																				
apple cinnamon																				
(Pop-Tarts) 1 pastry	210	3	9	5	*	12	—	7	*	*	10	*	*	10	*	10	10	10	—	10
blueberry																				
(Pop-Tarts) 1 pastry	210	3	9	5	*	12	—	9	*	*	10	2	2	10	*	10	10	10	—	10
brown sugar & cinnamon																				
(Pop-Tarts) 1 pastry	210	5	12	10	*	11	—	8	2	*	10	2	2	10	*	10	10	10	—	10
cherry																				
(Pop-Tarts) 1 pastry	210	3	9	5	*	12	—	9	2	*	10	2	2	10	*	10	10	10	—	10
chocolate graham																				
(Pop-Tarts) 1 pastry	210	5	9	10	*	12	—	9	2	*	10	2	2	10	*	10	10	10	—	10
strawberry																				
(Pop-Tarts) 1 pastry	210	3	9	5	*	12	—	8	2	*	10	2	2	10	*	10	10	10	—	10
frosted																				
blueberry																				
(Pop-Tarts) 1 pastry	200	3	8	5	*	12	—	9	*	*	10	2	2	10	*	10	10	10	—	10
brown sugar & cinnamon																				
(Pop-Tarts) 1 pastry	210	5	11	5	*	11	—	8	2	*	10	4	2	10	*	10	10	10	—	10
cherry																				
(Pop-Tarts) 1 pastry	200	3	8	5	*	12	—	9	*	*	10	2	2	10	*	10	10	10	—	10
chocolate fudge																				
(Pop-Tarts) 1 pastry	200	5	8	5	*	12	—	9	2	2	10	4	4	10	*	10	10	10	—	10
chocolate vanilla creme																				
(Pop-Tarts) 1 pastry	200	5	8	5	*	10	—	10	2	2	10	4	4	10	*	10	10	10	—	10
grape																				
(Pop-Tarts) 1 pastry	200	3	8	5	*	12	—	8	2	*	10	2	2	10	*	10	10	10	—	10
raspberry																				
(Pop-Tarts) 1 pastry	200	3	8	5	*	12	—	9	2	*	10	2	2	10	*	10	10	10	—	10
strawberry																				
(Pop-Tarts) 1 pastry	200	3	8	5	*	12	—	8	*	*	10	2	2	10	*	10	10	10	10	10
raisin bran																				
(Thomas') 1 pastry	100	2	5	5	3	6	4	7	2	*	2	—	—	*	*	6	6	4	—	—

	Calories	Protein	Fat	Sat. Fat	Cholesterol	Carbohydrates	Fiber	Sodium	Potassium	Calcium	Iron	Zinc	Magnesium	Vitamin A	Vitamin C	Thiamin	Riboflavin	Niacin	Vitamin B12	Folic acid
TOFU																				
raw																				
firm																				
1/2 cup	183	33	17	8	*	2	12	*	9	86	73	13	18	4	*	13	8	2	*	9
nigari																				
1/2 cup	183	33	17	8	*	2	12	*	9	26	73	13	30	4	*	13	8	2	*	9
regular																				
1/2 cup	94	17	9	5	*	*	4	*	4	43	37	7	9	2	*	7	4	*	*	5
nigari																				
1/2 cup	94	17	9	5	*	*	4	*	4	13	37	7	32	2	*	7	4	*	*	5
dried-frozen																				
3 oz	408	68	40	19	*	4	—	*	*	181	46	28	38	9	*	28	16	5	*	19
nigari																				
3 oz	408	68	40	19	*	4	—	*	*	31	46	28	13	9	*	28	16	5	*	19
fried																				
3 oz	230	24	26	13	*	3	12	*	4	82	23	11	20	*	*	10	2	*	*	6
nigari																				
3 oz	230	24	26	13	*	3	12	*	4	32	23	11	13	*	*	10	2	*	*	6
salted & fermented																				
3 oz	99	12	10	5	*	*	—	102	2	104	9	9	12	3	*	9	5	2	*	6
nigari																				
3 oz	99	12	10	5	*	*	—	102	2	4	9	9	11	3	*	9	5	2	*	6
TOM COLLINS																				
1 cocktail (7 1/2 oz)	122	*	*	*	*	*	—	2	*	*	*	*	*	*	*	*	*	*	*	*
TOMATILLO																				
raw																				
1/2 cup chopped	21	*	*	*	*	*	4	*	5	*	2	*	3	2	13	2	*	6	*	*
1 medium	11	*	*	*	*	*	4	*	3	*	*	*	2	*	7	*	*	3	*	*
TOMATO																				
green																				
raw																				
1 tomato	30	2	*	*	*	2	8	*	7	2	3	*	3	16	48	5	3	3	*	3
red																				
boiled w/ salt																				
1/2 cup	32	2	*	*	*	2	—	12	10	*	4	*	4	18	46	6	4	4	*	4
ripe boiled																				
1/2 cup	32	2	*	*	*	2	4	*	10	*	4	*	4	18	46	6	4	4	*	4
raw																				
1 tomato	26	2	*	*	*	2	4	*	8	*	3	*	3	15	39	5	3	4	*	5
raw																				
1 cup chopped	38	3	*	*	*	3	8	*	11	*	4	*	5	22	57	7	5	6	*	7
stewed																				
1/2 cup	40	2	2	*	*	2	4	10	4	2	3	*	2	7	16	4	3	3	*	2
TOMATO, CANNED																				
crushed																				
(Contadina) 1/2 cup	40	*	*	*	*	3	8	12	*	4	4	—	—	16	20	—	—	—	—	—
(Progresso) 1/2 cup	40	2	*	*	*	3	—	9	13	4	—	—	—	20	25	4	2	6	—	—
Angela Mia (Hunt's) 1/2 cup	35	2	*	*	*	2	2	11	11	4	5	—	—	*	22	5	4	6	—	—
Italian flavored (Hunt's) 1/2 cup	40	3	*	*	*	3	2	19	14	5	8	—	—	*	20	6	4	14	—	—
diced, peeled (Del Monte) 1/2 cup	25	2	*	*	*	2	8	7	—	2	2	—	—	10	25	—	—	—	—	—
Italian (Contadina) 1/2 cup	25	4	*	*	*	*	4	9	—	2	4	—	—	10	20	—	—	—	—	—
(Hunt's) 1/2 cup	20	2	*	*	*	2	2	13	7	4	2	—	—	*	12	4	2	4	—	—
stewed (Contadina) 1/2 cup	40	2	*	*	*	3	4	11	—	4	2	—	—	6	4	—	—	—	—	—
undrained (Progresso) 1/2 cup	18	2	*	*	*	*	4	10	9	*	—	—	—	15	20	*	*	6	—	—

	Calories	Protein	Fat	Sat. Fat	Cholesterol	Carbohydrates	Fiber	Sodium	Potassium	Calcium	Iron	Zinc	Magnesium	Vitamin A	Vitamin C	Thiamin	Riboflavin	Niacin	Vitamin B12	Folic acid
TOMATO, CANNED (continued)																				
Mexican style																				
stewed																				
(Contadina) 1/2 cup	40	2	*	*	*	3	4	9	—	4	2	—	—	6	4	—	—	—	—	—
peeled																				
choice-cut																				
(Hunt's) 1/2 cup	20	2	*	*	*	2	4	19	7	4	3	—	—	*	18	4	3	4	—	—
whole																				
(Del Monte) 1/2 cup	25	2	*	*	*	2	8	7	—	2	2	—	—	10	25	—	—	—	—	—
puree																				
(Contadina) 1/2 cup	40	*	*	*	*	3	—	*	*	*	4	—	—	20	30	—	—	—	—	—
(Del Monte) 1/2 cup	60	2	*	*	*	2	8	*	—	2	2	—	—	30	25	—	—	—	—	—
recipe ready																				
(Contadina) 1/2 cup	25	4	*	*	*	2	4	8	—	4	4	—	—	15	15	—	—	—	—	—
stewed																				
(Contadina) 1/2 cup	40	2	*	*	*	3	4	10	—	4	4	—	—	8	15	—	—	—	—	—
(Del Monte) 1/2 cup	35	2	*	*	*	3	8	15	—	2	2	—	—	10	25	—	—	—	—	—
(generic) 1/2 cup	33	2	*	*	*	3	—	14	9	4	5	*	4	14	28	4	3	5	*	2
(Hunt's) 1/2 cup	35	2	*	*	*	3	2	17	8	4	4	—	—	*	18	4	2	4	—	—
Cajun style																				
(Del Monte) 1/2 cup	35	2	*	*	*	3	8	19	—	2	2	—	—	10	25	—	—	—	—	—
chunky chili																				
(Del Monte) 1/2 cup	30	2	*	*	*	3	8	25	—	2	2	—	—	10	25	—	—	—	—	—
chunky pasta																				
(Del Monte) 1/2 cup	45	2	*	*	*	4	8	23	—	2	2	—	—	10	25	—	—	—	—	—
chunky pizza																				
(Del Monte) 1/2 cup	35	2	*	*	*	3	8	28	—	2	2	—	—	10	25	—	—	—	—	—
chunky salsa																				
(Del Monte) 1/2 cup	35	2	*	*	*	3	8	23	—	2	2	—	—	10	25	—	—	—	—	—
w/ green chili																				
(generic) 1/2 cup	18	*	*	*	*	*	—	20	4	2	2	*	3	9	12	3	*	4	*	3
Italian flavored																				
(Hunt's) 1/2 cup	40	3	*	*	*	3	2	15	7	4	5	—	—	*	20	6	4	14	—	—
Italian style																				
(Del Monte) 1/2 cup	30	2	*	*	*	3	8	18	—	2	2	—	—	10	25	—	—	—	—	—
Mexican style																				
(Del Monte) 1/2 cup	35	2	*	*	*	3	8	17	—	2	2	—	—	10	25	—	—	—	—	—
no salt added																				
(Del Monte) 1/2 cup	35	2	*	*	*	3	8	2	—	2	2	—	—	10	25	—	—	—	—	—
(Hunt's) 1/2 cup	35	2	*	*	*	3	2	*	8	5	4	—	—	*	18	4	2	4	—	—
wedges																				
1/2 cup	34	2	*	*	*	3	—	12	9	3	3	*	4	15	32	5	2	4	*	3
(Del Monte) 1/2 cup	35	2	*	*	*	3	8	16	—	2	2	—	—	10	25	—	—	—	—	—
whole																				
(Bush Bros) 1/2 cup	35	3	*	*	*	2	4	7	—	*	4	—	—	20	20	—	—	—	—	—
(Contadina) 1/2 cup	25	2	*	*	*	*	4	9	—	2	4	—	—	10	20	—	—	—	—	—
(generic) 1/2 cup	24	2	*	*	*	2	4	8	8	3	4	*	4	14	30	4	2	4	*	2
(Hunt's) 1/2 cup	20	2	*	*	*	2	3	14	7	4	2	—	—	*	12	4	2	4	—	—
Italian flavored																				
(Hunt's) 1/2 cup	25	2	*	*	*	2	3	17	7	4	2	—	—	*	20	9	5	14	—	—
low salt																				
(generic) 1/2 cup	24	2	*	*	*	2	8	*	8	3	4	*	4	14	30	4	2	4	*	2
no salt added																				
(Hunt's) 1/2 cup	20	2	*	*	*	2	3	*	7	4	4	—	—	*	18	4	2	4	—	—
TOMATO PASTE																				
(Contadina) 2 tbsp	30	3	*	*	*	2	4	*	—	*	4	—	—	10	10	—	—	—	—	—
(Del Monte) 2 tbsp	30	2	*	*	*	2	8	*	—	*	2	—	—	15	15	—	—	—	—	—
(generic) 1/2 cup	110	8	2	*	*	8	24	4	35	5	22	7	17	65	92	14	15	21	*	7
(Progresso) 2 oz	50	1	*	*	*	4	*	*	17	*	*	—	—	25	40	5	3	10	—	—

	Calories	Protein	Fat	Sat. Fat	Cholesterol	Carbohydrates	Fiber	Sodium	Potassium	Calcium	Iron	Zinc	Magnesium	Vitamin A	Vitamin C	Thiamin	Riboflavin	Niacin	Vitamin B12	Folic acid
TOMATO PASTE (continued)																				
w/ garlic (Hunt's) 2 oz	50	3	*	*	*	4	8	18	17	2	4	—	—	*	27	8	4	10	—	—
Italian (Contadina) 2 tbsp	40	2	2	*	*	2	4	13	—	*	6	—	—	6	10	—	—	—	—	—
Italian style (Hunt's) 2 oz	45	3	*	*	*	4	8	18	15	2	3	—	—	*	27	8	4	9	—	—
no salt added (Hunt's) 2 oz	45	3	*	*	*	4	8	*	15	2	10	—	—	*	28	8	4	8	—	—
plain (Hunt's) 2 oz	45	3	*	*	*	4	8	6	15	2	3	—	—	*	27	8	4	9	—	—
w/ salt (generic) 1/2 cup	110	8	2	*	*	8	24	43	35	5	22	7	17	65	92	14	15	21	*	7
TOMATO PUREE																				
(generic) 1/2 cup	51	4	*	*	*	4	12	*	15	2	7	2	8	34	74	6	4	11	*	7
(Hunt's) 1/2 cup	45	3	*	*	*	3	8	6	16	2	4	—	—	*	27	8	4	8	—	—
(Progresso) 1/2 cup	45	3	*	*	*	3	—	*	16	*	—	—	—	25	25	4	2	6	—	—
heavy concentrate (Progresso) 1/2 cup	50	3	*	*	*	4	—	*	16	*	—	—	—	35	35	4	4	10	—	—
w/ salt (generic) 1/2 cup	51	4	*	*	*	4	12	24	15	2	7	2	8	3	74	6	4	11	*	7
TOMATO SAUCE (see also PASTA SAUCE)																				
(Contadina) 1/2 cup	40	*	*	*	*	3	—	23	*	*	4	—	—	12	*	—	—	—	—	—
(Del Monte) 1/2 cup	40	3	*	*	*	2	6	28	—	*	4	—	—	8	16	—	—	—	—	—
(generic) 1/2 cup	37	3	*	*	*	3	8	31	13	2	5	2	6	24	27	5	4	7	*	3
(Hunt's) 1/2 cup	30	2	*	*	*	2	8	27	9	2	3	—	—	*	15	4	4	6	—	—
(Progresso) 1/2 cup	40	3	*	*	*	3	—	26	151	*	—	—	—	15	10	2	6	—	—
garlic (Hunt's) 1/2 cup	70	3	3	*	*	3	8	20	18	3	16	—	—	*	24	6	4	10	—	—
herb & cheese (generic) 1/2 cup	72	4	4	4	—	4	—	28	12	5	6	3	6	24	20	6	9	7	—	2
herb flavored (Hunt's) 1/2 cup	70	3	3	3	*	4	8	20	12	3	6	—	—	*	18	7	4	6	—	—
Italian (Contadina) 1/2 cup	30	*	*	*	*	3	8	27	*	*	4	—	—	12	20	—	—	—	—	—
(Hunt's) 1/2 cup	60	3	3	3	*	3	8	19	13	4	4	—	—	*	20	5	4	13	—	—
meatloaf fixn's (Hunt's) 1/4 cup	20	*	*	*	*	2	*	24	6	*	2	—	—	*	12	3	2	3	—	—
mushrooms (generic) 1/2 cup	43	3	*	*	*	3	—	23	13	2	6	2	6	23	25	6	8	8	*	3
(Hunt's) 1/2 cup	25	2	*	*	*	2	8	30	11	2	3	—	—	*	15	4	2	4	—	—
mushrooms & peppers (generic) 1/2 cup	50	2	*	*	*	4	16	28	14	2	5	2	6	20	27	5	9	7	*	4
no salt added (Del Monte) 1/2 cup	40	2	*	*	*	2	6	2	—	*	4	—	—	8	16	—	—	—	—	—
(Hunt's) 1/2 cup	35	2	*	*	*	3	8	*	10	*	4	—	—	*	27	4	2	6	—	—
onions (generic) 1/2 cup	51	3	*	*	*	4	—	28	14	2	6	2	6	21	26	6	10	8	*	7
(Hunt's) 1/2 cup	40	2	*	*	*	3	8	27	9	3	11	—	—	*	18	4	2	6	—	—
Spanish style (generic) 1/2 cup	41	3	*	*	*	3	—	24	23	2	24	3	6	24	18	6	5	8	*	4
special (Hunt's) 1/2 cup	35	2	*	*	*	3	8	12	8	*	3	—	—	*	15	4	2	6	—	—
thick & zesty (Contadina) 1/2 cup	30	*	*	*	*	3	8	27	*	*	8	—	—	20	20	—	—	—	—	—

	Calories	Protein	Fat	Sat. Fat	Cholesterol	Carbohydrates	Fiber	Sodium	Potassium	Calcium	Iron	Zinc	Magnesium	Vitamin A	Vitamin C	Thiamin	Riboflavin	Niacin	Vitamin B₁₂	Folic acid
TOMATO SAUCE (*continued*)																				
tomato bits																				
(generic) 1/2 cup	39	3	*	*	*	3	—	*	13	*	5	2	6	20	44	6	7	7	*	3
(Hunt's) 1/2 cup	30	2	*	*	*	2	8	26	8	*	2	—	—	3	18	4	2	6	—	—
TOMATO, SUN-DRIED																				
1/2 cup	70	6	*	*	*	5	12	24	26	3	14	4	13	5	18	9	8	12	*	5
4 tomatoes	21	2	*	*	*	*	4	7	8	*	4	*	4	*	5	3	2	4	*	*
packed in oil																				
1/2 cup	117	5	12	5	*	4	—	6	25	3	8	3	11	14	93	7	12	10	*	3
TOMATO JUICE COCKTAIL																				
(Campbell's) 6 fl oz	40	2	*	*	*	3	4	20	—	2	2	—	—	15	35	2	2	6	—	—
(Del Monte) 8 fl oz	50	3	*	*	*	3	4	32	—	4	6	—	—	35	100	—	—	—	—	—
(Del Monte Snap-E-Tom) 8 fl oz	50	3	*	*	*	3	6	21	—	*	10	—	—	50	20	—	—	—	—	—
(generic) 6 fl oz	31	2	*	*	*	3	4	*	11	2	6	2	5	—	55	6	3	6	*	9
(Hunt's) 6 fl oz	30	2	*	*	*	2	8	22	11	*	3	—	—	*	18	4	2	6	—	—
(V8) 6 fl oz	35	2	*	*	*	3	4	20	—	2	4	—	—	30	100	2	2	4	—	—
(Welch's) 6 fl oz	35	*	*	*	*	2	*	23	11	*	2	—	—	15	10	4	2	4	—	—
light 'n' tangy																				
(V8) 6 fl oz	40	2	*	*	*	3	4	10	—	2	6	—	—	45	100	2	4	6	—	—
low sodium																				
(V8) 6 fl oz	40	2	*	*	*	3	4	5	—	2	6	—	—	45	100	2	2	6	—	—
no salt added																				
(Hunt's) 6 fl oz	35	2	*	*	*	3	8	*	13	2	4	—	—	*	20	5	3	7	—	—
organic																				
(Knudsen) 8 fl oz	60	3	*	*	*	5	—	16	25	4	4	—	—	50	20	—	—	—	—	—
spicy hot																				
(V8) 6 fl oz	35	2	*	*	*	3	4	25	—	2	6	—	—	30	50	2	2	6	—	—
w/ salt																				
(generic) 6 fl oz	31	2	*	*	*	3	4	27	11	2	6	2	5	20	55	6	3	6	*	9
TOMATO-BEEF COCKTAIL																				
(generic) 3 1/2 oz glass	38	*	*	*	*	3	*	6	3	*	3	*	3	*	2	*	2	*	*	*
Beefamato																				
(Mott's) 8 fl oz	80	2	*	*	*	7	4	32	3	*	4	—	—	4	*	*	*	*	*	—
TOMATO-CLAM COCKTAIL																				
(generic) 12 fl oz can	163	4	*	*	*	13	*	59	9	4	12	26	20	15	24	9	6	3	1803	14
Clamato																				
(Mott's) 8 fl oz	100	2	*	*	*	8	8	30	2	*	4	—	—	2	2	*	*	*	*	—
Clamato caesar																				
(Mott's) 8 fl oz	100	*	*	*	*	8	*	32	5	2	8	—	—	10	2	*	*	*	*	—
TOMATOES & GREEN CHILES																				
bottled																				
(Old El Paso) 1/4 cup	11	2	*	*	*	*	4	20	—	*	2	—	—	*	*	*	*	2	—	—
TOMATOES & JALAPEÑOS																				
bottled																				
(Old El Paso) 1/4 cup	—	2	*	*	*	*	6	3	*	2	—	—	—	4	10	*	*	2	—	—
TONGUE see specific meats																				
TORTILLA																				
flour																				
(Old El Paso) 1	150	7	5	—	*	9	*	15	*	2	10	—	—	*	*	45	4	8	—	—
TORTILLA CHIP																				
(Bachman) 1 oz	150	3	9	5	*	7	7	4	—	6	4	—	—	*	*	—	—	—	—	—
(generic) 1 oz	142	4	12	7	*	6	8	6	3	5	3	3	6	*	—	*	3	2	—	*
baked																				
(Tostitos) 1 oz	110	5	2	*	*	8	8	6	—	—	—	—	—	—	—	—	—	—	—	—
cinnamon																				
(Tostitos) 1 oz	140	3	11	5	*	6	4	2	—	—	—	—	—	—	—	—	—	—	—	—
lime 'n' chili																				
(Tostitos) 1 oz	150	3	11	5	*	6	4	7	—	—	—	—	—	—	—	—	—	—	—	—

	Calories	Protein	Fat	Sat. Fat	Cholesterol	Carbohydrates	Fiber	Sodium	Potassium	Calcium	Iron	Zinc	Magnesium	Vitamin A	Vitamin C	Thiamin	Riboflavin	Niacin	Vitamin B$_{12}$	Folic acid
TORTILLA CHIP (continued)																				
nacho																				
light																				
(generic) 1 oz	126	4	7	4	*	7	—	12	4	5	3	—	7	2	—	4	5	*	—	2
ranch																				
(Baked Tostitos) 1 oz	120	3	5	3	*	7	4	7	—	—	—	—	—	—	—	—	—	—	—	—
(generic) 1 oz	134	4	11	7	*	6	—	7	4	4	3	3	7	2	*	2	4	2	—	*
restaurant style																				
(Tostitos) 1 oz	130	3	9	5	*	6	4	3	—	—	—	—	—	—	—	—	—	—	—	—
unsalted																				
(Tostitos) 1 oz	140	3	12	5	*	6	4	*	—	—	—	—	—	—	—	—	—	—	—	—
restaurant chips																				
(Santitas) 1 oz	140	3	9	5	*	6	4	3	—	—	—	—	—	—	—	—	—	—	—	—
restaurant strips																				
(Santitas) 1 oz	140	3	9	5	*	6	4	2	—	—	—	—	—	—	—	—	—	—	—	—
taco																				
(generic) 1 oz	136	4	11	7	*	6	—	10	4	5	3	3	6	5	*	5	4	3	—	2
unsalted																				
(Bachman) 1 oz	150	3	10	6	*	7	7	*	—	8	4	—	—	*	*	—	—	—	—	—
(Baked Tostitos) 1 oz	110	5	2	*	*	8	8	*	—	—	—	—	—	—	—	—	—	—	—	—
white corn																				
(Old El Paso) 1 oz	150	7	13	5	*	6	4	3	*	*	*	—	*	—	*	*	*	*	—	—
(Santitas) 1 oz	140	3	9	5	*	6	4	3	—	—	—	—	—	—	—	—	—	—	—	—
bite size																				
(Tostitos) 1 oz	140	3	12	5	*	6	4	5	—	—	—	—	—	—	—	—	—	—	—	—
round																				
(Tostitos) 1 oz	150	3	12	5	*	6	4	4	—	—	—	—	—	—	—	—	—	—	—	—
yellow corn																				
(Nachips) 1 oz	75	4	6	—	*	3	3	2	*	—	—	—	—	—	—	—	—	—	—	—
TOSCANA SAUCE																				
from mix																				
(Knorr) 1/2 cup	190	8	15	—	7	5	—	32	—	20	*	*	*	6	2	4	10	*	*	*
TOSTADA SHELL																				
(Old El Paso) 1	55	*	5	—	*	2	2	3	*	*	*	—	—	*	*	*	*	*	—	—
(Rosarita) 1 shell	60	2	5	11	*	3	*	*	*	*	4	—	—	*	*	11	5	6	—	—
TREE FERN																				
cooked																				
1/2 cup chopped	28	*	*	*	*	3	12	*	*	*	*	*	*	3	35	*	13	12	*	3
1 frond	12	*	*	*	*	*	4	*	*	*	*	*	*	*	15	*	5	5	*	*
cooked, salted																				
1/2 cup chopped	28	*	*	*	*	3	—	7	*	*	*	*	*	3	35	*	13	12	*	3
SEA TROUT																				
raw																				
1 fillet	248	66	13	12	66	*	*	6	23	4	4	7	18	5	*	10	24	29	119	*
broiled/baked																				
1 fillet	247	66	13	12	66	*	*	6	23	4	4	7	19	4	*	9	23	27	107	*
TROUT, RAINBOW																				
broiled/baked																				
1 fillet	120	29	8	8	16	*	*	*	9	*	—	2	6	4	4	11	3	31	59	*
wild																				
baked/broiled																				
1 fillet	215	55	13	12	33	*	*	3	18	12	3	5	11	*	5	14	8	41	150	*
TROUT, RIVER																				
broiled/baked																				
1 fillet	118	28	8	5	15	*	*	2	8	3	7	4	4	*	*	18	15	18	77	*
TUNA, BLUEFIN																				
raw																				
3 oz	122	33	6	6	11	*	*	*	6	*	5	3	11	37	*	14	13	37	133	*
baked/broiled																				
3 oz	156	42	8	7	14	*	*	2	8	*	6	4	14	43	*	16	15	45	153	*

	Calories	Protein	Fat	Sat. Fat	Cholesterol	Carbohydrates	Fiber	Sodium	Potassium	Calcium	Iron	Zinc	Magnesium	Vitamin A	Vitamin C	Thiamin	Riboflavin	Niacin	Vitamin B12	Folic acid
TUNA, SKIPJACK																				
raw 1/2 fillet	204	73	3	3	31	*	*	3	23	6	14	11	17	2	3	4	12	152	62	*
broiled/baked 1/2 fillet	203	72	3	3	31	*	*	3	23	6	14	11	17	2	3	4	11	144	56	*
TUNA, YELLOWFIN																				
raw 3 oz	92	33	*	*	13	*	*	*	11	*	3	3	11	*	*	25	2	42	7	*
broiled/baked 3 oz	118	42	2	*	16	*	*	2	14	2	4	4	14	*	*	28	3	51	8	*
TUNA, CANNED																				
light in oil (generic) 1/2 can	168	21	5	4	3	*	*	6	3	*	3	3	3	*	*	*	3	27	31	*
(Progresso) 1/3 cup	150	22	20	—	—	*	*	17	—	*	4	—	*	*	*	*	2	35	—	*
in water (Bumble Bee) 1/4 cup	60	26	1	0	10	*	*	10	—	*	2	*	*	*	*	—	—	20	20	*
(generic) 1/2 can	107	20	*	*	2	*	*	*	4	*	7	*	3	*	*	*	3	26	30	*
white in oil (generic) 1/2 can	162	20	6	4	5	*	*	7	4	*	2	*	4	*	*	*	2	26	33	*
in water (generic) 1/2 can	117	19	2	*	6	*	*	7	3	*	*	*	4	*	*	*	*	12	31	*
solid, in oil (Bumble Bee) 1/4 cup	90	47	5	3	8	*	*	10	—	*	*	—	*	*	*	*	*	25	15	*
TUNA ENTREE, FROM MIX																				
au gratin (Tuna Helper) 6 oz	280	23	17	—		10	—	40	7	10	8	—		6	*	40	15	25	—	
creamy mushroom (Tuna Helper) 7 oz	210	20	9	—		9	—	30	7	2	8	—		6	*	15	10	25	—	
creamy noodles (Tuna Helper) 8 oz	300	23	22	—		10	—	39	7	10	8	—		10	*	20	15	25	—	
Romanoff (Tuna Helper) 8 oz	280	23	12	—		13	—	33	7	4	8	—		2	*	20	15	25	—	
salad (Tuna Helper) 5 1/2 oz	410	42	42	—		10	—	37	5	2	8	—		*	*	15	6	25	—	
tetrazzini (Tuna Helper) 6 oz	230	23	12	—		9	—	32	6	8	8	—		*	*	30	10	25	—	
TUNA, FROZEN																				
pot pie (Tuna Helper) 5 oz	420	20	42	—		10	—	36	6	4	8	—		15	*	10	15	20	—	
w/ spinach noodles (Stouffer's Lean Cuisine) 9 3/4 oz	240	27	11	10	7	10	—	22	14	20	6	—		45	6	10	20	15	—	
tuna noodle casserole (Dinty Moore American Classics) 10 oz	240	27	11	20	22	9	—	53	*	6	10	—		2	6	6	15	15	—	
(Stouffer's) 10 oz	330	28	22	10	13	10	12	47	11	15	6	—		2	*	10	20	20	—	
(Weight Watchers) 9 1/2 oz	240	25	11	13	5	10	20	24	18	15	8	—		15	20	—	—	—	—	
TUNA SALAD																				
(generic) 1/2 cup	191	14	7	4	2	2	*	9	3	*	3	2	2	*	2	*	2	17	20	*
(Libby's) 2 oz	80	10	8	5	—	2	*	9	2	*	2	*	*	*	*	*	*	10	*	*
TURBOT																				
raw 1/2 fillet	194	55	9	8	33	*	*	13	14	4	4	3	26	*	6	9	10	22	75	*
broiled/baked 1/2 fillet	194	55	9	—	33	*	*	13	14	4	4	3	26	*	5	8	9	21	67	*

	Calories	Protein	Fat	Sat. Fat	Cholesterol	Carbohydrates	Fiber	Sodium	Potassium	Calcium	Iron	Zinc	Magnesium	Vitamin A	Vitamin C	Thiamin	Riboflavin	Niacin	Vitamin B$_{12}$	Folic acid
TURKEY																				
breast w/ skin roasted 3 oz	161	41	10	9	21	*	*	2	7	2	7	11	6	*	*	3	7	27	5	*
dark meat w/ out skin roasted 3 oz	159	40	9	11	24	*	*	3	7	3	11	25	5	*	*	4	12	16	5	2
dark meat w/ skin roasted 3 oz	188	39	15	15	25	*	*	3	7	3	11	24	5	*	*	3	12	15	5	2
fat 1 tbsp	115	*	20	19	4	*	*	*	*	*	*	*	*	*	*	*	*	*	*	*
giblets simmered 1 cup	242	64	11	11	202	*	*	4	8	2	54	36	6	175	4	4	77	33	578	125
gizzard simmered 1 cup	236	71	9	8	112	*	*	3	9	2	44	40	7	5	4	3	28	22	46	19
ground cooked 1 patty	193	37	17	14	28	*	*	4	6	2	9	16	5	*	*	3	8	20	4	2
heart simmered 1 cup	257	65	14	13	109	*	*	3	8	2	55	51	8	*	4	7	75	24	172	29
leg w/ skin roasted 3 oz	177	39	13	13	24	*	*	3	7	3	11	24	5	*	*	3	12	15	5	2
light meat w/ out skin roasted 3 oz	133	42	4	5	20	*	*	2	7	2	6	12	6	*	*	3	6	29	5	*
light meat w/ skin roasted 3 oz	167	40	11	10	22	*	*	2	7	2	7	12	6	*	*	3	7	27	5	*
liver simmered 3 oz	144	34	8	8	177	*	*	2	5	*	37	17	3	214	3	3	71	25	670	142
meat w/ out skin roasted 3 oz	145	42	6	7	22	*	*	2	7	2	8	18	6	*	*	4	9	23	5	2
meat w/ skin roasted 3 oz	177	40	13	12	23	*	*	2	7	2	8	17	5	*	*	3	9	22	5	2
neck w/ out skin simmered 3 oz	153	38	10	11	35	*	*	2	4	3	11	40	3	*	*	2	10	7	3	2
skin roasted 3 oz	376	28	52	44	32	*	*	2	4	3	8	12	3	*	*	*	7	11	3	*
wing w/ skin roasted 3 oz	195	39	16	15	23	*	*	2	6	2	7	12	5	*	*	3	7	24	5	*
TURKEY, CANNED																				
in broth (generic) 1/2 can	231	56	15	14	31	*	*	28	9	2	15	22	7	*	5	*	14	47	7	2
chunk (Hormel) 2 1/2 oz	80	22	5	5	15	*	—	17	8	1	5	11	—	*	1	1	10	21	—	—
chunk white (Swanson) 2 1/2 oz	80	35	2	—	—	*	—	11	—	*	2	—	—	*	*	*	2	20	—	—
TURKEY, COLD CUTS																				
bologna (generic) 1 1 oz slice	56	6	7	7	9	*	*	10	2	2	2	3	*	*	*	*	*	3	5	*	*
(Oscar Mayer) 1 slice	50	5	6	5	6	*	*	10	*	3	2	3	*	*	*	—	—	—	—	—

	Calories	Protein	Fat	Sat. Fat	Cholesterol	Carbohydrates	Fiber	Sodium	Potassium	Calcium	Iron	Zinc	Magnesium	Vitamin A	Vitamin C	Thiamin	Riboflavin	Niacin	Vitamin B12	Folic acid
TURKEY, COLD CUTS (continued)																				
breast																				
(Louis Rich) 1 slice	12	3	*	*	*	*	*	5	*	*	*	*	*	*	*	—	—	—	—	—
(Oscar Mayer Healthy Favorites) 1 slice	13	4	*	*	2	*	*	4	2	*	*	*	*	*	*	—	—	—	—	—
(Thorn Apple Valley) 1 slice	25	8	*	*	3	*	*	17	—	—	—	—	—	*	*	—	—	—	—	—
barbecue (Oscar Mayer) 1 slice	30	9	*	*	4	*	*	14	3	*	2	2	2	*	*	—	—	—	—	—
oven roasted (Bryan Thin Sliced) 1 oz	30	10	2	—	5	—	*	4	—	—	—	—	—	*	—	—	—	—	—	—
roasted (Oscar Mayer) 1 slice	13	4	*	*	2	*	*	6	*	*	*	*	*	*	*	—	—	—	—	—
skinless (Oscar Mayer) 1 slice	26	9	*	*	4	*	*	13	2	*	*	2	2	*	*	—	—	—	—	—
smoked (Bryan Thin Sliced) 1 oz	30	10	2	—	5	—	*	3	—	—	—	—	—	*	—	—	—	—	—	—
(Oscar Mayer) 1 slice	11	4	*	*	2	*	*	5	*	*	*	*	*	*	*	—	—	—	—	—
(Oscar Mayer Healthy Favorites) 1 slice	11	4	*	*	2	*	*	3	*	*	*	*	*	*	*	—	—	—	—	—
smoked, skinless (Oscar Mayer) 1 slice	28	9	*	*	4	*	*	15	2	*	*	2	2	*	*	—	—	—	—	—
breast meat																				
(generic) 1 1 oz slice	31	11	*	*	4	*	*	17	2	*	*	2	*	*	*	*	2	12	10	*
ham																				
(generic) 1 1 oz slice	36	9	2	3	5	*	*	12	3	*	4	6	*	*	*	*	4	5	*	*
(Oscar Mayer) 1 slice	23	6	*	*	5	*	*	10	2	*	2	3	*	*	*	*	—	—	—	—
(Thorn Apple Valley) 1 slice	30	7	2	—	5	*	*	15	—	—	—	—	—	*	*	—	—	—	—	—
chopped																				
(Oscar Mayer) 1 slice	42	8	4	*	7	*	*	12	2	*	2	6	*	*	*	*	—	—	—	—
honey cured																				
(Oscar Mayer) 1 slice	23	6	*	*	5	*	*	9	2	*	2	4	*	*	*	*	—	—	—	—
thigh meat cured																				
(generic) 2 slices (2 oz)	73	18	4	5	11	*	*	24	5	*	9	11	2	*	*	2	8	10	2	*
loaf																				
breast (generic) 2 slices (2 oz)	47	16	*	*	6	*	*	26	3	*	*	3	2	*	*	*	3	18	14	*
pastrami																				
(generic) 1 1 oz slice	40	9	3	3	5	*	*	12	2	*	3	4	*	*	*	*	4	5	*	*
roll																				
light & dark meat (generic) 1 1 oz slice	42	9	3	3	5	*	*	7	2	*	2	4	*	*	*	2	5	7	*	*
light meat (generic) 1 1 oz slice	42	9	3	3	4	*	*	6	2	*	2	3	*	*	*	2	4	10	*	*
salami																				
(generic) 1 1 oz slice	56	8	6	6	8	*	*	12	2	*	3	3	*	*	*	*	3	5	*	*
TURKEY, DICED																				
light & dark meat (generic) 1 oz	39	9	3	3	5	*	*	10	2	*	3	4	*	*	*	*	2	7	*	*
TURKEY DINNER, FROZEN																				
(Banquet Extra Helping) 17 oz	460	38	18	—	23	21	—	84	19	10	20	—	—	4	*	30	20	25	—	—
(Swanson) 11 1/2 oz	340	40	17	—	—	14	—	41	—	4	15	—	—	15	10	10	15	30	—	—
(Swanson Hungry-Man) 16 1/2 oz	510	60	25	—	—	20	—	51	—	8	25	—	—	30	20	25	35	50	—	—
breast (Healthy Choice) 10 1/2 oz	260	35	5	10	13	14	—	23	16	4	10	—	—	20	*	25	15	35	—	—
gravy & dressing (Healthy Choice Homestyle) 10 oz	270	45	6	10	17	10	—	22	17	6	10	—	—	15	*	20	20	40	—	—
grilled & glazed (Le Menu Dinner) 11 oz	410	42	17	—	—	17	—	37	—	8	15	—	—	25	15	10	25	35	—	—

	Calories	Protein	Fat	Sat. Fat	Cholesterol	Carbohydrates	Fiber	Sodium	Potassium	Calcium	Iron	Zinc	Magnesium	Vitamin A	Vitamin C	Thiamin	Riboflavin	Niacin	Vitamin B12	Folic acid
TURKEY DINNER, FROZEN (continued)																				
medallions and vegetables (Healthy Choice Homestyle) 12 1/2 oz	350	48	9	15	20	15	—	20	13	15	15	—	—	15	*	30	30	20	—	—
stuffed (Budget Gourmet Light & Healthy) 11 oz	250	35	9	10	12	10	—	24	15	*	8	—	—	60	100	15	15	40	—	—
w/ dressing & gravy (Dinty Moore American) 10 oz	290	47	8	5	13	11	—	38	16	6	11	10	10	*	*	9	18	51	—	—
pot pie (Swanson) 7 oz	390	20	32	—	—	7	—	30	—	2	10	—	—	30	*	15	10	15	—	—
(Swanson Hungry-Man) 14 oz	660	50	57	—	—	12	—	65	—	8	15	—	—	170	10	30	20	30	—	—
tetrazzini (Healthy Choice) 12 2/3 oz	340	38	9	15	13	16	—	20	15	10	10	—	—	*	120	15	20	20	—	—
vegetable w/ pot pie (Morton) 7 oz	420	23	43	—	13	9	—	31	7	4	10	—	—	4	*	20	15	25	—	—
TURKEY ENTREE, CANNED																				
(Libby's) 7 oz	180	18	11	8	12	6	8	35	—	2	6	—	—	*	*	—	—	—	—	—
TURKEY, FROZEN																				
breast																				
dressing (Stouffer's Lean Cuisine) 7 7/8 oz	200	25	9	5	10	7	—	22	11	4	8	—	—	60	8	10	10	25	—	—
mushroom sauce (Stouffer's Lean Cuisine) 8 oz	230	28	11	10	12	8	—	22	20	2	4	—	—	15	6	8	10	30	—	—
mushrooms in gravy (Healthy Choice) 8 1/2 oz	200	30	5	5	13	9	—	16	7	2	8	—	—	20	*	8	8	15	—	—
stuffed (Weight Watchers) 8 3/4 oz	240	30	12	15	7	9	4	25	15	8	8	—	—	20	15	—	—	—	—	—
dijon (Stouffer's Lean Cuisine) 9 1/2 oz	210	33	9	10	15	7	—	25	18	15	4	—	—	40	4	15	20	25	—	—
w/ dressing & gravy (Armour Classics) 11 1/2 oz	320	32	18	—	17	11	—	53	15	8	15	—	—	60	10	20	10	25	—	—
(Swanson) 9 oz	280	35	15	—	—	10	—	39	—	4	8	—	—	*	4	8	10	25	—	—
homestyle (Stouffer's) 7 7/8 oz	280	32	17	13	13	8	4	40	11	2	4	—	—	2	*	15	15	35	—	—
glazed (Budget Gourmet Light & Healthy) 9 oz	260	25	8	10	10	13	—	30	7	2	4	—	—	4	2	8	10	30	—	—
w/ gravy (generic) 15 oz package	95	14	6	6	9	2	*	33	2	2	7	7	3	*	*	2	11	13	6	*
lemon pepper (Turkey by George) 5 oz	160	47	6	5	20	*	—	35	28	2	4	7	9	*	5	5	11	62	—	—
medallions (Weight Watchers) 8 1/2 oz	190	20	2	*	5	11	16	20	8	2	6	—	—	10	10	—	—	—	—	—
pot pie (Stouffer's) 10 oz	530	27	51	45	22	12	12	43	9	10	8	—	—	30	4	20	25	20	—	—
pretzel sandwich (Weight Watchers) 4 oz	220	27	6	8	8	12	12	21	17	10	8	—	—	*	*	—	—	—	—	—
tetrazzini (Stouffer's) 10 oz	360	37	29	15	13	9	8	47	11	10	6	—	—	*	*	10	25	15	—	—
w/ vegetables, homestyle (Healthy Choice) 9 1/2 oz	230	40	5	5	12	9	—	20	5	6	8	—	—	60	8	20	15	20	—	—
w/ vegetables & pasta homestyle (Stouffer's Lean Cuisine) 9 3/8 oz	230	35	8	10	17	8	—	23	9	10	4	—	—	30	2	10	20	15	—	—
vegetable w/ pot pie (Banquet) 7 oz	510	27	48	—	13	13	—	36	7	4	10	—	—	4	*	20	15	25	—	—

	Calories	Protein	Fat	Sat. Fat	Cholesterol	Carbohydrates	Fiber	Sodium	Potassium	Calcium	Iron	Zinc	Magnesium	Vitamin A	Vitamin C	Thiamin	Riboflavin	Niacin	Vitamin B12	Folic acid
TURKEY GRAVY																				
canned																				
(Franco-American) 1/4 cup	30	*	3	—	—	*	*	12	—	*	*	—	—	*	*	*	*	*	—	—
(generic) 1/4 cup	31	3	2	—	—	*	*	14	2	*	2	3	*	*	*	*	3	4	*	*
seasoned																				
(Pepperidge Farm) 1/4 cup	30	2	2	—	—	*	*	13	—	*	—	—	*	*	*	*	4	2	*	*
TURKEY HAM see TURKEY, COLD CUTS																				
TURKEY HOT DOG see HOT DOG																				
TURKEY SALAD																				
canned																				
(Libby's) 2 oz	100	10	9	5	5	2	*	11	2	*	2	2	*	*	*	*	2	6	*	*
TURKEY SALAMI see TURKEY, COLD CUTS																				
TURKEY SPREAD																				
(Underwood) 2 1/8 oz	75	18	3	3	8	*	*	14	5	*	4	—	—	*	*	*	5	20	—	—
TURMERIC, GROUND																				
1 tbsp	24	*	*	*	*	*	4	*	5	*	16	2	3	*	3	*	*	2	*	*
TURNIP																				
raw																				
1/2 cup cubes	18	*	*	*	*	*	4	2	4	2	*	*	2	*	23	2	*	*	*	2
boiled																				
1/2 cup mashed	21	*	*	*	*	2	8	2	4	3	*	2	2	*	22	2	2	2	*	3
1/2 cup cubes	14	*	*	*	*	*	8	2	3	2	*	*	2	*	15	*	*	*	*	2
boiled, salted																				
1/2 cup cubes	14	*	*	*	*	*	8	9	3	2	*	*	2	*	15	*	*	*	*	2
TURNIP, FROZEN																				
boiled																				
3 oz	20	2	*	*	*	*	—	*	4	3	5	*	3	*	6	2	*	2	*	2
boiled, salted																				
3 oz	20	2	*	*	*	*	—	10	4	3	5	*	3	*	6	2	*	2	*	2
TURNIP GREENS																				
raw																				
1 cup chopped	15	*	*	*	*	*	4	*	5	10	3	*	4	84	55	3	3	2	*	27
boiled																				
1/2 cup chopped	14	*	*	*	*	*	8	*	4	10	3	*	4	79	33	2	3	*	*	21
boiled, salted																				
1/2 cup chopped	14	*	*	*	*	*	—	8	4	10	3	*	4	79	33	2	3	*	*	21
TURNIP GREENS, CANNED																				
(Bush Bros) 1/2 cup	25	3	*	*	*	*	8	12	—	10	5	—	—	65	15	—	—	—	—	—
solid & liquid																				
(generic) 1/2 cup	16	3	*	*	*	*	8	13	5	14	10	2	6	84	30	*	4	2	*	12
w/ turnips																				
(Bush Bros) 1/2 cup	30	2	*	*	*	2	8	16	—	15	6	—	—	70	25	—	—	—	—	—
TURNIP GREENS, FROZEN																				
boiled																				
(generic) 1/2 cup	25	5	*	*	*	*	—	*	5	12	9	2	5	131	30	3	4	2	*	8
w/ turnips																				
boiled																				
(generic) 3 oz	18	3	*	*	*	*	8	*	4	10	8	*	4	104	37	2	4	2	*	9
boiled w/ salt																				
(generic) 3 oz	14	3	*	*	*	*	—	9	2	8	6	*	3	88	13	2	3	*	*	5
TURNOVER																				
apple																				
(Pepperidge Farm) 3 1/4 oz	280	6	23	—	*	11	—	9	*	4	10	—	—	*	*	*	2	2	—	—
from refrigerated dough																				
(Pillsbury) 1	170	3	12	10	*	8	—	14	*	*	4	*	*	*	*	*	8	2	4	—
blueberry																				
(Pepperidge Farm) 3 1/4 oz	280	6	23	—	*	11	—	9	*	*	10	—	—	*	*	*	2	2	—	—
cherry																				
(Pepperidge Farm) 3 1/4 oz	290	6	26	—	*	11	—	9	*	*	10	—	—	*	*	*	8	2	2	—

	Calories	Protein	Fat	Sat. Fat	Cholesterol	Carbohydrates	Fiber	Sodium	Potassium	Calcium	Iron	Zinc	Magnesium	Vitamin A	Vitamin C	Thiamin	Riboflavin	Niacin	Vitamin B₁₂	Folic acid
TURNOVER (continued)																				
from refrigerated dough (Pillsbury) 1	170	3	12	10	*	8	—	14	*	*	4	—	—	*	6	8	2	4	—	—
peach (Pepperidge Farm) 1	310	4	28	—	*	11	—	11	*	*	2	—	—	6	60	2	2	2	—	—
raspberry (Pepperidge Farm) 3 1/4 oz	310	6	26	—	*	12	—	11	*	*	4	—	—	*	20	2	2	2	—	—
TUSCAN HERB SAUCE																				
from mix (Knorr) 1 1/2 oz	190	60	11	—	23	*	—	31	—	2	6	*	*	*	2	4	6	50	*	*
VANILLA EXTRACT																				
1 tsp	12	*	*	*	*	*	*	*	*	*	*	*	*	*	*	*	*	*	*	*
imitation 1 tsp	10	*	*	*	*	*	*	*	*	*	*	*	*	*	*	*	*	*	*	*
VEAL																				
arm																				
lean & fat braised 3 oz	200	47	14	17	42	*	*	3	8	2	7	33	6	*	*	5	16	43	24	4
roasted 3 oz	155	36	11	15	31	*	*	3	8	2	5	23	5	*	*	5	16	34	22	4
lean only braised 3 oz	170	50	7	7	44	*	*	3	8	2	7	35	6	*	*	5	17	46	26	4
roasted 3 oz	139	37	8	10	31	*	*	3	8	2	5	25	6	*	*	5	17	35	22	4
blade																				
lean & fat braised 3 oz	191	44	14	16	44	*	*	4	8	3	7	40	5	*	*	5	17	23	27	3
roasted 3 oz	158	35	11	15	33	*	*	4	8	2	5	32	5	*	*	5	17	24	29	2
lean only braised 3 oz	168	46	8	8	44	*	*	4	8	4	7	42	6	*	*	5	18	24	29	3
roasted 3 oz	145	36	9	11	34	*	*	4	8	2	5	32	5	*	*	5	18	25	29	2
brain																				
braised 3 oz	116	17	13	10	875	*	*	5	5	2	8	9	4	*	18	6	10	11	136	*
fried 3 oz	181	20	22	17	599	*	*	6	11	*	5	11	4	*	21	11	18	24	300	2
cubed																				
braised 3 oz	159	50	6	6	41	*	*	3	8	2	7	34	6	*	*	5	20	35	23	4
ground																				
broiled 3 oz	146	35	10	13	29	*	*	3	8	2	5	22	5	—	—	5	14	34	18	2
heart																				
braised 3 oz	158	41	9	8	50	*	*	2	5	*	20	13	4	*	14	26	47	21	203	*
kidney																				
braised 3 oz	138	38	8	8	224	*	*	4	4	2	14	24	5	4	11	14	99	20	519	5
leg																				
braised 3 oz	179	51	8	11	38	*	*	2	9	*	6	23	6	*	*	5	17	45	17	4
broiled 3 oz	194	38	12	14	32	3	*	*	11	*	146	*	53	*	*	12	17	44	17	4

	Calories	Protein	Fat	Sat. Fat	Cholesterol	Carbohydrates	Fiber	Sodium	Potassium	Calcium	Iron	Zinc	Magnesium	Vitamin A	Vitamin C	Thiamin	Riboflavin	Niacin	Vitamin B12	Folic acid
VEAL (continued)																				
fried																				
3 oz	179	45	11	14	30	*	*	3	11	*	5	18	7	*	*	5	17	51	20	3
roasted																				
3 oz	128	40	5	5	29	*	*	2	10	*	5	17	6	*	*	5	17	43	17	4
liver																				
braised																				
3 oz	140	31	9	11	158	*	*	2	5	*	12	54	4	456	44	10	97	36	514	161
fried																				
3 oz	208	42	15	18	93	*	*	5	11	*	25	44	5	319	31	19	167	72	900	68
loin																				
lean & fat																				
braised																				
3 oz	241	43	23	29	33	*	*	3	7	2	5	20	5	*	*	3	15	38	17	3
braised																				
3 oz	184	35	16	23	29	*	*	3	8	2	4	17	5	*	*	4	14	38	17	3
lean only																				
braised																				
3 oz	191	47	12	11	35	*	*	3	8	2	5	23	6	*	*	4	17	43	19	3
rib																				
lean & fat																				
braised																				
3 oz	213	46	17	21	39	*	*	3	8	2	7	32	5	*	*	4	14	32	20	4
roasted																				
3 oz	194	34	18	23	31	*	*	3	7	*	5	23	5	*	*	4	14	29	20	3
lean only																				
braised																				
3 oz	185	49	11	11	41	*	*	4	8	2	7	34	5	*	*	5	16	34	22	4
roasted																				
3 oz	150	36	10	9	32	*	*	4	8	*	5	26	5	*	*	5	14	32	23	3
shoulder																				
lean & fat																				
braised																				
3 oz	194	45	14	16	35	*	x	3	8	3	7	38	6	*	*	5	17	27	26	3
roasted																				
3 oz	156	36	11	14	32	*	*	3	8	2	5	29	5	*	*	5	17	27	26	2
lean only																				
braised																				
3 oz	169	47	8	8	37	*	*	4	8	3	7	40	6	*	*	5	17	29	27	4
roasted																				
3 oz	144	37	9	11	32	*	*	4	8	2	5	30	5	*	*	5	17	27	26	3
sirloin																				
lean & fat																				
braised																				
3 oz	214	44	17	23	31	*	*	3	8	2	6	25	6	*	*	4	17	28	21	3
roasted																				
3 oz	171	35	14	20	29	*	*	3	8	*	5	19	5	*	*	5	17	38	20	3
lean only																				
roasted																				
3 oz	143	38	8	11	29	*	*	3	9	2	5	20	6	*	*	5	19	40	21	4
sweetbreads																				
all types																				
braised																				
3 oz	148	44	5	7	132	*	*	2	8	*	10	17	4	*	104	5	8	9	31	*
pancreas																				
braised																				
3 oz	217	41	19	36	—	*	*	2	7	2	11	29	5	*	8	14	26	17	244	*
spleen																				
braised																				
3 oz	110	34	4	5	126	*	*	2	5	*	35	11	3	*	56	3	14	23	68	*

	Calories	Protein	Fat	Sat. Fat	Cholesterol	Carbohydrates	Fiber	Sodium	Potassium	Calcium	Iron	Zinc	Magnesium	Vitamin A	Vitamin C	Thiamin	Riboflavin	Niacin	Vitamin B12	Folic acid
VEAL (continued)																				
tongue																				
braised																				
3 oz	171	37	14	19	68	*	*	2	4	*	10	26	4	*	8	5	17	6	74	2
VEAL DINNER, FROZEN																				
parmigiana																				
(Armour Classics) 11 1/4 oz	400	30	34	—	18	11	—	55	15	15	20	—	—	20	45	20	20	15	—	—
(Le Menu)	320	40	23	—	—	10	—	31	—	10	10	—	—	25	60	10	15	20	—	—
(Swanson) 11 1/2 oz	400	40	28	—	—	13	—	45	—	15	15	—	—	15	15	10	15	25	—	—
(Swanson Hungry-Man) 18 1/4 oz	590	60	40	—	—	19	—	77	—	20	25	—	—	20	25	20	20	45	—	—
VEAL ENTREE, FROZEN																				
parmigiana																				
(Morton) 8 3/4 oz	30	15	11	—	10	10	—	55	11	2	10	—	—	60	4	10	8	8	—	—
(Swanson) 10 oz	320	40	18	—	—	11	—	41	—	10	15	—	—	8	10	10	10	20	—	—
w/ pasta alfredo (Stouffer's) 11 7/8 oz	420	47	29	20	25	14	24	50	22	10	10	—	—	15	10	20	30	30	—	—
VEGETABLE COMBINATION, CANNED																				
garden medley (Green Giant) 1/2 cup	35	2	*	*	*	3	4	15	4	*	2	—	—	40	*	*	2	2	—	—
mixed greens (Bush Bros) 1/2 cup	25	3	*	*	*	*	8	12	—	10	6	—	—	70	15	—	—	—	—	—
mixed vegetables (Bush Bros) 1/2 cup	40	3	*	*	*	2	12	10	—	2	4	—	—	100	*	—	—	—	—	—
(Del Monte) 1/2 cup	40	3	*	*	*	3	8	15	—	2	4	—	—	45	10	—	—	—	—	—
drained (generic) 1/2 cup	39	4	*	*	*	3	—	5	7	2	5	2	3	191	7	3	2	2	*	5
solid & liquid (generic) 1/2 cup	44	3	*	*	*	3	20	11	5	3	4	4	5	124	8	3	3	3	*	5
VEGETABLE COMBINATION, FROZEN																				
boiled, salted (generic) 1/2 cup	38	4	*	*	*	3	—	10	4	2	4	2	3	124	11	12	3	5	*	5
California style (Bird's Eye) 3 1/3 oz	90	5	8	10	3	3	8	10	—	2	6	—	—	70	20	10	4	4	—	—
(Green Giant American Mixtures) 1/2 cup	25	3	*	*	*	2	8	2	6	2	*	—	—	140	40	2	2	2	—	—
chop suey vegetables (La Choy) 1/2 cup	10	2	*	*	*	*	2	13	2	*	*	—	—	16	6	*	*	*	—	—
corn, green beans, carrots, & pasta in tomato sauce microwave (Green Giant) 1/2 cup	80	3	3	*	*	6	12	14	9	4	4	—	—	140	*	2	2	8	—	—
creamy cheddar vegetables (Green Giant Pasta Accents) 1/2 cup	90	7	5	5	2	5	8	12	4	6	2	—	—	30	4	2	4	4	—	—
fancy mix (La Choy) 1/2 cup	12	2	*	*	*	*	4	*	*	*	2	—	—	4	9	*	*	*	—	—
garden herb seasoning (Green Giant Pasta Accents) 1/2 cup	80	5	5	5	2	4	12	12	3	2	2	—	—	10	6	2	4	4	—	—
garlic seasoning (Green Giant Pasta Accents) 1/2 cup	100	5	6	10	2	5	8	11	4	2	2	—	—	20	2	*	4	4	—	—
green beans, potatoes & mushrooms in seasoned sauce microwave (Green Giant) 1/2 cup	60	2	5	3	*	3	10	18	4	*	4	—	—	6	4	*	2	4	—	—
heartland style (Green Giant American Mixtures) 1/2 cup	25	2	*	*	*	2	10	*	5	2	2	—	—	45	55	*	2	*	—	—
in butter sauce (Green Giant) 1/2 cup	60	3	3	3	4	8	12	4	2	4	—	—	80	6	4	*	6	—	—	

PERCENTAGE DAILY VALUE

	Calories	Protein	Fat	Sat. Fat	Cholesterol	Carbohydrates	Fiber	Sodium	Potassium	Calcium	Iron	Zinc	Magnesium	Vitamin A	Vitamin C	Thiamin	Riboflavin	Niacin	Vitamin B₁₂	Folic acid
VEGETABLE COMBINATION, FROZEN (continued)																				
Japanese style (Bird's Eye Deluxe) 1/2 cup	35	3	*	*	*	2	9	19	—	2	4	—	—	10	45	—	—	—	—	—
mandarin vegetables (Budget Gourmet Side Dish) 5 1/4 oz	160	4	17	—	3	4	—	18	5	4	4	—	—	90	25	4	6	4	—	—
Manhattan style (Green Giant American Mixtures) 1/2 cup	25	3	*	*	*	2	8	*	6	2	2	—	—	8	60	2	*	2	—	—
mixed vegetables (Bird's Eye) 1/2 cup	60	5	*	*	*	4	8	2	—	2	4	2	4	130	15	6	4	6	—	6
(Green Giant Harvest Fresh) 1/2 cup	40	3	*	*	*	3	8	5	4	*	2	—	—	80	10	4	2	4	—	—
microwave (Green Giant) 1/2 cup	35	2	*	*	*	3	4	12	3	2	*	—	—	100	*	*	*	6	—	—
New England recipe (Budget Gourmet Side Dish) 5 1/2 oz	230	8	20	—	8	7	—	16	6	4	4	—	—	15	25	8	8	10	—	—
New England style (Bird's Eye) 3 1/3 oz	110	5	9	10	4	8	10	—	2	2	—	—	15	25	4	2	2	—	—
(Green Giant American Mixtures) 1/2 cup	70	5	2	*	*	5	16	3	6	*	4	—	—	80	15	10	2	6	—	—
Oriental rice w/ vegetables (Budget Gourmet Side Dish) 5 3/4 oz	230	6	18	—	7	9	—	17	4	2	2	—	—	20	15	8	6	10	—	—
primavera (Green Giant Pasta Accents) 1/2 cup	110	8	6	10	2	5	10	8	3	6	4	—	—	4	8	2	6	8	—	—
San Francisco style (Green Giant American Mixtures) 1/2 cup	25	2	*	*	*	2	10	*	6	2	2	—	—	40	45	2	*	2	—	—
Santa Fe style (Green Giant American Mixtures) 1/2 cup	70	5	*	*	*	5	8	*	5	*	2	—	—	10	25	4	2	6	—	—
Seattle style (Green Giant American Mixtures) 1/2 cup	25	3	*	*	*	2	8	*	4	2	*	—	—	100	35	2	2	2	—	—
Spring vegetables in cheese sauce (Budget Gourmet Side Dish) 5 oz	130	8	12	—	7	3	—	15	6	15	4	—	—	60	50	6	10	2	—	—
Western style (Green Giant American Mixtures) 1/2 cup	60	3	3	*	*	4	8	*	7	2	2	—	—	8	20	4	2	2	—	—
VEGETABLE COMBINATION, PICKLED																				
garden mix hot & spicy (Vlasic) 1 oz	4	*	*	*	*	*	*	20	—	*	*	—	—	2	6	*	*	*	—	—
VEGETABLE, FROZEN see specific vegetables																				
VEGETABLE ENTREE																				
ratatouille (Homemade) 1 cup	265	4	38	—	4	—	14	14	6	7	3	8	16	69	9	3	6	*	9
VEGETABLE ENTREE, CANNED																				
beans & franks (Morton Entree) 8 1/2 oz	300	15	17	—	8	13	—	53	11	4	15	—	—	80	15	15	4	4	—	—
lentils w/ garden vegetables (Health Valley) 7 1/2 oz	120	15	*	*	*	6	62	9	10	9	30	—	—	150	*	12	12	6	—	—
vegetable stew (Dinty Moore) 8 oz	155	8	9	10	5	7	—	35	13	4	6	5	8	64	3	5	5	8	—	—
VEGETABLE, FROZEN																				
creamed spinach (Stouffer's Side Dishes) 9 oz	150	7	18	20	5	3	8	16	9	10	4	—	—	50	8	2	10	*	—	—

	Calories	Protein	Fat	Sat. Fat	Cholesterol	Carbohydrates	Fiber	Sodium	Potassium	Calcium	Iron	Zinc	Magnesium	Vitamin A	Vitamin C	Thiamin	Riboflavin	Niacin	Vitamin B12	Folic acid
VEGETABLE, FROZEN (continued)																				
creamy mushroom (Green Giant Garden Gourmet) 1 pkg (9 1/2 oz)	220	10	17	30	8	10	16	40	8	8	10	—	—	15	4	10	15	15	—	—
eggplant parmigiana (Mrs. Paul's) 5 oz	240	10	25	20	5	6	—	25	—	10	6	—	—	*	100	10	10	15	—	—
green bean mushroom casserole (Stouffer's Side Dishes) 9 1/2 oz	130	—	12	10	3	4	8	22	6	8	2	—	—	2	2	—	—	—	—	—
spinach souffle (generic) 1 cup	219	18	28	36	61	*	—	32	6	23	7	9	10	69	5	6	18	2	23	16
(Stouffer's Side Dishes) 12 oz	150	15	15	10	40	3	—	20	7	10	4	—	—	35	2	8	20	2	—	—
stuffed cabbage w/ meat in tomato sauce (Stouffer's Lean Cuisine Entrees) 9 1/2 oz	210	22	9	10	10	9	—	23	17	8	15	—	—	8	10	8	10	20	—	—
stuffed pepper (Stouffer's Entrees) 10 oz	200	17	12	8	8	8	4	37	15	2	8	—	—	4	20	15	10	15	—	—
VEGETABLE ENTREE, FROM MIX																				
creamy dill multi bran (Hain) 1 cup	150	20	9	—	*	7	20	15	2	2	8	—	—	4	*	8	4	8	—	—
Italian multi bran (Hain) 1 cup	120	17	11	—	*	6	20	16	2	4	8	—	—	10	*	8	4	10	—	—
salsa multi bran (Hain) 1 cup	130	13	11	—	*	6	20	16	2	*	4	—	—	10	*	6	2	10	—	—
VEGETABLE JUICE COCKTAIL (see also TOMATO JUICE COCKTAIL)																				
(Knudsen Very Veggie) 8 fl oz	50	5	2	5	*	3	*	25	27	4	4	—	—	30	4	—	—	—	—	—
(Mott's) 8 fl oz	48	2	*	*	*	4	7	26	16	2	5	—	—	112	4	*	*	*	—	—
hot & spicy (Smucker's) 8 fl oz	58	*	*	*	*	4	*	27	17	*	2	—	—	20	8	6	*	8	—	—
low sodium (Knudsen Very Veggie) 8 fl oz	50	5	2	5	*	3	*	*	27	4	4	—	—	30	4	—	—	—	—	—
organic (Knudsen Very Veggie) 8 fl oz	50	5	2	5	*	3	*	25	27	4	4	—	—	30	4	—	—	—	—	—
spiced (Knudsen Very Veggie) 8 fl oz	50	5	2	5	*	3	*	25	27	4	4	—	—	30	4	—	—	—	—	—
VEGETABLE OIL																				
(Crisco) 1 tbsp	120	*	22	8	*	*	*	*	*	*	*	*	*	*	*	*	*	*	*	*
(generic) 1 tbsp	124	*	22	8	*	*	*	*	*	*	*	*	*	*	*	*	*	*	*	*
(Puritan) 1 tbsp	120	*	22	5	*	*	*	*	*	*	*	*	*	*	*	*	*	*	*	*
(Wesson) 1 tbsp	120	*	22	10	*	*	*	*	*	*	*	—	*	*	*	*	*	*	*	—
VEGETABLE OYSTER see SALSIFY																				
VENISON																				
roasted 4 oz	179	57	6	7	42	*	*	3	11	*	28	21	7	*	*	14	40	38	—	—
VERA CRUZ SAUCE																				
microwave (Knorr) 3 1/3 oz	200	60	8	—	23	3	—	33	—	4	10	*	*	10	35	6	8	60	*	*
VIENNA SAUSAGE																				
(Hormel) 2 oz	69	10	11	10	5	*	*	9	2	*	4	3	*	*	5	*	2	3	—	—
barbecue sauce (Libby's) 2 1/2 oz	180	15	23	—	—	*	*	17	5	2	6	—	4	4	*	2	6	4	—	—
beef broth (Libby's) 3 links	130	8	18	13	17	*	*	12	—	2	4	—	—	*	*	—	—	—	—	—
beef & pork (generic) 7 2" sausages	315	19	44	53	20	*	*	45	3	*	6	12	2	*	*	7	7	9	19	*
chicken (Hormel) 2 oz	56	10	8	5	9	*	*	9	2	3	3	2	*	*	6	1	3	4	—	—
in beef broth (Libby's) 3 links	100	10	12	13	17	*	*	19	—	2	4	—	—	*	*	—	—	—	—	—

	Calories	Protein	Fat	Sat. Fat	Cholesterol	Carbohydrates	Fiber	Sodium	Potassium	Calcium	Iron	Zinc	Magnesium	Vitamin A	Vitamin C	Thiamin	Riboflavin	Niacin	Vitamin B12	Folic acid
VINEGAR																				
cider (generic) 1 tbsp	2	*	*	*	*	*	*	*	*	*	*	*	*	*	*	*	*	*	*	*
unpasteurized (Hain) 1 tbsp	2	*	*	*	*	*	*	*	*	*	*	*	*	*	*	*	*	*	*	*
red wine (Progresso) 1 tbsp	0	*	*	*	*	*	*	*	*	*	*	*	*	*	*	*	*	*	*	*
VINESPINACH																				
raw 3 oz	16	3	*	*	*	*	—	*	12	9	6	2	14	136	144	3	8	2	*	30
VODKA																				
1 1/2 fl oz	97	*	*	*	*	*	*	*	*	*	*	*	*	*	*	*	*	*	*	*
WAFFLE, FROZEN																				
(Downyflake) 2 waffles	120	5	5	5	*	7	—	13	*	*	10	—	—	*	*	20	10	10	—	—
(Hain) 2 waffles	150	30	2	—	*	7	20	28	5	4	10	—	—	*	*	10	8	6	—	—
(Nutri-Grain) 1 waffle	120	5	8	5	*	6	8	10	2	2	10	—	—	10	*	10	10	10	10	10
crisp & healthy (Downyflake) 2 waffles	160	14	3	*	*	11	8	15	6	*	50	—	—	30	40	20	40	60	—	—
jumbo (Downyflake) 2 waffles	170	7	6	5	*	10	—	18	2	*	15	—	—	*	*	30	15	15	—	—
apple & cinnamon (Eggo) 1 waffle	130	5	8	5	5	6	—	10	*	*	10	—	—	10	*	10	10	10	10	10
crisp & healthy (Downyflake) 2 waffles	160	14	3	*	*	11	8	15	6	*	50	—	—	30	40	20	40	60	—	—
blueberry (Aunt Jemima) 2 waffles	190	7	11	7	4	9	5	22	3	20	15	—	—	—	—	20	25	20	35	—
(Downyflake) 2 waffles	180	5	6	5	*	—	—	20	2	*	15	—	—	*	*	30	15	20	—	—
(Eggo) 1 waffle	130	5	8	5	5	6	—	10	*	*	10	—	—	10	*	10	10	10	10	10
buttermilk (Aunt Jemima) 2 waffles	220	7	12	—	*	7	—	27	3	10	10	—	—	*	*	10	10	10	—	—
(Eggo) 1 waffle	120	5	8	5	5	5	—	10	*	*	10	—	—	10	*	10	10	10	10	10
jumbo (Downyflake) 2 waffles	160	7	6	5	*	9	—	20	*	*	15	—	—	*	*	30	20	15	—	—
homestyle (Eggo) 1 waffle	120	5	8	5	5	5	—	10	*	*	10	—	—	10	*	10	10	10	10	10
hot-n-buttery (Downyflake) 2 waffles	180	7	9	5	—	9	—	26	2	2	20	—	—	*	*	25	10	15	—	—
low fat (Aunt Jemima) 2 waffles	160	8	2	*	*	11	5	23	4	15	25	—	—	—	—	25	25	25	30	—
mini (Eggo) 4 waffles	90	3	5	5	3	5	—	8	*	*	10	—	—	10	*	10	10	10	10	10
multi-bran (Nutri-Grain) 1 waffle	110	3	8	5	*	6	12	9	—	2	10	—	—	10	*	10	10	10	10	10
nut & honey (Eggo) 1 waffle	130	5	9	5	5	6	—	10	2	2	10	—	—	10	*	10	10	10	10	10
oat bran (Eggo Common Sense) 1 waffle	110	5	6	5	*	5	8	9	2	2	10	—	—	10	*	10	10	10	10	10
fruit & nut (Eggo Common Sense) 1 waffle	120	5	8	5	*	6	8	9	—	2	10	—	—	10	*	10	10	10	10	10
raisin & bran (Nutri-Grain) 1 waffle	120	5	8	5	*	6	8	10	—	2	10	—	—	10	*	10	10	10	10	10
Special K (Kellogg's) 1 waffle	80	5	*	*	*	5	—	5	*	2	10	—	—	10	*	10	10	10	10	10
strawberry (Eggo) 1 waffle	130	5	8	5	5	6	—	10	*	2	10	—	—	10	*	10	10	10	10	10
whole grain (Roman Meal) 2 waffles	280	8	22	10	7	11	12	28	4	40	40	—	—	*	*	40	40	40	—	—

WAFFLE MIX see PANCAKE & WAFFLE MIX

	Calories	Protein	Fat	Sat. Fat	Cholesterol	Carbohydrates	Fiber	Sodium	Potassium	Calcium	Iron	Zinc	Magnesium	Vitamin A	Vitamin C	Thiamin	Riboflavin	Niacin	Vitamin B₁₂	Folic acid
WALNUT																				
black																				
1 oz	172	12	25	5	*	*	4	*	4	2	5	6	14	2	2	4	2	*	*	5
English																				
1 oz (14 halves)	182	7	27	8	*	2	4	*	4	3	4	5	12	*	2	7	2	*	*	5
WALNUT OIL																				
1 tbsp	120	*	22	6	*	*	*	*	*	*	*	*	*	*	*	*	*	*	*	*
WALNUT TOPPING																				
(Smucker's) 2 tbsp	130	3	2	—	*	9	*	*	—	*	22	*	*	*	*	2	2	*	—	*
WATER																				
(Perrier) 6 1/2 fl oz bottle	0	*	*	*	*	*	*	*	*	3	*	*	*	*	*	*	*	*	*	*
(Poland Spring) 8 fl oz	0	*	*	*	*	*	*	*	*	*	*	*	*	*	*	*	*	*	*	*
WATER BUFFALO																				
roasted																				
4 oz	148	51	3	4	23	*	*	3	10	2	13	19	9	—	*	2	17	36	33	3
WATER CHESTNUT																				
Chinese																				
raw																				
1/2 cup slices	66	*	*	*	*	5	8	*	10	*	*	2	3	*	4	6	7	3	*	3
4 nuts	38	*	*	*	*	3	4	*	6	*	*	*	2	*	2	3	4	2	*	2
canned																				
sliced																				
(La Choy) 1/4 cup	18	*	*	*	*	*	2	*	*	*	2	—	*	*	*	*	*	*	—	—
solid & liquid																				
1/4 cup slices	18	*	*	*	*	2	4	*	*	*	2	*	*	*	*	*	*	x	x	x
4 nuts	14	*	*	*	*	*	4	*	*	*	*	*	*	*	*	*	*	*	*	*
whole																				
(La Choy) 4 nuts	14	*	*	*	*	*	2	—	—	*	*	*	*	*	35	*	*	*	*	*
WATERCRESS																				
raw																				
1/2 cup chopped	2	*	*	*	*	*	*	*	2	2	*	*	*	16	12	*	*	*	*	*
1 sprig	0	*	*	*	*	*	*	*	*	*	*	*	*	3	2	*	*	*	*	*
WATERMELON																				
1 cup cubed	51	2	*	*	*	4	4	*	5	2	*	2	*	12	26	9	2	2	—	*
1/16 fruit	154	5	3	—	*	12	8	*	16	4	5	2	13	35	77	26	6	5	—	3
WATERMELON SEED																				
dried																				
1 oz	158	13	21	14	*	*	—	*	5	2	11	19	37	*	*	4	2	5	*	4
WAX BEAN, CANNED																				
(Bush Bros) 1/2 cup	25	3	*	*	*	*	8	17	—	4	6	—	*	*	4	—	—	—	—	—
(Del Monte) 1/2 cup	20	2	*	*	*	*	8	15	—	2	2	—	*	*	10	—	—	—	—	—
WAXGOURD																				
raw																				
1/2 cup cubes	9	*	*	*	*	*	8	3	*	*	3	2	*	*	14	2	4	*	*	*
boiled																				
1/2 cup cubes	11	*	*	*	*	*	4	4	*	2	2	3	2	*	15	2	*	2	*	*
boiled w/ salt																				
1/2 cup cubes	11	*	*	*	*	*	—	12	*	2	2	3	2	*	15	2	*	2	*	*
WELSH RAREBIT see CHEESE ENTREE																				
WHEAT FLOUR																				
all purpose																				
(Ballard) 1 cup	366	19	*	2	*	26	9	*	3	2	19	—	—	*	*	50	25	22	—	—
bleached																				
(Gold Medal) 1 cup	400	18	2	*	*	29	—	*	4	2	25	—	—	*	*	45	25	30	—	—
(Pillsbury Best) 1 cup	364	20	2	*	*	25	9	*	9	2	25	—	—	*	*	63	19	17	—	—
(Red Band) 1 cup	390	17	2	*	*	28	—	*	3	2	25	—	—	*	*	45	25	30	—	—
(Robin Hood) 1 cup	400	22	2	*	*	28	—	*	3	2	25	—	—	*	*	45	25	30	—	—

	Calories	Protein	Fat	Sat. Fat	Cholesterol	Carbohydrates	Fiber	Sodium	Potassium	Calcium	Iron	Zinc	Magnesium	Vitamin A	Vitamin C	Thiamin	Riboflavin	Niacin	Vitamin B12	Folic acid
WHEAT FLOUR (continued)																				
bread																				
(Gold Medal) 1 cup	400	23	2	*	*	28	—	*	3	2	25	—	—	*	*	45	25	30	—	—
(Pillsbury Best) 1 cup	358	23	4	3	*	24	10	*	2	2	23	—	—	*	*	60	29	12	—	—
drifted snow																				
(Red Band) 1 cup	400	18	2	*	*	29	—	*	4	20	25	—	—	*	*	45	25	30	—	—
la pina																				
(Red Band) 1 cup	400	17	2	*	*	29	—	*	5	2	25	—	—	*	*	45	25	30	—	—
self-rising																				
(Gold Medal) 1 cup	380	17	2	*	*	28	—	63	4	20	25	—	—	*	*	45	25	30	—	—
(Red Band) 1 cup	380	15	2	*	*	28	—	63	4	20	25	—	—	*	*	45	25	30	—	—
(Robin Hood) 1 cup	380	17	2	*	*	28	—	*	43	20	25	—	—	*	*	45	25	30	—	—
bleached																				
(Pillsbury Best) 1 cup	330	14	*	3	*	24	7	47	3	29	16	—	—	*	*	41	22	25	—	—
unbleached																				
(Pillsbury Best) 1 cup	330	14	*	3	*	24	7	47	3	29	16	—	—	*	*	41	22	25	—	—
shake & blend																				
(Pillsbury Best) 1 cup	357	20	*	*	*	26	—	*	3	2	14	—	—	*	*	37	19	24	—	—
Softasilk																				
(Red Band) 1 cup	100	13	*	*	*	8	—	*	3	.5	6	—	—	*	*	10	6	8	—	—
unbleached																				
(Gold Medal) 1 cup	400	18	2	*	*	29	—	*	4	2	25	—	—	*	*	45	25	30	—	—
(Pillsbury Best) 1 cup	368	21	2	*	*	25	11	*	4	20	4.5	—	—	*	*	.74	.41	5.78	—	—
(Robin Hood) 1 cup	400	22	2	*	*	28	—	*	4	2	25	—	—	*	*	45	25	30	—	—
whole wheat																				
(Gold Medal) 1 cup	350	27	3	*	*	26	40	*	12	2	25	—	—	*	*	35	8	30	—	—
(Pillsbury Best) 1 cup	359	28	3	2	*	23	47	*	12	3	22	—	—	*	*	26	11	33	—	—
whole wheat blend																				
(Gold Medal) 1 cup	380	23	3	—	*	28	—	*	10	2	25	—	—	*	*	40	15	25	—	—
Wondra																				
(Red Band) 1 cup	400	18	2	*	*	29	—	*	4	2	25	—	—	*	*	45	25	30	—	—
WHEAT GERM																				
original																				
(Kretschmer) 1 oz	100	15	3	1	*	4	13	*	9	*	10	4	20	*	*	30	10	6	—	25
toasted																				
(generic) 1 cup	432	55	19	11	*	19	60	*	30	5	57	125	90	—	11	—	54	32	*	100
toasted w/ sugar																				
(generic) 1 cup	426	41	14	8	*	23	20	*	23	4	43	94	68	*	—	94	41	24	*	75
WHEAT GERM OIL																				
1 tbsp	120	*	22	13	*	*	*	*	*	*	*	*	*	*	*	*	*	*	*	*
WHEATNUTS																				
1 oz	177	7	25	13	*	2	4	6	3	*	4	6	4	*	*	6	5	2	*	10
WHELK																				
raw																				
3 oz	116	34	*	*	18	2	*	7	8	5	24	9	18	*	6	*	5	4	128	*
steamed/poached																				
3 oz	234	68	*	*	37	4	*	15	17	10	47	18	37	3	10	3	11	8	256	*
WHEY, ACID																				
dried																				
1 tbsp	10	*	*	*	*	*	*	*	2	6	*	*	*	*	*	*	*	*	*	*
fluid																				
1 cup	59	3	*	*	*	4	*	5	10	25	*	7	6	*	*	7	*	*	7	*
WHEY, SWEET																				
dried																				
1 tbsp	26	2	*	*	*	2	*	3	4	6	*	*	3	*	*	3	*	*	3	*
fluid																				
1 cup	66	3	*	3	2	4	*	5	11	12	*	2	5	*	*	6	*	*	11	*

Item	Calories	Protein	Fat	Sat. Fat	Cholesterol	Carbohydrates	Fiber	Sodium	Potassium	Calcium	Iron	Zinc	Magnesium	Vitamin A	Vitamin C	Thiamin	Riboflavin	Niacin	Vitamin B_{12}	Folic acid
WHISKEY																				
1 1/2 fl oz	105	*	*	*	*	*	*	*	*	*	*	*	*	*	*	*	*	*	*	*
WHISKEY SOUR																				
bottled 2 fl oz	54	*	*	*	*	5	*	3	*	*	*	*	*	*	*	*	*	*	*	*
canned 6 3/4 oz can	249	*	*	*	*	9	*	4	*	*	*	*	*	*	*	2	*	*	*	*
from mix 2 oz mix + 1 1/2 oz whiskey	158	*	*	*	*	5	*	3	*	*	*	*	*	*	*	*	*	*	*	*
homemade 1 cocktail (3 fl oz)	122	*	*	*	*	2	*	*	*	*	*	*	*	*	*	13	*	*	*	*
WHITE BEAN																				
1/2 cup	363	38	2	*	*	22	—	*	47	19	46	20	49	*	*	53	13	7	*	104
regular cooked salted 1/2 cup	125	15	*	*	*	8	24	*	14	8	18	8	14	*	*	7	2	*	*	18
unsalted 1/2 cup	125	15	*	*	*	8	—	9	14	8	18	8	14	*	*	7	2	*	*	18
small cooked salted 1/2 cup	128	13	*	*	*	8	—	*	12	7	14	7	15	*	*	14	3	*	*	31
unsalted 1/2 cup	128	13	*	*	*	8	—	9	12	7	14	7	15	*	*	14	3	*	*	31
WHITE BEAN, CANNED																				
1/2 cup	153	16	*	*	*	10	24	*	17	10	22	10	17	*	*	8	3	*	*	21
WHITE BREAD see BREAD																				
WHITE SAUCE																				
from mix (generic) 1/2 cup	178	5	12	—	—	5	4	40	3	19	*	2	3	*	2	4	7	*	4	*
(Knorr) 1/2 cup	120	8	12	—	6	4	—	18	—	16	*	*	*	*	*	4	12	*	*	*
homemade medium 1/2 cup	184	8	20	18	3	4	*	18	6	15	2	3	4	14	2	6	14	3	6	2
thick 1/2 cup	233	8	27	22	2	5	*	19	5	14	3	3	4	17	*	7	14	4	5	2
thin 1/2 cup	131	8	13	14	3	3	*	17	6	16	*	3	5	10	2	5	14	2	6	2
WHITEFISH																				
raw 1 fillet	265	63	18	9	40	*	*	4	18	5	4	13	16	5	*	18	14	30	33	*
broiled/baked 1 fillet	265	63	18	9	39	*	*	4	18	5	4	13	16	4	*	18	14	30	25	*
smoked 3 oz	92	33	*	*	9	*	*	36	10	2	2	3	5	3	*	2	5	10	46	*
WHITING																				
raw 1 fillet	83	28	2	*	21	*	*	3	7	4	2	5	5	2	*	3	2	6	35	*
baked/broiled 1 fillet	83	28	2	*	20	*	*	4	9	4	2	3	5	2	*	3	3	6	31	*
WHOLE WHEAT BREAD see BREAD																				
WINE																				
dessert dry 3 1/2 oz glass	130	*	*	*	*	*	*	*	3	*	*	*	*	2	*	*	*	*	*	*
red 3 1/2 oz glass	74	*	*	*	*	*	*	*	3	*	2	*	3	*	*	*	2	*	*	*
rosé 3 1/2 oz glass	73	*	*	*	*	*	*	*	3	*	2	*	3	*	*	*	*	*	*	*
white 3 1/2 oz glass	70	*	*	*	*	*	*	*	2	*	2	*	3	*	*	*	*	*	*	*

	Calories	Protein	Fat	Sat. Fat	Cholesterol	Carbohydrates	Fiber	Sodium	Potassium	Calcium	Iron	Zinc	Magnesium	Vitamin A	Vitamin C	Thiamin	Riboflavin	Niacin	Vitamin B12	Folic acid
WINGED BEAN																				
raw																				
1/2 cup slices	11	3	*	*	*	*	—	*	*	2	2	*	2	*	7	2	*	*	*	4
2 pods	16	4	*	*	*	*	—	*	2	3	3	*	3	*	10	3	2	*	*	5
tuber																				
raw																				
3 oz	135	16	*	*	*	8	—	*	14	3	9	8	5	*	*	21	7	7	*	4
boiled																				
1/2 cup	12	3	*	*	*	*	—	*	2	2	2	*	2	*	5	2	*	*	*	3
boiled w/ salt																				
1/2 cup	12	3	*	*	*	*	—	3	2	2	2	*	2	*	5	2	*	—	*	—
cooked																				
1/2 cup	126	15	8	4	*	4	—	*	9	7	12	21	8	12	*	17	7	4	*	2
salted																				
(generic) 1/2 cup	126	15	8	4	*	4	—	*	7	12	21	8	12	*	17	7	4	*	2	
WINTER SQUASH see SQUASH																				
WOLFFISH																				
raw																				
1/2 fillet	147	45	6	3	23	*	*	5	13	*	*	8	11	11	*	18	7	16	52	*
broiled/baked																				
1/2 fillet	146	44	6	3	23	*	*	5	13	*	*	8	11	10	*	16	7	15	46	*
WORCHESTERSHIRE SAUCE																				
(Heinz) 1 tsp	0	*	*	*	*	*	*	2	—	*	*	*	*	*	*	*	*	*	*	*
(Lea & Perrins) 1 tsp	5	*	*	*	*	*	*	3	—	2	*	*	*	*	*	*	*	*	*	*
YAM																				
raw																				
1/2 cup cubes	89	2	*	*	*	7	12	*	17	*	2	*	4	*	21	6	*	2	*	4
boiled or baked																				
1/2 cup cubes	79	2	*	*	*	6	12	*	13	*	2	*	3	*	14	4	*	2	*	3
boiled w/ salt																				
1/2 cup cubes	79	2	*	*	*	6	12	7	13	*	2	*	3	*	14	4	*	2	*	3
YAM, CANNED																				
(Bush Bros) 1/2 cup	110	2	*	*	*	9	8	*	—	*	6	—	—	25	4	—	—	—	—	
YAM, MOUNTAIN																				
raw																				
1/2 cup cubes	46	2	*	*	*	4	—	*	8	2	2	*	2	*	3	5	*	2	*	2
1 large	281	9	*	*	*	23	—	2	50	11	10	8	13	*	18	29	5	10	*	15
steamed																				
1/2 cup cubes	59	2	*	*	*	5	—	*	10	*	2	2	2	*	*	4	*	*	*	2
steamed, salted																				
1/2 cup cubes	59	2	*	*	*	5	—	7	10	*	2	2	2	*	*	4	*	*	*	2
YAMBEAN																				
raw																				
1 cup slices	46	*	*	*	*	4	24	*	5	*	4	*	4	*	40	2	2	*	*	4
boiled																				
3 oz	32	*	*	*	*	2	—	*	3	*	3	*	2	*	20	*	*	*	*	2
boiled w/ salt																				
3 oz	32	*	*	*	*	2	—	9	3	*	3	*	2	*	20	*	*	*	*	2
YARDLONG BEAN																				
raw																				
1 cup slices	43	4	*	*	*	3	—	*	6	5	2	2	10	16	29	6	6	2	*	14
boiled																				
1 cup slices	49	4	*	*	*	3	—	*	9	5	6	2	11	9	28	6	6	3	*	12
boiled w/ salt																				
1 cup slices	49	4	*	*	*	3	—	10	9	5	6	2	11	9	28	6	6	3	*	12
YELLOW BEAN																				
raw																				
1/2 cup	17	2	*	*	*	*	4	*	3	2	3	*	3	*	15	3	3	2	*	5
boiled																				
1/2 cup	22	2	*	*	*	2	4	*	5	3	4	*	4	*	10	3	4	2	*	5

	Calories	Protein	Fat	Sat. Fat	Cholesterol	Carbohydrates	Fiber	Sodium	Potassium	Calcium	Iron	Zinc	Magnesium	Vitamin A	Vitamin C	Thiamin	Riboflavin	Niacin	Vitamin B₁₂	Folic acid

PERCENTAGE DAILY VALUE

YELLOW BEAN (continued)

	Calories	Protein	Fat	Sat. Fat	Cholesterol	Carbohydrates	Fiber	Sodium	Potassium	Calcium	Iron	Zinc	Magnesium	Vitamin A	Vitamin C	Thiamin	Riboflavin	Niacin	Vitamin B12	Folic acid
boiled w/ salt 1/2 cup	22	2	*	*	*	2	4	6	5	3	4	*	4	*	10	3	4	2	*	5
cooked 1/2 cup	127	13	2	*	*	7	4	9	8	5	12	6	16	*	3	11	5	3	*	18
salted 1/2 cup	127	13	2	*	*	7	4	*	8	5	12	6	16	*	3	11	5	3	*	18
YELLOW BEAN, CANNED																				
drained 1/2 cup	14	*	*	*	*	*	4	7	2	2	3	*	2	*	5	*	2	*	*	5
solid & liquid 1/2 cup	18	2	*	*	*	*	4	18	3	3	6	2	4	2	8	2	4	*	*	5
YELLOW BEAN, FROZEN																				
1/2 cup	20	2	*	*	*	2	4	*	3	3	3	*	2	13	4	3	2	*	*	2
boiled 1/2 cup	19	2	*	*	*	*	8	*	2	3	3	2	4	2	5	2	4	*	*	4
boiled w/ salt 1/2 cup	19	2	*	*	*	*	8	7	2	3	3	2	4	2	5	2	4	*	*	4
YELLOWEYE BEAN, CANNED *(B & M)* 8 oz	250	23	8	—	2	17	44	34	20	9	40	—	—	*	*	6	6	6	—	—
YELLOW SQUASH see SQUASH																				
YELLOWTAIL																				
raw 1/2 fillet	273	72	15	12	34	*	*	3	22	4	5	6	14	4	9	18	4	64	40	*
broiled/baked 1/2 fillet	273	72	15	—	35	*	*	3	22	4	5	7	14	3	7	17	4	64	30	*
YOGURT																				
all fruit flavors low fat *(generic)* 1 container	239	18	5	11	4	14	*	6	14	38	*	12	9	3	3	6	*	*	20	6
banana (La Yogurt) 6 oz	190	10	4	9	4	11	*	4	—	25	4	—	—	2	8	—	—	—	—	—
(Yoplait) 6 oz	180	12	5	—	5	10	—	5	10	25	*	—	—	*	*	4	15	*	6	—
blueberries & creme (Weight Watchers Ultimate) 1 cup	90	13	*	*	2	5	12	6	7	25	*	—	—	*	*	—	—	—	—	—
blueberry (Yoplait) 6 oz	180	13	3	—	—	11	—	5	12	25	*	—	—	*	*	6	20	*	6	—
fat free (Yoplait) 6 oz	160	13	*	*	2	11	—	5	9	25	*	—	—	*	*	6	15	*	20	—
light (Dannon) 6 oz	100	15	*	*	2	7	*	6	13	35	2	—	—	*	6	—	—	—	—	—
light, sweetened w/ aspartame (Yoplait) 6 oz	80	10	*	*	*	4	—	4	8	20	*	—	—	*	*	4	15	*	6	—
blueberry/ vanilla (Yoplait) 6 oz	200	13	5	—	—	11	—	5	14	25	*	—	—	*	*	4	20	*	6	—
boysenberry (Yoplait) 6 oz	180	13	3	—	—	11	—	5	12	25	*	—	—	*	*	6	20	*	6	—
cappucino (Weight Watchers Ultimate) 1 cup	90	13	*	*	2	5	*	6	7	25	*	—	—	*	*	—	—	—	—	—
cherry (Yoplait) 6 oz	180	13	3	—	—	11	—	5	12	25	*	—	—	*	*	6	20	*	6	—
fat free (Yoplait) 6 oz	160	13	*	*	2	11	—	5	9	25	*	—	—	*	*	6	15	*	20	—
light, sweetened w/ aspartame (Yoplait) 6 oz	80	10	*	*	*	4	—	4	8	20	*	—	—	*	*	4	15	*	6	—
cherry almond breakfast yogurt *(Yoplait)* 6 oz	210	15	3	—	—	14	—	4	11	25	2	—	—	*	*	6	15	*	8	—

YOGURT (continued)

	Calories	Protein	Fat	Sat. Fat	Cholesterol	Carbohydrates	Fiber	Sodium	Potassium	Calcium	Iron	Zinc	Magnesium	Vitamin A	Vitamin C	Thiamin	Riboflavin	Niacin	Vitamin B₁₂	Folic acid
cherry jubilee (Weight Watchers Ultimate) 1 cup	90	13	*	*	2	5	*	6	8	25	*	—	—	*	*	—	—	—	—	—
cherry/vanilla (Yoplait) 6 oz	200	13	5	—	—	11	—	5	14	25	*	—	—	*	*	4	20	*	6	—
coffee (Breyer's) 6 oz	220	17	5	10	7	13	*	6	—	35	*	—	—	2	*	—	—	—	—	—
cranberry raspberry (Weight Watchers Ultimate) 1 cup	90	13	*	*	2	5		6	—	25	*									
lemon (Dannon) 6 oz	210	17	5	10	5	12	*	7	15	10	*	—	—	4	4	—	—	—	—	—
lemon (Yoplait) 6 oz	180	13	3	—	—	11	—	5	12	25	*	—	—	*	*	6	20	*	6	—
lemon chiffon (Weight Watchers Ultimate) 1 cup	90	13	*	*	2	5	4	6	9	25	*	—	—	*	*	—	—	—	—	—
mixed berry (Dannon) 6 oz	240	15	5	8	5	15	4	6	13	35	*	—	—	2	10	—	—	—	—	—
mixed berry (Yoplait) 6 oz	180	13	3	—	—	11	—	5	12	25	*	—	—	*	*	6	20	*	6	—
breakfast yogurt (Yoplait) 6 oz	200	13	3	—	—	13	—	5	11	25	2	—	—	*	*	6	20	*	8	—
orange (Yoplait) 6 oz	180	13	3	—	—	11	—	5	12	25	*	—	—	*	*	6	20	*	6	—
peach (Breyer's) 6 oz	250	13	4	8	5	*	*	5	—	30	*	—	—	*	*	—	—	—	—	—
peach (Weight Watchers Ultimate) 1 cup	90	13	*	*	2	5	*	6	—	25	*	—	—	*	*	—	—	—	—	—
peach (Yoplait) 6 oz	180	13	3	—	—	11	—	5	12	25	*	—	—	*	*	6	20	*	6	—
peach fat free (Yoplait) 6 oz	160	13	*	*	2	11	—	5	9	25	*	—	—	*	*	6	15	*	20	—
peach light, sweetened w/ aspartame (Yoplait) 6 oz	80	10	*	*	*	4	—	4	8	20	*	—	—	*	*	4	15	*	6	—
peach/vanilla (Yoplait) 6 oz	200	13	5	—	—	11	—	5	14	25	*	—	—	*	*	4	20	*	6	—
pina colada (Yoplait) 6 oz	180	13	3	—	—	11	—	5	12	25	*	—	—	*	*	6	20	*	6	—
pineapple (Yoplait) 6 oz	180	13	3	—	—	11	—	5	12	25	*	—	—	*	*	6	20	*	6	—
plain (Dannon) 6 oz	140	20	6	11	6	5	*	6	15	35	*	—	—	4	4	—	—	—	—	—
plain (generic) 1 container	139	13	11	24	10	4	*	4	10	27	*	9	7	6	2	4	*	*	14	4
plain (Weight Watchers Ultimate) 1 cup	90	13	*	*	2	5	*	6	9	30	*	—	—	*	*	—	—	—	—	—
plain (Yoplait) 6 oz	120	17	3	—	5	5	—	6	15	35	*	—	—	*	*	6	30	*	15	—
plain fat free (Yoplait) 6 oz	120	16	*	*	3	6	—	7	17	45	*	—	—	*	*	10	40	*	35	—
plain low fat (generic) 1 container	144	20	5	12	5	5	*	7	15	41	*	13	10	3	3	7	*	*	21	6
plain skim (generic) 1 container	127	22	*	*	*	6	*	7	17	45	*	15	11	*	3	7	*	*	23	7
raspberries & creme (Weight Watchers Ultimate) 1 cup	90	13	*	*	2	5	*	6	6	25	*	—	—	*	*	—	—	—	—	—
raspberry (Whitney's) 6 oz	190	10	8	15	7	10	*	4	—	25	—	—	—	4	2	—	—	—	—	—
raspberry (Yoplait) 6 oz	180	12	5	—	5	10	—	5	10	25	*	—	—	*	*	4	15	*	6	—
raspberry fat free (Yoplait) 6 oz	160	13	*	*	2	11	—	5	9	25	*	—	—	*	*	6	15	*	20	—

PERCENTAGE DAILY VALUE

	Calories	Protein	Fat	Sat. Fat	Cholesterol	Carbohydrates	Fiber	Sodium	Potassium	Calcium	Iron	Zinc	Magnesium	Vitamin A	Vitamin C	Thiamin	Riboflavin	Niacin	Vitamin B₁₂	Folic acid
YOGURT (continued)																				
light, sweetened w/ aspartame (Yoplait) 6 oz	80	10	*	*	*	4	—	4	8	20	*	—	—	*	*	4	15	*	6	—
strawberry (Weight Watchers Ultimate) 1 cup	90	13	*	*	2	5	8	6	8	25	*	—	—	*	*	—	—	—	—	—
(Yoplait) 6 oz	180	13	3	—	—	11	—	5	12	25	*	—	—	*	*	6	20	*	6	—
fat free (Yoplait) 6 oz	160	13	*	*	2	11	—	5	9	25	*	—	—	*	*	6	15	*	20	—
light (Dannon) 6 oz	100	15	*	*	2	6	*	6	13	35	2	—	—	*	10	—	—	—	—	—
light, sweetened w/ aspartame (Yoplait) 6 oz	80	10	*	*	*	4	—	4	8	20	*	—	—	*	*	4	15	*	6	—
strawberry almond breakfast yogurt (Yoplait) 6 oz	200	15	3	—	—	13	—	4	11	25	2	—	—	*	*	6	20	*	8	—
strawberry/banana (Weight Watchers Ultimate) 1 cup	90	13	*	*	2	5	8	6	9	25	*	—	—	*	*	—	—	—	—	—
(Yoplait) 6 oz	180	13	3	—	—	11	—	5	12	25	*	—	—	*	*	6	20	*	6	—
breakfast yogurt (Yoplait) 6 oz	200	13	3	—	—	13	—	5	10	25	2	—	—	*	*	6	15	*	8	—
fat free (Yoplait) 6 oz	160	13	*	*	2	11	—	5	9	25	*	—	—	*	*	6	15	*	20	—
light, sweetened w/ aspartame (Yoplait) 6 oz	80	10	*	*	*	4	—	4	8	20	*	—	—	*	*	4	15	*	6	—
strawberry fruit cup (La Yogurt) 6 oz	180	10	4	8	4	11	*	4	—	25	*	—	—	4	10	—	—	—	—	—
strawberry/vanilla (Yoplait) 6 oz	200	13	5	—	—	11	—	5	14	25	*	—	—	*	*	4	20	*	6	—
tropical fruit breakfast yogurt (Yoplait) 6 oz	220	13	5	—	—	14	—	5	11	25	2	—	—	*	*	6	20	*	8	—
vanilla (Weight Watchers Ultimate) 1 cup	90	13	*	*	2	5	*	6	7	25	*	—	—	*	*	—	—	—	—	—
(Yoplait) 6 oz	170	15	3	—	3	10	—	5	12	30	*	—	—	*	*	6	20	*	6	—
fat free (Yoplait) 6 oz	180	14	*	*	3	11	—	7	14	40	*	—	—	*	*	8	35	*	10	—
ZABAGLIONE																				
from mix (Knorr) 1/2 cup	70	2	5	—	2	4	—	*	—	*	*	*	—	*	*	*	2	*	*	4
ZUCCHINI																				
baby raw 1 medium	2	*	*	*	*	*	—	*	*	*	*	*	*	*	*	*	6	*	*	*	*
raw 1/2 cup slices	9	*	*	*	*	*	4	*	5	*	2	*	4	4	10	3	*	*	*	4
boiled 1/2 cup slices	14	*	*	*	*	*	4	*	6	*	2	*	5	4	7	2	2	2	*	4
boiled w/ salt 1/2 cup slices	14	*	*	*	*	*	—	9	6	*	2	*	5	4	7	2	2	2	*	4
ZUCCHINI, CANNED																				
(generic) 1/2 cup	33	2	*	*	*	3	—	18	9	2	4	2	4	12	4	3	3	3	*	9
in tomato sauce (Del Monte) 1/2 cup	30	2	*	*	*	2	4	20	—	*	4	—	—	6	15	—	—	—	—	—
Italian style (Progresso) 1/2 cup	50	2	3	3	*	3	8	22	9	2	—	—	—	6	20	4	*	4	—	—
ZUCCHINI, FROZEN																				
boiled 1/2 cup	19	2	*	*	*	*	—	*	6	2	3	*	4	10	7	3	3	2	*	2

INDEX